《中医实用预防康复学：汉英对照》编委会

主　审　郭永章　昆明医科大学

主　编　李　青　昆明医科大学第二附属医院
　　　　宋精玲　昆明医科大学

副主编　张济周　温州市中医院
　　　　杨梁梓　深圳市第三人民医院（南方科技大学第二附属医院）
　　　　吕路艳　云南省曲靖市第一人民医院
　　　　姚　璐　昆明医科大学

编　译　董　妍　云南开放大学
　　　　刘德周　云南师范大学外国语学院
　　　　朱　明　北京博颐文化科技有限公司

编　委（排名不分先后）

贝立民	昆明医科大学第二附属医院	夏秀宏	昆明医科大学第二附属医院
琚　坚	昆明医科大学第二附属医院	孙　敏	昆明医科大学第二附属医院
张家骅	昆明医科大学第二附属医院	张嘉諝	昆明医科大学第二附属医院
朱　萍	昆明医科大学第二附属医院	朱　丹	云南省音乐家协会小提琴分会
朱雪玲	昆明医科大学第二附属医院	农征雪	昆明医科大学第二附属医院
吕　琳	昆明医科大学第二附属医院	杨建华	昆明医科大学第二附属医院
杨　杰	昆明市第一人民医院	刘礼媛	昆明市第一人民医院
吴鹏兰	昆明医科大学第二附属医院	闫　滨	昆明医科大学第二附属医院
吴丽华	昆明医科大学第二附属医院	李晓玲	成都军区昆明总医院
李　群	昆明医科大学第一附属医院	李斗艳	昆明医科大学第二附属医院
李启芬	昆明医科大学第二附属医院	李　奕	云南省疾病预防控制中心
李锦鸣	昆明医科大学第二附属医院	李慈春	昆明医科大学第二附属医院
李　晓	云南中医药大学第一附属医院	何渝熙	云南中医药大学第一附属医院
肖云霞	昆明医科大学第二附属医院	陈安宝	昆明医科大学第二附属医院
陈沛卓	昆明医科大学第二附属医院	陈丽秋	昆明医科大学第二附属医院
邵琪琦	温州市中医院	张　林	昆明医科大学第二附属医院
张　栩	昆明医科大学第二附属医院	张芝春	云南省曲靖市马龙区中医院
范　围	昆明医科大学第二附属医院	林　萍	昆明医科大学
赵燕菲	昆明医科大学第二附属医院	赵国厚	昆明医科大学第二附属医院
袁开芬	昆明医科大学第二附属医院	赵柏玲	昆明医科大学第二附属医院
王晓琼	昆明医科大学第二附属医院	姜妤杰	昆明医科大学第二附属医院
熊芳华	昆明普健金福地医院	戴　睿	昆明医科大学
樊　瑾	昆明医科大学第二附属医院	洪　霞	昆明医科大学第二附属医院
杨春燕	昆明医科大学第二附属医院	段宇珠	昆明医科大学第二附属医院

主编助理

　　　　王丽娜　昆明农业发展投资有限公司
　　　　李　冉　云南广播电视台
　　　　施　韵　云南科技出版社

云南高校学术文库
Yunnan Gaoxiao Xueshu Wenku

汉英对照

中医实用预防康复学

Practical Preventive and Rehabilitative Therapies of Traditional Chinese Medicine

主　编◎李　青　宋精玲
副主编◎张济周　杨梁梓
吕路艳　姚　璐
编　译◎董　妍　刘德周
朱　明

云南大学出版社
YUNNAN UNIVERSITY PRESS

图书在版编目（CIP）数据

中医实用预防康复学：汉英对照 / 李青，宋精玲主编；董妍，刘德周，朱明编译. -- 昆明：云南大学出版社，2019
（云南高校学术文库）
ISBN 978-7-5482-1843-2

Ⅰ. ①中… Ⅱ. ①李… ②宋… ③董… ④刘… ⑤朱… Ⅲ. ①中医学—康复医学—汉、英 Ⅳ. ①R247.9

中国版本图书馆CIP数据核字（2013）第321744号

策　　划：朱　军
责任编辑：蒋丽杰
装帧设计：刘　雨

云南高校学术文库
Yunnan Gaoxiao Xueshu Wenku

中医实用预防康复学

汉英对照

Practical Preventive and Rehabilitative Therapies of Traditional Chinese Medicine

主　编◎李　青　宋精玲 / 副主编◎张济周　杨梁梓　吕路艳　姚　璐
编　译◎董　妍　刘德周　朱　明

出版发行：云南大学出版社
印　　装：昆明理煋印务有限公司
开　　本：889mm×1194mm　1/16
印　　张：24.875
字　　数：754
版　　次：2019年4月第1版
印　　次：2019年4月第1次印刷
书　　号：ISBN 978-7-5482-1843-2
定　　价：88.00元

社　　址：云南省昆明市一二一大街182号（云南大学东陆校区英华园内）
邮　　编：650091
电　　话：（0871）65033244　65031071
网　　址：http://www. ynup. com
E-mail：market@ynup. com

主编简介

◎ 李　青

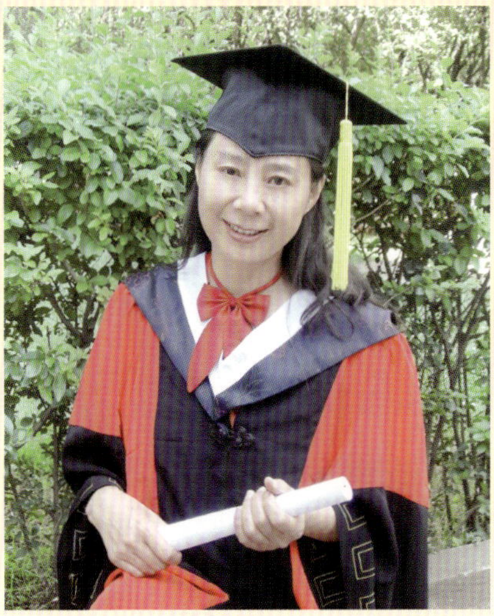

李青，女，教授，主任医师、硕士生导师，师从国家级名中医詹文涛教授。昆明医科大学第二附属医院中西医结合科原主任、中国中西医结合学会教育工作委员会委员、养生与康复医学专业委员会委员、云南省中西医结合学会常务理事、中医药国际交流专家库专家、国家中医药管理局中医药科技咨询与评审专家库专家、科技重大专项课题评审专家、云南省中西医结合学会养生专业委员会主任委员、云南省中西医结合消化病研究中心主任。从事中西医结合临床教学科研工作三十余年，发表论文六十余篇，获云南省科技进步三等奖四项、云南省卫生科技教育管理协会卫生科技成果奖励二等奖一项，获第二届“中西医结合贡献奖”。主编、参编多部医学著作，多次参加国内外学术会议，先后赴瑞典、芬兰、丹麦、新加坡、泰国、法国、西班牙等国讲授中医知识。

Professor Li Qing，female，chief physician，tutor of postgraduate students，learned from Professor Zhan Wentao，a nationally famous Traditional Chinese Medicine（TCM）doctor. She holds quite a few academic positions and titles which include：director of Integrated Traditional Chinese Medicine & Western Medicine Department，the Second Affiliated Hospital of Kunming Medical University，member of Education Committee of Chinese Association of Integrative Medicine，managing director of Yunnan Association of Integrative Medicine，expert of International Exchange Expert Base of TCM，expert of TCM Technology Consulting and Evaluation，State Administration of Traditional Chinese Medicine of the People’s Republic of China，evaluation expert of national key Science and Technology Special Projects，chairperson of Health Preservation Committee of Yunnan Association of Integrative Medicine，director of Digestive Disease Research Center of Yunnan Integrative Medicine. She has conducted clinical teaching and researches of integrative medicine for over thirty years and has published over sixty academic papers. Professor Li has won many awards which include 4 Third Award of Yunnan Science and Technology Progress，1 Second Award of Health Science and Technology Achievements of Yunnan Health Science and Technology Education and Management Association，Contribution Award of Second Integrative Medicine. She participated in the edition of many medical monographs and medical books. She participated in many international conferences and has been to Sweden，Finland，Denmark，Singapore，Thailand，France and Spain etc. to give lectures on traditional Chinese medicine.

◎ 宋精玲

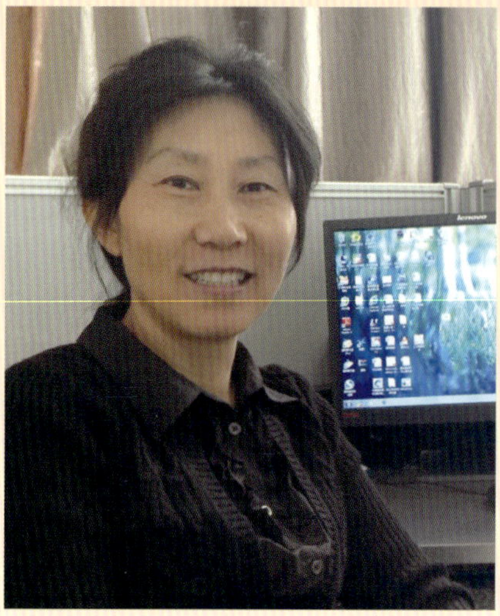

宋精玲，女，昆明医科大学病理学副教授。从事病理、超微病理教学研究三十余年，对中西医结合养生有一定研究；发表论文四十余篇，主编《中西医结合医学》，并参编多部医学教材。

Song Jingling, female, associate professor of Kunming Medical University, is the chief editor of Chinese and Western Integrative Medicine. She has conducted pathological and ultrastructural pathological teaching and researches for over thirty years. She has published over forty academic papers, and participated in editing several texts books.

副主编简介

◎ 张济周

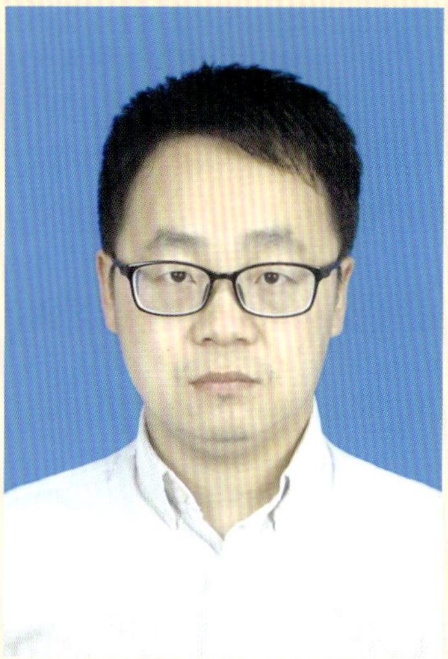

张济周，男，副主任，中医师，医学博士，中共党员。温州市中医院科教科副科长，浙江省中青年临床名中医，温州市“551”人才，温州市青年联合会委员，温州市卫生局“雄鹰计划”人才，中国老年学和老年医学学会肿瘤康复分会（CSGOR）青年委员，浙江省中医药学会肿瘤康复分会青年委员，中国中医药信息学会委员，中国抗癌协会临床肿瘤学协作专业委员会（CSCO）会员。现就职于温州市中医院，主要从事中医药系列研究及恶性肿瘤的相关研究，先后主持两项省部级课题、四项厅局级课题，参与一项国家级课题及多项省、市级课题，参编《中西医结合医学》等三部著作。对内科常见病、疑难杂症及肺癌、胃癌、乳腺癌、大肠癌等肿瘤的发病与中西医结合治疗有较深入的研究，在国内外核心期刊发表论文十余篇。

Zhang Jizhou, male, deputy chief physician, doctor of Medicine(MD), member of Communist Party of China. As the deputy chief of the Department of Science and Education, Wenzhou Hospital of Traditional Chinese Medicine, he is a famous clinical TCM doctor of Zhejiang Province, candidate of Wenzhou 551 Talent Program, member of the Wenzhou Youth Federation, talent of Wenzhou Municipal Health Bureau Eagle Program, youth member of Chinese Society of Gerontology and Geriatrics (CSGOR), youth member of Zhejiang Cancer Rehabilitation Branch of Chinese Medicine Society, member of Information Society of Traditional Chinese Medicine, member of the Coordinating Committee of Chinese Society of Clinical Oncology (CSCO) of China Anti–Cancer Association. He is now working in Wenzhou Hospital of Traditional Chinese Medicine. He has been conducting a series of researches on traditional Chinese medicine and related researches on cancer. He has presided over 2 provincial and ministerial research projects and 4 department–level and municipal research projects; he also participated in 1 national research projects and a number of provincial and municipal research projects, and the compilation of three books, including “Integrated Traditional Chinese Medicine and Western Medicine” etc. He has deep understanding of the attack of the common diseases of internal medicine, difficult and difficult miscellaneous diseases, lung cancer, gastric cancer, breast cancer, large intestine cancer and the treatment of these diseases by adopting Integrated Traditional Medicine and Western Medicine. He has published more than 10 academic papers in the core periodicals at home and abroad.

◎ 杨梁梓

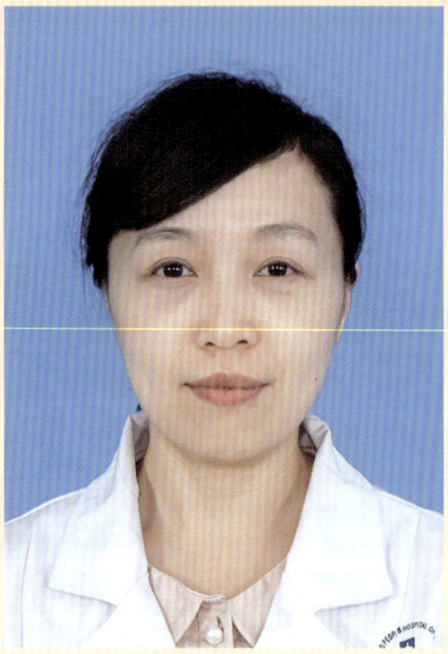

杨梁梓，女，硕士，主治医师。现就职于深圳市第三人民医院肺病医学部肺病三科，深圳医学会结核病专业委员会委员兼秘书、深圳市胸科医师学会会员、“三名工程”刘又宁教授团队青年骨干。从事临床医疗工作七年，擅长呼吸系统疾病中西医结合诊治预防及康复。曾到中国医学科学院肿瘤医院及美国加州大学尔湾分校医疗中心进修。参与两项课题，发表多篇医学文章。参编医学著作《中西医结合医学》。

Yang Liangzi, female, master of medicine, is an attending physician of Pulmonary Disease Department at Shenshen Third People's Hospital. She is a committee member and academic secretary of Shenzhen Medical Association Tuberculosis Branch, as well as member of Shenzhen Chest Physicians Association and a core member of Liu Youning's team. Having 7 years' experience of clinical medicine, Dr. Yang is good at diagnosis, prevention, treatment and rehabilitation of respiratory diseases by using integrated Traditional Chinese Medicine and Western medicine. She engaged in advanced study at Cancer Hospital of Chinese Academy of Medical Science and University of California Irvine Medical center. She participated in two medical research projects, writing of one medical book (Integrated Traditional Chinese Medicine and Western Medicine) and she has published many academic articles.

◎ 吕路艳

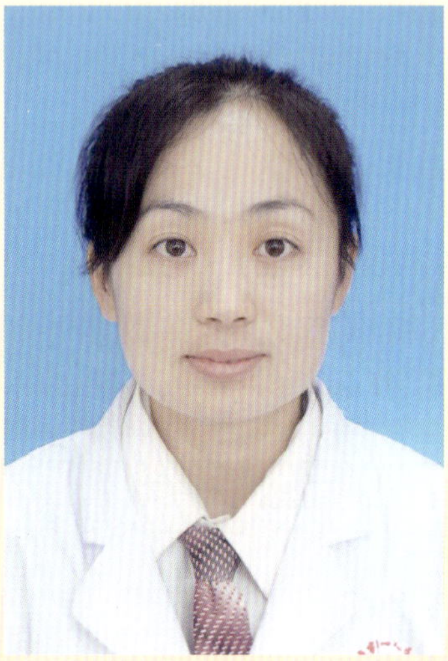

吕路艳，女，硕士，主治医师。2008 年本科毕业于昆明医科大学临床医学专业。2012 年 6 月硕士毕业于昆明医科大学中西医结合临床医学专业，师从昆明医科大学第二附属医院李青教授。在校期间主要从事中西医结合心肺疾病的基础及临床研究。现就职于云南省曲靖市第一人民医院老年病科。

Lv Luyan, female, master of medicine, attending physician, graduated from clinical medicine major of Kunming Medical University in 2008. From September 2009 to June 2012, she attended master program at Kunming Medical University, majoring in Integrated Traditional Chinese Medicine and Western Medicine.

During this period of time, she had Professor Li Qing as her tutor at the Second Affiliated Hospital of Kunming Medical University. During the postgraduate period, she mainly engaged in the basic and clinical research on the integration of Traditional Chinese Medicine and Western Medicine for the treatment of cardiopulmonary diseases. Since August 2012, she has been working in the department of geriatrics of the First People's Hospital of Qujing Municipality, Yunnan Province.

◎ 姚 璐

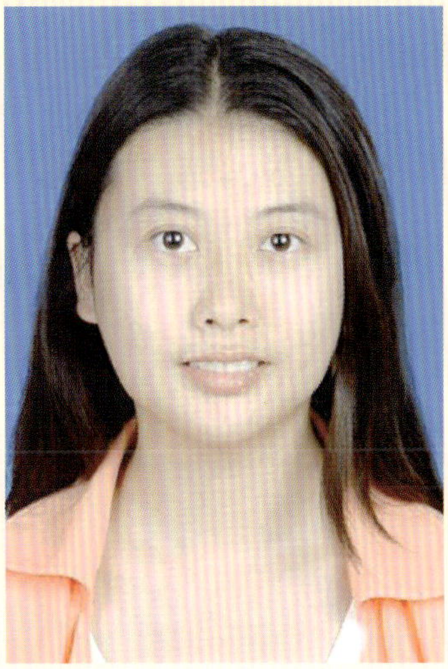

姚璐，女，在职研究生，昆明医科大学临床技能中心助教。2013年7月本科毕业于大理学院临床医学专业。2014年9月至2015年7月在昆明医科大学第二附属医院进行住院医师规范化培训。现就职于昆明医科大学临床技能中心，主要从事临床技能教学工作。主持完成昆明医科大学教研教改课题一项。参与云南省教育厅课题项目一项，同时在国内期刊发表论文三篇。

Yao Lu, female, on-the-job graduate student, teaching assistant of clinical skills center of Kunming Medical University, majored in clinical medicine and graduated from Dali University in July 2013. She particpated in resident standardization training in the Second Affiliated Hospital of Kunming Medical University from September 2014 to July 2015. Since September 2015, she has been working in the Clinical Skill Center of Kunming Medical University, mainly engaging in clinical skills teaching. Since she began to work in Kunming Medical University, she has presided and finished one teaching research and reform project of Kunming Medical University, and she has participated in a project funded by Yunnan Provincial Department of Education. She has published three academic papers in domestic journals.

翻　译

◎ 董　妍

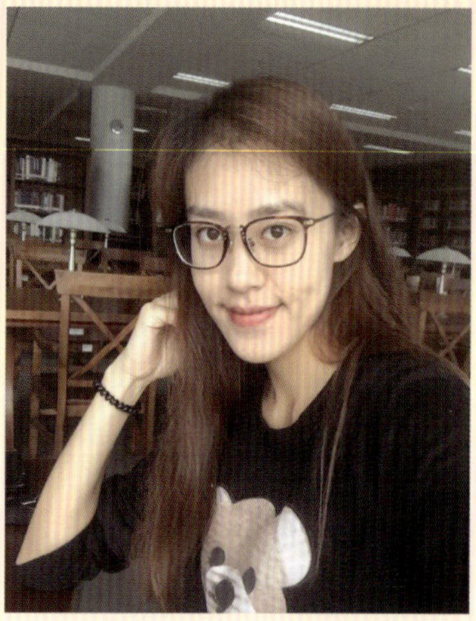

董妍，女，云南开放大学助教。硕士研究生毕业于澳大利亚 Monash 大学 TESOL 专业，现为在读博士，主要研究方向为认知语言及语言政策与规划。

Dong Yan, female, master of education, teaching assistant of Yunnan Open University, graduated from Monash University, and she is a PhD candidate in cognitive linguistics and language policy.

◎ 刘德周

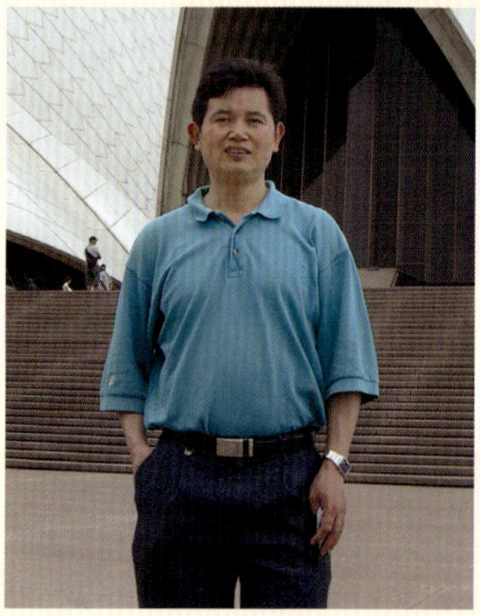

刘德周，男，硕士，云南师范大学外国语学院教授，英语语言文学及翻译专业硕士研究生导师，研究方向为英汉对比语言学及翻译学。对自然疗法等养生、保健知识有一定研究，在校内开设自然疗法方面的选修课程，深受学生欢迎。为国际会议、国际培训、中外合作国际项目、中外合作 MBA 项目等担任过数百场同声传译和交替传译工作。撰写有专著两部，参编教材多部，发表文章数十篇。

Liu Dezhou, male, professor of the School of Foreign Languages and Literature, Yunnan Normal University, is a tutor of the Master Program of English Language & literature and Master Program of Translation and Interpretation. His academic interests include English-Chinese Comparative Linguistics, translation & interpretation, natural therapy and health care etc. He has been giving lectures on natural therapy in the university for years, which is warmly welcomed by students. He has made simultaneous interpretation and consecutive interpretation for hundreds of international conferences, international training workshops, international cooperative projects, MBA programs etc. He has published two monographs and dozens of academic articles and participated in editing several texts books.

◎ 朱 明

朱明，男，北美精算师，《青铜兵器》第二作者兼主译。

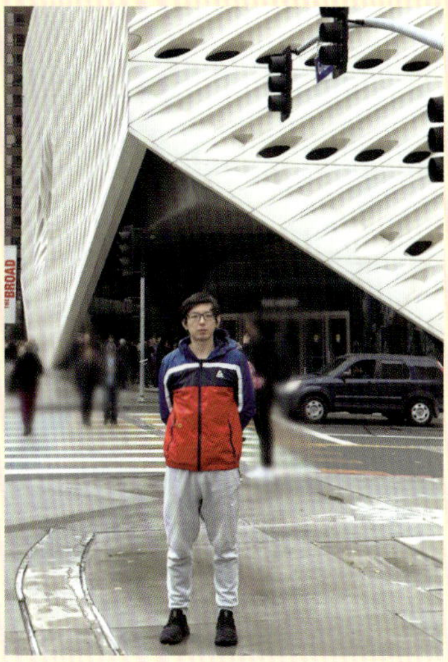

Zhu Ming, male, member of Society of Actuary, Co-author of “Bronze Weapons” and translator of the book.

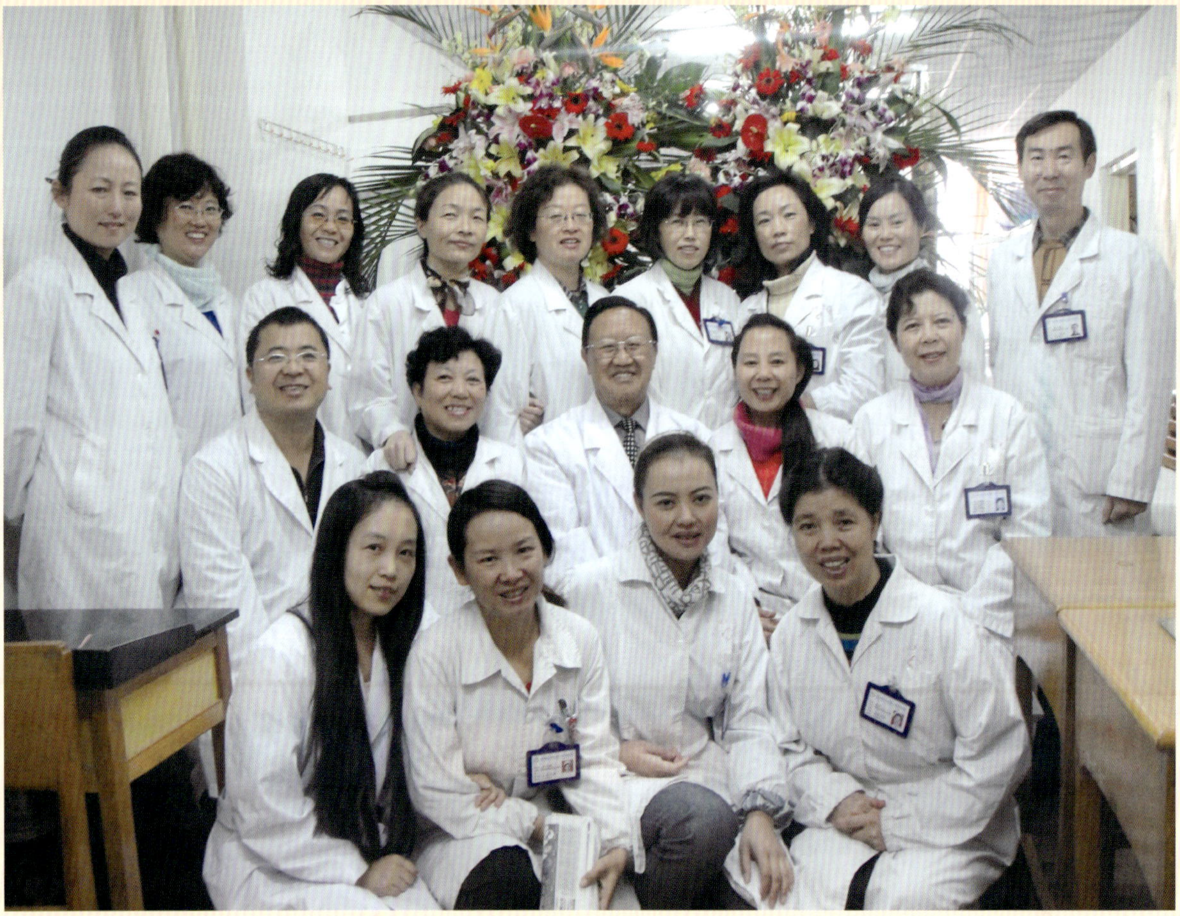

编委会部分成员合影

A Group Photo of Some Members of the Editorial Committee

前 言

世界上最宝贵的是生命，珍惜生命、追求健康长寿是古今中外人们的共同愿望，上至帝王将相，下至黎民百姓，概莫能外。生命像花儿一样美丽，生命像阳光一样灿烂，生命像烟花一样绚丽，她是那么美好，却又那般短暂。对于生命，我们应该怀着敬畏和感恩的心去呵护她、保护她、爱护她，让其轨迹得以延续，完善灿烂、绚丽的一生。而预防养生、卫生保健则是维护生命的基础。

在21世纪，“人人享有卫生保健”是世界卫生工作面临的重要任务。要实现“人人享有卫生保健”的宏伟目标，需要包括传统医药学在内的多种医学学科团队相互协作、共同努力。近年来，世界卫生组织越来越重视传统医药学的发展，并为推动其发展做出了卓有成效的工作。目前，疾病谱正在发生变化，疑难杂症不断增多，化学药品的毒副作用日益显现，日趋沉重的医疗负担困扰着各国政府和民众。中医药学是世界传统医学体系中最完整的传统医学，其独到的学科理论和突出的临床疗效，较符合当前人类社会解决上述难题的需要。因此，科学有效地发挥中医药学的医疗保健作用，成为21世纪世界卫生工作的重点之一。

在现代医学形成之前，人类一直依赖草药和一些传统疗法治病强身，从而发展出许多有理论、有实践价值的传统医学。例如，中医学、印度医学、阿拉伯医学等。中医学是世界上林林总总的传统医学中的瑰宝，并衍生了朝鲜传统医学和日本汉方医学。

在21世纪的今天，古老的传统医学依然散发着活力，非但没有因现代医学的发展而式微，其影响还有增无减，人们对传统医学的价值也有了更深刻的体会和认识。在许多第三世界国家，大多数农村人口仍依赖传统医学疗法和传统医务工作者来满足他们对初级卫生保健的需求。在现代医学占主导地位的许多国家，传统医学及其他一些“另类疗法”，如顺势疗法、整骨疗法、自然疗法等，也越来越为人们所接受。

伴随着世界各地经济、文化和生活的变革以及世界人口的老龄化，世界疾病谱发生了变化，新疾病所引起的新需求以及现代医学的局限使传统医学又重新得到重视与应用，绽放出夺目光彩。

Preface

Human lives are the most important thing in the world. Cherishing lives and pursuing health and longevity are the common wish of people in the past and present, in China and abroad; emperors, generals, ministers of states and the common are no exception. Lives are as beautiful as flowers, as bright as sunlight, and as magnificent as fireworks. Lives are fine but short. For lives, we should care them, protect them and love them with awesome and grateful heart, so that paths of lives can be extended and everyone will have a perfect, bright and magnificent life.

In the 21st century, "health for all" is an important task for world health to accomplish in the new century. The realization of "health for all" requires mutual cooperation and concerted efforts of various medical sciences, including traditional medicine. In recent years, WHO has increasingly emphasized the development of traditional medicine and has made fruitful efforts to promote its development. Currently the spectrum of diseases is changing and an increasing number of diseases are difficult to cure. The side effects of chemical drugs have become more and more evident. Furthermore, both the governments and peoples in all countries are faced with the problem of heavy burden of medical treatment. Traditional Chinese Medicine (TCM), a complete system of traditional medicine in the world with unique theory and excellent clinical curative effects, can basically meet the needs to solve such problems. Therefore, bringing TCM into full play in medical treatment and healthcare will certainly become one of the features in the world medical business in the 21st century.

Before the existence of the modern medicine, human beings depended on herbal medicines and other traditional therapeutic methods to treat diseases and preserve health. Such practices gave rise to the establishment of various kinds of traditional medicine with unique theories and practices, such as Traditional Chinese Medicine, Indian Medicine and Arabian Medicine, etc. Among these traditional systems of medicine, Traditional Chinese Medicine is a treasure from which traditional Korean medicine and traditional medicine in Japan are derived.

Even in the 21st century, traditional medicines are still of great vitality. In spite of the fast development of modern medicine, traditional medicines are disseminated far and wide, and people have more profound understanding and recognition of the value of traditional medicines. In many developing countries, most of the people in the rural areas still depend on traditional medicines and traditional medical practitioners to meet the need for primary healthcare. Even in the countries with dominant modern medicine, more and more people accept traditional medicines and other therapeutic methods, such as homeopathy, osteopathy and naturopathy, etc.

With the change of economy, culture and living styles in various regions as well as the aging in world population, the disease spectrum has changed. The new requirements initiated by the new diseases and the achievements and limitations of modern medicine have attracted people's attention and reapplication of traditional medicines. Therefore, traditional medicines are blooming with dazzling glamor again.

目 录

Contents

第一章　中医预防康复学概论

预防即康复疗法，是指合理选用养精神、调饮食、练形体、慎房事、适寒温等保健方法，通过长期的锻炼和修习，达到保养身体、减少疾病、增进健康、延年益寿的目的。中医预防学，是在中医理论的指导下，探索和研究中国历代心理、生理保健以及增强体质，预防疾病以延长寿命的实用科学。

治疗即康复，是指采用精神调节、合理饮食、体育锻炼、针灸推拿、药物等各种措施，对先天或后天各种因素造成的机体功能衰退或障碍进行恢复，达到提高或改善病残者生命质量的目的。它主要适用于病残、伤残患者。中医康复学，则是在中医学理论指导下，研究借鉴和吸收现代康复医学基本理论、医疗方法及其应用而形成的一门学科。

1.1　基本理念

中医养生康复学是从几千年实践经验中总结出来且不断有所发展的一门学科，其内容包括预防医学、心理医学、行为医学、保健医学、天文气象学、地理医学、社会医学等学科知识，中医养生康复学是以健康长寿为目的的综合学术体系。

1.1.1　天人相应

中医学认为，人生活在宇宙之间，生命活动必然会受到自然界物质运动规律的影响。因此，人体的所有活动必然与自然息息相关。人体生命活动与自然、社会的关系，必须是和谐有序的，否则，会对健康不利。这就是“天人相应”“形神合一”的思想。因此中医养生学和中医康复学特别强调人与自然环境和社会环境的协调。

1.1.2　和谐平衡

中医理论强调和谐、平衡，认为体内的物质代谢必须有升有降，心理与生理应该相互协调，心理疾病可以通过脏腑活动来调整，生理疾病也可以运用心理疗法来治愈。

中医养生、康复遵循自然变化的规律，使生命过程的节奏随着时间、空间的移易和四时气候的改变而进行调整。情绪保健要求不卑不亢，中和适度；睡眠不能偏多偏少；性生活不可无也不可多；形体需要劳动但不能疲倦等，都是立足于健康长寿的独特理论和方法。

1.1.3　身心互养

中医养生和康复的方法很多，但强调综合调理，不可以偏执偏信于一方一法。同时还要持之以恒，从自然环境到衣食住行，从生活爱好到精神卫生，从药饵强身到运动保健等，进行较为全面、综合的防病保健和功能康复。

中医基础理论中有因人、因时、因地制宜的原则。这也同样适用于养生活动和康复医疗。人有男女老幼之不同，时有春夏秋冬之四季，地有南北高低之悬殊，都不可一概而论。要根据个体，区别异同，合理运用不同的养生、康复措施，以达到最佳效果。

1.2 生命基础

1.2.1 精、气、神

中医经典著作《黄帝内经》认为，生命是由“气”所构成的，“气”属古典哲学中的物质范畴，指构成世间万物的基本元素。内环境的平衡协调、内环境与外界环境的整体统一，是人体得以生存的基础。在正常情况下，人通过自我调节可使其内环境与外界自然环境的变化相适应，以保持正常的生理功能。如果人的活动违反自然变化的规律，或外界自然环境发生反常的剧变，而人的自我调节功能又不能与之相适应，因内、外环境的相对平衡遭到破坏而导致疾病。因此，“顺应自然”是养生的首要条件。

精、气、神是生命活动所需的基本物质。

精，是构成人体及促进人体生长发育的基本物质，有“先天之精”与“后天之精”之分。“先天之精”来自父母；人出生之后，从饮食中获得的营养精华称为“后天之精”，先天、后天之精相互转化，相互补充，成为生命活动的动力基础。精的不足或亏虚，可导致生命活动减退，或导致早衰多病。

气，也是构成生命的重要物质。人体生命力的强弱、生命的寿夭，在于气的盛衰。生命现象，就是气机的升降出入。

神，是机体生命活动的总称，也是人体生命活动的外在表现，包括精神意识、思维活动、运动、知觉等。神以精血为物质基础，精、气充盈，神就健旺。所以，生命的健康与否，可以通过神的状况来判断。

由此可见，生命活动，是由精、气、神以及脏腑功能状态决定的。精、气、神充足，脏腑气血平衡，人体才会健康无病，不易衰老，寿命才能得以延长。

1.2.2 长寿基石

中国古代将人的寿命称为“天年”，意指先天赋予的“寿数”。古代医家认为，正常人的寿命在100~120岁。按照生物学的原理，哺乳动物的寿命是其生长期的5~7倍，人的生长期是以最后一颗牙齿长出来的时间（20~25岁）来计算，因此人的寿命应该是120岁左右。但由于天灾人祸、贫病横夭，大多会折损年寿，达不到预期寿命。中国人的平均寿命为70岁左右，比理论寿命少了50岁左右。

寿命的长短由人体的健康状况所决定，而影响健康的主要因素是衰老和疾病，所以维护健康、恢复健康是长寿的必要条件。

人体健康与否，可通过对“神”的观察来判断。“有神”的标志为形体壮实，肥瘦恰当；须发润泽，黑亮有光；面色红润，表情欢畅；眼睛有神，灵气荡漾；呼吸从容，不急不慢；食欲旺盛，美食三餐；牙齿坚固，不蛀不伤；听觉灵敏，耳内不响；声音洪亮，气息悠长；腰腿灵便，不痛不酸；二便通利，排放正常；舌红苔薄，脉象匀缓。

以上健康状态包括生理和心理两部分。实际上，中医自古以来就认为心理健康与生理健康同样重要。病因学说中的“七情”理论，要求情志调和，精神愉快，这也是脏腑功能良好的外在表现。

1.2.3　早衰因素

衰老是人类正常生命活动的自然规律，合理的养生和康复措施，可以延缓生理性衰老，阻断病理性衰老的进程，从而延长人的寿命。早衰的主要原因有如下几方面：

1.2.3.1　精气不足

精藏于肾，“肾为先天之本”，肾精匮乏，生命就会早衰。造成精气不足的原因主要有先天不足、性生活过度、疾病消耗、过度疲劳等。

1.2.3.2　营养不良

饮食是人体获取养料的来源。营养不良，包括营养摄入不足和营养吸收不良两方面。现代人营养摄入不足已很少见，而营养吸收不足则较多见，若人体所需要的营养得不到及时补充，便会影响机体健康，加速衰老，甚至导致死亡。

1.2.3.3　五脏受损

心藏神，主血脉，是生命活动的主宰。心脏患病，会影响血脉的运行及神志功能，从而加速衰老。肝藏血，主疏泄，调节情志，帮助消化，又有贮存和调节血量的作用。肝脏患病会影响到血液、情志、消化等众多方面的生理功能，导致人体衰老。肺主一身之气，肺气虚损或肺气阻塞，全身功能都会受到影响，出现不耐劳作、呼吸及血液循环功能逐渐减退等衰老表现。

1.2.3.4　情志过激

长期持久的精神刺激或突然受到剧烈的精神创伤，超过人体生理活动所能调节的范围，就会引起体内阴阳气血失调，脏腑经络功能紊乱，从而加速衰老。

1.2.3.5　劳逸失度

过劳或者过逸都对健康不利。过劳，不仅指脑力劳动、体力劳动过于繁重，也包括不正常的生活方式，如过于频繁的性生活、过度的饮食和娱乐等。反之，过于舒适的生活，也不利于健康长寿。

1.2.3.6　遗传禀赋

衰老和遗传有密切关系。先天禀赋强则身体壮盛，精力充沛，不易衰老。反之，先天禀赋弱则身体虚弱，精神萎靡，衰老就会提前或加速。

1.2.3.7　社会环境

社会地位的急剧变化，会给人带来精神和形体的损伤，从而导致早衰。先富后贫、先尊后卑者，会导致早衰甚至早夭。不合理的社会制度、不良的社会习俗、落后的意识形态、紧张激烈的生存竞争与复杂的人际关系，都可使人体代谢功能紊乱，导致早衰。

1.2.3.8　自然环境

气候寒冷的高山地区，居民寿命相对较长；平原或低洼以及南方常年高温的地区，居民寿命相对短些。此外，城市的环境污染比乡村严重，会危害健康，导致早衰。

1.2.4 养生渊源

中国是世界上人均寿命较长的国家，研究长寿理论和方法有两千多年的历史。每一个不同的历史时期都有著名的长寿典型，他们不仅自己能够得以长生，而且累积了很多健体延寿的经验。

1.2.4.1 老子："清静无为"

春秋战国时期，道家鼻祖老子提出了"清静无为""返璞归真""顺应自然""贵柔""动形达郁"的养生观。其主要精神是：心神宁静，少私寡欲，这样，人的精神才能得到润养，精气才能内藏而健康长寿。"清静无为以养神长寿"的思想，一直为历代养生家所重视，是中医养生理论的源头之一。传说老子寿命达160岁以上。

1.2.4.2 孔子："仁爱多寿"

孔子是儒家学术的奠基人。在养生长寿方面，孔子提倡道德养生，强调精神调摄，尽量减少物质欲望，以社会准则来规范人的行为。其"仁爱""中庸"的哲学观念，也体现在养生实践之中，如"君子三戒"（戒色、戒斗、戒得）。此外，注意生活规律，不过劳过逸；在饮食上，要求营养丰富，新鲜洁净，烹调精细，味道鲜美。孔子生活在战乱时代，其寿命亦达72岁。另一位善养"浩然正气"的儒家代表人物孟子则享年83岁。

1.2.4.3 华佗："动则不衰"

汉代名医华佗，从理论上阐述了动形养生的道理，认为"动"能够消化食物，流通血脉。"流水不腐，户枢不蠹"，所以健康长寿。在此基础上，他创编了著名的"五禽戏"，即模仿虎、鹿、熊、猿、鸟五种动物动作的健身体操，方法简便，行之有效。

1.2.4.4 陶弘景："调神养形"

南朝的著名养生家陶弘景，精于医学，通晓佛、道，所著《养性延命录》一书，为中国现存最早的养生学专著。书中论述的养生法则和方术甚多，大致有顺四时、调情志、动诸节、调气息、节饮食、宜小劳、慎房事等，其中"调神养形"是其主导思想。陶弘景享年80岁。

1.2.4.5 孙思邈："养性摄生"

唐代大医学家、养生家孙思邈，有巨著《千金方》存世，另著有《摄养枕中方》等养生专著。其养生术采用综合调理的方法，诸如食疗调养、房中补益（性生活对健康的促进作用）、调神动形、推拿按摩等，内容丰富。这些养生方法的使用，建立在"养性"（调摄情志，未病先防）学说的基础上。孙思邈高龄至101岁。

1.2.4.6 李东垣："调理脾胃"

金元四大家中"补土派"的李东垣，强调维护脾胃功能是延年益寿的重要原则：一是调节饮食护养脾胃；二是调摄情志保护脾胃；三是防病治病顾护脾胃。该理论为养生学，尤其是为老年养生奠定了基础。李东垣年寿71岁。

1.2.4.7 朱丹溪："养护阴气"

朱丹溪对人体健康状态有一个著名的理论——"阳常有余，阴常不足"，在养生上特别强调保护阴精，尤其对性生活损伤阴气的现象一再告诫。具体措施为强调顺四时以调养神气，饮食清淡以免升火助湿，节欲保精以熄相火欲念。朱丹溪寿至77岁。

1.2.4.8　李时珍："耐劳增年"

明代名医李时珍不仅以《本草纲目》而闻名，而且对养生术的综合运用甚有心得，论述药饵和食养的内容极为丰富，收集了很多食疗方法。李时珍主张老年人应培补元气，调理脾胃，用温补之剂延年益寿。他自己身体力行的健身术则是"耐劳增年"，不辞劳苦，跋山涉水，一方面寻求医药资料，另一方面也强健了体格，寿至75岁。

1.2.4.9　张景岳："阴阳互根"

明代医学家张景岳认为，阳气、阴精的根本在肾，养生必须强肾，阴阳兼顾。他创立了一批阴阳互动的补益方剂，流传至今。此外，他还提出了"中年修理"（重视中年人的养生保健）的理论，对于防止早衰、预防老年病具有积极的意义。张景岳年寿77岁。

1.3　适应自然

在中医理论体系中，顺应自然是整体观念的重要内容，无论是养生保健还是疾病的康复，所有的方法和机能，都体现着与自然相适应的特点。

1.3.1　人与自然相适应

中医认为人生于天地之间，一切生命活动都与大自然息息相关，必须随时随地与其保持和谐一致，这就是"天人相应"的思想。在养生、康复实践中，只有遵循这一基本法则，才能取得良好的养生、康复效果。

1.3.1.1　适应季节

四季的气候变化对人体的影响最大。春夏阳气发泄，气血易趋向于表，故皮肤松弛，疏泄多汗；秋冬阳气收藏，气血易趋向于里，表现为皮肤致密，少汗多溺。因此，有"春夏养阳，秋冬养阴"的理论，在康复医疗中，也要根据季节变化来增减药物，以获得较好的康复效果。

季节对五脏六腑、经络腧穴有直接的影响，不同的脏腑经络在不同的季节会出现气血偏旺的情况，如"肝旺于春""心旺于夏""脾旺于长夏""肺旺于秋""肾旺于冬"。合理运用这一规律来养生或康复，可收到事半功倍的效果。针灸、推拿康复治疗时的辨证选穴，也应在应用时体现这一原理。

1.3.1.2　顺从地理

中国的地理环境具有东方多湿、南方多热、西方多燥、北方多寒的特点。地域不同，人的体质和易患疾病也不一样。因此，要根据日常养生、疾病康复的具体情况，进行不同的处理。

1.3.1.3　顺应社会

中国历代养生家都认为健康和长寿之人能用乐观的、积极的态度看世界，而不以悲观的、消极的态度看待社会。无论何时何地，社会上都会存在利益的冲突，存在不稳定或不平衡的事件。如果以悲观的态度看社会，天天都会生气，会对健康造成不好的影响。若是以乐观的态度看社会，就会形成一种良好的精神环境，有利于养生和康复。俗语有"知足者常乐"，古籍《养生要语》中则说："笑一笑，少一少；恼一恼，老一老。乐一乐，瘦一瘦；让一让，壮一壮。"

1.3.2　形神共养

形，指形体，即肌肉、血脉、筋骨、脏腑等组织器官，是人的物质基础；神，指情志、意识、思维等精神活动，又指生命活动的全部外在表现，是人体功能的反映。

1.3.2.1　形为基础

形是神的物质基础，中医的“五神”（神、魂、魄、志、意）、“五志”（怒、喜、思、忧、恐）分别由五脏（心、肝、脾、肺、肾）所生成。神需要大量的气血精微濡养，如果神志方面出现疾患，要从五脏论治，这就是中医形神统一、形为基础观的具体体现。

1.3.2.2　神为统帅

人体起统帅和协调作用的是心神。生命活动表现出的整体特性、整体功能、整体行为、整体规律，都由神志管理、协调、统一。因此，养生时要以“养性”“调神”为先，而情志康复法也可以用于形体疾病的治疗。

1.3.2.3　形神共养

形神共养，既要注意形体的保养和复健，又要注意精神的摄养和康复，两者相辅相成，相得益彰，身体和精神都得到均衡统一的发展。

1.3.3　动静兼修

1.3.3.1　阳动阴静

脏腑器官属阴，以静为特征；功能活动属阳，以动为特征。人体有关饮食的吸收、运化，水的代谢，气血的循环贯注，代谢废物的传导排泄，其物质和功能的相互转化等，都是在机体内脏功能动静协调之下完成的。因此，保持适当的动静协调状态，才能使各器官充满活力，从而推迟各器官的衰老改变。

1.3.3.2　动静相济

中国历代养生家有的偏重于运动，有的偏重于静养，但大多数养生家提倡动静结合，根据不同对象和情况各有侧重。动静兼修、动静适宜，运动和静养并重，是中国传统养生和康复的重要原则。

1.3.4　协调平衡

协调人体自身的生理功能状态及其与外在环境之间的相互关系，平衡机体各系统和组织器官间的正常功能，以及机体与外界的物质交换，也是中国养生、康复学的重要内容。

1.3.4.1　元素平衡

五行元素的“生克制化”维持着自然界的生态平衡和人体生理的协调平衡。人体还必须与自然界化学元素平衡协调。例如，缺碘导致甲状腺肿、缺锌可致不育。依照中医元素平衡的观念，必须纠正体内元素的失调，维持体内各种元素的协调平衡。

1.3.4.2　调节平衡

人体的功能失调、对称失衡、状态失稳，是人体生理功能低下和早衰、疾病的重要原因。中医养生学和康复技术手段中有调节平衡的理论和方法，如针灸、推拿中的“上病下取”“下病上取”“左病右取”“右病左取”等方法，养生学中的“体脑交替”“动静交替”等。

1.3.5　培补正气

“先天之本在肾，后天之本在脾”，脾、肾两脏产生的营养精微，是全身脏腑功能的动力。因此，正气为本的观念，首先要落实在脾、肾两脏。

培补正气是补肾的关键，增强运化是健脾的关键，两者还有相互促进、相互补充的作用。在所有的养生、康复活动中，脾肾功能的维护和促进，是不可忽视的重要内容。

1.4　整体观念

1.4.1　整体原则

人体是一个有机的整体，中医养生康复学应指导或帮助患者与自然、社会融为一个整体，还要使人体各个组成部分之间协调统一，形体与精神协调统一，这就是中医养生康复学的整体原则。

1.4.1.1　注重协调

在进行养生保健和康复医疗时，对局部的功能障碍要使之能与整体统一，还要时时注意调整形体与精神之间的关系，使之恢复统一协调的状态。

1.4.1.2　与自然同步

中医养生和康复活动要顺应季节气候的变化及地理条件的差异等。注意“因地制宜”“因时制宜”的原则，目的就是顺从四时气候、地域差异的变化规律，来调理脏腑、调畅气血、调摄精神，以适应自然界的生、长、收、藏的变化，保持人体内外阴阳的相对平衡，从而达到健康长寿的目的。

1.4.1.3　与社会适应

社会环境的变化也会影响人体的生理功能及病理变化，如社会发展的工业化和都市化趋势的加快，导致环境（包括空气、土壤、噪声）污染，引发一些新的疾病；生活方式的改变、工作压力的增大，使“现代文明病”日益严重。当今时代大量流行的疾病，如冠心病、高血压、消化性溃疡、支气管哮喘等的发生，都与社会环境有关。因此，帮助患者适应社会环境的变化，纠正其不良生活方式与行为，加大对环境污染的治理与防护等，也都属于中医康复学的重要内容。

1.4.2　辨证观念

辨证论治是中医学最大的特色。养生措施和康复医疗必须根据辨证的结果来确定相应的养生、康复原则和方法。在辨证论治理论的指导下，病同证异，康复亦异；病异证同，康复亦同。此外，还要兼顾辨证与辨病相结合的原理来指导康复医疗。

1.4.3　功能观念

人体生理活动，是气机的“升降出入”有序。养生学要求维护生理功能；康复医疗的目的是恢复正常的功能状态，它注重功能训练，运动形体，促使精气流通，使脏腑组织的生理功能得以协调，最大限度地恢复个人生活、家庭和社会生活以及职业工作的适应能力。

1.4.3.1　脏腑功能重在协调

康复患者，伤残病后余邪未尽，正气尚虚，脏腑功能未完全恢复正常，必须针对其病理特点，采取综合措施，促使脏腑功能尽快恢复，并且能与其他脏腑协调。如肝病患者康复期不仅要消除其肝经湿热，也要顾及脾胃功能的损伤。

1.4.3.2　生存能力重在质量

生存能力主要指日常生活能力和职业工作能力。要采取多种方式进行功能训练，保存和恢复其身体运动、感知、言语交流等方面的功能，提高生活质量。

Chapter 1 The Theoretical basis of Prevention and Treatment of Diseases in TCM

Prevention of diseases is life cultivation. Life cultivation is to achieve the purposes of conserving health, preventing diseases, enhancing health and prolonging life span by means of various health care measures such as cultivating the mind, regulating the diet, exercising the body, moderating sexual life and adapting oneself to cold and heat, etc. Disease Prevention of TCM, a practical science, is to explore and study Chinese psychological and physiological health care measures through the ages as well as enhancement of physique, prevention of diseases and prolongation of life under the guidance of TCM theories.

Rehabilitation. Rehabilitation is to improve the life quality of patients and the handicapped by rehabilitating the functional decline or dysfunction of body caused by various congenital or postnatal factors by way of mental regulation, proper diet, physical training, acupuncture and massage, medicine as well as bathing, recreation, etc. It is mainly applicable to the pathogenically handicapped and maimed patients. Rehabilitation of TCM is a science to study and absorb the basic theories, therapeutic methods and the application of modern rehabilitation medicine under the guidance of TCM theories.

1.1 Basic Concepts

TCM Life Cultivation and Rehabilitation is a science based on the summarization of the practical experiences of thousands of years. As a comprehensive academic system with health and longevity as its purposes, it includes multidisciplinary knowledge like preventive medicine, psychological medicine, behavioral medicine, medical health care, astrometeorology, geomedicine and social medicine etc.

1.1.1 Correspondence between man and universe

TCM believes that man lives amidst the universe and his activities are inevitably influenced by the natural laws of material movement. Therefore, all the activities of the human body inevitably has close relationship with nature. The relationship between activities of the human body and nature as well as society should be harmonious and orderly. Otherwise it is not good for health. This is the thought of "correspondence between man and universe" and "unity of physique and spirit". Accordingly special emphasis is placed on the harmony between man and natural and social environments.

1.1.2 Harmony and balance

The theories of TCM stress the significance of harmony and balance. They hold that the substance metabolism of the human body should include ascension and descension, that psychological conditions and physiological conditions should be mutually harmonious and that psychological disorders may be regulated with visceral movement while body diseases may be cured with psychological therapeutic methods.

TCM life cultivation and rehabilitation follows the patterns of natural changes so that the pace of life process is accordingly adjusted with the changes of time, space, four seasons and climate. For example, emotional healthcare should be neutral and moderate rather than humble or arrogant; we should neither sleep excessively nor insufficiently; sexual life should neither be ignored nor be excessive; the body needs labor but should not be exhausted, etc. All these are based on the unique theories and methods of health and longevity.

1.1.3 Mutual regulation of physiological health and mental health

TCM has numerous life cultivation and rehabilitation methods, but it emphasizes comprehensive regulation so that people should not focus on or have partiality to one method only. Meanwhile, perseverance is required to achieve more overall and comprehensive prevention of diseases and health care as well as functional rehabilitation from natural environment to food, clothing, shelter and transportation, from hobbies to mental hygiene, from enhancement of physique with drugs to health care through sports, etc.

In basic TCM, there is a principle that treatment should suit individual physique, seasonal conditions and local conditions. It is also applicable to health preservation activities and rehabilitation treatment. People differ in gender and age; season differs in spring, summer, autumn and winter while geography varies in south and north as well as altitude. All these should not be lumped together. Different methods of health preservation and rehabilitation should be reasonably adopted on the basis of individual condition.

1.2 Basis of Life

1.2.1 Essence, Qi and sprit

TCM classic *Huangdi Neijing* holds that life consists of "Qi" (In classic philosophy "Qi" belongs to material category, referring to the basic elements which constitute everything in the world). The balance and harmony of the internal environment of the human body, the unity of the human body and the external surroundings are the foundation for man to live and exist. In normal cases, the adjustment of the human body can adapt the internal environment to the changes of the external natural environment to maintain normal physiological functions. When human activities violate the laws of natural changes, when abnormal and violent changes occur in the external natural surroundings and the regulatory function of the human body fail to adapt itself to the situation, the relative balance of the internal and external surroundings may be destroyed, which give rise to disease. Therefore, "conforming to nature" is the first requirement for health preservation.

Essence, Qi and spirit are the basic substances essential to vital activities.

Essence is the basic material constituting the human body and promoting the growth and development of the human body. Essence is divided into "congenital essence" and "acquired essence". Congenital essence is inherited from the parents. After birth, the nutrition derived form the diet is called acquired essence. Congenital essence and acquired essence can be transformed into each other and supplement mutually to form the dynamic foundation of vital activities. If essence is deficient, vital activities will decline, causing premature ageing and susceptibility to diseases.

Qi is the important substance constituting life, too. The sufficiency or deficiency of Qi determines the strength of life and life span. The vital phenomena are the ascending, descending, coming - in and going - out of the functional activities of Qi.

Spirit is a general term for vital activities of body and also the outward manifestation of vital activities of the human body. It includes mentality, consciousness, thinking, movement and perception etc. Essence and blood are the material foundation of spirit. And sufficient essence and Qi bring on prosperous spirit. Therefore, whether life is healthy or not can be judged by inspecting the state of spirit.

It can be seen from the above that vital activities are determined by the conditions of essence, Qi, spirit and visceral functions. Abundant essence, Qi and spirit, the balance of visceral Qi and blood ensure good health and freedom from diseases, insusceptibility to ageing, and extension of life span.

1.2.2 Foundation of longevity

In ancient China, life span was called "tian nian", which means "the life span endowed by Heaven for existence in the world". Ancient medical professionals believed that the normal human life span is 100 years to 120 years. According to the biological laws, the life span of mammals is 5 times to 7 times of the period of growth. The growth period of human being is calculated according to the time of dentition of the last tooth (at the age of 20 to 25). Accordingly, the life span of human beings should be 120 or so. However, due to natural and man-made calamities, poverty and diseases, most people suffer from shorter life and cannot reach the normal life expectancy. The average life span of the Chinese is about 70, 50 years shorter than theoretical life span.

Life span is determined by the human health conditions while the main factors affecting health are ageing and diseases. Accordingly, preserving and restoring health are the essential requirements for longevity.

Inspecting "spirit" can judge whether the human body is healthy or not. The signs of "having spirit" are as follows: the general appearance is sturdy, neither fat nor thin; the beard and hair are black, bright and lustrous; the complexion is ruddy with delightful expression; the eyes are expressive and full of vividness; the respiration is calm and neither rapid nor slow; the appetite is good with three meals deliciously eaten; the teeth are hard and firm without caries and injury; the sense of hearing is acute without tinnitus; the voice is loud and clear with long breath; the waist and legs are flexible without pain and soreness; the urination and defecation are smooth with normal discharges; the tongue is red with thin fur while the pulse is even and slow.

The above discussion includes the two parts of physiological and psychological health states. In fact, TCM has held that psychological health is as important as physiological health since ancient times. The theory of "seven emotions" in the etiology requires emotional regulation and spiritual happiness. This is also the external manifestation of good visceral functions.

1. 2. 3 Factors of premature aging

Aging is the natural law of normal human vital activities. Reasonable health preservation and rehabilitation measures may delay the occurrence of physiological aging and block the progress of pathological aging so as to prolong human life span. Premature aging mainly includes the following causes:

1. 2. 3. 1 Deficiency of essence and Qi

Essence is stored in the kidney. "The kidney is the congenital base of life." If renal essence is deficient, life will age prematurely. The deficiency of essence and Qi mainly originates from congenital insufficiency, excessive sexual life, exhaustion caused by diseases, physical overstrain etc.

1. 2. 3. 2 Malnutrition

The diet is the source for the human body to obtain nutrients. Malnutrition includes the two aspects of insufficient ingestion and malabsorption. Insufficient ingestion is seldom seen in modern people while malabsorption is more common. If the nutrients required by the human body cannot be instantly supplemented, this will affect the health of human body, speed up aging, and even result in death.

1. 2. 3. 3 Impairment of the five Zang organs

The heart stores spirit and controls blood circulation. It is the dominator of vital activities. If the heart suffers from diseases, it will affect blood circulation and mental functions, consequently accelerating aging. The liver stores blood, governs smoothing, regulates emotions, promotes digestion as well as regulates blood volume. If the liver suffers from diseases, it will affect various physiological functions of blood, emotions, digestion, etc. accordingly giving rise to aging of the human body. The lung dominates Qi of the general body. Deficiency and impairment or obstruction of the lung may affect the functions of the general body. In these cases, aging manifestations like lack of durance to physical labor, gradual functional decline of respiration and blood circulation will occur.

1. 2. 3. 4 Excessive emotional stimuli

If persistent emotional stimuli or sudden violent psychic trauma occur beyond the range of adjustment of physiological activities of the human body, it will cause disorders of Qi and blood inside the human body, functional disturbances of viscera, meridians and collaterals, thus speeding up aging.

1. 2. 3. 5 Maladjustment of work and rest

Overstrain and too much rest are both harmful to health. The so-called overstrain refers to not only excessive and heavy mental labor and physical labor, but also abnormal life style such as too frequent sexual life, excessive food ingestion and recreation, etc. On the contrary, excessively comfortable life is not good for health and longevity, either.

1. 2. 3. 6 Heredity

Aging is closely related to heredity. Good heredity results in strong physique full of vigor and insusceptibility to aging. Conversely, poor heredity brings on wan and sallow complexion and listlessness consequently; aging will occur early or acceleratively.

1. 2. 3. 7 Social environment

Dramatic changes in social position may bring about mental and physical impairment to people. Thus, premature aging will appear. Besides, when rich life is replaced by poverty or respectable status is followed by low one, both may result in premature aging, and even death at a young age. Also, irrational social systems, unhealthy social customs, backward ideology, intense and acute competition for existence as well as complicated interpersonal relationships may all result in metabolic disorders of the human body, giving rise to premature aging.

1.2.3.8 Natural surroundings

Residents in mountainous areas with cold climate possess relatively long life; dwellers have relatively short life in flatlands and low-lying lands as well as in the south with high temperature throughout the year. Besides, environmental pollution in cities is more serious than that in rural areas; this can affect health and promote premature aging.

1.2.4 Origins of life cultivation and life prolongation

China is a country with longer average life span in the world and a history of studying the theory and methods of longevity for more than 2,000 years. During each historical period, there exist famous typical longevous masters. They have not only lived a long life, but also accumulated much experience in strengthening health and prolonging life.

1.2.4.1 Lao Zi: "Cherish no worries and keep away from fame and gain"

During Spring and Autumn Period and the Warring States Period, Lao Zi, the originator of Taoism, put forward his ideas about life cultivation: "Cherish no worries and keep away from fame and gain" "Man restores the pure and innocent nature of the ancients" "Conform to nature" "cherish mild character" and "train the body to remove depression". The chief gist of these ideas lies in mental tranquilization and abstinence from improper personal desires. Only in this way, can human spirit be cultivated essence and Qi internally stored. Consequently health and longevity can be obtained. Experts on life cultivation throughout the ages have attached importance to the thought on life cultivation of "cherishing no worries and keeping away from fame and gain". It is the theoretical source of TCM life cultivation. According to the record of historical literature, the life span of Lao Zi exceeded more than 160 years.

1.2.4.2 Confucius: "Be benevolent to achieve longevity"

Confucius was the academic founder of Confucianism. As far as life cultivation and longevity are concerned Confucius advocated moral life cultivation, stressed the importance of cultivation of the mind, that material desires should be reduced as much as possible and that human behavior should be restrained by social norms. Of these social norms, the philosophical concepts of "benevolence" and "the doctrine of the mean" were also embodied in his life cultivation practice such as "three kinds of abstinence for gentlemen (Namely: abstinence from sexual life, abstinence from fights, abstinence from worrying about personal gains and losses)". In addition, people should live a regular life and avoid overstrain and overrest; dietary requirements should be nutritious, fresh, clean, meticulously cooked and delicious. Though Confucius lived in an age of chaos caused by war, his life span also reached 72 years. Another representative figure of Confucianism, was good at cultivating noble spirit, and he died at the age of 83.

1.2.4.3 Hua Tuo: "Ageing does not occur with the movement of the body"

Hua Tuo, the noted doctor in the Han Dynasty, theoretically expounded life cultivation with the bodily movement. He thought "movement" promotes easy digestion and smooth blood circulation, and that in this way, people can enjoy long life just as "Running water is never stale and a door hinge never gets worm-eaten". On this basis, he invented the famous "Wuqinxi", or the five mimic-animal games. It is an easy, convenient and effective keeping-fit exercise which imitates the motions of the five animals of tiger, dear, bear, monkey and bird.

1.2.4.4 Tao Hongjing: "Cultivate the mind to nourish the body"

Tao Hongjing, the famous expert on life cultivation in the Southern Dynasty, had a good command of medicine and was well versed in Buddhism and Taoism. His book *Records on Cultivating Character and Prolonging Life* is the earliest extant treatise on life cultivation in China. The book discusses a great number of life cultivation principles and methods, the main ones of which include conformity to seasonal changes, regulation of emotions, movement of every joint, regulation of respiration, moderate amount of food intake, light physical labor, proper sexual life, etc. Of all the principles and methods, "cultivate the mind to nourish the body" is the dominant idea. Tao Hongjing also died at the age of 80.

1.2.4.5 Sun Simiao: "Cultivate the disposition to preserve health"

Sun Simiao, a great expert on medicine and life cultivation, wrote a great work *Qian Jin Fang* or *Valuable Prescriptions*, which has been handed down. Besides, he wrote treatises on life cultivation such as *Sheyang Zhen-Zhong Fang* or *Handy Prescriptions for Life Cultivation*. The comprehensive, regulation methods are adopted in his life cultivation techniques such as dietary therapy for life cultivation, promotion of health with moderate sexual life (Sexual life promotes health), regulation of the mind for promotion of activities, massage, etc. The content is very rich. The application of these life cultivation methods is based on the theory of "cultivation of disposition" (regulating emotions, taking prevention before the onset of diseases). Sun Simiao lived to the age of 101.

1.2.4.6 Li Dongyuan: "Regulate the spleen and stomach"

Li Dongyuan, the founder of the School of Nourishing Earth (Spleen) of the four medical schools in the Jin and Yuan Dynasties, also emphasized that the protection of splenogastric functions is the important principle for prolonging life. This means, firstly, regulation of diet protects and nourishes the spleen and stomach; secondly, emotional regulation protects the spleen and stomach; thirdly, in preventing and treating diseases, protection of the spleen and stomach should be taken into consideration. This theory has laid a foundation for health preservation, especially for senile life cultivation. Li Dongyuan died at the age of 71.

1.2.4.7 Zhu Danxi: "Nourish and protect yin"

Zhu Danxi put forth a well-known theory concerning the human health— "Yang is usually in excess while yin is constantly insufficient in the human body." He especially emphasized the importance of protecting essence. Particularly, he warned people time and again of the impairment of yin due to excessive sexual life. The specific measures for protecting yin include conforming to seasonal variations to regulate and nourish the mind and Qi, eating bland diet to avoid promoting fire and promoting dampness, abstinence from sexual desires for conservation of essence to extinguish renal fire and eliminate lust. Zhu Danxi died at the age of 77.

1.2.4.8 Li Shizhen: "Stand hard work to extend life span"

Li Shizhen of the Ming Dynasty is not only famous for *Bencao Gangmu* or *Compendium of Materia Medica*, but also had a good command of the comprehensive application of life cultivation techniques. He had very rich discussions concerning life cultivation with drugs and the diet and he collected many dietary therapeutic methods. Li Shizhen advocated that senior people should reinforce and tonify primordial Qi, regulate the spleen and stomach, use prescriptions with warming and tonic actions to prolong life. He himself earnestly practiced his advocation of "standing hard work to prolong life". On the one hand, he made nothing of hardships, traveled across mountains and rivers to seek for medical materials. On the other hand, he also strengthened his constitution in this way. Li Shizhen lived to be 75.

1.2.4.9 Zhang Jingyue: "The interdependence of yin and yang"

Zhang Jingyue, a medical expert of the Ming Dynasty, believed that yang Qi and yin essence are rooted in the kidney. Therefore, he advocated that life cultivation should concentrate on enhancing the kidney with simultaneous consideration of yin and yang. And he also established a set of tonic prescriptions with the actions of mutual tonification of yin and yang which have been handed down up to now. In addition, he also put forward the theory of "life cultivation in the middle-age" (which attaches importance to life cultivation in middle-aged people). This has a positive significance for prevention of premature aging and senile diseases. He died at the age of 77.

1.3 Conforming to Nature

Conforming to nature is the important content of the concept of holism in Chinese medical system. All the methods and functions in life cultivation and health care and the rehabilitation of diseases are embodied in the feature of Conforming to nature.

1.3.1 Man's adaptation to nature

TCM believes man and universe, all vital activities and nature are closely related to each other, and man should keep harmony with nature at any time anywhere. This is the thought of "man's relevant adaptation to nature". Only when the concept of man's harmony and unity with nature is constantly observed, can good effects of life cultivation and rehabilitation be achieved.

1.3.1.1 Adaptation to seasons

Seasonal variations influence the human body greatly. In spring and summer, yang Qi releases and Qi and blood easily tend to reach the surface. Therefore, the skin is loosened and sweat comes out. In autumn and winter, yang Qi turns constricted and stored. At this time, Qi and blood tend to reach the interior. Thus, it manifests as tight skin, scanty sweat and profuse urine. Because of the above points, there exists the theory of "nourishing yang in spring and summer, and yin in autumn and winter". Seasonal changes should also be taken into account in modifying drugs to achieve better effects in rehabilitation.

Seasons have direct influences on the five Zang organs and six Fu organs. Relative excess of Qi and blood may occur in different viscera, meridians and collaterals in different seasons. For example, "relative excess of Qi and blood exists in the liver in spring" "relative excess of Qi and blood exists in the heart in summer" "relative excess of Qi and blood exists in the spleen in late summer" "relative excess of Qi and blood exists in the lung in autumn" and "relative excess of Qi and blood exists in the kidney in winter". Reasonable application of this principle may get twice the result with half the effort in life cultivation or rehabilitation. This principle can also be applied in selecting acupoints according to the syndrome differentiation in acupuncture and massage.

1.3.1.2 Conforming to geography

Dampness prevails in the east; heat in the south; dryness in the west and cold in the north in the Chinese geographical environment. People in different regions differ from one another in physique and susceptibility to diseases. Accordingly, different treatment should be based on specific situations during the daily life cultivation and rehabilitation of diseases.

1.3.1.3 Conforming to society

Chinese life cultivation experts throughout the history believe that healthy and longevous people view the world optimistically and positively. They do not approach society pessimistically and negatively. There exist conflicts of interests, unstable or unfair affairs in society everywhere anytime. If viewing society pessimistically, people may get angry every day. This has bad effects on health. If approaching society optimistically, people may form a good spiritual environment. This is beneficial to life cultivation and rehabilitation. A Chinese saying goes like this "One is always happy if one is content with one's lot". The classic *Yang Sheng Yao Yu* or *Essential Words for Life Cultivation*, says: "If one smiles, he will become a little younger; if one is angry, he will become a little older; if one becomes a little happy, he will get a little thinner; if one yields, he will become a little stronger."

1.3.2 Unity of physique and spirit

Physique refers to the configuration and constitution of the human body consisting of the tissues and muscle, blood vessels, tendons, bones, viscera, etc. as the material base of man; spirit refers to the mental activities such as emotions, consciousness and thinking. It also denotes the outward manifestations of all vital activities as the reflections of the functions of the human body.

1.3.2.1 Physique as the base

"Physique" is the material base of "spirit". TCM believes "the five types of spirit" (vitality, soul, vigor, will, consciousness) and five emotions (anger, joy, sorrow, anxiety, fear) are produced by the five Zang organs (the heart, liver, spleen, lung and kidney) respectively. "Spirit" requires the nourishment of Qi, blood and food essence. In case of spiritual disorders, the treatment should be based on the five Zang organs. This is the specific manifestation of unity of physique and spirit, and physique as the material base of spirit.

1.3.2.2 Spirit as the commander

The spirit functions as the commander and coordinator of the human body. The wholeness of characteristics, functions, behavior and principles reflected in vital activities are all managed, coordinated and unified by spirit. Thus, there exist the measures of putting "cultivation of disposition" and "regulation of the mind" first in life cultivation. These methods of life cultivation with regulation of the mind are also applicable to physical diseases.

1.3.2.3 Simultaneous cultivation of spirit and physique

This means that people should not only pay attention to conserving their physique, but also to the cultivation of spirit. The two aspects supplement each other and promote mutually to achieve the harmonious and unified development of the body and spirit.

1.3.3 Interdependence of movement and motionlessness

1.3.3.1 Movement of yang and motionlessness of yin

Viscera belong to yin, characterized by motionlessness. Functional activities pertain to yang, marked by movement. The coordination of movement with motionlessness of visceral functions of organism completes all the absorption, transportation and transformation of food, the circulation and metabolism of water, the flow of Qi and blood, the transportation and excretion of digested stuff, mutual transformation of material and function, etc. Proper harmony between movement and motionlessness can make every organ function vigorously. As a result, the aging and changes of each organ are delayed.

1.3.3.2 Coordination between movement and motionlessness

Of Chinese experts on life cultivation in successive dynasties, some relatively attached importance to movement, and some to tranquility. However, most of them advocated the combination of movement and motionlessness. According to different people and situations, relative emphasis is placed on one aspect to gain the effect of simultaneous nourishment of physique and spirit. Life cultivation with concurrent movement and motionlessness, proper adjustment of movement and motionlessness and equal stress on both are the important principles of traditional Chinese life cultivation and rehabilitation.

1.3.4 Coordination and balance

Coordination of physiological functional states of the human body and the relationships with the external environment, balance of the normal functions of each system and tissues and organs of the organism as well as exchanges of material between functions of organism and nature are the important academic content of traditional Chinese life cultivation and rehabilitation.

1.3.4.1 Balance of elements

The interpromotion and restraint of the five elements maintain ecological balance in nature and the physiological coordination and balance of the human body. Besides, the human body should have the balance and coordination of chemical elements in nature. For instance, iodine deficiency gives rise to thyroid enlargement and zinc deficiency to infertility. According to the concept of balance of elements in TCM, imbalance of elements inside the human body should be remedied to keep the coordination and balance of various elements inside the body.

1.3.4.2 Coordinative balance

Dysfunctions, loss of symmetry and unstable states of the human body are the important causes giving rise to physiological hypofunction, premature aging and diseases of the human body. There exist the theory and methods of coordinative balance in the medical techniques of life cultivation and rehabilitation in

TCM. For example, there are such methods as "treating diseases in the upper part by managing the lower" "treating diseases in the lower part by managing the upper" "treating diseases in the left by managing the right" and "treating diseases in the right by managing the left" in acupuncture and massage as well as "alternation of physical labor and mental one" and "alternation of movement and motionlessness" in life cultivation.

1.3.5 Healthy Qi as the base

"The congenital base lies in the kidney and the postnatal base in the spleen." The nutritional essence coming from the two Zang organs of the spleen and kidney is the motive power of the visceral functions of the whole human body. Thus, the concept of healthy Qi as the base should first aim at the two Zang organs of the spleen and kidney.

Reinforcing essence and Qi is the key to the tonification of the kidney, and strengthening transportation and transformation is the key to enhancement of the spleen, both of which promote and supplement mutually. Of all activities of life cultivation and rehabilitation, the conservation and promotion of functions of the spleen and kidney are the important content which cannot be ignored.

1.4 The Concept of Wholism

1.4.1 Principle of wholism

The human body is an organic whole. The medicine of TCM life cultivation and rehabilitation should guide or help patients to be in harmony with nature and society. Besides, it should also make all parts of the human body harmonious and unified, physique and spirit harmonious and unified. These are the principles of wholism in the science of life cultivation and rehabilitation.

1.4.1.1 Attach importance to coordination

During rehabilitation, local dysfunctions should be unified with the organic whole. In addition, attention should be constantly paid to the regulation of relationships between physique and spirit to restore the unified and harmonious states.

1.4.1.2 Conform to natural change

The activities of life cultivation and rehabilitation should conform to seasonal and climatic changes as well as geographical differences, etc. This book constantly pays attention to principles of "treatment in accordance with geographical conditions" and "treatment in accordance with seasonal conditions", the purposes of which are to conform to the laws of seasonal and climatic changes and regional differences during regulation of viscera, promotion of Qi flow and blood circulation and cultivation of the mind. In doing so, people can adapt themselves to the natural changes of germination, growth, reaping and storing so as to keep the relative balance of yin and yang inside and outside the human body. As a result, the aim of health and longevity will be reached.

1.4.1.3 Adapt to social changes

Social environments may also influence physiological functions and pathological changes of the human body. For example, due to the social development, industrialization and urbanization speed up. This causes environmental pollution (including air pollution, soil pollution and noise pollution). As a result, some new diseases occur. The changes of life style and increase of work pressure give rise to more and more "modern civilization diseases". A large number of the currently widespread diseases, such as coronary heart disease, hypertension, peptic ulcer and bronchial asthma, are associated with social environments. Therefore, guiding patients to adapt themselves to changes of social environments, correcting their bad life styles and behaviors, greatly enhancing the control over and prevention of environmental pollution, belong to the important content of the science of TCM rehabilitation as well.

1.4.2 Principle of syndrome differentiation

Differentiating syndrome to decide treatment is the greatest characteristic of TCM. During life cultivation and rehabilitation, the result of syndrome differentiation should be applied to determine the corresponding principles and methods of life cultivation and rehabilitation. Under the guidance of differentiating syndrome to decide treatment, same disease with different syndromes is rehabilitated differently while different diseases with the same syndrome are rehabilitated in the same way, too. Besides, the principle of combination of syndrome differentiation with disease differentiation should be concurrently taken into consideration to guide rehabilitation.

1.4.3 Principle of functions

The physiological activities of the human body are the ascending, descending, exiting and entering of the functional activities of Qi. The science of life cultivation requires that these normal functional states should be maintained and restored in rehabilitation. Besides, attention should be paid to functional training, movement of physique to promote circulation of healthy Qi, and harmonization of physiological functions of viscera and tissues. In this way, patients' abilities to adapt themselves to their individual life, family and social life as well as professional work can be restored to the greatest extent.

1.4.3.1 Normal visceral functions mainly lie in coordination

Convalescent patients still suffer from residual pathogenic factors and deficiency of healthy Qi after recovery from wounds, handicap and diseases. Their visceral functions are not completely restored. Comprehensive measures should be taken to restore visceral functions as quickly as possible, and to coordinate other viscera according to the pathological features. For instance, as for a patient with liver disease during convalescence, not only dampness and heat in the liver meridian should be cleared away, but also the injury of the spleen and stomach should be taken into account.

1.4.3.2 The significance of viability mainly lies in quality

Viability chiefly refers to daily living ability and professional working ability. Various ways should be adopted to train, conserve and restore functions in the fields of bodily movement, perception, lingual communication, etc. to improve the life quality.

第二章 养生康复疗法

2.1 精神疗法

中国古代医学家们很早以前就指出：健康的人体，不仅是没有疾病和虚弱现象，而且还要有良好的精神状态和社会适应能力。现代社会中，精神因素引起的身心疾患越来越普遍，21世纪，精神类疾病将成为人类的多发病和流行病。

在正常情况下，七情活动对五脏生理功能起着协调作用，但若七情太过，超过人体自身调节的范围，脏腑气血紊乱，则导致疾病。

2.1.1 制 怒

“怒”是历代养生家最忌讳的一种情绪，它不仅伤肝脏，还可伤心、伤胃、伤脑等，导致各种疾病。因此，怒是养生、康复最应节制的不良情绪。

制怒，就是要以理性克服感情上的冲动，平时遇到可怒之事，要想到不良后果，以理智驾驭并控制粗暴的情绪反应。如古今明理之人常在案头悬挂“制怒”“息怒”之类警句，提醒自己戒怒。

2.1.2 发 泄

在遭遇挫折，或蒙受冤屈，或遇见烦闷、悲愤之事时，应采取适当的方式发泄不良情绪。如遇到不幸事件，悲痛万分时，在无人处大哭一场；遭逢挫折，心情压抑时，去空旷处大声喊叫，将郁结情绪发泄出来。

2.1.3 疏 导

出现不良情绪时，相约两三个知心朋友，宣泄心中郁闷，并接受友人的劝解疏导，可以借此化解或排遣不良情绪。

2.1.4 移 情

移情，即排遣情思，改变情绪的指向性，以排除内心杂念和抑郁，改变不良情绪和习惯。当遇到情绪郁闷时，不妨“看书解闷、听曲消愁”，利用琴棋书画来转移情志，陶冶性情。

2.1.5 运 动

精神刺激造成的不良情绪，可以通过运动发散出去，也可以转移自己的注意力，调整机体平衡。如打球、散步、爬山、打拳、舞剑等，都可转移或释放精神上的紧张不适。尤其传统的体育运动锻炼，动静结合，能使形神舒畅，对消除不良情绪有效。此外，还可以参加适当的体力劳动，用形体的运动去消除精神的紧张、恼怒和悲伤。

2.1.6 暗 示

暗示疗法是通过暗示手段促使患者康复的一种方法。古代“杯弓蛇影”的成语就是典型的暗示实例。中国古代的祝由术也包含暗示疗法的成分。

暗示有积极暗示和消极暗示两类：积极暗示是不管别人的意见正确与否，都无条件、无分析、无批判地加以全盘接受，它对人的身心产生积极作用；消极暗示则是全盘否定和拒绝，它对人的身心起消极作用。暗示疗法正是利用暗示的积极作用促使人体身心的康复，同时应注意避免暗示的消极作用。

暗示疗法可在两种场合下进行：一种是不经任何催眠过程，而在完全觉醒状态下进行；另一种是先使患者进入催眠状态，然后予以暗示。后者的效果优于前者。此外，患者还可以进行积极的自我暗示，反复强化“身体健康、疾病痊愈”的意识，从而引导脏腑功能向有序的方向发展。

2.1.7 色 彩

根据色彩对人体神志的影响，选定一定的色彩，通过眼睛直接作用于精神情志，即“悦目爽神”，还可以通过色调、色温等调节精神。

该法以“五色配五脏、五志”的理论为指导，在病人居住环境，如居室、用具、陈设、衣被、窗帘、灯光以及与病人接触的康复医护人员的衣着上，按需要的颜色布置和穿戴，或者在医院或疗养院设置色彩疗法康复室和“颜色仪”，来对适合的病种进行康复调理。色彩及其适应证如下：

2.1.7.1 暖色

红色、橙色，具有温暖的感觉，有使人兴奋、喜乐的功效。适用于郁证、癫证、嗜睡、痴呆症等。

2.1.7.2 冷色

青色、蓝色、紫色、绿色，任选其中一、二、三色均可，有清凉、镇静的作用。适用于烦躁易怒、失眠惊恐诸证以及狂证、痛证等。

2.1.7.3 喜色

红色、粉红色，使人喜悦，有制悲之效。适用于情绪低落、易悲善泣、抑郁不乐者。

2.1.7.4 悲色

黑色为主，亦可用白色，有制怒之功。适用于易怒、过喜者等。

2.1.7.5 恐色

黑色，有制止过喜的功效。适用于狂证、喜笑不休等。

2.1.7.6 思色

黄色、浅蓝、淡绿，有制恐和利于思维的功效。适用于惊恐、思想不集中等。具体应用时可据病情需要适当配伍，或用单色、或用复色、或淡色、或浓色，灵活选择。

2.1.8 以情制情

以情制情是两千多年前《素问·阴阳应象大论》提出的方法，其内容是：怒伤肝，悲胜怒；喜伤心，恐胜喜；思伤脾，怒胜思；忧伤肺，喜胜忧；恐伤肾，思胜恐。这种“以情制情”的方法，基于“以偏救偏”的原理。金元医家张子和对它进行具体的介绍：“以悲制怒，以怆恻苦楚之言感之；以喜治悲，以谑浪戏狎之言娱之；以恐治喜，以恐惧死亡之言怖之；以怒制思，以污辱欺罔之言触之；以思治恐，以虑彼忘此之言夺之。”

2.1.8.1 恐胜喜

这是通过恐惧因素来收敛耗散的心神，克制大喜伤心，恢复心神功能。本法常用于喜笑不休、心气涣散的病症以及因过喜而致的情志失调。

2.1.8.2 怒胜思

这是通过愤怒因素来克制思虑太多，恢复心脾功能。本法常用于思虑太多，伤脾耗神所致的郁证、失眠、癫痫等病症。

2.1.8.3 喜胜悲

这是通过喜乐因素来消除太过悲哀的方法。本法常利用轻松浪漫、妙趣横生的语言和滑稽可笑的表演、说笑话、听相声、观喜剧，乃至医者有意的荒唐诊断来满足患者急切的愿望，以解救患者的困境，从而收到以喜制悲的效果。临床多用于悲哭证、脏躁证以及由悲哀过度所致的病症。

2.1.8.4 悲胜怒

这是通过悲哀因素来克制愤怒太过。本法常用于其他病症兼有情绪亢奋者，如眩晕、狂证、痫证等。

2.1.8.5 思胜恐

这是通过思虑因素来克制惊恐太过。本法常用于惊恐证的康复医疗，以消除患者的恐惧情绪。

在运用“以情制情”方法时，要注意情志刺激的强度，使之超过或压倒致病的情志因素。如采用突然的刺激，或是采用持续不断的强化刺激。此外，现代人领会上述方法的精神实质，可以采用其他相应方法，不可简单地生搬硬套。

2.2 日常疗法

起居养生法，主要探讨外环境对人类健康的影响，对其日常生活中的衣食住行、站立坐卧、苦乐劳逸等各个方面进行科学的安排并采取一系列健身措施，以达到祛病强身、延年益寿的目的。

2.2.1 环 境

环境包括自然环境和人工环境。自然环境包括地球上的空气、水、土壤、岩石和生物等；人工环境指人类为从事社会聚居生活而建立的城乡生活居住环境。室内环境包括在人工环境中。

中国古代的风水术，是一种探讨如何创造有益于延年益寿、养生保健的理想环境的理论。它强调人与自然的和谐相处，是集地质学、地理学、生态学、建筑学、伦理学、美学等于一体的综合性的古代建筑规划设计理论。综合其中要点，它认为人类适宜的自然环境应该具有洁净而充足的水源、新鲜的空气、充沛的阳光、良好的植被以及幽静秀丽的景观等。这种自然环境不仅能满足人类基本的物质生活需求，还适应人类特殊的心理需求。

某些地方因地理条件而出现“山区多瘿瘤”“岭南多瘴气”等地方病，中医学很多专著对此早有论述。还有人体必需的微量元素，在不同地理条件下分布亦不同，如缺碘地区易患地方性甲状腺肿，缺氟引起龋齿。另外，某些放射性物质对人体也是有害的，如铀矿、磷矿等。若有强烈的放射源，可造成当地居民贫血以及白血病、癌症的发病率增高。

因此，应尽量避开不利于人体健康的地区、矿藏，避开高压线、强磁场和有超声波、放射线的地方营建生活区。

此外，治理大气、水源、噪声污染，是保证人体健康的基本条件，需要政府、社会、家庭与个人的努力，以营造健康长寿的环境。

2.2.2　起　居

2.2.2.1　作息规律

中医养生的一个基本要求是“起居有常”，即起居作息、日常生活要有规律，这是强身健体、延年益寿的重要原则。

若起居作息毫无规律，恣意妄行，则会导致适应能力减退、抵抗能力下降、发病率增加等老化现象的出现，进而引起早衰，甚至影响寿命。

对养生长寿最有帮助的正确生活方式：安排合理的生活作息制度，做到每日定时睡眠、定时起床、定时用餐、定时工作学习、定时锻炼身体、定时排出大小便、定期洗澡等。但所有“定时”“定期”，仍需根据具体情况（如年龄、季节、地域、体质等）加以灵活掌握，切勿过于机械。

2.2.2.2　劳逸适度

古人主张劳和逸的标准是“中和”，有常有节，不偏不过。只有动静结合，劳逸适度，才能活动筋骨，通畅气血，强健体魄，增强毅力，保持生命活力的旺盛。劳和逸，不仅包括体力的消耗，还包括用脑适度。应提倡善于用脑，劳而不倦，保持大脑常用不衰。经常性合理用脑，可以预防衰老，增强智力，尤其是能够预防老年性痴呆。

劳逸适度的标准因人而异，一般可借鉴以下做法：①体力劳动要轻重相宜。②脑力劳动要与体力劳动相结合。③休息保养多样化，除了采用睡眠形式的休息，也可选用听音乐、聊天、下棋、散步、观景、钓鱼、赋诗作画、打拳等休息方式。

2.2.2.3　科学睡眠

在人的一生中，睡眠占有极为重要的地位。要想健康长寿，就要采用合理的睡眠方法，保证睡眠质量、消除机体疲劳、养蓄精神，从而达到防病治病、强身益寿的目的。睡眠对健康长寿的作用表现在以下五个方面：①消除疲劳，恢复体力。②保护大脑，维护智力。③增强免疫，增加抵抗力。④促进儿童发育，增长身高。⑤健美皮肤，排除废物。如果睡眠异常，则上述五个方面就会出现不良改变，从而影响人体健康和长寿。

1. 睡眠时间。中国养生家创造了不少有益的睡眠养生方法，简便易行，而且卓有成效。例如，“子午觉”就是睡眠养生法之一。其法为：每天于子时（23 时 ~ 1 时）、午时（11 时 ~ 13

时）两次入睡。原因：子午之时，阴阳交接，极盛及衰，体内气血阴阳极不平衡，此时静卧，可避免气血受损。实践证明，子、午两时睡眠的质量和效率都好，老年人还可以降低心脑血管疾病的发病率，符合养生道理。在睡眠时间上，要训练良好的睡眠规律。

古人将睡眠的时间规律总结为“春夏宜早起，秋冬任晏眠，晏忌日出后，早忌鸡鸣前”。

2. 睡眠姿势。在睡眠姿势方面，要求“卧如弓”。这是一种对人体有益的卧姿。古今医学家都选择右侧卧为最佳卧姿。右侧卧时心输出量增多，食物的消化和营养物质的吸收与代谢得到加强，人自身感觉也比较舒适。

对于女性来说，不宜仰卧和俯卧，因为俯卧会增加颜面皱纹，仰卧对盆腔血液循环不利，易致各种月经病。正常人宜右侧卧，而孕妇宜取左侧卧，因为右侧卧会压迫腹部下腔静脉，影响血液回流，不利于胎儿发育和分娩。而左侧卧有利于胎儿生长，可以大大减少妊娠并发症。

对婴幼儿来说，应该在大人的帮助下经常地变换体位。因为长时间一侧卧或仰卧、俯卧，易使头颅发育不对称，或面部五官畸形。一般每隔 1 ~ 2 小时翻一次身。

对于心衰病人及咳喘发作病人宜取半侧位或半卧位，同时将枕与后背垫高。对于肺病造成的胸腹积液患者，宜取侧卧位。有瘀血症状的心脏病人，如肺心病人等一般不宜取左侧卧或俯卧，以防心脏负荷过重。头低足高位置睡觉，易得肾脏疾患。

应该指出的是，上述睡眠姿势虽然有利于养生保健，但并不要求睡着后姿势永远不变，因为这是无法做到的。

3. 卧具选择。

（1）枕头。枕高以稍低于肩至同侧颈部距离为宜，过高影响肝脉疏泄，还会诱发脑缺氧、打鼾和落枕；过低则影响肺气宣降，还会使头部充血，易造成眼睑和颜面浮肿。枕头不宜过宽，以 15cm ~ 20cm 为好，但稍长不妨。枕芯应选质地松软之物，软硬适度，稍有弹性。

中医有使用药枕养生、康复的习惯。药枕是采用不同药物加工制成枕芯做成的枕头。这种枕头既有治疗作用，又具保健作用。常用的单味药枕有：

菊花枕：适用于头痛目赤、头晕或患风火赤眼、虚烦失眠及高血压病患者。

薄荷枕：适用于头痛、牙痛、鼻炎、咽喉炎、高血压等疾病患者，并有防暑降温作用。

桑叶枕：适用于头痛、眩晕、高血压等疾病患者。

茶叶枕：用饮后晒干的茶叶装枕。适用于防治高血压、神经衰弱、暑热头晕等。

荞麦枕：适用于失眠、头痛眩晕、小儿夜啼等病症。

绿豆枕：适用于防治头痛、头风，可令人明目开窍，解暑除烦。

灯芯枕：适用于失眠、心烦、健忘、小儿夜啼等证，并有益智作用。

决明子枕：适用于便秘、目疾、高血压和小儿夜啼等。

侧柏叶枕：适用于口鼻经常出血、慢性咽炎、咽部充血、慢性咳嗽及轻度脱发者。

蚕沙枕：适用于头风、落枕、颈椎关节痛及下颌关节痛。

以上为单味药制成的药枕，若根据病症情况适用复方药枕，则疗效更佳。

失眠用枕：用黑豆、磁石粉装枕芯。

鼻炎（鼻炎、鼻窦炎）用枕：白芷、辛夷各等分装枕。

青光眼、眼胀痛用枕：夏枯草、荷叶、白芷、草决明子各等分装枕。

高血压患者用枕：①用草决明子、菊花装入枕芯。②菊花 100g、川芎 100g、牡丹皮 100g、白芷200g，装枕。

解暑枕：绿豆衣200g、扁豆衣200g、荷叶150g、薄荷200g、荞麦壳100g，装枕。

明目枕：荞麦皮200g、黑豆皮200g、决明子80g、菊花150g，装枕。

安眠枕：夜交藤200g，合欢花60g，酸枣仁、柏子仁、五味子各30g，装枕。

此外，古代道家有一著名的延年益寿药枕方，名为“丁公仙枕”：川椒、秸梗、荆实子、柏子仁、姜黄、吴茱萸、白术、薄荷、肉桂、川芎、益智仁、枳实、当归、川乌头、千年健、五加皮、白蒺藜、羌活、防风、辛夷、白芷、附子、白芍药、藁本、苁蓉、北细辛、猪牙皂、芜荑、甘草、荆芥、菊花、杜仲、乌药、半夏各30g。

以上药物粉碎成粗末，装入布袋或绢袋，充为枕芯，每夜枕之。一剂药料可用半年左右。

药枕对头面、五官、肩颈等部位的疾病疗效较好，而胸、腹及肢体疾患则不宜用。如患者对药物过敏，应停止使用。

（2）床上用品。被里宜柔软，可选细棉布、棉纱、细麻布等，不宜用腈纶、尼龙、的确良等带静电荷的化纤品。被胎宜选棉花、丝绵、羽绒为最好。被宜轻不宜重，宜宽大；褥宜软而厚，随天气冷暖变化加减。

（3）睡衣、睡帽等。睡衣宜宽大无领无扣，秋冬宜棉绒、毛巾布，春夏宜丝绸、薄纱。老人冬日睡卧宜戴棉布睡帽，以能遮盖住整个头顶为宜；不论冬夏，睡卧时宜穿肚兜，70岁以上老人更应如此。

睡眠“十忌”。一忌仰卧；二忌忧虑；三忌睡前恼怒；四忌睡前进食；五忌睡卧言语；六忌睡卧对灯光；七忌睡时张口；八忌夜卧覆首；九忌卧处当风；十忌睡卧对炉火。

4. 服饰选择。

中医养生学对四季服饰的增减方面有较多经验。它要求脱、添衣服时必须不失四时之节。如春季阴寒未尽，阳气渐生，早春宜减衣不减裤，以助阳气的升发。夏季尽管阳热炽盛，仍需适当穿着衣服，才能固护正气。秋季气候转凉，亦要注意增衣，但要避免一次添衣过多。俗有“春捂秋冻”之说，即春季宁稍暖，秋季可稍凉。冬季衣物要随寒冷而渐增，不能“一步到位”，穿着过厚。

穿衣不宜过暖过寒，否则机体缺乏耐受风寒的能力，而使抗邪防病之力减弱。老人和身体虚弱的人对寒热的耐受性较差，应尽量慎重脱、添衣物，以免风寒暑湿之侵。

大汗之时忌当风脱衣，否则易受风寒之邪侵袭而致病。汗湿之衣不得久穿，因为汗后腠理虚，湿衣不易干，汗湿滞留肌肤，伤害人体阳气，易产生风寒湿之类的病变。

5. 注意排便。

养成良好的二便卫生习惯，对健康长寿具有重要意义。

（1）保持大便通畅。古代养生家对保持大便通畅极为重视。如果老人一天中有规律地正常排便两次，被认为是长寿的征象。如果大便经常秘结不畅，则会导致浊气上扰，气血逆乱，脏腑功能失调，产生或诱发多种疾病，如头痛、牙痛、肛肠病、冠心病、高血压病、脑血管意外、肠癌等。保持大便通畅的方法主要有：①要养成定时排便的习惯。②排便要顺其自然，有便不强忍，大便不努责。③按摩通便。顺时针按摩可以增强肠胃功能和消化排泄功能，经常进行腹部按摩有助通便。④注意肛门卫生和便后调理。所用手纸要薄而柔软。晚上睡觉前，用温水清洗一下肛门。经常以热水坐浴，保持肛门清洁和良好的血液循环。

在食物中，燕麦粥通大便较好，尤其适宜老年人。因为燕麦不仅有通便作用，还能降低胆固醇、三酰甘油，也有减肥效果。

便后保健亦不能忽视。如饱食后大便，便后宜稍喝一些汤或饮料，以助胃气而利消化。若在饥饿时大便，则排便时宜取坐位，便后稍进食物，还可做提肛动作3～5次，以补固正气。

（2）维持小便清利。古代养生家十分重视小便卫生。保持小便清洁、通利，是维持身体健康的重要内容。其具体方法主要有：①合理饮食。少食、素食、食后不要立即饮水、感到口渴才饮水等，是古人从实践中得出的保证小便清利的经验。②按摩利尿。按摩腰：取端坐位，两手置于背后，上下推搓30～50次，上至背部，下至骶尾，以腰背部发热为佳，可在晚上就寝时和早晨起床时进行练习。按摩腹：取仰卧位，调匀呼吸，将掌搓热，置于下腹部，先推摩下腹部两侧，再推下腹部中央，各做30次。动作要由轻渐重，力量要和缓均匀。早晚练习。③切忌忍尿。有尿时要及时排出，忍尿会损伤肾与膀胱之气，引起病变。

此外，情绪、房事、运动对小便的清利也有一定的影响，要保持情绪乐观、节制房事和适当运动。

2.3 饮食疗法

2.3.1 饮食养生

2.3.1.1 补充身体的营养供给，强身防病

例如，食用动物肝脏，既可养肝，又能预防夜盲症；食用海带，既可补充碘及维生素，又可预防甲状腺肿；食用水果和新鲜蔬菜，既可补充营养，又可预防坏血病等。还可以发挥某些食物的特异作用，可直接用于某些疾病的预防。例如，用大蒜预防外感和腹泻；用绿豆汤预防中暑；用葱白、生姜预防伤风感冒等。

2.3.1.2 延年益寿，抗衰防老

很多食物都具有防老抗衰作用。例如，芝麻、桑葚子、枸杞子、桂圆肉、胡桃、蜂王浆、山药、人乳、牛奶、甲鱼等，经常食用，有利于健康、长寿。

2.3.2 饮食康复

2.3.2.1 辨证用膳

根据临床所辨证型，施以不同的饮食。如外感风寒表证，有头痛、鼻塞、畏寒、全身酸痛、无汗等表现，应选用生姜、葱白、红糖等温热食品煎汤热服，或吃大蒜末拌热面、芫荽黄豆汤发汗解表以散寒。若肾阳不足证，见腰酸膝软、肢冷畏寒、少腹拘急、尿频或不利等症状，应选用狗肉、雀肉、羊肉等食品，或白羊肾羹、冬虫夏草鸡等益火消阴的膳食。

2.3.2.2 辨病用膳

在辨证施食的基础上，还应根据病种不同而选用不同的饮食。如心悸怔忡，可选用当归、人参煮猪心；夜盲，可选多种动物肝脏与枸杞子、桑葚子等同用；肺虚咳嗽，可选用麻油炒猪肺或猪肺粥；肾虚腰痛可选用杜仲蒸猪腰；阿尔茨海默病，可选用猪骨髓、猪脑粉或桃仁粥；糖尿病，可选用猪胰脏；骨质疏松，可多食牛乳等。

2.3.2.3　科学用膳

科学用膳，可以用谚语“有粗有细不甜不咸，三四五顿七八分饱”来表述。前一句指中医养生提倡粗粮与细粮搭配，粗粮如玉米、黄豆、红薯之类，细粮则是粳米、面粉之类。后一句中，“三四五顿”是指每天吃的餐数，“七八分饱”则是经过历史检验的长寿经验。

古今中外，“七八分饱”饮食方式，是公认的有效的延年益寿办法。与现代的“低热量膳食”原理相近。所谓七八分饱，有两种衡量方法：一是离开饭桌时还有点饿，还想吃；二是未到下次进食时间就有饥饿感。中医养生格言“若要身体安，常带三分饥和寒”，已被无数长寿者所证实。

2.3.3　常用食疗处方

2.3.3.1　补益正气类处方

这类处方有滋补强壮、抗衰益寿的作用，适用于久病体虚，正气亏损者。

1. 补气类。

黄芪膏：生黄芪12g，生石膏12g，鲜白茅根12g，甘草细末6g，山药细末10g，蜂蜜30g。先将黄芪、石膏、鲜茅根煎煮十余沸，去渣澄清汁2杯，再调入甘草、山药细末同煮，并不断搅拌，以免药粉沉底。煮一沸其膏即成，再调入蜂蜜，煮令沸即可。分3次食用，1日服完。

补虚正气粥：炙黄芪30～60g，人参3～5g（或党参15～30g），白糖少许，粳米100g。先将黄芪、人参（或党参）切成薄片，用冷水浸泡半小时，煎取药汁，分早晚2次同粳米煮粥服食。

人参莲肉粥：人参10g，莲子10g，冰糖30g。以常法熬粥食用。

2. 补血类。

当归炖母鸡：当归15g，党参15g，母鸡1只（约重1500g），葱、生姜、料酒、食盐各适量。宰杀母鸡后，去净毛及内脏，洗净，将当归、党参置鸡腹内，放入砂锅中，加入葱、姜、料酒、食盐及适量清水，置灶上先武火煮沸，再改文火慢煎，直至烂熟即成。吃肉、喝汤。

红枣黑木耳汤：红枣5个，黑木耳15g，炖烂食用。

枸杞粥：鲜枸杞子100g，粳米60g，煮粥，粥成以咸豆豉佐餐食用。

3. 气血双补类。

桂圆参蜜膏：党参250g，北沙参120g，桂圆肉120g，先将这些原料以适量水浸泡，发透以后加热煎煮，沸腾后再煎30分钟，煎煮3次，合并3次煎汁，以文火浓缩，至成稠膏状时加入1倍量的蜂蜜，再煎沸即可停火，待冷后装瓶备用。每服1汤匙，以沸水冲化，顿服，每日3次。

龙眼肉粥：龙眼肉15g，茯苓10g，红枣3～5枚，粳米100g，同煮为粥，可加白糖少许食用。

4. 补阴类。

枸杞子酒：枸杞子200g，白酒600mL，将枸杞子用清水洗净，剪碎放入瓶中，加白酒约400mL，瓶口密封，每日振摇1次，浸泡一星期以后即可供饮用。每日晚餐或临睡前饮用10～20mL。瓶中酒可边饮边加（约共加200mL），枸杞子可拌糖食用。

玄参炖猪肝：玄参15g，猪肝500g，菜油、姜、葱、酱油、黄酒、豆粉各适量。将猪肝洗净，与玄参同置锅内，加水适量煮1小时，取出猪肝切成薄片备用。另将葱、姜加菜油稍炒，放入猪肝片中，再将酱油、白糖、料酒少量，兑加煮玄参、猪肝之原汤少许，收汁，勾入豆粉，使汁液透明，倒入猪肝片中，拌匀即成。

二母元鱼：元鱼（鳖）1只（约重500g），贝母、知母、前胡、柴胡、杏仁各5g，黄酒适量，食盐少许，宰杀元鱼，去头、内脏，洗净切块，加入贝母、知母、前胡、柴胡、杏仁及适量黄酒、少许食盐，加水没过肉块，置蒸锅中蒸1小时，于蒸熟后趁热食用。

百合粥：干百合研粉30g（鲜品加倍），粳米100g，加冰糖适量，煮粥早晚服食。

5. 补阳类。

鹿茸酒：鹿茸3～6g，山药30～60g，白酒500mL。将鹿茸、山药浸入酒中，封固，不定期地振摇，7天后即可供饮用。每晚临睡前饮服10mL。

白羊肾羹：肉苁蓉50g，荜拨10g，草果10枚，陈皮5g，胡椒10g，白羊肾2对，白羊脂200g，食盐、葱、酱油、发酵面等，如常法作羹。食用时，吃单肾、喝羹。

冬虫夏草鸡：公鸡1只，冬虫夏草5～10枚，姜、葱、食盐少许。宰杀公鸡。去净毛及内脏，洗净后放锅中，加入冬虫夏草及姜、葱、食盐、适量水，用小火慢炖，直至鸡肉烂熟即可供食用。

2.3.3.2　养心健脑类处方

这类处方有养心安神、健脑益智的功效。

核桃仁粥：核桃仁50g，粳米适量。将核桃仁捣碎，粳米淘洗干净，加水适量，如常法煮粥。

甘麦大枣汤：小麦30g，大枣10枚，甘草6g。先将大枣洗净，将小麦淘洗干净。再与甘草一同煎煮2～3次，去渣取汁，每日早晚饮用，或代茶饮用。

桂圆肉粥：桂圆肉15g，红枣3～5枚，粳米100g，同煮为粥，可加白糖少许食用。

2.3.3.3　生津止渴类处方

这类处方有清热除烦、滋阴润燥、生津止渴的作用，有益于消渴病人的康复。

五汁饮：梨汁、荸荠汁、藕汁、麦门冬汁、鲜芦根汁。将生梨去皮核，荸荠去皮，鲜藕去皮节，鲜芦根、麦门冬洗净，切碎或剪碎，以洁净纱布绞挤取汁，供饮用。不拘时、量饮服。若不喜凉，可水浴令温饮服。

猪胰汤：猪胰1具，生薏苡仁30g，黄芪60g，山药120g。先将猪胰洗净，入群药煎煮作汤供用。煮汤，盛汁饮用，不拘时。

清蒸茶鲫鱼：鲫鱼、绿茶。取500g重鲫鱼1条，去鳃、肠、内脏（留下鱼鳞），腹内装满绿茶，置盘中，放蒸锅内清蒸，熟透即可供用，食肉。

2.3.3.4　蠲痹止痛类处方

这类处方主要用于风寒湿痹、关节不利、痉挛急痛者。

木瓜汤：木瓜4个，白沙蜜1000g。先将木瓜蒸熟去皮，研烂如泥。另将白沙蜜炼净。再将两者调和均匀，放入洁净瓷器中盛贮备用，每日晨起空腹，用沸水冲调1～2汤匙，食用。

五加皮酒酿：五加皮50g，元米500g，酒曲适量，先将五加皮洗净，加适量水泡透后煎煮，煮沸后每30分钟滤取煎液1次，共取煎液两次。合并两次煎液，与淘净元米共烧元米饭。待冷，加适量酒曲，搅拌均匀，发酵成酒酿。每日适量。

川乌粥：生川乌头3～5g，粳米30g，姜汁约10滴，蜂蜜适量。先将生川乌头捣碎，碾为极细粉末。另将粳米煮粥。待粥沸，即加入川乌粉，并改文火缓慢熬煮。粥熟加入生姜汁，调入蜂蜜，搅匀，再稍煮1～2沸即可。早晚温服。热证及孕妇忌服，不可与半夏、贝母、瓜蒌、白及、白蔹等同用。

2.3.3.5 行气活血类处方

这类处方有行气活血、化瘀通络的作用，适用于心肌梗死、卒中后遗症等心脑血管病患者的康复期。

薤白粥：薤白10～15g（鲜品30～45g），粳米100g。取薤白、粳米一同煮粥，可供早点、晚餐服食用，温热食之。

丹参酒：丹参60g，好酒500mL。将丹参洗净晾干打碎，放入酒内泡1个月即可。

山楂粥：山楂30～40g（鲜品60g），粳米100g，砂糖10g。先将山楂用砂锅煎取浓汁，去渣，再入粳米、糖煮粥。

2.3.3.6 潜阳熄风类处方

这类处方有平肝潜阳，育阴熄风的作用，适用于高血压病、癫狂、震颤麻痹综合征等病症患者的康复期。

玉竹粥：玉竹15～20g（鲜品30～60g），冰糖少许，粳米100g。先将玉竹洗净切碎，煎取浓汁后去渣，入粳米煮为稀粥，放入冰糖，稍煮1～2沸即可，早晚服食。

荷叶粥：新鲜荷叶1大张，洗净煎取汁约500mL，加粳米100g，白糖适量煮粥，早晚服食。

葛粉面：葛粉250g，荆芥穗50g，淡豆豉150g。先煮荆芥穗、淡豆豉6～7沸，去渣滤取煎汁。将葛粉做成面条，放入芥穗、豆豉汤中煮熟。空腹食用。

2.3.3.7 止咳、祛痰、平喘类处方

这类处方具有止咳、祛痰、平喘等作用，可用于呼吸道疾患的保健康复。

燕窝汤：燕窝3g，冰糖30g。将燕窝放入碗内，加温水泡至松软，拣净杂入的金丝燕毛，复以清水冲洗，使洁净。沥去水，细撕如条，置净碗中。将冰糖压碎加入锅中，加清水250g，文火令沸使冰糖溶解，捞去浮沫并滤除杂质，倾入另锅中，再加入燕窝，加热令沸，盛入净碗备用。每日早晚各服1次。

银耳羹：银耳5g，鸡蛋1个，冰糖60g，猪油适量。将银耳以适量温水泡发，发透后，摘除蒂头，洗令洁净，加适量水，武火煮令沸。改用文火慢炖2～3小时，至银耳烂如泥。另器加适量水，放入冰糖，文火令沸使糖溶化，滤除杂质。又取鸡蛋清加少许清水搅匀后加入糖水锅中，加热令沸，捞去浮沫，将此汁倒入银耳锅中。出锅时加入猪油，即得。早晨或睡前服用。

枇杷叶粥：枇杷叶10～15g，粳米50g，冰糖适量。先将枇杷叶用布包起，水煎，去渣取浓汁，或将鲜枇杷叶30～60g刷尽毛绒，切丝水煎，去渣取汁，加入粳米煮粥，粥将成时加入冰糖，稍煮，供用。每日早、晚食用。

2.3.3.8 导滞除满、健脾和胃类处方

这类处方有消积导滞、清胃降逆、开郁除满、健脾燥湿等作用。适用于消化系统的保健和康复。

梅花粥：白梅花（绿萼梅）5g，粳米100g。先煮粳米，将成粥时，加入白梅花煮2～3沸即可，每日分2次空腹食用，3～5日为1个疗程。

橘皮粥：橘皮15～20g（鲜者30g），粳米50～100g。先把橘皮煎取药汁去渣，然后加入粳米煮粥。或将橘皮晒干研为细末，每次用3～5g，调入已煮沸的稀粥中，再同煮为粥。

益脾饼：白术30g，干姜6g，鸡内金15g，熟枣泥250g，面粉500g。白术、鸡内金、干姜生用取粉，熟枣泥（红枣煮熟收汁，将去核枣肉压拌成泥）中加少量水，和入药粉及面粉制小饼，

烙熟供用。不拘时、量，可常食。

2.3.3.9　润燥通便类处方

这类处方多适用于便秘病人的康复。

桑葚子醪：鲜桑葚子1000g，元米500g。鲜桑葚子洗净捣烂取汁（或干桑葚子300g煎煮去渣取汁），将桑葚子汁与淘净元米共煮米饭，待凉，加适量酒曲，拌匀发酵为酒酿，供服食。

柏子仁粥：柏子仁15g，蜂蜜适量，粳米100g。先将柏子仁去尽皮壳杂质，稍捣烂，同粳米煮粥，待粥将成时，兑入蜂蜜，稍煮1~2沸即可。

苁蓉羊肉粥：肉苁蓉10~15g，精羊肉100g，粳米100g，细盐少许，葱白2茎，生姜3片。先用砂锅煎苁蓉取汁，去渣，入羊肉、粳米同煮，待煮沸后再加入盐、姜、葱，煮为稀粥。

2.3.3.10　温肾固涩类处方

这类处方多适用于便秘、尿频、尿失禁等病人的康复。

芡实粉粥：芡实粉30~60g，粳米100g。取芡实粉与淘洗干净的粳米一同如常法煮粥。早、晚食用。

山萸肉粥：山萸肉15~20g，粳米100g，白糖适量。山萸肉去核洗净，与淘净的粳米一同如常法煮粥，早、晚食用。

2.3.4　饮食保健

进食时应该从容缓和，专心致志，细嚼慢咽。这样有利于食物消化吸收，保护肠胃。进食时，播放轻柔欢快的乐曲，有利于增进食欲及加强消化功能。进食之后，为了帮助消化食物，可以做一些必要的护理活动。

2.3.4.1　食后摩腹

顺时针方向按摩腹部，可连续做二三十次不等。这样有利于腹腔血液循环，促进胃肠消化，对全身健康也有好处。

2.3.4.2　食后散步

“饭后百步走，能活九十九。”散步有利于胃肠蠕动，促进消化吸收。亦可边散步边摩腹，效果更佳。

2.3.4.3　食后漱口

食后漱口可使口腔保持清洁，牙齿坚固，并能防治口臭、龋齿等疾病。

2.4　运动疗法

运用传统的体育运动方式进行锻炼，有畅达经络、疏通气血、和调脏腑、祛除疾病、延年益寿的功效，尤其对恢复肢体功能有着独特的作用，适用于偏瘫、痿证、痹证、颈椎病、骨折、伤筋等肢体功能障碍性疾病的康复。此外，它还能促进机体代偿功能，对病伤和残疾的机体功能障碍，能最大限度地发挥机体的代偿能力，对多种慢性病也能起到良好的辅助治疗作用。

2.4.1　中医运动健身的特点和运用原则

2.4.1.1　中国传统运动的特点

1. 在中医学理论指导下进行。传统运动健身法，是以中医的阴阳、脏腑、气血、经络等理论为基础，以养精、炼气、调神为运动的基本要点。所以，要认真学习中医理论，并正确运用于运动锻炼。

2. 注重意守、调息和动形的谐调统一。意守指意念专注，调息指呼吸调节，动形指形体运动。三者之间要协调配合，要达到形、神一致，意、气相随，形、气相感，使形体内外和谐，动静得宜，方能起到养生、康复的作用。

2.4.1.2　运动养生、体育康复的运用原则

1. 形神统一。运动养生和体育康复的要领就是意守、调息、动形的统一。三者的关系：以意领气，以气动形，使内外和谐、气血周流，整个机体可得到全面锻炼。

2. 合理适度。要强调适量的锻炼，循序渐进，不可急于求成、操之过急，否则欲速则不达。

3. 持之以恒。“流水不腐，户枢不蠹。”只有坚持不懈，才能收到养生、康复效果。传统体育运动不仅是身体的锻炼，也是意志和毅力的锻炼。

2.4.2　古典运动养生、康复法举隅

2.4.2.1　五禽戏

五禽戏是一种模仿虎、鹿、熊、猿、鸟五种禽兽动作的古典体操，自古至今一直是中国人防病治病、延年益寿的方法。

虎戏：模仿虎的形象，取其神气、善用爪牙和摇首摆尾、鼓荡周身的动作。要求意守命门，有益肾强腰、壮骨生髓的作用，可以通督脉、祛风邪。

鹿戏：模仿鹿的形象，取其长寿而性灵，善运尾闾。要求意守尾闾，可以通经络、行血脉、舒展筋骨。

熊戏：模仿熊的形象，熊体笨力大，外静而内动。要求意守中宫（脐内），着重于内动而外静。

猿戏：模仿猿的形象，猿机警灵活，好动无定。要求意守脐中，以求形动而神静。

鸟戏：又称鹤戏，即模仿鹤的形象，动作轻翔舒展。练此戏要意守气海，可以调达气血，疏通经络，活动筋骨关节。

五禽戏既有形体动作，又要求排除杂念，意守丹田及呼吸配合，能调理阴阳、流通气血、扶正祛邪，故有较好的养精神、调气血、益脏腑、通经络、活筋骨、利关节的作用，临床则常用于偏瘫、截瘫、痹证、痿证、骨质疏松证、震颤麻痹综合征等患者的康复治疗。

2.4.2.2　易筋经

“易”指移动、改变；“筋”，泛指肌肉、筋骨；“经”，指常道、规范。“易筋经”就是活动肌肉、筋骨，使全身经络、气血通畅，从而增进健康、祛病延年的一种传统健身康复法。

易筋经中所设动作都是由仿效古代的各种劳动姿势演化而成的。例如，舂谷、载运、进仓、收囤和珍惜谷物等动作，均以劳动的各种动作为基础形态。其具体内容为捣杆舂粮，扁担挑粮，扬风净粮，换肩扛粮，推袋垛粮，牵牛拉粮，背牵运粮，盘箩卸粮，围茓囤粮，扑地护粮，屈体

捡粮，弓身收粮。十二式的活动以形体屈伸、俯仰、扭转为特点，以达到“伸筋拔骨”的锻炼效果。因此，对于青少年来说，这种方法可以纠正身体的不良姿态，促进肌肉、骨骼的生长发育；对于年老体弱者来讲，可以防止老年性肌肉萎缩，促进血液循环，调整和加强全身的营养和吸收，对慢性疾病的恢复，以及延缓衰老都很有益处。临床常用于痿证、废用综合征等病人的康复期。

2.4.2.3　八段锦

八段锦是由八种不同动作组成的运动，故名“八段”。因为这种健身运动可以强身益寿、祛病除疾，其效果甚佳，有如展示给人们一幅绚丽多彩的锦缎，故称为“锦”。由于八段锦不受环境场地限制，随时随地可做，术式简单易记易学，运动量适中，老少皆宜，既可用于强身保健，又可用于多种慢性病的康复治疗，故一直流传至今，是广大群众所喜爱的健身方法。

其内容被编为广为流传的七言歌诀，从中可以看出各种动作的不同养生效果：两手托天理三焦，左右开弓似射雕；调理脾胃须单举，五劳七伤往后瞧；摇头摆尾去心火，两手攀足固肾腰；攒拳怒目增气力，背后七颠百病消。

2.4.2.4　太极拳

太极拳是一种顺应自然的养生、康复方法。它要求呼吸、意识、动作三者紧密结合，达到内外合一、浑然无间的境地。目前比较流行的套路是简化太极拳（二十四式），其动作由简到繁，从易到难，循序渐进，便于普及和掌握。还有四十八式太极拳、八十八式太极拳等，运动量依次增大，动作也相应变得更复杂。

太极拳以“太极”哲理指导拳路，拳路的一招一式又构成了太极图形。拳形为“太极”，拳意亦在“太极”，以太极之动而生阳，静而生阴，激发人体自身的阴阳气血达到“阴平阳秘”的状态，使生命保持旺盛的活力。

坚持练习太极拳，能协调脏腑、调畅气机、调理阴阳、强壮身体，故有较好的康复医疗作用。临床常用于高血压、低血压、心肌梗死、慢性阻塞性肺疾患、胃下垂、慢性肝炎等病人的康复治疗。

2.5　娱乐疗法

2.5.1　音　乐

音乐疗法是让病人通过欣赏音乐颐养身心、促进身心康复的方法。早在两千多年前，《乐记》《内经》等古籍中就有关于音乐能增进健康的记载。

2.5.1.1　养生、康复原理

音乐通过曲调的节奏、旋律、响度、和声四大要素，对人的心理和生理产生作用。在心理方面，它通过艺术感染力影响人们的情绪和行为，以情导理，以调摄情志。节奏鲜明的音乐能使人振奋，旋律柔和优美的音乐能使人轻松愉快和平静，深沉哀愁的音乐能使人抑郁忧愁。不同的音阶亦有不同的作用。在生理方面，音乐是一定频度的声波振动，它作用于人体，使各器官节奏协调一致。音响还对听觉器官和听觉神经起作用，进而影响肌张力、血液循环及其脏器活动。总之，音乐能调摄情志，协调脏腑功能，促进气血正常运行，以达到养生、康复的目的。

2.5.1.2　常用音乐处方

1. 抒情解郁。选用节奏明快、旋律流畅、情调欢乐、优美动听的曲目，如《步步高》《喜洋洋》《莫愁啊，莫愁》《金水河》《假日的海滩》等，可用于情志郁结所致的各种病症者。

2. 宁心安神。选用节奏缓慢、旋律婉转的曲目，如《春江花月夜》《平沙落雁》以及《平湖秋月》《江南好》等。具有安神宁心、镇静除烦之功效，可用于与情志焦躁烦恼有关的各种病症者。

3. 振奋激昂。选用节奏鲜明有力、旋律高亢激昂、曲调雄壮或悲壮一类的乐曲，如《黄河大合唱》《马赛曲》等。具有激昂情绪、增强魄力、振奋勇气之功效，可用于与低沉消极、悲观失望有关的各种病症者。

4. 抑躁制怒。选用节奏缓慢、旋律低沉、曲调凄切悲凉的乐曲，如《江河水》《哀乐》《葬花》《天涯歌女》《汉宫秋月》等。具有抑制狂躁、愤怒，减轻情绪亢奋之功效，可用于情志偏激易怒以及喜笑不休证、狂躁证者。

5. 增进智力。少儿增智选用情绪欢乐、旋律飘逸、节奏较快的乐曲，如《赛马》《快乐的罗素》《梦幻曲》《新疆之春》《杜鹃圆舞曲》等。可用于弱智儿童、智残、痴呆的康复医疗。中老年增智则选用听者幼时和年轻时熟悉或喜欢的乐曲，具体曲目因人而异。诱导听者边听边回忆。可推迟患者大脑的衰老，唤起失去的记忆，并有助于痴呆病人的康复。

音乐疗法每日2~3次，每次30~60分钟。音量适中，环境应雅静舒适，没有噪声干扰。在条件许可的情况下，可配相应的灯光、色彩、花卉等，以增强效果。

在有条件的情况下，可以鼓励患者采用主动方法，即演奏、演唱、创作音乐作品。

2.5.2　歌　咏

歌咏疗法是让病人通过歌咏，以促进养生、康复的方法。歌咏需要集中注意力和想象力，以便进入意境，同时需调节身体姿势，运气发声，对脏腑是有益的“按摩”。歌咏疗法除了陶冶情操、强身健体外，还可以用于伤病、残疾之后情绪抑郁、消极者以及与之有关的各种病症者。还适用于哮喘的康复期，因为唱歌可畅通气道，加强胸膈运动，有利于痰涎的排出和呼吸功能的提高。此外，它还可以锻炼和恢复咽喉、唇腭、声带的生理功能，故用于连舌、舌强、面瘫、言謇语塞等病症，以及腭上举困难者等。

所唱歌曲，应根据患者自己的音乐修养、爱好等予以选择。

2.5.3　舞　蹈

舞蹈能娱情畅志，用于情志养生和情志病症的康复，如情绪忧郁、悲伤、烦恼者，或智障者、痴呆、神经衰弱者；其次是舒筋活血，用于锻炼肢体和形体病症的康复，诸如痿证、痹证、五软、伤筋的康复期以及肥胖、骨质疏松和废用综合征。

不同的舞蹈，其节奏和动作也有所不同，故应根据患者的具体情况，在当地流行舞种中灵活选择。

2.5.4　戏　剧

戏剧有角色，有情节，既可使人捧腹大笑，又可使人悲哀涕泣；既可使人情绪激昂，又可使人心情愉悦，故长于调节情志，用于情志养生。对于情绪异常的康复患者，要针对病人的具体情况选择不同的剧种和戏剧内容。凡情绪抑郁、消沉一类的病人，应选择轻松愉快，或热烈激昂的剧种和戏剧内容，如喜剧等；而情绪烦躁、亢奋一类的病人，则应选择恬静优雅的剧种和戏剧内容，如各种正剧。

2.5.5 琴棋书画

琴棋疗法是让病人通过弹琴、弈棋促进身心健康的方法。由于手指的精细动作与协调运动是在大脑的指挥下进行的，因此，琴棋书画对预防脑动脉硬化、阿尔茨海默病等有积极的作用。

2.5.5.1 弹琴

其养生作用是通过怡情悦志和运指健脑两方面实现的。弹琴时的专心致志和恬愉优美的音乐享受，使人心情舒畅，轻松愉快，故有畅娱神情的作用；同时，它有练习指掌，使之灵活自如，帮助手指关节恢复活动功能的功效。对于卒中后遗症、痿证、痹证、烧伤、伤筋等病症所致手指拘挛、屈指不利等，可通过弹琴以消除手指功能障碍。

2.5.5.2 弈棋

弈棋是一项促进智力发展的养生方法和康复疗法。弈棋时，心神集中，意守棋局，杂念尽消，故适合注意力分散、精力不易集中者。弈棋还有助于解除郁闷，愉快心情。可用于小儿智力发育迟缓及老人智力衰减。

弈棋亦要注意适度，不能耗神太多，也不能过于计较输赢，应以遣情益智为要。

2.5.5.3 书画

书画疗法是让病人通过观看、习练书画，促进身心健康的方法。由于观、作书画之前，要排除杂念，再调节呼吸，运气于指、腕、臂、腰，调动全身之力于笔端，实际上已内蕴调心、调息、调形之义。其养生、康复的机理在于：

1. 调节情志。观赏和习练书画能陶冶性情，舒发郁气，故情绪烦躁、愤怒、抑郁者，或七情逆乱者，均可选用。古人认为书写或观赏不同的字体有不同的怡情作用。

（1）楷书，有静气安神、消除烦恼和急躁情绪的作用，适用于烦躁、愤怒致病者。

（2）隶书，凝重稳健，清幽恬静，易使人产生沉稳安定的情绪，亦适用于烦躁、愤怒致病者，并常与楷书配合使用，以静制动。

（3）行书、草书，潇洒活泼，似行云流水，能使人情绪高昂、胸怀舒畅，故对情志抑郁低沉之患者尤为适宜。

2. 锻炼形体。书画时，臂、肘、腕、指要进行精细活动，能使周身筋骨肌肉（尤其是上肢）得到锻炼而获调畅气血、舒筋活络之效。凡卒中后遗症、痿证、痹证、烧伤、伤筋所致手腕肘臂拘挛或屈伸不利者，可习书画以消除障碍，恢复功能。

书画还能通过集中思维、巧运手指而达到激发灵感、增进智力的目的，对弱智儿童、老年健忘、痴呆等可行书画康复疗法。现代研究也表明，绘画对弱智儿童的康复效果颇佳。

2.6　沐浴疗法

沐浴疗法，是利用水、日光、空气、泥沙等有形的或无形的天然物理因素祛病健身的方法。

不同的沐浴方式，可分别起到发汗解表、祛风除湿、行气活血、舒筋活络、调和阴阳、振奋精神等作用。沐浴形式较多，如温泉浴、热水浴、日光浴、海水浴、桑拿浴、冷水浴、药浴、泥浆浴、沙浴、森林浴等，现介绍具有中医特色的三种沐浴法。

2.6.1　药　浴

用一定浓度的药液，洗浴或浸泡全身，使药物中的有效成分直接作用于病变部位，起杀菌、止痛、止痒、消炎的作用，同时通过皮肤吸收进入血液循环，到达人体各个组织器官，发挥药物的治疗作用。

2.6.1.1　药浴的养生、康复机理

药浴与温泉浴、热水浴、桑拿浴一样，其物理效应可使皮肤血管扩张、充血、新陈代谢加快，汗腺分泌增强，大量排汗，排出代谢产物及毒素。温热又可以降低神经系统的兴奋性，产生镇静作用，有利于睡眠。水的温热作用又可降低肌肉的张力，缓解肌肉疼痛与痉挛。而药浴液中的药物与身体直接接触，所产生的药理作用是其他沐浴疗法所不具备的。

药浴可应用于高血压、局部软组织损伤、神经官能症、风湿性关节炎、类风湿性关节炎、腰腿痛、坐骨神经痛、脑血管意外后遗症、肥胖病、银屑病、皮肤瘙痒等疾病的康复治疗。

洗浴前先将药物浸泡半小时以上，煎煮成药汁，再兑入洗澡水中，水温在40℃～50℃左右，每次浸浴15～20分钟（手足癣等传染性皮肤病只浸泡患处），每日1次，或隔日1次，或视病情而定，以午后或晚间进行为宜。每剂药物可煎煮2次。浴后用干毛巾拭干，盖被静卧片刻。但需注意，药物不能对皮肤有刺激和腐蚀性；老、幼、病重者药浴需有人护理，避免发生意外；皮肤破损、饥饱过度、月经期、妊娠期不宜药浴。

2.6.1.2　常用药浴方剂

中医的药浴方剂数量庞大，现简要介绍几则，以供参考：

1. 皮肤瘙痒症药浴方。干荷叶、藁本、甘松、白芷、威灵仙、苍耳草、忍冬藤、盐各90g。

2. 皮肤湿疹药浴方。鲜川楝皮100g，七叶一枝花、龙骨、炉甘石各30g，土茯苓、苦参、地肤子、虎杖各25g，黄连、黄芩、黄檗、生大黄、白鲜皮、花椒、地榆各20g，赤小豆、百药煎、刘寄奴、丹皮各15g，车前子、冰片各10g。

3. 小儿发育不良药浴方。苦参、茯苓皮、苍术、桑白皮、白矾各15g，葱白5g。

4. 热毒疮疖药浴方。防风、白芷、细辛、苦参、吴茱萸、苦楝子、藜芦、荞草、麻黄根各30g，川椒15g，盐60g。

5. 治疗手足癣。苦参、桃仁、蛇床子、乌梅、连翘、大黄各30g，甘草20g，芒硝40g。

6. 关节炎、痛风药浴方。老鹳草、五加皮、伸筋草各等分。

7. 补壮元阳、治疗性功能减退方。丁香、肉桂、紫梢花、蛇床子各30g，苍术、杜仲各60g。以上均为粗末。每用30g，加水煎煮，沐浴时熏洗脐、腹部。

2.6.2 泥浆浴

某些有温泉的地方，由于受矿泉的长期滋润，在泉水的中心地带形成了特有的天然热矿泥，其温度在42℃～65℃，并有大量的胶体物质、盐类和气体等。用这样的热矿泥进行全身或局部埋浴、擦浴，能刺激和调节机体的神经和体液，具有消炎、止痛和美容等作用。

在地热资源比较丰富的地方，会有天然的或人工建造的泥浆浴室。浴者先在浴池的泥巴中浸泡三五分钟或者十来分钟，然后到沙滩上躺下，待身上的泥浆晒干后一块块自然剥落，再用清水洗净身体。泥浆浴对治疗皮肤病和风湿性关节炎有特效，健康的人在泥浆池内泡上一段时间，也有消除疲劳的益处。

中国古代还有一种泥浴疗法，但不是用地热产生的热泥浆，而是用井底挖出的冷泥浆，称之为“井底泥”。唐代的《千金要方》《证类本草》等医书中都记载了这种方法，认为能治疗妊娠胎热导致的胎动不安，以及风热头痛等疾病。这种方法，实际上就是现代所说的腐殖酸钠浴，除了井底泥以外，沼泽地里的泥浆也有同样的作用。

腐殖酸是有机物腐败后生成的物质，具有调节机体内分泌、抑制各种有害酶、加速人体血液循环、促进新陈代谢、提高人体免疫力的功能。

泥浆浴对治疗类风湿性关节炎、四肢关节疼痛、皮肤紫斑、机体软组织损伤、消化道溃疡、某些妇产科疾病、高血压均有较好的疗效。尤其对因比赛或训练而扭伤者，有消除肿胀、恢复体力的疗效。

2.6.3 沙 浴

沙浴，就是以沙为媒介，与身体接触，向体内传热，以达到治疗效果的方法。沙浴对风湿性关节炎、运动系统疾病有非常好的疗效。

沙浴的机理，主要是利用磁疗（沙子中含有的磁性物质）、理疗（干燥高温和红外辐射）、推拿按摩、日光浴等综合疗效，可通经脉、舒筋骨、祛痼疾，有促进血液循环、增强新陈代谢之功效。

沙浴的方法，是将除头以外的整个身体或身体的局部埋入太阳晒热的沙子之中。上有烈日，下有烫沙，上下夹攻，使患者大汗淋漓，热不可耐。沙疗正是通过这种热效应来治疗疾病的。风湿性关节炎、坐骨神经痛、神经系统障碍等患者，往往一两次沙疗就能拔除病根。对于慢性消化道疾病、自主神经功能紊乱等疾病也有治疗作用。

根据气温、沙子的温度，每次沙浴时间10～15分钟，10天为1个疗程。

2.7 中医养生康复方法简介

2.7.1 按摩推拿疗法

按摩是一种保健手法，以各种手法技巧或器械为作用力，直接作用于人体表面的特殊部位（筋络穴位），调节气血，达到保健的作用。

2.7.2　针灸疗法

针灸疗法是中国独特的养生方法之一，不仅可用于强身保健，也可用于久病体虚之人的康复。所谓针灸，就是在身体某些特定穴位上施灸，以达到和气血、调经络、养脏腑、延年益寿的目的。

2.7.3　刮　痧

刮痧是以中医经络腧穴理论为指导，通过特制的刮痧器具和相应的手法，蘸取一定的介质，在体表进行反复刮动、摩擦，使皮肤局部出现红色粟粒状，或暗红色出血点等“出痧”变化，从而达到活血透痧的作用。因其简、便、廉、效的特点，临床应用广泛，适合医疗及家庭保健。还可配合针灸、拔罐、刺络放血等疗法使用，具有加强活血化瘀、驱邪排毒的效果。

2.7.4　拔罐法

拔罐法是以罐为工具，利用燃烧排除罐内空气，造成负压，使之吸附于腧穴或应拔部位的体表，产生刺激，使被拔部位的皮肤充血、淤血，以达到防治疾病的目的。

2.7.5　中药疗法

任何疾病的发生和发展都是由致病因素作用于人体，由此引起机体发生阴阳失调、邪正消长或脏腑功能失常等病理现象。中药治病就是利用药物的特性来去除病因、消除病邪，或恢复脏腑功能的协调，从而纠正阴阳的偏盛偏衰，使疾病得以痊愈。

中药的性能是以中医的阴阳、脏腑、经络、治疗法则等理论为基础，从医疗实践中予以归纳总结出来的，是分析药物及临床用药的基本依据。中药药性理论主要有四气五味、升降浮沉、归经及毒性等。

Chapter 2 Therapeutitc Methods of Life Cultivation and Rehabilitation

2.1 Regulating Emotions

Ancient Chinese medical staff pointed out long ago that health means not only freedom from diseases and weakness, but also sound mental condition and social adaptive capacity. In modern society, psychic factors give rise to more and more psychosomatic diseases. Psychological diseases will become the frequent and widespread diseases of human beings in the 21st century.

Under normal circumstances, seven emotional activities play a role of coordinating the physiological functions of the five Zang organs. But excessive seven emotions beyond the scope of the self-adjustment of the human body can cause disturbance of visceral Qi and blood. Consequently, diseases occur.

2.1.1 Abstaining from anger

"Anger" has been the emotional taboo for experts on life cultivation throughout the history. It impairs not only the liver, but also the heart, stomach and brain etc., which leads to various diseases. Accordingly, anger is the worst emotion which should be controlled in life cultivation and rehabilitation.

Restraining one's anger means that one should rationally overcome emotional impulses. When anything irritating comes up, one should first think of its bad consequence so as to rationally restrain and control one's bad and violent emotions. For instance, ancient and modern wise people often hang up aphorisms such as "restraining anger" and "ceasing to be angry" over their desks to remind them of abstinence from anger.

2.1.2 Giving vent to depression

One may adopt proper methods to give vent to one's bad emotions when meeting setbacks, or being wronged, or confronting troublesome and grief affairs. For instance, one may cry aloud in a place where there are no other people when meeting with a misfortune or being extremely grieved; one may go to an open field and shout loudly to let off his depression and emotions when encountering setbacks and feeling depressed.

2.1.3 Counseling

When bad emotions occur, one could find two or three intimate friends to air his depression and follow friend's advice, eventually to overcome bad emotions.

2.1.4 Diverting emotions

Diverting emotions means overcoming emotions and changing the directionality of emotions to get rid of distracting thoughts and depression and to change bad emotions and habits. When meeting with depression, one might as well "read books to divert oneself from boredom, listen to music to dispel melancholy". In addition, the musical instrument, chess, painting and calligraphy may be utilized to divert emotions and mould one's temperament.

2.1.5 Sports

Bad emotions caused by mental stimuli can be let off by sports activities, by diverting one's attention, or by regulating the balance of the human body. Various activities such as playing balls, walking, mountaineering, practicing Taijiquan and performing a sword dance can all divert or let off mental stress and discomfort. Especially, traditional physical training emphasizes the combination of movement with motionlessness, which can make the body comfortable and people happy. It is very effective for eliminating bad emotions. In addition, people may also take part in physical labor to get rid of mental tension, anger and grief with physical exercises.

2.1.6 Implication

Implication therapy is a method to promote the patients' rehabilitation by means of implication. The ancient Chinese idiom "mistaking the reflection of a bow in the cup for a snake" is a typical example of this implication. The ancient Chinese pray for recovery also includes some elements of implication therapy.

Implication is divided into positive implication and negative implication. Positive implication means that the patient accepts other people's ideas completely, unconditionally, uncritically and without analysis, no matter whether the ideas are correct not. It exerts positive effects on psychosomatic health. Negative implication, however, denotes that the patient thoroughly negates and rejects other people's ideas. It has negative effects on psychosomatic health. Implication therapy makes use of the positive effects of implication to promote psychosomatic health of the human body. Meanwhile, attention should be paid to avoiding the negative effects of implication.

Implication therapy may be conducted on two occasions: one is performed in complete waking state without hypnotization; the other means of implication is given to the patient after he or she enters hypnosis. The latter excels the former in effects. Besides, the patient may also perform positive self implication and repeatedly intensify the consciousness of "excellent health and recovery from the disease". In this way, visceral functions can be consequently induced to develop along an orderly direction.

2.1.7 Colors

According to the effects of colors on the human body and emotions, certain colors are selected to exert direct effects on the mind and emotions via eyes. This is the so-called "pleasing the eyes and refreshing the mind". Besides, the color tones, color temperatures, etc. may also be used to regulate emotions.

The method, under the guidance of the theory of "the five colors corresponding to the five Zang organs and five emotions", is used to arrange the colors of the patient's living surroundings such as living rooms, utensils, furnishings, clothes, quilts, window curtains and lights as well as the dresses of doctors and nurses of rehabilitation according to the requirements. Also, rooms of rehabilitation with colors and "color instruments" are installed in hospitals and sanitariums to rehabilitate the corresponding diseases. Colors and their indications are as follows:

2.1.7.1 Warm colors

Red and orange, with warm feeling, possess the actions of making people excited and joyful. The colors are applicable to depression, depressive psychosis, lethargy and dementia etc.

2.1.7.2 Cold colors

Among indigo blue, blue, purple and green, one may select one, two, or three colors. The colors have the actions of cooling, tranquilizing and making people restrained. Cold colors are applicable to dysphoria, irascibility, insomnia, terror and fear as well as mania and epilepsy etc.

2.1.7.3 Joyful colors

Red and pink make people happy and have the effect of restraining grief. The colors are applicable to people with low spirits, susceptibility to grief and cry, and depression.

2.1.7.4 Sad colors

Black is mainly applied or white may also be used to restrict anger. Both colors are applicable to susceptibility to anger and overjoy etc.

2.1.7.5 Fearful color

Black has the effect of restricting overjoy. The color is applicable to mania, endless laughing, etc.

2.1.7.6 Anxious colors

Yellow, light blue and light green possess the effect of restricting fear and benefiting thinking. The colors are applicable to terror, fear, distraction, etc. The flexible selection of either single color or multiple colors, either light colors or rich colors, is used to form the proper compatibility according to the requirement of the patients in applying the colors.

2.1.8 Checking one emotion with another

This is the method mentioned more than 2000 years ago in *Plain Questions. Discussion on Principles of Yin-Yang Doctrine and Its Relations with Natural Things and Phenomena*. The content includes "anger impairs the liver while grief restricts anger"; "joy impairs the heart while fear restricts joy"; "anxiety impairs the spleen while anger restricts anxiety"; "melancholy impairs the lung while joy restricts melancholy" and "fear impairs the kidney while anxiety restricts fear". This method of checking one emotion with another is based on the principle of excess curing excess. Zhang Zihe, a medical expert of the Jin and Yuan Dynasties, introduced it specifically as follows: "Checking anger with grief means using sorrowful words to move one; checking grief with joy using crack jokes to please one; checking joy with fear using fear and death to frighten one; checking anxiety with anger using insulting language to excite one; checking fear with anxiety using worrying words to make one forget the fear."

2.1.8.1 Fear restricts joy

This is a method to restrain great joy impairing the heart and restore mental functions by applying fearful factors to astringe the dissipated cardiac spirit. The method is often applicable to diseases of scattered cardiac qi due to endless laughing as well as emotional disorders due to excessive joy.

2.1.8.2 Anger restricts anxiety

This is a method to restore functions of the heart and spleen by using irritating factors to restrain excessive anxiety. The method is often applicable to melancholia, insomnia, epilepsy, etc. caused by impairment of the spleen and consumption of spirit due to excessive anxiety.

2.1.8.3 Joy restricts grief

This is a method to overcome excessive grief by utilizing funny factors. The method often makes use of romantic, very witty and humorous language, and amusing performance, telling jokes, listening to xiangsheng (a traditional Chinese comic dialogue) and watching plays. And even sometimes, the doctor intentionally makes a ridiculous diagnosis to satisfy the patient's eagerness. In doing these, the purposes are to free the patient from the difficult positions and consequently achieve the effect of joy restricting grief. The method is often clinically applicable to crying with grief and hysteria as well as diseases due to excessive grief.

2.1.8.4 Grief restricts anger

This is a method to restrain excessive anger by making use of grievous factors. The method is commonly applicable to other diseases with accompanying emotional excitement such as vertigo, mania and epilepsy.

2.1.8.5 Anxiety restricts fear

This is a method to restrain fright and fear by adopting anxious factors. The method is commonly applied in rehabilitation to get rid of the patient's fearful mood.

In applying the method of "checking one emotion with another", pay attention to the intensity of emotional stimuli. The intensity has to exceed that of the pathogenic emotional factors. For instance, sudden stimuli or continuous intensification of stimuli may be applied. Moreover, modern people may adopt other relevant methods as long as they grasp the essence of the above-mentioned methods. Mechanical application of these methods is not advisable.

2.2 Environments, Daily Life and Clothing

The life and cultivation methods of environments, daily life and clothing mainly discuss the environmental influences on human health, the scientific arrangement of daily life, including food, clothing, shelter and transportation, standing, lying, suffering, enjoyment, strain, rest, etc. as well as adoption of a set of measures, the purposes of which are to eliminate diseases, strengthen health and prolong life.

2.2.1 Environments

Environments include natural environments and artificial environments. Natural environments include air, water, soil, rocks, living things, etc. on the earth; artificial environments refer to the urban and rural living residential environments built by man for collective life. The indoor environment is included in the artificial environments.

The ancient Chinese fengshuishu (geomancy) was the theory which studies how to establish an ideal environment beneficial to prolonging life and life cultivation. It was the comprehensive theory of ancient architectural planning and design integrating geology, geography, ecology, architecture, ethics, aesthetics, etc. into an organic whole. Synthesizing the essentials of the above aspects, the ancient Chinese fengshuishu believes that the natural environment suitable for man is one with clean and plentiful water source, fresh air, sufficient sunlight, good vegetation as well as a quiet secluded and beautiful landscape. This type of natural environment not only satisfies the basic human need of material life, but also suits the special human psychological requirement.

Because of geographical causes in certain places, "goiter prevails to the mountain area" and "malaria prevails to the south of the Five Ridges (the area covering Guangdong and Guangxi") etc. Many TCM treatises have realized these phenomena long ago. In addition, the trace elements essential for the human body also distribute differently under different geographical conditions. For example, endemic goiter easily occurs in iodine deficiency areas while fluorine deficiency gives rise to dental caries, etc. Apart from the above, certain radioactive substances, such as uranium ore and phosphorus ore are also harmful to the human body. Powerful radioactive sources may give rise to increased incidences of anemia, leukemia and cancer in local people.

Therefore, people should try their best to avoid the areas and ores, which are not beneficial to human health, high tension lines and strong magnetic field as well as the locally built living areas with supersonic waves and radioactive rays.

Besides, harnessing pollution of air, water sources and noises is the basic conditions to ensure health. It needs the joint efforts of the government, society, families and individuals for the establishment of an environment beneficial to health and longevity.

2.2.2 Daily life

2.2.2.1 Regular work and rest

One basic requirement of TCM life cultivation is normal daily life "which means regular work, rest and daily life". This is an important principle for strengthening health and prolonging life.

If there exist irregular daily life, work and rest and unscrupulous behavior, aging phenomena may occur such as declined adaptive capacity and body resistance. As a result, premature aging may occur to affect life span.

The most helpful and correct life style for life cultivation and longevity is the reasonable arrangement of daily life, work and rest which requires that people should sleep, get up, eat, work, study, exercise the body, defecate, urinate, bathe, etc. at fixed time. However, the so-called "at fixed time" should still be flexibly handled according to the specific conditions (the differences in ages, seasons, regions and physiques) and mechanical application should be avoided.

2.2.2.2 Proper balance between work and rest

The ancients advocated that the criteria for work and rest were "moderation", regular and moderate adjustment without excess in either one. Only when the integration of movement and motionlessness, and moderation of work and rest are adopted, can tendons and bones be exercised, Qi and blood flow smooth, physique become strong, willpower be enhanced and vigorous life-force be conserved. Work and rest include not only the consumption of physical strength, but also the moderate use of the brain. In other words, the use of the brain should include moderation of work and rest and the advocation of scientific use of the brain. Mental labor without tiredness keeps the constant use of the brain without decline. Regular and reasonable use of the brain can prevent aging, increase intelligence, especially prevent senile dementia.

The criteria for moderation of work and rest vary in persons. In general, the following may be used for reference: ①Physical labor should be proper in intensity. ②Mental labor should be integrated with physical activities. ③Rest and health conservation should be various. Not only should rest in sleeping way be adopted, but also rest in other ways should be applied, such as listening to music, chatting, playing chess, walking, enjoying the sight of scenery, fishing, composing poems, painting and practicing Taijiquan.

2.2.2.3 Scientific sleeping

Sleeping plays an extremely important role in one's life time. If one wants health and longevity, he or she should adopt reasonable sleeping habits to ensure sleeping quality, restore the body from fatigue, store up energy to prevent and treat diseases, and strengthen health and benefit longevity. The effects of sleeping on health and longevity manifest in the following five fields: ①Eliminating fatigue to restore strength. ② Protecting brain to conserve intelligence. ③ Strengthening immunity to increase body resistance. ④Promoting infantile development. ⑤Beautifying skin and excreting the waste. In the case of abnormal sleeping, the above-mentioned five aspects may change for the worse and affect the health of human body and longevity.

1. Sleeping time. Chinese life cultivation experts have created quite a number of beneficial and very effective sleeping methods for life cultivation which are simple and convenient and easy to practice. For instance, "Sleeping at Midnight and Noon" is one of the sleeping methods for life cultivation. The method is as follows: Go to sleep at midnight (11 p.m. to 1 a.m.) and noon (11a.m. to 1 p.m.) respectively, because midnight and noon are the time for the alternation of yin and yang, the moments yin and yang change from excess to extreme deficiency or from extreme deficiency to excess, and Qi and blood, yin and yang inside the body are extremely imbalanced. At this time, peaceful lying can avoid the impairment of Qi and blood. It has been proved by practice that the quality and efficiency of sleeping at midnight and noon are both good. As for old people, the sleeping method can also reduce the incidence rates of cardiovascular and cerebrovascular diseases. It conforms to the principle of life cultivation.

Good sleeping regularity should be developed in sleeping time. The ancients summarized the regularity in sleeping as: "Man should rise early in spring and summer and late in autumn and winter, but not as early as before the cock crows in the morning or as late as after the sun rises."

2. Sleeping postures. "Sleeping like a bow" is the requirement of sleeping posture. This is a beneficial sleeping posture for the human body. Medical experts both in the past and at present have chosen the right lateral position. The right lateral position can increase cardiac output, strengthen digestion of food, absorption of nutrients and metabolism. Besides, man himself feels more comfortable, too.

As for females, supination and prone position are not advisable, because pronation may increase facial wrinkles and supination is harmful to pelvic blood circulation which easily gives rise to emmeniopathy. Right lateral position is suitable for normal people while left lateral position is advisable for pregnant women, because right lateral position may constrict veins of lower abdominal cavity and affect blood return, which is harmful to fetal development and delivery. Nevertheless, left lateral position is beneficial to fetal growth and may greatly reduce complications of pregnancy.

As far as infants are concerned, the posture should be constantly changed with the help of adults, because prolonged lateral position or supination and prone position easily cause asymmetrical development of skull, or deformity of five sense organs of the face. Generally, infants should be turned over once every 1 to 2 hours.

Semilateral position or semi-sitting position is advisable for patients with heart failure and patients with attack of cough and asthma. Meanwhile, the pillow and postdorsal region are high padded. Lateral position is suitable for patients with thoracoabdominal dropsy due to pulmonary diseases. Left lateral position or prone position is not suitable for patients with heart diseases with symptoms of blood stasis. The same is true of patients with pulmonary heart disease in case cardiac load is too heavy. Lying position with low head and high feet easily results in renal diseases.

It should be pointed out that though the above sleeping postures are beneficial to life cultivation and health care, keeping the postures unchanged after falling asleep is not required, for it is impossible to realize this.

3. Sleeping articles.

(1) Pillow. The pillow should be slightly lower than the distance from the shoulder to the neck of the same side. If it is too high, it may affect the smoothing and regulating functions of the liver meridian, and also induce cerebral anoxia, snoring and stiff neck; if it is too low, it may affect the dispersing and descending of the lung Qi and also cause congestion of the head of resultant edema of eyelids and the face. The pillow is not advisably much wider than 15 to 20cm. But being slightly longer is not harmful. The material of loose and soft texture with proper hardness and slight elasticity should be selected for pillow core.

There exists the habit of using medicinal pillows for life cultivation and rehabilitation in TCM. A medicinal pillow is the one with the medicinal core prepared with different traditional Chinese drugs. This type of pillows has therapeutic and health care actions. The commonly-used medicinal pillows with one ingredient include:

Pillow padded with chrysanthemums: It is applicable to patients with headache, conjunctival congestion and dizziness or acute catarrhal conjunctivitis, insomnia with asthenic dysphoria as well as hypertension.

Pillow padded with peppermint leaves: It is applicable to headache, toothache, rhinitis, laryngopharyngitis, hypertension, etc. and it also has the actions of preventing summer-heat and lowering the temperature.

Pillow padded with mulberry leaves: It is applicable to headache, vertigo and hypertension etc.

Pillow padded with tea leaves: The pillow is padded with the used and dried tea leaves. It is applicable to the prevention and treatment of hypertension, neurasthenia and dizziness due to summer-heat etc.

Pillow padded with buckwheat: It is applicable to insomnia, headache, vertigo and infantile night cry etc.

Pillow padded with mung beans: It is applicable to the prevention and treatment of headache and wind syndrome of the head, and improves sight, induces resuscitation, removes summer-heat and dysphoria.

Pillow padded with Juncus effusus: It is applicable to insomnia, vexation, amnesia, and infantile night cry etc. and benefits intelligence.

Pillow padded with Semen Cassiae: It is applicable to constipation, ocular diseases, hypertension, and infantile night cry etc.

Pillow padded with Oriental arborvitae leaves: It is applicable to persistent oral and nasal bleeding, chronic pharyngitis, congestion of throat, chronic cough and patients with mild baldness.

Pillow padded with Silkworm excrement: It is applicable to wind syndrome of the head, stiff neck, arthritis of cervical vertebrae and mandible.

The above are the medicinal pillows made of a single ingredient. If made into compound medicinal pillows, they have better therapeutic effects:

Insomnia: The pillow core is padded with black beans and powder of magnetite.

Rhinitis and nasosinusitis: The pillow core is padded with equal shares of Baizhi (RadixAngelicae Dahuricae) and Xinyi (Flos Magnoliae).

Glaucoma and distending ocular pain: The pillow core is padded with equal shares of Xiakucao (Spica Prunellae), Heye (Folium Nelumnbinis), Baizhi (Radix Angelicae Dahuricae) and Caojueming (Semen Cassiae).

Pillow for hypertension. ①The pillow core is padded with Caojueming (Semen Cassiae) and Juhua (Flos Chrysanthemi). ②The pillow core is padded with 100g of Juhua (Flos Chrysanthemi), 100g of Chuanxiong (Rhizoma Ligustici Chuanxiong), 100g of Mudanpi (Cortex Moutan Radicis) and 200g of Baizhi (Radix Angelicae Dahuricae).

Pillow for Eliminating Summer-heat. The pillow core is padded with 200g of the covering of Lüdou (Semen Phaseoli Radiati), 200g of the covering of Biandou (Semen Dolichoris), 150g of Heye (Folium Nelumbinis), 200g of Bohe (Herba Menthae) and 100 g of Qiaomaike (the shell of Semen Fagopyri Esculenti).

Sight-Improving Pillow: The pillow core is padded with 200g of the covering of buckwheat, 200g of the covering of Heidou (Semen Sojae Nigrum), 80g of Caojuemingzi (Semen Cassiae) and 150g of Juhua (Flos Chrysanthemi).

Soporific pillow: The pillow core is padded with 200g of Yejiaoteng (Caulis Polygoni Multiflori), 60g of Hehuanhua (Flos Albiziae), 30g of Suanzaoren (Semen Ziziphi Spinosae), 30g of Baiziren (Semen Biotae) and 30g of Wuweizi (Fructus Schisandrae).

Besides, the ancient Taoists had a well-known medicinal pillow for longevity called the "Revered Mr. Ding's Celestial Pillow". The prescription is composed of 30g of Chuanjiao (Pericarpium Zanthoxyli), Jiegeng (Citri Reticulatae Fructus), Jingshizi (Herba Schizonepetae), Baiziren (Semen

Biotae), Jianghuang (Rhizoma Curcumae Longae), Wuzhuyu (Fructus Evodiae), Baizhu (Rhizoma Atractylodis Macrocephalae), Bohe (Herba Menthae), Rougui (Herba Cistanchis), Chuanxiong (Rhizoma Ligustici Chuanxiong), Yizhiren (Fructus Alpiniae Oxyphyllae), Zhishi (Fructus Aurantii Immaturus), Danggui (Radix Angelicae Sinensis), Chuanwutou (Radix Aconiti), Qiannianjian (Rhizoma Homalomenae), Wujiapi (Cortex Acanthopancis Radicis), Baijili (Fructus Tribuli), Qianghuo (Rhizoma seu Radix Notopterygii), Fangfeng (Radix Ledebouriellae), Xinyi (Flos Magnoliae), Baizhi (Radix Angelicae Dahuriae), Fuzi (Radix Aconiti Praeparata), Baishaoyao (Radix Paeoniae Alba), Gaoben (Rhizoma Ligustici), Congrong (Herba Cistanchis), Beixixin (Herba Asari Mandshurici), Zhuyazao (Fructus Gleditsiae Abnormalis), Wuyi (Flos Magnoliae), Gancao (Radix Glycyrrhizae), Jingjie (Herba Schizonepetae), Juhua (Flos Chrysanthemi), Duzhong (Cortex Eucommiae), Wuyao (Radix Linderae) and Banxia (Rhizoma Pinelliae) respectively.

All the above ingredients are ground into powder. Then fill the pillow with the powder. Use the pillow every night. One pillow can be used for about half a year.

The medicinal pillow has better therapeutic effects on diseases of the head, face, five sense organs, shoulders and neck etc. but it is not applicable to diseases of the chest, abdomen and limbs. The application should be stopped if the patient is allergic to the drugs.

(2) Bedding. Soft materials such as fine cotton cloth, cotton yarn and fine gunny cloth are preferred for the underneath side of the quilt while the materials of chemical fibre with electrostatic charge such as acrylic fibres, nylon and dacron are not advisable. It is best to select cotton, silk floss and eiderdown for the wadding of the quilt. Light and big quilt is preferable, but heavy one is not suitable. Soft and thick mattress is advisable. The modification is made with the changes of temperature.

(3) Night clothes and nightcap. The large night clothes without collars and buttons are preferable. Cotton velvet and towelling are advisable in autumn and winter while silk and muslin are suitable in spring and summer. In winter, it is suitable for old people to wear the cotton nightcap, the size of which is proper to cover the whole head. Wearing the belly band is advisable for old people, no matter whether it is in winter or summer, especially for old people above the age of 70.

"Ten forbidden points" for sleeping. Our Chinese ancients had ten forbidden points for sleeping which include: First, supination; Second, anxiety; Third, anger before bed time; Fourth, ingestion before bed time; Fifth, speaking during sleeping; Sixth, facing the lamplight; Seventh opening the mouth during sleeping; Eighth, covering the head during sleeping; Ninth, facing the draught during sleeping; Tenth, facing the stove during sleep.

4. Clothing articles.

TCM life cultivation has accumulated a lot of experiences in the modification of clothing in the four seasons. It demands that dressing and undressing should keep with seasonal changes. For example, in spring, cold does not disappear completely and yang Qi increases gradually. Accordingly, it is advisable to wear less upper garments and usual trousers to promote the rising of yang Qi. In summer, though yang Qi and heat are excessive, people still need proper dressing to consolidate and protect healthy Qi. In autumn, it turns cool and people should pay attention to the addition of clothing. However, too many garments at a time should be avoided. As the saying goes: "muffle the body in spring and freeze the body in autumn." This means that man should keep himself warm in spring and wear less so as to feel a bit cool in autumn. In winter, more clothing should be added with the increasing intensity of cold. The "once and for all" in dressing cannot be reached and excessively heavy clothing should be avoided.

Keeping the body extremely warm or excessively cold is not advisable. Otherwise, the body will lose its ability to endure wind and cold, consequently causing the declined body resistance against pathogenic factors and weakened ability to prevent diseases. As for old people and people with weak physique, their tolerance of cold and heat is relatively poor. Thus, undressing or dressing should be as cautious as possible to avoid the invasion of wind, cold, summer-heat and dampness.

In the case of profuse sweating, undressing should be shunned from wind. Otherwise, the body is susceptible to be attacked by pathogenic wind and cold which consequently gives rise to diseases. Wet clothes with sweat should not be worn long, for after perspiration, the striae of skin are loose and the wet garments are not easily dried. If the sweat and dampness stay on the skin long, they will impair the yang Qi of the human body, easily giving rise to pathological changes of wind, cold and dampness.

5. Defecation and urination.

Cultivating good habits of defecation and urination is of great significance for health and longevity.

(1) Keeping free movement of the bowels. The ancient life cultivation experts attached extreme importance to smooth movement of the bowels. It is regarded as a symbol of longevity that an old person defecates regularly two times a day. Constant constipation may cause the ascending of turbid Qi, adverse and disorderly Qi flow and blood circulation, and visceral dysfunctions, consequently giving rise to or inducing many diseases such as headache, toothache, anal and intestinal diseases, coronary heart disease, hyperten-sion cerebrovascular accident and intestinal cancer. The methods of keeping smooth movement of the bowels include: ① Cultivating the habit of defecation at fixed time; ② defecating naturally without forced control if there exists stool and no forced defecation if there is no stool; ③ catharsis with massage; clockwise massage can enhance enterogastric functions, digestive and excretory functions while massaging abdominal region regularly promotes catharsis; ④ Paying attention to the perianal hygiene and recuperation after defecation. The toilet paper used should be thin and soft. Every night before bed time, the anus is washed with warm and clean water. Sitz bath with warm water is adopted to keep the anus clean and to maintain good blood circulation.

As for food, oats gruel is helpful for catharsis, especially for old people. Oats not only relieves constipation but also reduces cholesterol and triglyceride. Therefore, it has slimming effect as well.

Healthcare after defecation should not be ignored, either. For example, it is advisable to eat some soup or drink some beverage in the case of defecation after overeating to strengthen the stomach Qi and promote digestion. In the case of hunger, sitting position is advisable for defecation. Ingestion of a small amount of food is proper after defecation. Besides, drawing up anal muscle may be conducted for 3 to 5 times, the purpose of which is to supplement and consolidate healthy Qi.

(2) Maintaining clear and smooth urination. The ancient life cultivation experts attached great importance to hygiene of urination. Maintaining clean urine and smooth urination is the important content of

conserving health of the body. The specific methods are mainly as follows: ①Reasonable diet: Small amount of ingestion, vegetarian diet, no immediate drinking after meal and drinking in the case of thirst etc. are the experience of the ancients for ensuring clean urination. ②Diuresis with massage. Massage of the waist: Assume erectly sitting position. Place the hands on the back to push and rub upwards to the back and downwards to the sacrococcygeal region for 30 to 50 times until the back gets warm. It may be performed at bed time at night and at the time to get up in the morning. Massage of the abdomen: Assume the supine position and regulate breathing. Rub the palms against each other until they get warm. Then, place the palm on the abdomen. Firstly, push and rub the two sides of the abdomen; then, push the middle of the lower abdomen, both of which are done for 30 times. The movements should shift gradually from gentle ones to forceful ones and the force should be mild, slow and even. It is performed in the morning and at night. ③Forced control over urination should be avoided. Urination should be timely when there exists urine. Forced control over urination may impair the kidney and the urinary bladder Qi, causing pathological changes.

In addition, emotions, sexual life and sports also influence urination to a certain degree. Therefore, people should keep optimistic, regulate sexual life and exercise properly.

2.3 Food Therapy

2.3.1 Life cultivation with the diet

2.3.1.1 Supplementing the supply of nutrients in the human body to strengthen health and prevent diseases

For example, eating animal livers can nourish the liver and prevent night blindness; ingestion of kelp can not only supplement iodine and vitamin, but also prevent goiter; intake of fruit and fresh vegetables can supplement nutrition and prevent scurvy etc. Besides, the special function of certain food may be directly utilized to prevent certain diseases. For instance, garlic is used to prevent affection by exopathogen and diarrhea; green gram soup is applied to prevent summer-heat; Congbai (Bulbus Allii Fistulosi) and Shengjiang (Rhizoma Zingiberis Recens) are adopted to prevent common cold due to invasion by wind, etc.

2.3.1.2 Prolonging life, resisting and preventing aging

Many types of food have the anti-aging functions, such as sesame, mulberry, Gouqizi (Fructus Lycii), Guiyuanrou (Arillus Longan), Hutao (Semen Juglandis), bee milk, Rhizoma Dioscoreae, human milk, milk, soft-shelled turtle, the regular ingestion of which is beneficial to health and longevity.

2.3.2 Principles of rehabilitation with the diet

2.3.2.1 Differentiating syndrome to decide the diet

Different diets are selected for different syndromes. For example, in the case of the exterior syndrome of affection by exogenous wind and cold with the manifestations such as headache, nasal obstruction, aversion to cold, general pain, anhidrosis, warm-and hot-natured food such as Shengjiang (Rhizoma

Zingiberis Recens), Congbai (Bulbus Allii Fistulosi) and brown sugar should be selected and decocted. Take it while the decoction is warm. Or minced garlic shredded with warm noodles, or soup of coriander and soybean may be ingested to induce diaphoresis, relieve the exterior syndrome and expel cold. In the case of renal Yang deficiency with the symptoms such as lassitude in loins and legs, cold limbs, aversion to cold, cramping sensation of the lower abdomen, frequent or unsmooth urination, diets of supplementing fire to remove Yin should be Selected such as dog meat, sparrow meat and mutton, or renal soup of a white sheep and chicken cooked with Dongchongxiacao (Cordyceps).

2.3.2.2 Differentiating disease to decide the diet

Different diets should be selected according to the differences of diseases on the basis of differentiating syndrome to decide the diet. For instance, in the case of palpitation, Danggui (Radix Angelicae Sinensis) and Renshen (Radix Ginseng) may be selected to be cooked with the pork heart; in the case of night blindness, various animal livers may be decocted with Gouqizi (Fructus Lycii), and Sangshenzi (Semen Mori) etc. for oral administration; the pork lung fried with sesame oil or soup of the pork lung may be used for cough due to pulmonary asthenia; pork kidney steamed with Eucommia bark may be selected for lumbago due to deficiency of the kidney; bone marrow and cerebral marrow powder of the pig or gruel of Taoren (peach kernel gruel) may be selected for senile dementia; the pig pancreas may be selected for diabetes mellitus; more milk may be drunken for osteoporosis.

2.3.2.3 Scientific selection of diets

The scientific use of diets can be defined by the proverb "The diet should include coarse and fine food grains without being too sweet and salty. People should have three, or four or five meals a day with being 70 to 80 percent full". The first sentence refers to the advocation of a proper proportion between coarse and fine food grains in TCM life cultivation. Coarse food grains include maize, soybean, sweet potato and the like; fine food grains include nonglutinous rice, flour and so on. In the second sentence, "three, four or five meals" means the times people should have meals a day; "70 to 80 percent full" is the experience of becoming longevous which has been proven by history.

The dietary style of being "70 to 80 percent full" has proven to be the effective method of promoting longevity by the public at all times and in all countries. This is similar to the modern theory of "low caloric diet". There are two methods to measure the so-called "70 to 80 percent full": one is that people feel a little hungry and still want to eat when leaving the dinning table; the other is that people have the sense of hunger when it is not the time for the next meal yet. There exists a saying in TCM life cultivation: "If you want to be healthy, you should always feel 30 percent cold and hungry." This has already been verified by numerous longevous people.

2.3.3 The commonly-used dietary prescriptions for life cultivation

2.3.3.1 Prescriptions for supplementing healthy Qi

These prescriptions have tonic, roborant, anti-aging and life-prolonging actions. They are applicable to patients with weak constitution and deficiency of healthy Qi due to prolonged diseases.

1. Prescriptions for supplementing Qi.

Paste of Huangqi (Radix Astragaliseu): 12g of Shenghuangqi (fresh Radix Astragali), 12g of

Shengshigao (Gypsum Fibrosum), 12g of Xianmaogen (fresh Radix Curculiginis), 6g of the fine powder of Gancao (Radix Glycyrrhizae), 10g of the powder of Huaishanyao (Rhizoma Dioscoreae) and 30g of honey. At first, decoct Huangqi (Radix Astragali seu Hedgsari), Shigao (Gypsum Fibrosum) and Xianmaogen (fresh Radix Curculiginis) until the decoction boils for more than 10 times. Then, remove the dregs to leave two cups of the clear decoction. At this time, add Gancao (Radix Glycyrrhizae) and Rhizoma Dioscoreae powder to the decoction and stir the decoction constantly to prevent the sedimentation of the medicinal powder. Boil the decoction for one more time and the paste forms. Next, pour the honey into the decoction. The whole process comes to an end when the decoction boils. Take all the paste in 3 divided times within a day.

Gruel for strengthening healthy Qi: 30 to 60g of prepared Huangqi (Radix Astragaliseu Hedgsari), 3 to 5g of Renshen (Radix Ginseng) or 15 to 30g of Dangshen (Radix Codonopsis Pilosulae), a small amount of white sugar and 100g of Jingmi (non-glutinous rice). At first, cut Huangqi (Radix Astragali seu Hedgsari) and Renshen (Radix Ginseng) or Dangshen (Radix Codonopsis Pilosulae) into slices and soak them in cold water for half an hour. Then, decoct the ingredients to get the decoction. Use the decoction to cook gruel with Jingmi (non-glutinous rice) and take it in two divided times in the morning and evening for ingestion.

Gruel of Renshen (Radix Ginseng) and Lianrou (Semen Nelumbinis): 10g of Renshen (Radix Ginseng), 10g of Lianzi (Semen Nelumbinis) and 30g of Bingtang (Saccharum). The common method is used to cook gruel for ingestion.

2. Prescriptions for tonifying blood.

Hen Stewed with Danggui (Radix Angelicae Sinensis): 15g of Danggui (Radix Angelicae Sinensis), 15g of Dangshen (Radix Codonopsis Pilosulae), one hen (roughly 1500g), proper amount of green onion, fresh ginger, cooking wine and salt respectively. After butchering the hen, remove the feather and internal organs. Then, wash the hen clean. Next, put Danggui (Radix Angelicae Sinensis) and Dangshen (Radix Codonopsis Pilosulae) into the abdomen. At this time, add green onion, ginger, cooking wine and a proper amount of clear water. At first, boil the water with strong fire. Afterwards, change the fire into slow fire to decoct until the meat is thoroughly cooked. Eat the meat and drink the soup.

Soup of Chinese dates (Fructus Ziziphi Jujubae) and Black Edible Fungus: Five Chinese dates (Fructus Ziziphi Jujubae) and 15g of black edible fungus. Stew the two thoroughly to be eaten.

Gruel of Gouqi (Fructus Lycii): 100g of fresh Gouqizi (Fructus Lycii) and 60g of Jingmi (non-glutinous rice). The two are used to cook gruel. Drink the gruel with salty fermented soybeans as the assistant food.

3. Prescriptions for supplementing Qi and tonifying blood.

Paste of Guiyuan Shenmi (Paste of Arillus Longan, Radix Codonopsis Pilosulae and honey): 250g of Dangshen (Radix Codonopsis Pilosulae), 120g of Beishashen (Radix Glehniae) and 120g of Guiyuanrou (Arillus Longan). At first, soak the above ingredients in a proper amount of water until they thoroughly wet. Decoct the drugs for 30 minutes after the water boils. Decoct the ingredients in 3 different times. Then, mix the decoctions got in 3 times. Next, decoct the mixed decoction to be condensed with slow fire until the paste forms. At this time, add double amount of honey. Afterwards, decoct them until boiling appears again. Finally, stop decocting and wait until the paste is cold. Store the paste in a bottle for later use. Dissolve a spoonful of the paste in boiling water to be taken each time, three times a day.

Gruel of Longyanrou (Arillus Longan): 15g of Longyanrou (Arillus Longan), 10g of Fuling (Poria), 3 to 5 Chinese dates and 100g of Jingmi (non-glutinous rice). All the ingredients are used to cook gruel. Add a bit of white sugar to the gruel to be eaten.

4. Prescriptions for nourishing yin.

Wine of Gouqizi (Fructus Lycii): 200g of Gouqizi (Fructus Lycii) and 600mL of white spirit. First, wash Gouqizi (Fructus Lycii) clean in clear water. Then, cut the ingredient into small pieces to be kept in a bottle. Afterwards, add about 400mL of white spirit into the bottle. Next, keep the mouth of the bottle airtight. Vibrate and shake the bottle once every day. The wine can be drunk after a week's soakage. Drink 10 to 20mL before supper or bed time every day. The wine in the bottle may be added continuously (altogether about 200mL). Gouqizi (Fructus Lycii) may be mixed with sugar for eating.

Pork Liver Stewed with Xuanshen (Radix Scrophulariae): 15g of Xuanshen (Radix Scrophulariae), 500g of pork liver, a proper amount of rapeseed oil, ginger, green onion, soy sauce, yellow rice wine and bean powder respectively. At first, wash the pork liver clean, and place it and Xuanshen (Radix Scrophulariae) together in a pot. Then, add a proper amount of water to the pot and cook the ingredients for an hour. Next, take out the pork liver and cut it into slices for later use. In addition, parch the green onion and ginger with a bit of rapeseed oil and put them into the slices of the pig liver. Afterwards, put the soy sauce, white sugar and a small amount of cooking wine into the above decoction and cook the decoction with these ingredients again. After that, put some bean powder into the decoction to make the decoction transparent. Finally, pour the slices of pork liver into the juice and stir the juice evenly. Now, it is ready for use.

Soft-Shelled Turtle Steamed with Ermu (Bulbus Fritillariae and Rhizoma Anemarrhenae): One softshelled turtle (approximately 500g), 5g of Beimu (Bulbus Fritillariae), Zhimu (Rhizoma Anemarrhenae), Qianhu (Radix Peucedani), Chaihu (Radix Bupleuri) and Xingren (Semen Armeniace Amarum) respectively, a proper amount of yellow rice wine and a bit of salt. At first, butcher the soft-shelled turtle and remove head and internal organs. Then, wash the turtle clean and it cut into cubes. Next, add Beimu (Bulbus Fritillariae), Zhimu (Rhizoma Anemarrhenae), Qianhu (Radix Peucedani), Chaihu (Radix Bupleuri) and Xingren (Semen Armeniacae Amarum) as well as a proper mount of yellow rice wine and a bit of salt. Add water to inundate the meat cubes. Finally, all the ingredients are steamed in a steamer for an hour. Eat the meat while it is still warm.

Gruel of Baihe (Bulbus Lilii): 30g of the powder of dried Baihe (Bulbus Lilii) (doubled in case of fresh one), 100g of Jingmi (non-glutinous rice) and a proper quantity of Bingtang (Saccharum). All the ingredients are used to cook gruel. Eat it in the morning and in the evening respectively.

5. Prescriptions for strengthening yang.

Wine of Lurong (Cornu Cervi Pantotrichum): 3 to 6g of Lurong (Cornu Cervi Pantotrichem), 30 to 60g of Rhizoma Dioscoreae and 500mL of white spirit. Soak Lurong (Cornu Cervi Pantotrichum) and Huaishanyao (Rhizoma Dioscoreae) in the spirit. Keep the container airtight. Vibrate and shake the container occasionally. It may be drunk in 7 days. Drink 10mL every night before bed time.

Kidney Soup of White Sheep: 50g of Roucongrong (Herba Cistanchis), 10g of Biba (Fructus Piperis Longi), Caoguo (Fructus Tsaoko) (ten in number), 5g of Chenpi (Pericarpium Citri Reticulatae), 10g of Hujiao (Fructus Piperis Nigri Seu Albi), two pairs of white sheep kidneys, 200g of white sheep fat, salt, green onion, soy sauce and fermented flour etc. The common methods are adopted to cook soup with the above ingredients. Eat one sheep kidney and drink some soup each time.

Chicken Stewed with Dongchongxiacao (Cordyceps): 1 cock, Dongchongxiacao (Cordyceps) (5 to 10 in number), a bit of ginger, green onion and salt respectively. At first, butcher the cock. Then, get rid of the feathers and internal organs to be washed clean. Afterwards, put the cock into a pot and add the Dongchongxiacao (Cordyceps), ginger, green onion, salt as well as a proper quantity of water. Finally, stew all the above together until the meat is thoroughly cooked for eating.

2.3.3.2 Prescriptions for nourishing the heart and tonifying the brain

These prescriptions have the actions of nourishing the heart, tranquilizing the mind and tonifying the brain to benefit intelligence.

Gruel of Hetaoren (Semen Juglandis): 50g of Hetaoren (Semen Juglandis) and a proper amount of Jingmi (non-glutinous rice). Pound the Hetaoren (Semen Juglandis) into pieces. Then, wash the rice clean. Next, add a proper quantity of water. All the ingredients are used to cook gruel in the common ways. The gruel is used as assistant food.

Ganmai Dazao Decoction (Decoction of Radix Glycyrrhizae, Wheat and Chinese Dates): 30g of wheat, 10 Chinese dates and 6g of Gancao (Radix Glycyrrhizae). First, wash the Chinese dates and wheat clean. Then, decoct the two together with Gancao (Radix Glyrhizae) for 2 to 3 times. Remove the dregs to get the decoction. Take the decoction in the morning and in the evening, or drink it as tea.

Gruel of Guiyuanrou (Arillus Longan): 15g of Guiyuanrou (Arillus Longan), 3 to 5 Chinese dates and 100g of Jingmi (non-glutinous rice). The ingredients are used together to cook gruel. A bit of white sugar may be added for eating.

2.3.3.3 Prescriptions for promoting the production of body fluids to quench thirst

These prescriptions possess the functions of clearing away heat, removing dysphoria, nourishing yin, moistening dryness, promoting the production of body fluids to quench thirst, benefiting the rehabilitation of patients with diabetes.

Five-Juice Drink: The juice of pear, juice of water chestnut, juice of lotus root, juice of Maimendong (Radix Ophiopogonis) and juice of fresh Lugen (Rhizoma Phragmitis). First, peel the pear (with the kernel removed), water chestnut and fresh lotus root. Then, wash the fresh Lugen (Rhizoma Phragmitis) and Maimendong (Radix Ophiopogonis) and cut them into pieces. Next, wrap the five ingredients in a piece of clean gauze to squeeze the juice for drinking. The drinking time and quantity may not be fixed. If the patient doesn't prefer cool drink, just warm it with hot water.

Decoction of Pig Pancreas: One pig pancreas, 30g of fresh Yiyiren (Semen Coicis), 60g of Huangqi (Radix Astragali seu Hedysari) and 120g of Huaishanyao (Rhizoma Dioscoreae). Wash the pig pancreas clean. Then, all the ingredients are decocted together for use. Cook the decoction. Drink the clear decoction. The time may not be fixed for drinking.

Crucian Carp Steamed with Tea: Crucian carp and green tea leaves. Take one crucian carp with the weight of 500g. Then, remove the gills, intestines and internal organs (with the scales remained). Next, fill the abdomen with green tea leaves. Afterwards, place the crucian carp in a dish and put it in a steamer. Finally, steam the crucian carp until it is thoroughly cooked. Eat the bland meat.

2.3.3.4 Prescriptions for rheumatic and rheumatoid arthralgia

These prescriptions are mainly applicable to patients with arthralgia due to wind, cold and dampness, inflexible movement of joints, clonic spasm and contracture of muscle.

Decoction of Chinese Flowering Quince: 4 Chinese flowering quinces and 1000g of white honey. First, steam the Chinese flowering quinces until they are cooked. Then, grind them into paste. Besides, refine the white honey clean. Finally, mix the two evenly to be stored in a clean chinaware for later use. Mix the prepared paste with boiling water, 1 to 2 spoonfuls each time. Drink the soup with an empty stomach every morning after getting up.

Wine of Wujiapi (Cortex Acanthopancis): 50g of Wujiapi (Cortex Acanthopancis), 500g of Glutinous rice and a proper amount of yeast. First, wash Wujiapi (Cortex Acanthopancis) clean. Then, decoct the drug after soaking it thoroughly in a proper quantity of water. Take out the decoction 30 minutes after boiling. Altogether, take out the decoction for two times. Mix the two decoctions. The decoction and clean-washed Jingmi (non-glutinous rice) are used to cook rice. When the rice is cool, add a proper amount of yeast and stir the two evenly. Finally, fermented glutinous rice is ready after fermentation. Take it every day in a proper amount.

Gruel of Chuanwu (Radix Aconiti): 3 to 5g of raw Chuanwutou (Radix Aconiti), 30g of Jingmi (non-glutinous rice), 10 drops of ginger juice and a proper amount of honey. First, pound the raw Chuanwutou (Radix Aconiti) into pieces and grind them into very fine powder. Then, use the Jingmi (non-glutinous rice) to cook gruel. When the gruel boils, add the powder of Chuanwutou (Radix Aconiti) and change into slow fire to cook. When the gruel is ready, add the juice of fresh ginger and honey and stir them evenly. The gruel is finished after another 1 to 2 times of boiling. Drink the warm gruel in the morning and in the evening. It is contraindicated for heat syndromes and pregnant women as well as the simultaneous use with Banxia (Rhizoma Pinelliae), Beimu (Bulbus Fritillariae), Gualou (Fructus Trichosanthis), Baiji (Rhizoma Bletillae) and Bailian (Radix Ampelopsis) etc.

2.3.3.5 Prescriptions for promoting qi flow and activating blood circulation

These prescriptions have the actions of promoting qi flow and activating blood circulation, removing blood stasis and activating collaterals. They are applicable to patients with cardiovascular and cerebrovascular diseases such as myocardiac infarction and the sequelae of apoplexy during the stage of recovery.

Gruel of Xiebai (Bulbus Allii Macrostemi): 10 to 15g (or 30 to 45g fresh ones) of Xiebai (Bulbus Allii Macrostemi) and 100g of Jingmi (non-gltinous rice). The two are used together to cook gruel. The warm gruel may be used for breakfast and supper.

Spirit of Danshen (Radix: Salviae Miltiorrhizae): 60g of Danshen (Radix Salviae Miltorrhizae) and 500mL of high quality spirit. Danshen (Radix Salviae Miltiorrhizae) is washed clean and pounded into pieces. Then, put the piece into the spirit. The spirit is finished after a month of soakage.

Gruel of Shanzha (Fructus Crataegi): 30 to 40g (or 60g fresh ones) of Shanzha (Fructus Crataegi), 100g of Jingmi (non-glutinous rice) and 10g of granulated sugar. First, decoct Shanzha (Fructus Crataegi) in an earthenware pot. Then, take out the thick decoction and remove the dregs. Finally, add Jingmi (non-glutinous rice) and granulated sugar to the decoction to cook gruel.

2.3.3.6 Prescriptions for suppressing hyperactive yang to eliminate wind

These prescriptions possess the actions of calming the liver and suppressing hyperactive yang, nourishing yin and eliminating wind. They are applicable to patients with hypertension, mental disease and Parkinson's syndrome etc. at the stage of recovery.

Gruel of Yuzhu (Rhizoma Polygonati Odorati): 15 to 20g (or 30 to 60g fresh ones) of Yuzhu (Rhizorna Polygonati Odorati), a bit of crystal sugar and 100g of Jingmi (non-glutinous rice). First, wash Yuzhu (Rhizoma Polygonati) clean and cut it into pieces. Then, decoct the pieces to keep the decoction and to remove the dregs. Next, add Jingmi (non-glutinous rice) into the decoction to cook thin gruel. Finally, add crystal sugar to the gruel. The gruel is finished after one to two times of boiling. Drink the gruel in the morning and in the evening.

Gruel of Lotus Leaf: A large lotus leaf. Wash it clean and decoct it. Then, take out about 500mL of the decoction. Next, add 100g of Jingmi (non-glutinous rice) and a proper quantity of white sugar to the decoction to cook gruel. Drink the gruel in the morning and in the evening.

Noodle of Gefen (powder of Radix Puerariae): 250g of Gefen (powder of Radix Puerariae), 50g of Jingjiesui (Spica Schizonepetae) and 150g of Dandouchi (Semen Sojae Praeparatum). First, decoct Jingjiesui (Spica Schizonepetae) and Dandouchi (Semen Sojae Praeparatum) until decoction boils for 6 to 7 times. Then, remove the dregs to take out decoction. Next, make Gefen (powder of Radix Puerariae) into noodles. Afterwards, put the noodles into the decoction and decoct it. Eat it with an empty stomach.

2.3.3.7 Prescriptions for relieving cough and asthma and eliminating phlegm

These prescriptions possess the functions of relieving cough and asthma and eliminating asthma etc. They may be applicable to the health care and rehabilitation of diseases of respiratory tract.

Soup of Yanwo (Nidus Collocaliae): 3g of Yanwo (Nidus Collocaliae) and 30g of crystal sugar. First, put Yanwo (Nidus Collocaliae) into a bowl. Then, add warm water and soak Yanwo (Nidus Collocaliae) in the bowl until it becomes soft. Secondly, remove all the golden swallow feathers mixed in Yanwo (Nidus Collocaliae). Thirdly, wash Yanwo (Nidus Collocaliae) again to make it clean with clear water. Fourthly, remove the water and tear it into thin strips and place the strips in the bowl. Fifthly, crush the crystal sugar to pieces and put the pieces into a pot with 250g of clear water. Dissolve the crystal sugar in boiling water with slow fire. Sixthly, scoop up the floating foam and filter the liquid to remove impurities. Seventhly, pour the liquid into another pot and add Yanwo (Nidus Collocaliae) to the liquid. Eighthly, heat the pot until the liquid boils. Finally, fill a clear bowl with the soup for later use. Drink the soup once in the morning and in the evening respectively.

Thick Soup of Yin'er (Tremella): 5g of Yin'er (Tremella), an egg, 60g of crystal sugar and a proper amount of lard. Firstly, soak Yin'er (Tremella) in a proper amount of warm water to make it thoroughly soaked. Secondly, remove the base and wash the drug clean. Thirdly, add a proper amount of water to decoct the drug until the water boils. Fourthly, shift to slow fire to stew Yin'er (Tremella) slowly for 2 to 3 hours until it becomes paste. Fifthly, add water to another pot and put the crystal sugar into it. Sixthly, heat the pot until the water boils with slow fire to dissolve the crystal sugar. Seventhly, filter the liquid to remove impurities. Eighthly, take out the egg white and add a bit of clear water to it. Stir the egg white and water evenly and then add the egg white to the pot with crystal sugar water. Ninthly, heat the pot until the water boils and scoop up the floating foam. At this time, pour the water into the pot with Yin'er (Tremella). The Thick Soup of Yin'er (Tremella) is finished by adding the lard to the pot with Yin'er (Tremella). Drink the soup in the morning and before bed time.

Gruel of Pipaye (Folium Eriobotryae): 10 to 15g of Pipaye (Folium Eriobotryae), 50g of Jingmi (non-glutinous rice) and a proper amount of crystal sugar. First, wrap Pipaye (Folium Eriobotrgae) in a piece of cloth. Secondly, decoct it to remove dregs and to keep the thick decoction. Or brush off the villi of 30 to 60g of fresh Pipaye (Folium Eriobotryae). Then, cut it into thin slivers and decoct it. Next, remove the dregs and keep the decoction. At this time, add Jingmi (non-glutinous rice) to the decoction to cook gruel. Finally, add the crystal sugar to the gruel when it is done. Again, cook the gruel slightly for later use. Drink the gruel every day in the morning and in the evening.

2.3.3.8 Prescriptions for removing food retention and flatulence, strengthening the spleen and stomach

These prescriptions have the actions of promoting digestion to remove food retention, clearing away heat from the stomach and lowering the adverse flow of the stomach qi, eliminating food retention to get rid of flatulence, strengthening the spleen, and drying dampness etc. They are applicable to the health care and rehabilitation of the diseases of digestive system.

Gruel of Meihua (Flos Mume Albus): 5g of Baimeihua (Flos Mume Albus) and 100g of Jingmi (non-glutinous rice). First, use Jingmi (non-glutinous rice) to cook gruel. Then, add Baimeihua (Flos Mume Albus) to the gruel and heat the gruel until it boils for 2 to 3 times. Eat the gruel twice a day with an empty stomach. Three to five days constitute a course of treatment.

Gruel of Jupi (Pericarpium Citri Reticulatae): 15 to 20g (or 30g in case of fresh ones) of Jupi (Pericarpium Citri Reticulatae) and 50 to 100g of Jingmi (non-glutinous rice). First, decoct Jupi (Pericarpium Citri Reticulatae) to keep the decoction and to remove the dregs. Then, add Jingmi (non-glutinous rice) to the decoction to cook gruel. Or dry Jupi (Pericarpium Citri Reticulatae) in the sun and grind it into fine powder. Mix 3 to 5g of the powder with the boiling gruel each time. Finally, cook the gruel again.

Spleen-Benefiting Cake: 30g of Baizhu (Rhizoma Atractylodis Macrocephalae), 6g of dry ginger, 15g of Jineijin (Endothelium Corneum Gigeriae Galli), 250g of cooked jujube paste and 500g of flour. Grind Baizhu (Rhizoma Atractylodis Macrocephalae), Jineijin (Endothelium Corneum Gigeriae Galli) and dried ginger into powder. Then, add a small amount of water to the cooked jujube paste (Decoct the jujube until it is down. Then, keep the decoction and remove the pit. Finally, crush it to paste). Next, mix the paste with the powder and flour and make them into small cakes. Bake the cakes until they are done. The cakes may be eaten at any time without definite quantity.

2.3.3.9 Prescriptions for moistening bowels to relieve constipation

These prescriptions are applicable to the rehabilitation of patients with constipation.

Fermented glutinous Rice with Sangshenzi (Fructus Mori): 1000g of fresh Sangshenzi (Fructus Mori) and 500g of Glutinous rice. Wash the fresh Sangshenzi (Fructus Mori) clean and pound it into paste to keep the juice [or decoct 300g of dry Sangshenzi (Fructus Mori) and remove the dregs and keep the decoction]. Then, cook rice with the juice or decoction and Glutinous rice. When the rice is cool, add yeast to it and stir the two evenly. After fermentation, the fermented glutinous rice forms. It is ready for taking.

Gruel of Baiziren (Semen Biotae): 15g of Baiziren (Semen Biotae), a proper amount of honey and 100g of Jingmi (non-glutinous rice). First, remove the peel, shell and impurities of Baiziren (Semen Biotae). Then, slightly pound it into paste. Next, use the paste and Jingmi (non-glutinous rice) to cook gruel. When the gruel is to become done, add the honey to the gruel. Finally, decoct the gruel until it boils for one or two times. The gruel is finished now.

Gruel of Roucongrong (Herba Cistanchis) and Mutton: 10 to 15g of Roucongrong (Herba Cistanchis), 100g of fine mutton, 100g of Jingmi (non-glutinous rice), a bit of fine salt, three segments of scallion stalk, three slices of ginger. First, decoct Roucongrong (Herba Cistanchis) in an earthenware pot and keep the decoction and remove the dregs. Then, add mutton and Jingmi (non-glutinous rice) to decoction and decoct them together. When the decoction boils, add the salt, ginger and scallion stalk. Decoct all the ingredients together again and the gruel is finished.

2.3.3.10 Prescriptions for warming the kidney to induce astringency

These prescriptions are mostly applicable to the rehabilitation of patients with constipation, frequent urination, and urinary incontinence etc.

Gruel of Powder of Qianshi (Semen Euryales): 30 to 60g of powder of Qianshi (Semen Euryales) and 100g of Jingmi (non-glutinous rice). Use the powder of Qianshi (Semen Euryales) and clean-washed Jingmi (non-glutinous rice) to cook gruel in the common ways. Eat the gruel in the morning and evening.

Gruel of Shanyurou (Fructus Corni): 15 to 20g of Shanyurou (Fructus Corni), 100g of Jingmi (non-glutinous rice) and a proper amount of white sugar. Remove the pit of Shanyurou (Fructus Corni) and wash it clean. Use the ingredient and the clean-washed Jingmi (non-glutinous rice) to cook gruel in the common ways. Eat it in the morning and in the evening.

2.3.4 Health care with diet

Ingesting food should be unhurried, moderate, careful in chewing and slow in swallowing. Doing so is beneficial to the digestion and absorption of food, and the protection of the intestine and stomach. When people ingest food, listening to light and lively music is advantageous to improving appetite and enhancing digestive function. People can perform the following nursing activities after ingesting food.

2.3.4.1 Abdominal massage after meals

Massaging the abdomen clockwise for 20 to 30 times continuously is beneficial to abdominal blood circulation, the promotion of gastrointestional digestive functions as well as general health.

2.3.4.2 Taking a walk after meals

"Taking a hundred-step walk after meals can make one live to 99." Taking a walk helps enterogastric peristalsis and promotes digestion and absorption. Besides, taking a walk while massaging the abdomen has better effects.

2.3.4.3 Rinsing the mouth after meals

Rinsing the mouth can make the oral cavity remain clean, teeth firm and prevent diseases such as foul breath and caries.

2.4 Therapies with Sports

The application of physical training with traditional sports activities has the actions of activating meridians and collaterals, promoting Qi flow and blood circulation, regulating viscera, eliminating diseases and prolonging life. It possesses unique effects on the restoration of limb functions in particular. The method is applicable to the functional disturbances of limbs such as hemiplegia, flaccidity syndrome, arthralgia syndrome, cervical spondylosis, paraplegia, fracture and injury of the muscle and tendon. In addition, it can promote the metabolism of the organism, bring the compensation of the organism into full play. The method has good accessory therapeutic effects on many chronic diseases as well.

2.4.1 The characteristics and applying principles of enhancing health with sports activities in TCM

2.4.1.1 The main characteristics of traditional Chinese sports activities

1. Being under the guidance of TCM theories. The methods of strengthening health with traditional sports activities are based on TCM theories of yin and yang, viscera, Qi and blood, meridians and collaterals etc. The basic essentials of these sports activities include nourishing essence, training Qi and regulating the mind. Therefore, people should study TCM theories carefully and apply the theories to the practice of physical training.

2. Attaching importance to the harmony and unity of mental concentration, regulating breathing and exercising the body. Mental concentration refers to highly concentrated mind, regulating breathing to regulation of respiration, and exercising the body to training the body, the three of which should be harmonious and cooperative to achieve unity between the body and spirit, interflow of mind and Qi, and

interaction between the body and Qi. Only when the interior and exterior of the body are harmonious, movement and motionlessness are moderate, can the effects of life cultivation and rehabilitation be gained.

2. 4. 1. 2 Applying principles of life cultivation and rehabilitation with sports activities

1. Unity of the body and spirit. The main points of life cultivation and rehabilitation with sports activities are the unity of mental concentration, regulating respiration and exercising the body. The relationships among the three are as follows: direct Qi with the mind and move the body with Qi, the purposes of which are to achieve the harmony between the interior and exterior, general flow of qi and blood, and overall training of the whole organism.

2. Being reasonable and moderate. Emphasis should be placed on moderation and orderly and gradual advancement, whereas seeking success impatiently should not be allowed. Otherwise, acting with undue haste may lead to the consequence of more haste, less speed.

3. Persevering in one's efforts. "Running water is never stale and a door hinge never gets worm-eaten." Only when one perseveres in one's effort can better effects of life cultivation and rehabilitation be achieved. Traditional sports activities train not only the body, but also will and stamina.

2. 4. 2 Examples of life cultivation and rehabilitation with classical sports activities

2. 4. 2. 1 The five mimic-animal games

It is a classical physical exercise which imitates the motions of the five animals of tigers, deer, bears, monkeys and birds. The exercise has been the method for Chinese people to build up health and to prolong life since the ancient times.

The game of mimic-tiger. It imitates the tiger's image, adopts the tiger's air and its perfect utilization of its paws as well as its motions of shaking the head and wagging the tail, bulging and vibrating the whole body. The game requires concentration of the mind on Mingmen (GV4). It has the functions of strengthening the kidney and waist, enhancing the bone and promoting the production of marrow. The exercise may remove obstruction of governor vessel and eliminate pathogenic wind.

The game of mimic-deer. It imitates the deer's image, adopts the animal's longevity and intelligence as well as its perfect use of the coccyx. The game requires concentration of the mind on the coccyx. It can remove obstruction of meridians and collaterals, promote blood circulation, limber up muscles and joints.

The game of mimic-bear. It imitates the bear's image of being clumsy in bodily movement and great in physical strength, static in exterior and dynamic in interior. The game requires concentration of the mind on Zhong-gong (within the navel), and puts emphasis on being dynamic in the interior and static in exterior.

The game of mimic-monkey. It imitates the monkey's image of being alert, dexterous and quick in action, and liable to movement. The game requires concentration of the mind on the navel to seek for physical movement and mental peace.

The game of mimic-bird. It is also called the game of mimic-crane which imitates the crane's image of being lithe in flying and unfolding in action. Practicing this games requires concentration of the mind on Qihai (CV6). It can regulate and promote Qi flow and blood circulation, dredge meridians and collaterals, limber up the tendons, bones and joints.

The five mimic-animal games not only include bodily movements, but also requires elimination of all distracting thoughts, concentration of the mind on Dantian as well as the cooperation of respiration. The games can regulate yin and yang, promote qi flow and blood circulation, strengthen the body resistance to eliminate pathogenic factors. Therefore, they have very good actions of nourishing the mind, regulating Qi flow and blood circulation, strengthening viscera, dredging meridians and collaterals, limbering up muscles and joints, and facilitating flexible movement of joints. Clinically, the game is commonly applicable to patients with hemiplegia, paraplegia, arthralgia syndrome, flaccidity syndrome, osteoporosis and Parkinson's syndrome etc. at the stage of recovery.

2.4.2.2 Yijinjing (tendon-exercising technique)

"Yi" means movement and change; "jin", in general sense, refers to the muscle, tendon and bone; "jing" denotes the general law and norm. "Yijinjing" means the technique that exercises the muscle, tendon and bone, makes general meridians and collaterals, qi flow and blood circulation unobstructed. As a result, it strengthens health, eliminates diseases and prolongs life. The technique is a traditional method of enhancing health and rehabilitation.

All the movements of Yijinjing imitate the various ancient postures of physical labor and have evolved from them. For example, the actions of husking grain with a mortar and pestle, carrying grain, putting grain in storage, harvesting crops and storing grain and cherishing grain etc. all of which are the basic forms based on various movements of physical labor. The specific content includes husking grain with a mortar and pestle, carrying grain on a carrying pole, winnowing impurities from grain, carrying grain on the alternate side of the shoulder, pushing a cart with sacks of grain and piling them up, leading an ox to carry grain, carrying grain on the back, unloading grain with the square-bottomed bamboo basket, enclosing grain for storage with the mat, bending over to protect grain and bending down to pick up grains and bending low to gather crops. The twelve movements are marked by bodily flexion and extension, bending and lifting as well as torsion to achieve the training effect of "limbering up joints". Therefore, this method can remedy the bad postures, promote the growth and development of muscles and skeleton for teenagers; as far as old and weak people are concerned, the method can prevent senile muscular atrophy, promote blood circulation, adjust and strengthen general nutrition and absorption; it is very beneficial to the rehabilitation of patients with hemiplegia diseases as well as delaying aging. Clinically, the method is commonly applied to patients with flaccidity syndrome, disuse syndrome and so on at the stage of recovery.

2.4.2.3 Eight-section brocade

Eight-section brocade consists of eight different movements, hence the name "eight-section". This gymnastic activity strengthens health, prolongs life and eliminates diseases. Its effect is very excellent, just like a piece of bright and colorful brocade presenting itself before people's eyes, hence the name "brocade". Practicing eight-section brocade is not limited by the surroundings and place. Thus, it can be performed at any time and in any place. Besides, the postures are easy to memorize and learn. Meanwhile, its amount of exercise is moderate. The exercise is suitable for both the old and the young. It is not only used for strengthening health, but also for the rehabilitation of many chronic diseases. Accordingly, eight-section brocade has been handed down from ancient times to the present and still has been the popular keep-fit method among the vast number of the Chinese masses.

The content of eight-section brocade has been written in the form of seven-character verse, from which the different effects of different movements on life cultivation can be seen. The verse reads: Both hands stretch upwards to regulate triple energizer, bend a bow with alternate hands to shoot at a vulture; stretch one hand upwards to regulate gastrosplenic functions, look round to remove seven types of impairment and five kinds of consumptive diseases; shake the head and move the low back to eliminate the heart fire, both hands reach for feet to reinforce the kidney and lumbus; clench fists with round eyes to enhance physical strength, hold the neck with interlocked hands and jolt to prevent all diseases.

2. 4. 2. 4 Taijiquan

It is a method of life cultivation and rehabilitation conforming to nature. It requires the close integration of breathing, consciousness and movements to achieve the state of integrating the exterior with interior into one in perfect harmony. The present popular school of Taijiquan is the simplified Taijiquan (24-posture style). The movements vary from simple ones to complicated ones, from easy ones to difficult ones, proceeding in an orderly way and step by step. Accordingly, it is convenient to spread and master. In addition, there are 48-posture Taijiquan and 88-posture Taijiquan etc. the amount of exercises of which increases in proper order, and the movements of which are more complicated correspondingly.

The course of Taijiquan is under the guidance of the philosophical theory of Taiji (infinite void). Every stroke and every posture forms the Taiji diagram. The shape of Taijiquan is "Taiji" and the intention of Taijiquan also lies in "Taiji". The movement of Taiji generates yang, while the motionlessness of Taiji generates yin, with both of which stimulate qi and blood of the human body itself to reach the state of "yin is even and well while yang is firm" and to make life brimming with exuberant vigor.

Persevering in practicing Taijiquan can coordinate viscera, promote qi activities, regulate yin and yang and strengthen health. Thus, it has very good rehabilitation effect. Clinically, it is commonly applicable to patients with hypertension, hypotension, myocardial infarction, chronic obstructive pulmonary disease, gastroptosis and chronic hepatitis etc. at the stage of recovery.

2. 5 Therapies with Recreation

2. 5. 1 Musical therapy

Musical therapy is a method to recuperate health and cultivate the mind for the promotion of somatopsychic rehabilitation by asking patients to appreciate music. As early as over two thousand years ago, classics such as *YueJi* or *Records of Music* and *Neijing* or *Canon of Medicine* carried the account of promoting health with music.

2. 5. 1. 1 Principles of life cultivation and rehabilitation with music

Music exerts effects on the human psychology and physiology through the four major elements of the tune, rhythm, melody, loudness and harmony. Psychologically, music influences people's emotions and behavior by means of artistic appeal. It straightens people out with sentiments to regulate emotional activities. Music with strongly accented rhythms can inspire people; beautiful music with gentle melodies can make people light-hearted, happy and calm; deep and sad music can make people depressed and worried. Physiologically, different scales have different actions as well. Music, the sound wave vibration with given frequency, exerts effects on the human body to make the rhythm of every organ harmonized. Besides, sound exerts effects on the auditory organ and auditory nerve. It further influences the muscle tension, blood circulation and visceral activities. In short, music can regulate emotions, coordinate visceral functions, promote normal Qi flow and blood circulation to achieve the purpose of life cultivation and rehabilitation.

2.5.1.2 Commonly-used musical prescriptions

1. Prescriptions for expressing emotions and removing worries: Select beautiful songs with lively rhythms, smooth melodies and happy emotional appeal. For instance, *Bubugao* (*Higher and Higher*), *Xiyangyang* (*Jubilance*), *Don't Worry, Don't Worry*, *The Golden Water River*, and *Sea Beach During the Holiday*, etc. This type of songs may be applicable to various diseases due to emotional depression.

2. Prescriptions for tranquilizing the mind: Select songs with slow rhythms, mild and sweet melodies and gentle emotional appeal. For example, *The Night of Spring River with Flowers and the Moon*, *Wild Geese Fly down the Sandy Beach* as well as *Calm Lake with the Autumnal Moon*, *How Wonderful the South of the Yangtze is*, etc. This kind of songs has the actions of relieving mental stress, tranquilizing the mind and removing worries. These songs are applicable to various diseases concerning restlessness with anxiety and vexation.

3. Prescriptions for inspiring and arousing people: Select songs with strongly accented and forceful rhythms, sonorous and arousing melodies, majestic or solemn and stirring tunes. For example, *The Yellow River Cantata*, *March of the Volunteers* and so on. This type of songs possesses the actions of arousing emotions, increasing courage and inspiring people. These songs can be applicable to various diseases concerning low-spiritedness, pessimism and disheartenedness.

4. Prescriptions for inhibiting mania and anger: Select songs with slow rhythms, deep melodies, mournful and sorrowful tunes. For instance, *River Water*, *Dirge*, *Burying Flowers*, *the Homeless Singing Girl*, and *the Han Palace Below the Autumnal Moon*, etc. This kind of songs has the actions of inhibiting mania and anger, and relieving emotional excitement. They are applicable to patients with extreme emotional activities, irascibility, endless laughing and mania.

5. Prescriptions for improving intelligence: Select songs with happy emotions, elegant melodies and quick rhythms to improve children's and juvenile intelligence. For example, *Horse Race*, *Happy Russell*, *Fantasia*, *Spring of Xinjiang*, and *Cuckoo Waltz* etc. These songs may be used for the rehabilitation of children with weak intelligence and patients with intelligence disability or dementia. Select songs which people were familiar with or loved when they were infants or young to improve mid-aged and old people's intelligence. The songs may vary in people. Guide people to listen and recall something. These songs may delay cerebral aging of patients, evoke the lost memories and help the rehabilitation of patients with dementia.

Musical therapy can be conducted twice or thrice a day, 30 to 60 minutes each time. The volume should be moderate. The environment should be elegant, peaceful and cozy, free from the interference of noises. If the conditions permit, the effects can be improved with the corresponding cooperation of light, colors, and flowers etc.

If the conditions permit, patients may be encouraged to adopt active methods such as playing musical instruments, singing and composing musical works.

2.5.2 Singing therapy

Singing therapy is a method to promote life cultivation and rehabilitation by asking patients to sing songs. Singing songs requires concentration of the mind and imagination in order to enter the artistic conception. Meanwhile, regulating bodily postures is needed to direct air and produce sounds. Therefore, singing is the "massage" beneficial to viscera. Besides, moulding sentiments and enhancing health, singing therapy may be applicable to emotional depression and pessimism after being wounded, ill and handicapped as well as various diseases concerning these factors. In addition, it may be applicable to asthma at the stage of recovery, because singing songs can remove the obstruction of air passage, enhance thoracic and diaphragmatic movement, and thus it is beneficial to the discharge of sputum and saliva as well as the enhancement of respiratory function. Moreover, singing songs can train and restore the physiological functions of the throat, lips, palates and vocal cords. Accordingly, it is applicable to diseases such as ankyloglossia, stiff tongue, facial paralysis and dysphasia as well as difficulty in raising the palate upwards etc.

The songs should be selected on the basis of the patient's musical accomplishment, hobbies and national customs etc.

2.5.3 Dancing therapy

It is applicable to life cultivation of emotions and emotional disorders such as emotional depression, sorrow, vexation, hypophrenia, dementia and neurasthenia. Besides, it relaxes muscles and tendons to promote blood circulation. The therapy is applicable to exercising limbs and the rehabilitation of bodily diseases such as flaccidity syndrome, arthralgia syndrome, five types of flaccidity and injury of muscles and tendons at the stage of recovery as well as obesity, osteoporosis and disuse syndrome.

Different dances have different rhythms and movements. Therefore, flexible selection of dances among the local popular dances should be based on the patient's specific conditions.

2.5.4 Drama therapy

There are roles and plots in dramas. Dramas can not only set people roaring with laughter, but also make people grieved and cry; dramas can not only arouse people's feeling, but also make people have a light heart. Accordingly, drama therapy is good at regulating emotional activities and applicable to life cultivation of emotional disorders. Different types and contents of dramas should be selected for the rehabilitation patients with abnormal emotions on the basis of the patient's specific conditions. Light and merry, or lively and inspiring types and contents of dramas such as comedies, should be selected for patients with depression and pessimism; peaceful and elegant types and contents of dramas such as various orthodox dramas should be selected for patients with dysphoria and emotional excitement.

2.5.5 Therapies with a musical instrument and chess, practicing paintings and calligraphy

Therapies with a musical instrument and chess are the methods to promote somatopsychic health by asking patients to play a musical instrument and chess. The fine movement and coordination of the fingers are under the control of the brain. Thus playing a musical instrument and chess, practicing painting and calligraphy have positive effects on the prevention of cerebral arteriosclerosis and Alzheimer's disease, etc.

2.5.5.1 Playing a musical instrument

Its effects on life cultivation are realized by means of "keeping relaxed and happy" and "exercising fingers to tonify the brain". The single-hearted devotion and the appreciation of peaceful, cheerful and beautiful music during playing a musical instrument make people happy and relaxed. Thus, it has the action of making people have ease of mind and a light heart. Meanwhile, playing a musical instrument can exercise fingers and palms, make them flexible in movements and help finger joints to restore active functions. Playing a musical instrument can be used to eliminate finger dysfunctions such as finger spasm and inflexible finger flexion due to sequelae of apoplexy, flaccidity syndrome, arthralgia syndrome, burn, and injury of muscles and tendons etc.

2.5.5.2 Playing chess

It is a method of life cultivation and rehabilitation to promote intelligence development. When playing chess, people concentrate the mind on the chessboard and get rid of all distracting thoughts. Therefore, playing chess is applicable to people with distractibility and difficulty in concentrating the mind. Besides, playing chess helps to remove depression and have a light heart. It can be applicable to infantile retarded intelligence development and declining intelligence in old people.

Playing chess should be moderate, too. People should not spend too much energy and should not be too particular about the result. The most important aspect is always to while away the time for a light heart and to benefit intelligence.

2.5.5.3 Therapy with painting and calligraphy

Therapy with painting and calligraphy is a method to promote somatopsychic health by asking the patients to watch and practice painting and calligraphy. People should get rid of distracting thoughts before watching and practicing painting and calligraphy. Then, they regulate breathing and direct qi to fingers, wrists, arms and waist to bring all the force of the body onto the pen point or tip of a writing brush. Actually, this already includes regulation of the mind, breathing and bodily movement. Its mechanism lies in the following aspects.

1. Regulating emotions. Appreciating and practicing painting and calligraphy can mould temperament, soothe and disperse stagnated Qi. Therefore, the method is applicable to patients with impetuosity, anger and depression, or patients with disorders of seven emotions. Ancients believed that watching and writing different forms of characters may have different effects on moulding temperament.

(1) Regular script: It has the actions of tranquilizing qi and the mind, removing vexation and impetuosity. Regular script is applicable to diseases due to dysphoria and anger.

(2) Official script: It is imposing and firm, quiet and beautiful, which easily makes people

emotionally stable. Official script is also applicable to diseases due to dysphoria and anger. Besides, it is cooperatively used with regular scrip to check activity with tranquility.

(3) Running hand and cursive hand: Both are natural, unrestrained and lively, like floating clouds and flowing water, which can make people in high spirits and have ease of mind. Accordingly, running hand and cursive hand are particularly applicable to patients with depression and pessimism.

2. Training the body. When practicing painting and calligraphy, people have fine movements of arms, elbows, wrists and fingers. These fine movements can train general tendons, bones and muscles (especially the upper limbs) to regulate and promote Qi flow and blood circulation, relax muscles and tendons and activate collaterals. Practicing painting and calligraphy is used to eliminate dysfunctions and restore functions such as spasm or unsmooth flexion of hands, wrists, elbows and arms due to sequelae of apoplexy, flaccidity syndrome, arthralgia syndrome, burn and injury of muscles and tendons.

Practicing painting and calligraphy can also achieve the purposes of arousing inspiration and improving intelligence by focusing on thinking and cleverly applying fingers. It may be applicable to the rehabilitation of children with hypophrenia, senile amnesia and dementia etc. Modern researches also indicate practicing painting has satisfactory effects on rehabilitation of feeble-minded children.

2.6 Loutrotherapy

Loutrotherapy is a method to eliminate diseases and strengthen health by applying visible or invisible natural physical factors such as water, sunlight, air, mud and sand.

Different bathing forms may relieve exterior syndromes by means of diaphoresis, remove wind and dampness, promote Qi flow and blood circulation, relax muscles and tendons, activate collaterals, regulate yin and yang, and inspire enthusiasm etc. respectively. Bathing forms are numerous, such as hot spring bath, hot water bath, sunbath, seawater bath, sauna, cold water bath, medicated bath, mud bath, sand bath and forestry bath. Because of limited space, this section only introduces the three bathing methods with TCM characteristics.

2.6.1 Medicated bath

Medicated liquid with a certain concentration is used to bathe or soak the whole body. In this way, the active ingredients of the drugs can exert direct effects on the region of pathological changes to destroy bacteria, kill pain, check itching and relieve inflammation. Meanwhile, by means of skin absorption, the active ingredients enter blood circulation to reach every tissue and organ of the human body, and to bring the therapeutic effects into full play.

2.6.1.1 The mechanism of life cultivation and rehabilitation with medicated bath

Medicated bath, like hot spring bath, hot water bath and sauna, can make skin blood vessels dilated and congested, accelerate metabolism and strengthen syringadenous excretion to promote profuse sweating and discharge of metabolite and toxin. Heat can reduce the excitability of nervous system to produce tranquilization and to be beneficial to sleeping, too. The heat of water can reduce muscular tension to relieve muscular pain and spasm as well. Moreover, the drugs in the medicated liquid reach the body directly. Therefore, it can produce a pharmacological action which does not exist in other bathing therapies.

Medicated bath may be applicable to the rehabilitation of hypertension, local soft tissue injury, neurosis, rheumatic arthritis, rhematoid arthritis, lumbago, pain of legs, ischias, sequelae of cerebrovascular accident, obesity, psoriasis and skin itching etc.

Before bathing, soak the drug for more than half an hour. Then, decoct the drugs into decoction. Next, mix the decoction with bathing water. The temperature of the water is 40℃ to 50℃. The bathing lasts 15 to 20 minutes (soak only the affected part in the case of contagious skin diseases such as tinea manuum and tinea pedis) each time, once a day or once every other day. It is advisable to take the medicated bath after noon or in the evening according to the specific patient's conditions. Each dose can be decocted twice. After bathing, wipe the body dry with a towel. Then, cover the body with a quilt and lie in bed peacefully for a while. However, be cautious not to select the drugs which irritate and corrode the skin; old, very young and seriously sick patients should be nursed to avoid accidents; medicated bath is not advisable in the case of skin injury, excessive starvation, overfeeding, menstrual period and pregnant stage.

2. 6. 1. 2 The commonly-used prescriptions for medicated bath

TCM possesses a large number of prescriptions for medicated bath handed down from the ancient times. Here is a brief introduction only for your reference.

1. Prescription for skin itching: 90g of Ganheye (dry Folium Nelumbinis), Gaoben (Rhizoma Ligustici), Gansong (Rhizoma Nardostachyos), Baizhi (Radix Angelicae Dachuricae), Weilingxian (Radix Clematidis), Cangercao (Herba Xanthii), Rendongteng (Caulis Lonicerae) and salt respectively.

2. Prescription for skin eczema: 100g of fresh Chuanlianpi (Pericarpium Meliae Toosendan), 30g of Qiyeyizhihua (Cortex Actinodaphnes Obovatae), Longgu (Os Draconis) and Luganshi (Calamina) respectively, 25g of Tufuling (Rhizoma Smilacis Glabrae), Kushen (Radix Sophorae Flavescentis), Difuzi (Fructus Kochiae) and Huzhang (Rhizoma Polygoni Cuspidati) respectively, 20g of Huanglian (Rhizoma Coptidis), Huangqin (Radix Scutellariae), Huangbai (Cortex Phellodendri), Shengdahuang (Radix et Rhizoma Rhei), Baixianpi (Cortex Dictamni Radicis), Huajiao (Pericarpium Zanthoxyli) and Diyu (Radix Sanguisorbae) respectively, 15g of Chixiaodou (Semen Phaseoli), Baiyaojian (Massa Gallae et Thei Fermentata), Liujinu (Herba Artemisiae Anomalae) and Danpi (Cortex Moutan Radicis) respectively, 10g of Cheqianzi (Semen Plantaginis) and Bingpian (Borneolum Syntheticum) respectively.

3. Prescription for infantile malnutrition: 15g of Kushen (Radix Sophorae Flavescentis), Fulingpi (Epidemis Poriae), Cangzhu (Rhizoma Atractylodis), Sangbaipi (Cortex Mori Radicis) and Baifan (Alumen) respectively and 15g of Congbai (Bulbus Allii Fistulosi).

4. Prescription for sore and scabies due to toxic heat: 30g of Fangfeng (Radix Ledebouriellae with the tip removed), Baizhi (Radix Angelicae Dahuriae), Xixin (Herba Asari), Kushen (Radix Sophorae Flavescentis), Wuzhuyu (Fructus Evodiae), Kulianzi (Fructus Meliae Toosendan), Lilu

(Radix et Rhizorma Veratri) with the tip removed, Mangcao (Folium Illicii Lanceolati) and Mahuanggen (Radix Ephedriae) respectively, 15g of Chuanjiao (Pericarpium Zanthoxyli) and 60g of salt.

5. Prescription for tinea manuum and tinea pedis: 30g of Kushen (Radix Sophorae Flavscentis), Taoren (Semen Persicae), Shechuangzi (Fructus Cnidii), Wumei (Fructus Mume), Lianqiao (Fructus Forsythiae) and Dahuang (Radix et Rhizoma Rhei) respectively, 20g of Gancao (Radix Glycyrrhizae) and 40g of Mangxiao (Natrii Sulfas).

6. Prescription for arthritis and gout: Equal amount of Laoguancao (Herba Erodii seu Geranii), Wujiapi (Cortex Acnthopancis Radicis), and Shenjincao (Herba Lycopodii) respectively.

7. Prescription for strengthening renal yang and sexual function: 30g of Dingxiang (Flos Caryophylli), Rougui (Cortex Cinnamomi), Zishaohua (Spongillae Fragillae), and Shechuangzi (Fructus Cnidii) respectively, 60g of Cangzhu (Rhizoma Atractylodis) and Duzhong (Cortex Eucommiae) respectively. All the above ingredients are ground into coarse powder. 30g of the powder is decocted each time for use. Fumigate and wash the navel, abdomen and Dantian with the decoction.

2.6.2 Mud bath

Unique natural hot mineral mud forms in the central zone of the hot spring in some places with the hot spring due to prolonged moistening of spring water. The temperature of the mud remains at 42℃ to 65℃ and the mud contains a large amount of colloidal substances, salts, and gases etc. Applying such hot mineral mud to bury and clean the body generally or locally can stimulate and regulate the nerves and body fluid of the organism. This has anti-inflammatory, pain-checking and cosmetic actions, etc.

There are natural or artificial mud bath rooms in places with rich geothermal resources. Bathers soak themselves in the mud of the bathing pool for 3 to 5 minutes or about 10 minutes. Then, they go to the sandy beach to lie down. When the mud on the body dries up in the sun and peels off one lump after another, wash the body clean with clear water. Mud bath has specific therapeutic effects on skin diseases and rheumatic arthritis. For healthy people, it also removes fatigue after they are soaked in the mud pool for a period of time.

There existed a kind of mud therapy in the ancient China. However, it was not the hot mud produced by terrestrial heat, but the cold mud dug from the well called "well mud". Medical books in the Tang Dynasty carried this method, such as *Qianjin Yaofang*, or *Valuable Prescriptions* and *Zhenlei Bencao*, or *Classified Materia Medica for Emergency*. It was used to cure diseases such as threatened abortion due to fetal heat at pregnant stage as well as headache due to wind and heat. This method, in fact, is the so-called humic acidic natrium bath. Besides well mud, the mud in marshland also has the same effects.

Humic acid is the substance produced by putrefied organic substances. It has the actions of regulating the endocrine of the organism, inhibiting various harmful enzymes, accelerating blood circulation, promoting metabolism and increasing the immunity of the human body.

Mud bath has very good therapeutic effects on rheumatoid arthritis, arthralgia of limbs, skin purpura, soft tissue injury of the organism, ulcer of digestive tract, certain obstetrical and gynecological diseases as well as hypertension. It has the therapeutic actions of relieving swelling and restoring physical strength, especially in the people with sprain due to competitions or training.

2.6.3 Sand bath

Sand bath is the method to achieve the therapeutic effects by means of heat transmission into the body with sand directly contacting the body as the medium. It has very good therapeutic effects on rheumatic arthritis and diseases of motor system.

The mechanism of sand bath mainly lies in the comprehensive therapeutic effects of magnetic therapy (the sand contains magnetic substances), physical therapy (dryness, high temperature and infrared radiation), massage, and sunbath etc. Sand bath can remove obstruction of meridians, relax muscles, tendons and bones, eliminate intractable diseases, promote blood circulation and enhance metabolism.

The method of taking a sand bath is burying the whole body except the head, or part of the body in the hot solarized sand. With the scorching sun overhead and the burning sand around the body, patients perspire all over the body and the heat is almost unendurable. Sand bath just makes use of such thermal effect to cure diseases. In general, taking sand bath once or twice can eliminate the diseases for patients with rheumatic arthritis, ischias, and disturbances of nervous system etc. It also has therapeutic effects on diseases such as chronic diseases of digestive tract and dysfunctions of autonomic nerve.

Sand bath lasts 10 to 15 minutes each time in accordance with the air temperature and the sand temperature. 10 days constitute one course of treatment.

2.7 Professional Therapies of Life Cultivation in TCM

2.7.1 Therapies with massage

Massage (called "an mo" in ancient times) is a rehabilitation method in which different manipulations are applied on the certain parts of the patient's body to dredge meridians and regulate qi and blood for the promotion of health by means of manual techniques or apparatus.

2.7.2 Therapies with acupuncture and moxibustion

Acupuncture is one kind of unique life cultivation in China. It can not only build people's body but also promote the rehabilitation of weak patients with prolonged diseases. By needling or cauterizing the acupoints, acupuncture and moxibustion can regulate Qi, blood and collateral, nourish the viscera and prolong life.

2.7.3 Scraping therapy

Scraping therapy is guided by TCM theories of meridian and acupoint. Use specially made ware and corresponding technique to dip certain medium and then scrape or rub the surface of human body until some red or marroon appear, which is also called acture diseases), so as to invigorate the circulation of blood. It is widely used in clinic and family health care due to its simple, convenient, cheap and effective feature. When combined with acupuncture, moxibustion, cupping, blood – letting therapy, scraping therapy can promote blood circulation to remove blood stasis, and drive out evil and toxin.

2.7.4 Cupping

In cupping therapy, cups are used as devices and flaming alcohol sponges are used to create negative pressure inside cups; the cups are attached over selected acupoints or spots for some time until congestion appear on the skin, so as to prevent and treat diseases.

2.7.5 Therapies with Chinese herbs

The occurrence and development of all kinds of diseases are caused by pathogenic factors acting on human body, which result in the pathologic phenomena such as imbalance between yin and yang, growth of pathogenic factors and reduction of healthy Qi, and the disorders of Zang organs and Fu organs. The basic principle of treating diseases with Chinese medicinal herbs is to eliminate causes of disease, dispel pathogenic factors or restore the coordination of the functions of zang and fu organs so that excess and deficiency of yin or yang can be corrected and the diseases can be cured.

The properties and actions of Chinese medicinal herbs, which are the essential basis of the analyses and clinical usage of Chinese medicinal herbs, are summarized in medical practice and on the basis of the theories of yinyang, ZangFu, meridians, and therapeutic principles of traditional Chinese medicine etc.

第三章　推拿按摩法

推拿是人类最早掌握的医疗方法之一。推拿手法是推拿治疗的基本手段。

3.1　手法分类

中医推拿素以历史悠久、流派众多、手法丰富、技巧性强，适应证广、疗效显著而著称于世。根据目前统计，我国有文字记载的推拿手法已有200余种，而流传于民间尚未定型的手法可能更多。手法虽然繁多，但可以根据其外力作用方式而划分为两门，即《内经》所言的“按”和“蹻”。根据唐代医家王冰的注释，“按”为“抑按皮肉”，“蹻”为“捷举手足”。前者的手法力直接作用于接触部位，而后者的外力间接作用于远离接触部位的关节、肌肉、筋膜。每一门手法又可根据动作特点而分为若干类，每一类手法又包括若干种基本手法，每一基本手法还可根据其接触部位、动作变化而分为若干种变法。若从手法的主要作用途径分类，其则可以分为刺激性手法、矫正性手法和松动性手法。

各类手法间的相互关系如图3－1所示：

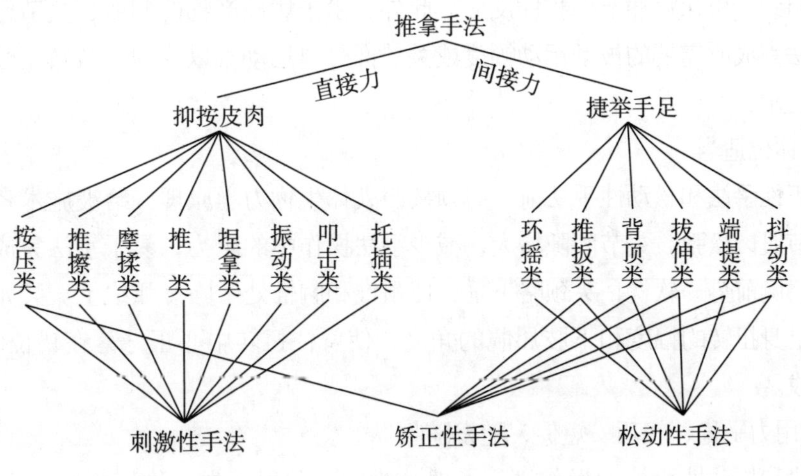

图3－1　各类手法间的相互关系

3.2　推拿手法

推拿手法的本质是一种外力，手法外力可直接引起关节位置的改变，肌肉、筋膜等软组织的形变、撕裂而纠正人体病理状态，治愈疾病。但更重要的是，手法外力作为一种刺激因素，激活了经络系统的调整功能，使机体趋于康复。

3.2.1 刺激性手法的技术要求

抑按皮肉类手法中，大多数为刺激性手法，刺激性手法并不是以本身直接的力改变人体的病理状态而发挥治疗效应，而是手法作用于经络系统，再通过经络系统的中介，激发人体固有的调整与自愈功能，进而防病治病。故刺激性手法必须符合持久、有力、均匀、柔和、深透等技术要求。

所谓“持久”，是指手法能严格按照特定操作规范持续运用一段时间而不走样，使手法的刺激量积累到临界点，足以推动经络系统的调整作用，改变病理状态。例如，小儿推拿的“推三关”和“退六腑”手法对某些病情严重的患儿必须连续操作半小时以上才能发挥显著的解表发汗或退热作用。所谓“有力”，就是指手法应具有恰当的力量。在一定范围内，手法力的大小与对经络系统的刺激强度成正比，但超过这个限度，反而造成组织损伤，或成为一种超限抑制信号。手法力的大小也并不是固定不变的，必须根据施术部位、病理特点、患者体质等具体情况而调整力的大小。根据临床具体情况而施加恰当的手法力，需经过长期的实践才能掌握。所谓“均匀”，是指手法动作要有节奏性，速度不可时快时慢，压力不可时轻时重。所谓“柔和”，是指手法的用力方式，平稳而缓慢变化的力要比急剧变化的爆发力柔和，以柔软易变形的掌面着力要比以坚硬而不易变形的骨突着力柔和。所谓“深透”，是指通过运用各种富于技巧性的手法，降低人体组织的张力，减少对外力传递的阻抗而使手法作用达到组织深层。

3.2.2 矫正性、松动性手法的技术要求

矫正性手法和松动性手法统称“关节运动性手法”。矫正性手法和松动性手法通常作用于已存在运动障碍的关节，而手法的完成又必须突破关节的病理运动限制范围或生理运动限制范围，必然刺激病变组织，引起疼痛及保护性反应。此外，由于病理产物的刺激，关节运动肌群处于痉挛状态，使手法完成所需要的被动运动幅度或关节面分离运动难以实现。故矫正性、松动性手法必须遵循以下要求：

3.2.2.1 体位适当

在运用矫正性手法和松动性手法前，必须按照人体生物力学原理，给被施术者摆好合适的体位，使病变关节肌肉松弛，关节间隙增大，减少手法操作中的阻力，易于手法完成。如矫正上胸段椎骨错缝时，胸前垫一软枕，头颈略下垂，使颈椎和胸椎处于同一弧线上。又如矫正腰椎椎骨错缝时，调整上身扭转的幅度和下肢屈髋的角度，使脊柱扭转中心正好落在错位的运动单元上，手法就容易完成。

3.2.2.2 用力平稳、轻巧、短促，随发随收

矫正性手法和松动性手法的操作过程一般分为两个阶段：先平稳地将关节运动到某一限制位，然后做一轻巧、短促的突发动作，扩大关节运动幅度，随即停止用力，使关节恢复中立位。

3.2.2.3 把握正确的用力方向

操作过程中，必须考虑到关节面的形态、关节瞬时运动中心的位置、关节面互相错移的方向，而把握正确的用力方向。否则，难以完成手法目标。例如，骶髂关节错位有后错（髂后上棘隆凸）和前错（髂后上棘低陷）两型，前者应按髂后上棘向前外下用力，按骶骨下端向上方用力；而后者应按坐骨结节向前外上用力，按骶骨上端向前下方用力。若用力方向不对，就不能达

到复位的目的。

3.3　常用推拿

3.3.1　按压类手法

所谓按压类手法是指把操作者的掌、指或身体其他部位置于患者体表后，沿体表垂直方向向深部用力的一类手法。

3.3.1.1　代表手法：按法

按法以拇指指端或指腹接触，为指按法；用掌根部接触，称掌按法。既可单手操作，又可两手相叠，增加按压力量，协同操作。

1. 指按法。

拇指伸直，其余四指自然弯曲，食指与拇指相靠，助拇指指力；用前臂的力量，逐渐向下按压，用力由轻而重，使刺激充分深透到机体组织深部后，逐渐减轻压力，再重复以上按压过程（图3－2）。欲增加按压力量，可将另一手拇指重叠于指骨间关节上，两指协同向下按压（图3－3）。

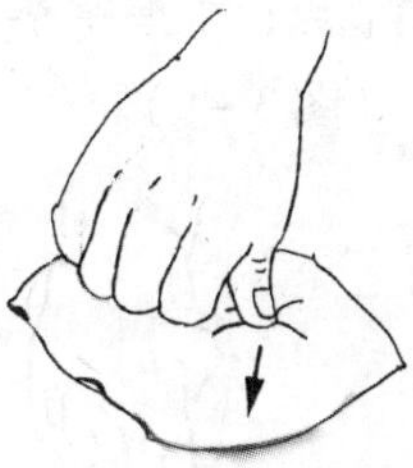

图3－2　指按法

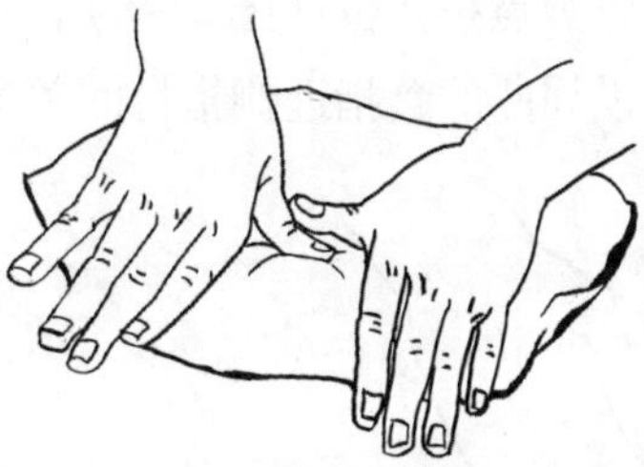

图3－3　叠指按

指按法接触面积小而集中，刺激强弱容易控制，适用于全身各部的穴位与反应点、压痛点，具有较好的止痛作用，常用于各种痛症的治疗。

2. 掌按法。

掌按法以两手操作居多。操作时，手指自然伸直，腕关节背伸，一手掌根部接触体表，另一手掌重叠其上，上肢伸直；然后以肩部或躯干发力，逐渐增加按压力量，使力沿伸直的上肢纵轴传达到按压部位；待刺激充分深透后再逐渐减小按压力量。重复以上操作（图3－4）。

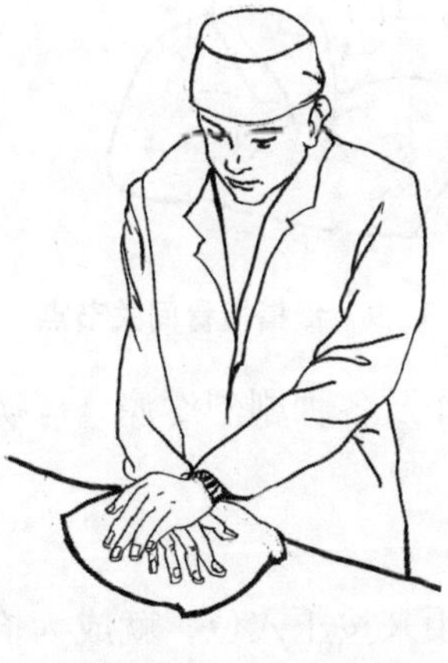

图3－4　掌按法

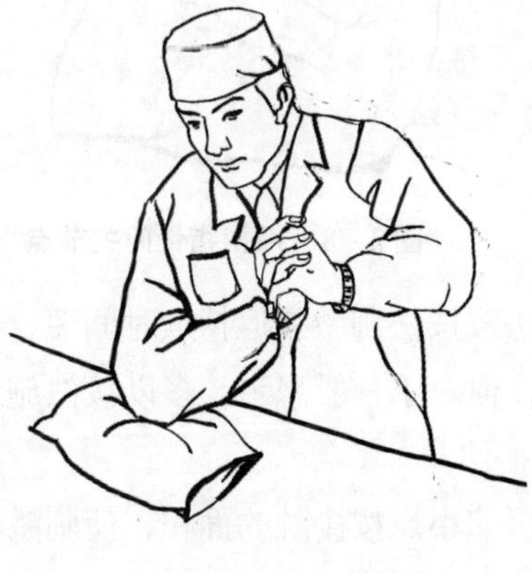

图3－5　肘压法

掌按法按压力量大，接触面积也大，适用于腰背部、臀部、大腿、小腿和肩部，具有较好的放松痉挛肌组织的作用，常用于治疗急慢性腰腿痛、肩关节周围炎等病症。

3.3.1.2　按法的衍化

1. 肘压法。

“按”是指手法的动作形态，“压”是指手法所引起的压缩效应，故通常按压混称。若严格区分两者，则“按”偏于动，“压”偏于静；按的压力持续时间短，压的刺激持续时间长；按的压力小，刺激轻；压的力量大，刺激强。用肘部按压习惯称为“肘压法”，肘压操作时，肘关节屈曲，以肘尖置体表某部，用上肢与躯干发力，垂直向下按压（图3－5）。肘压法刺激强烈，一般仅用于肌肉发达厚实的下腰部、臀部，治疗顽固性腰腿痛、腰肌僵硬等病症。

2. 点法。

如欲得到比指按法刺激更强的穴位刺激，则可减小按压时的接触面积，称为点法。点法有4种操作方式：①中指点：拇、食、中三指自然伸直，拇指置中指掌侧，食指置中指背侧，挟持中指助力；然后利用腕、肘、肩关节力量，以中指端点按穴位，使刺激深入组织深部，然后将手指抬起（图3－6）。②剑指点：食、中二指伸直成剑指，然后仿中指点操作方式，利用腕、肘、肩关节的力量，以食、中二指指端点按穴位（图3－7）。③拇指指骨间关节点：手握空拳，以屈曲的拇指指骨间关节骨突点按穴位（图3－8）。④食指指骨间关节点：手握空拳，用拇指尺侧缘抵住食指指甲，然后以屈曲的食指近侧指骨间关节骨突点按穴位（图3－9）。

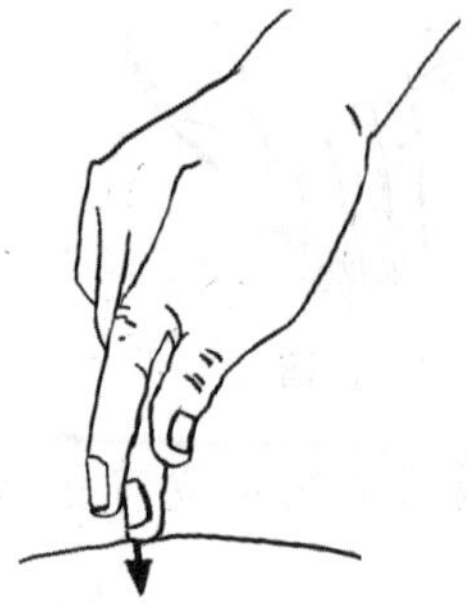

图3－6　中指点法

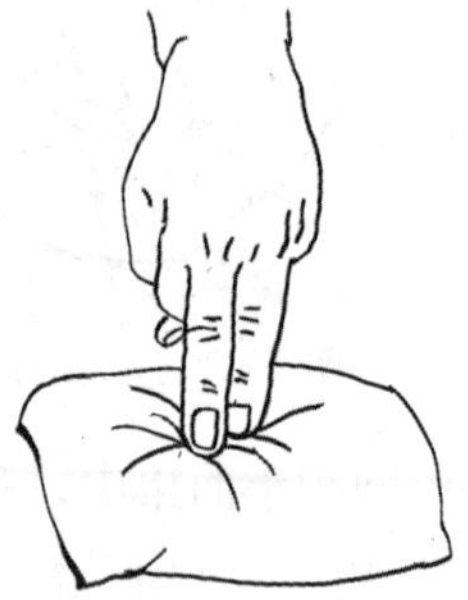

图3－7　剑指点法

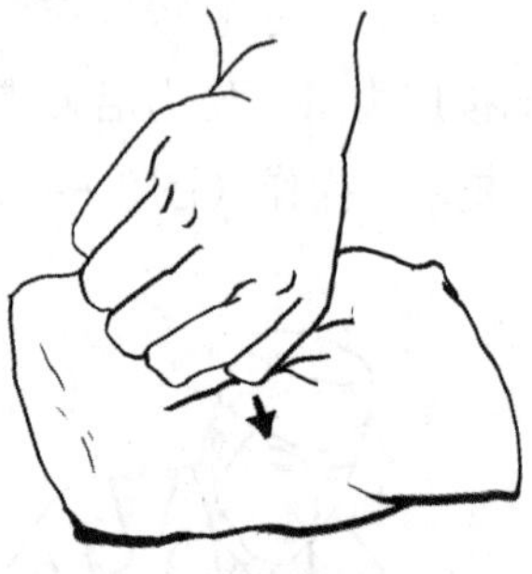

图3－8　拇指指骨间关节点

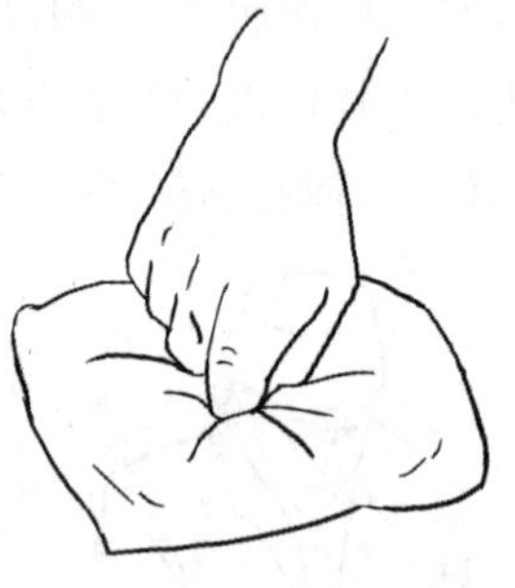

图3－9　食指指骨间关节点

点法较按法刺激强但持续时间短，适用于骨缝关节处穴位操作及各种剧烈疼痛、瘫痪等病症的治疗，但对于一般患者，多以按法施之。

3. 掐法。

如再缩小点按接触的面积，使刺激更为强烈尖锐，则可用指甲来按压穴位，就成为掐法。又称爪法或切法（图3－10）。掐法刺激强烈，常用于水沟、素髎、内关、中冲、老龙等急救穴位的操作，有开窍解痉的作用，以治疗昏迷、惊风、休克等危急症。有时为了缓解掐法所形成的锐痛，在应用掐法之后，再用揉法和之。

4. 押法。

在指按法的基础上，减轻向下按压的力量，以手指螺纹面按于穴位而不动，称押法（图3-11）。押法常用于探求穴位得气。

5. 掩法、扪法。

在掌按法的基础上，减轻向下按压的力量，以手掌轻按于胸腹部不动，称掩法；若按于胸腹前，先将手掌擦热，则称扪法（图3-12）。但在目前临床中，已不再细分，统称为掌按法。

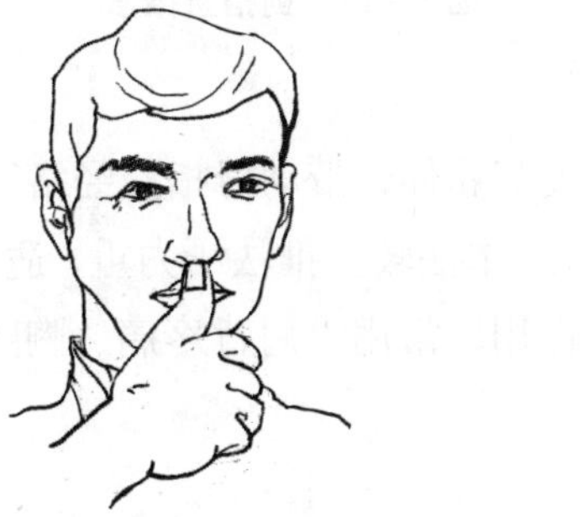

图3-10 掐法

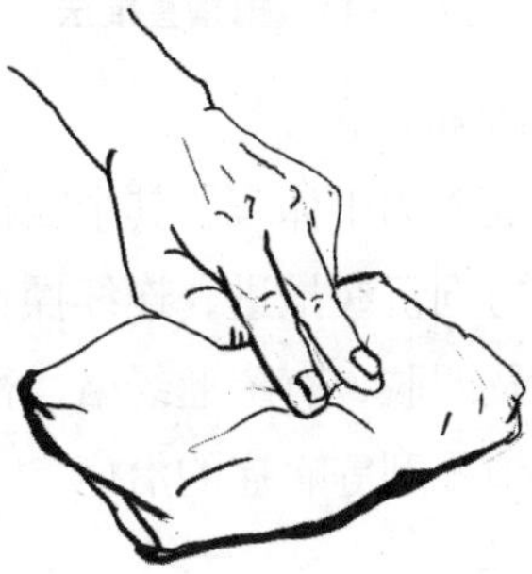

图3-11 押法

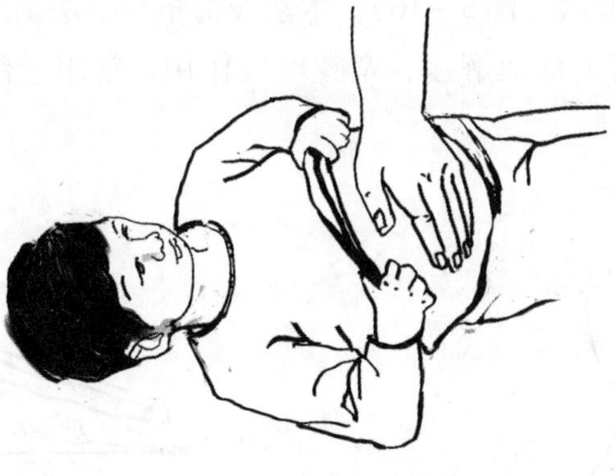

图3-12 掩法、扪法

3.3.2 推擦类手法

所谓推擦类手法是指操作者以指、掌或身体其他部位置于患者体表，在保持一定垂直压力下，做直线或弧线运动的一类手法。

3.3.2.1 代表手法：推法

1. 拇指直推法。

手指伸直，拇指在后，以桡侧缘触及皮肤，位于所推穴位的起点；四指在前，指尖触及所推穴位的终点；然后虎口快速一合一张，用拇指做单方向轻快推动（图3-13）。频率为每分钟200~240次。

2. 剑指直推法。

食指、中指伸直成剑指状，以螺纹面轻触皮肤，然后前臂快速摆动，带动手指轻快地做单方向推动（图3-14）。频率为每分钟200~240次。直推法是压力最轻的推法，要求操作时皮肤不变形，操作后皮肤不发红。推时需蘸姜汁或清水，保持皮肤湿润。直推法用于小儿推拿操作，如“推三关”“退六腑”等，其作用由所推穴位及方向决定。

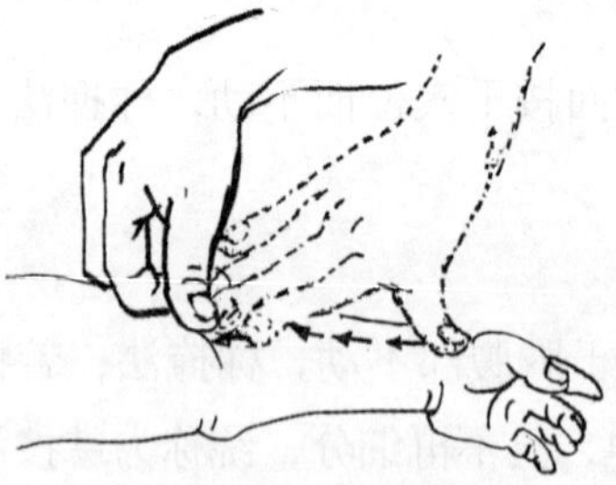
图 3－13　拇指直推法

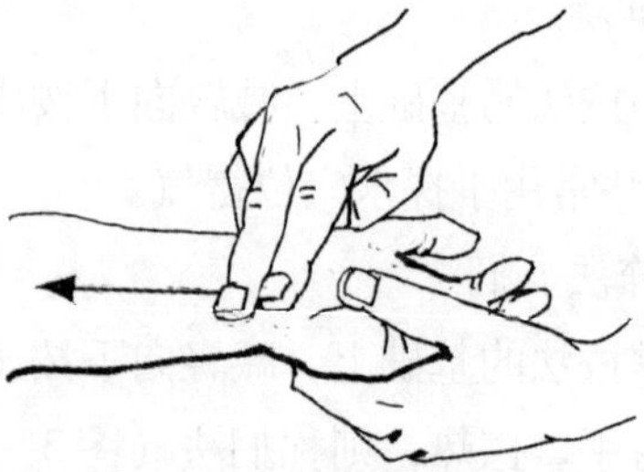
图 3－14　剑指直推法

3. 拇指平推法。

以拇指面着力于体表，其余四指分开助力，然后用肘关节屈伸，带动拇指沿经络循行或肌纤维方向做单方向沉缓推进，连续操作 5～15 次（图 3－15）。本法较直推法压力重，适用于肩背、胸腹、腰臀及四肢，有疏通经络、行气活血、理筋止痛等作用，常用于肩背疼痛、胸闷腹胀、痉挛拘急、关节不利等病症的治疗。

4. 掌平推法。

以掌根部着力于体表，手指伸直；然后用肘关节屈伸运动，带动掌面沿经络循行路线做单方向沉缓推进，连续操作 5～10 次（图 3－16）。本法较拇指平推法刺激缓和，适用于腰背、胸腹、大腿等平坦部位，具有较好的活血解痉、宽胸理气作用，常用于治疗腰背酸痛、胸腹胀闷等病症。

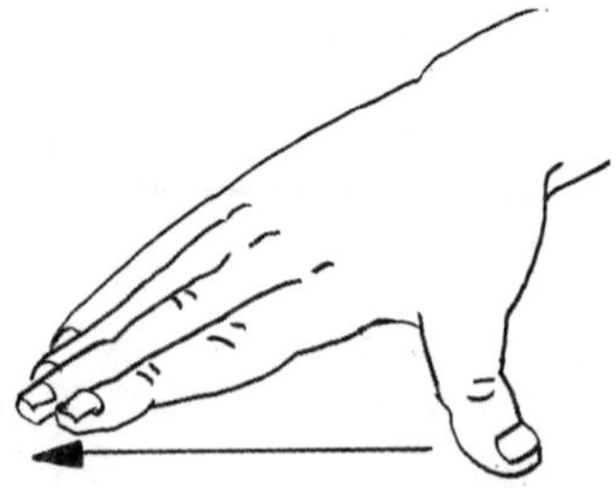
图 3－15　拇指平推法

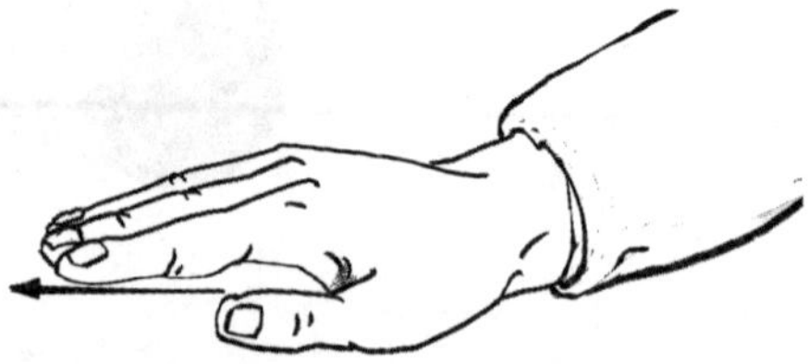
图 3－16　掌平推法

5. 刨推法。

用一手轻握患肢，然后以肘关节屈伸运动带动手掌沿肢体纵轴做单方向推动，连续操作 5～10 次（图 3－17）。本法刺激缓和，适用于四肢，有舒筋活血、消肿止痛的作用，常用于四肢软组织损伤、关节痹痛的治疗。

6. 拳平推法。

握拳，以食指、中指、无名指、小指四指的指间关节突起处着力于体表，向一定方向推动，连续操作 5～10 次（图 3－18）。本法刺激强烈，适用于肩、背、臀、腿肌肉厚实处操作，对陈伤及风湿痹痛而又感觉迟钝者，较为适用。

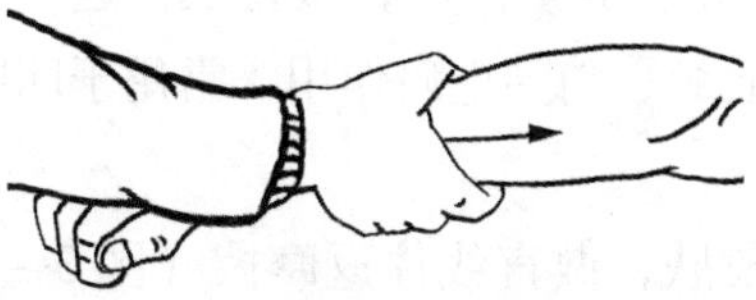

图 3－17　刨推法

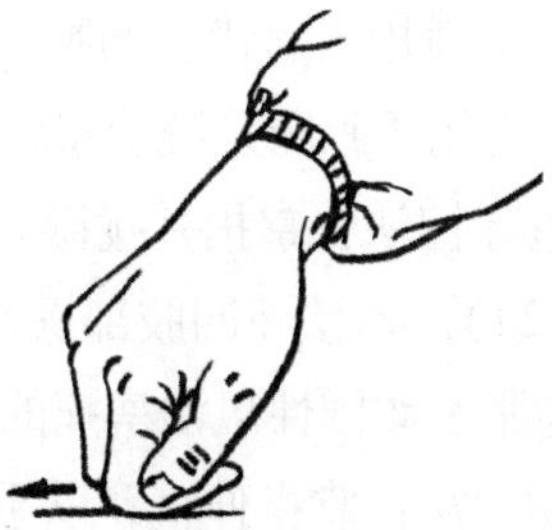

图 3－18　拳平推法

7. 肘平推法。

屈肘，以鹰嘴突着力于体表，向一定方向推动，连续操作 5～10 次（图 3－19）。本法在推法中刺激最强，仅对身体壮实者使用。适用范围同拳平推法。

8. 分推法与合推法。

以两手同时操作，自肢体中轴线向两侧推动，称分推法；自肢体两侧向中轴线推动为合推法。分推法和合推法在不同部位操作有不同名称，如分（合）腕阴阳（图 3－20）、分膻中（图 3－21），适合小儿推拿治疗；“八”字分推法（图 3－22），适合腰背疾患治疗等。

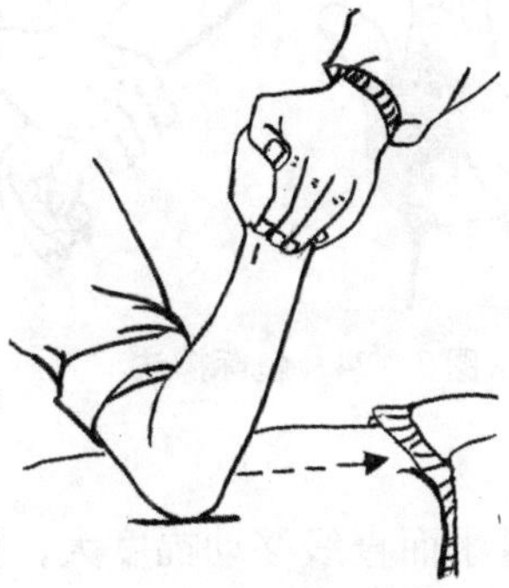

图 3－19　肘平推法

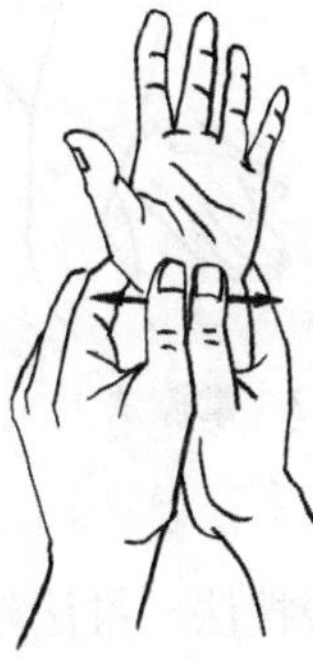

图 3－20　分（合）腕阴阳

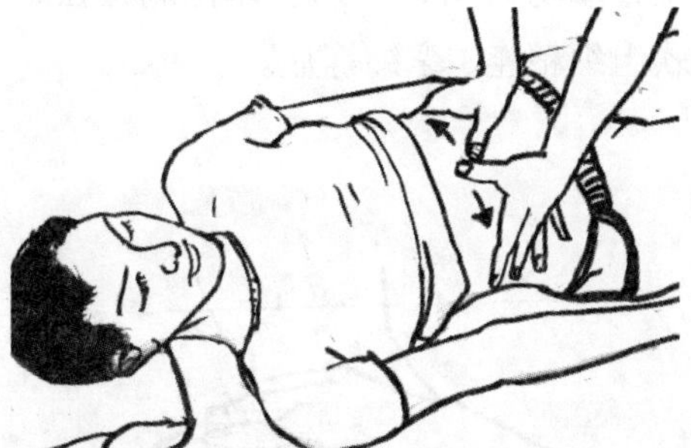

图 3－21　分膻中

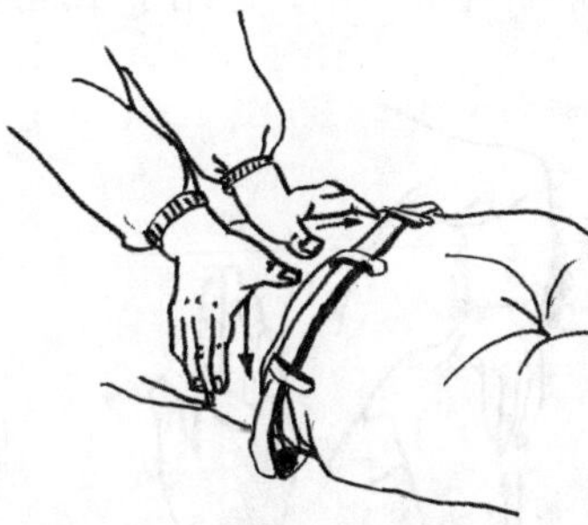

图 3－22　“八”字分推法

3.3.2.2　推法的衍化

1. 擦法。

推法的用意是推动气血在经脉中运行，故推法是单方向的推动。擦法的用意是使手掌与皮肤间及组织各层间的相互摩擦转化为热能，故擦法须往返操作。擦法的压力不能过大，以摩擦时皮肤不起皱叠为宜；擦法的移动速度较平推法快，一般掌握在每分钟 100～120 次。

（1）掌擦法。类似掌平推法，但压力较平推法轻，做直线往返摩擦，以深部透热为度（图

3－23）。本法适用于肩背、胸腹等平坦部位的操作，有温经通络、宽胸理气、调理脾胃、强壮身体的作用，常用于呼吸系统疾患、消化系统疾患及体质虚弱者的治疗。

（2）鱼际擦法：掌指并拢微屈成虚掌，以大鱼际及掌根紧贴皮肤，做直线往返摩擦，透热为度（图3－24）。本法在四肢部操作较为平稳，有活血通经、消肿止痛作用，常用于四肢软组织损伤、关节肿胀及顽固性风湿痹痛的治疗。

（3）侧擦法：掌指伸直，以手掌小鱼际部位紧贴皮肤，做直线往返摩擦（图3－25）。本法温热作用较强，适用于腰背、骶部、小腹等处操作，有温经散寒、补肾强身、活血祛风作用，常用于治疗腰背疼痛、筋脉拘急、小腹冷痛、体质虚弱等。擦法操作时，可在局部涂少许润滑剂，既可保护皮肤，又可使热量深透。擦法使用后，皮肤可能轻度损伤，故擦法多在其他手法之后应用。不可在擦法之后再在局部应用其他手法，以免破皮。

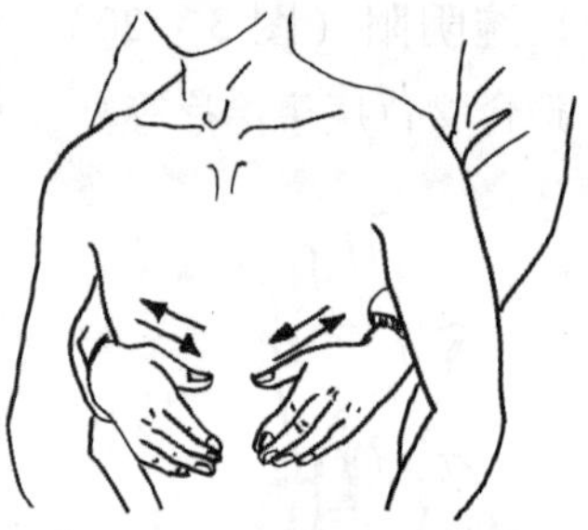

图3－23　掌擦法

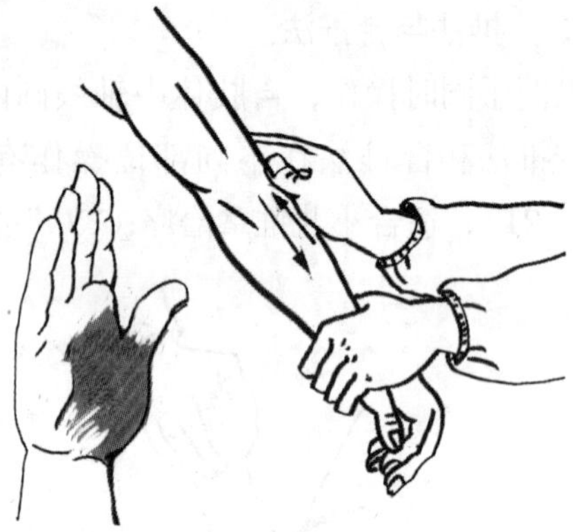

图3－24　鱼际擦法

2. 拨法。

拨法，又称弹拨法。推法与擦法操作时，垂直按压力量小而直线移动幅度大，操作者手与患者体表间产生相对摩擦。拨法操作时，垂直按压力量大而直线移动幅度小。以拇指端按在治疗部位上，做短距离直线拨动，使深层组织之间产生相互错移摩动（图3－26）。本法刺激强烈，有分离粘连、舒筋解痉的作用，适用于压痛点操作，治疗软组织粘连、挛缩等症。

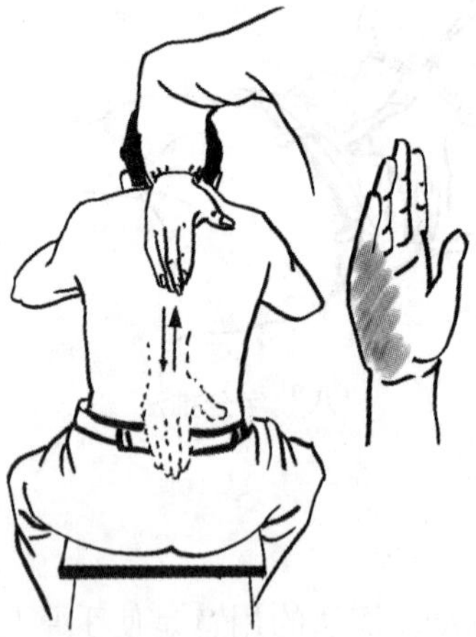

图3－25　侧擦法

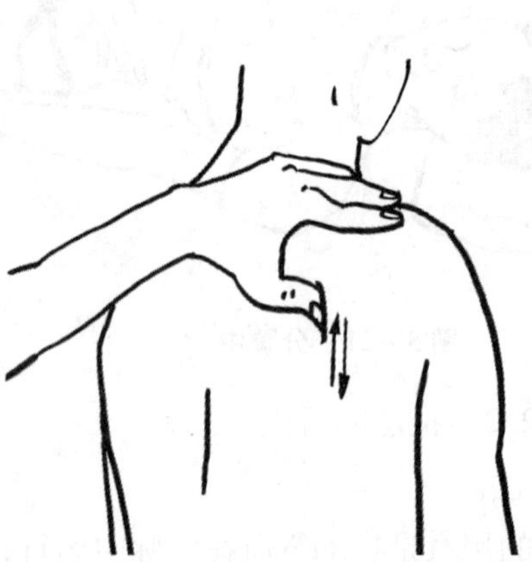

图3－26　拨法

3. 抹法。

以拇指平推法或掌平推法在头面部按固定程序操作，称抹法。抹法操作方式是：医生面对病人站立，用双手轻扶患者头部两侧，两拇指自印堂穴交替向上抹至前额，往返15次；随后两拇指自印堂分抹至两侧太阳穴并揉太阳穴数次，仍合推至印堂，往返15次；再从印堂沿眼眶周围反复抹动15次；最后，从印堂沿鼻柱两侧、颧骨下缘分抹至两耳前听宫穴，并返回印堂，往返15次（图3－27）。以上动作要连续不断，一气呵成。结束后患者顿觉眼目清亮，头脑清醒。抹头面具有祛风醒目、宁神降压的作用，常用于治疗感冒、头痛、失眠、高血压等症。

4. 扫散法。

医生以一手轻轻扶住患者头部，另一手指伸直，以拇指桡侧面及其余四指指端，同时贴于头颞部，稍用力在耳上后方（胆经循行部位）自前上向后下做弧形单向摩动（图3－28）。本法具有平肝潜阳、祛风止痛作用，常用于头痛、眩晕、高血压等症。

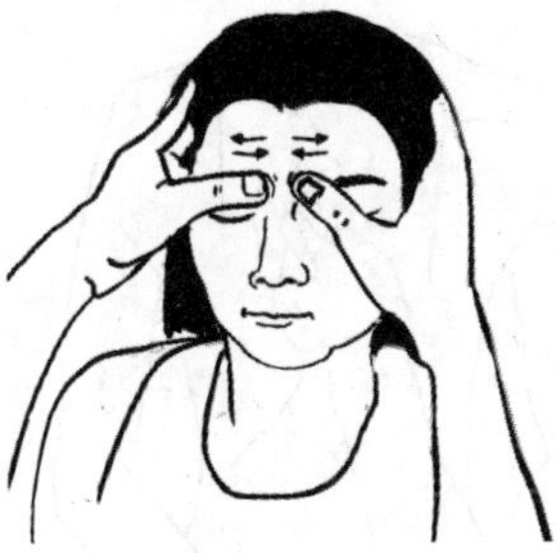

图3－27　抹法

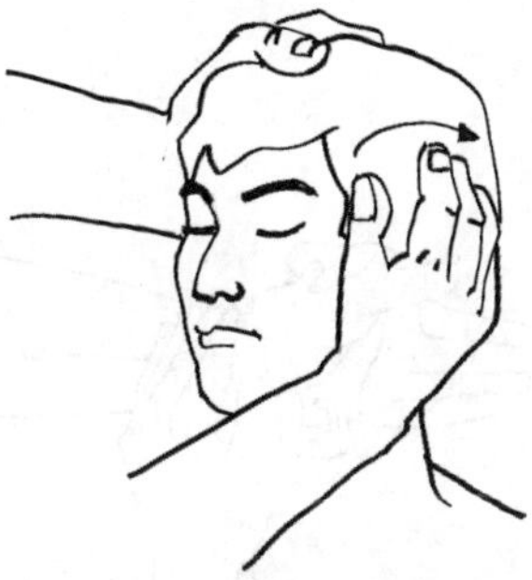

图3－28　扫散法

5. 钩法。

与扫散法相似，但操作者位于患者后面操作。两拇指按在枕骨两侧，把两手其他指并拢微屈成钩状，以食指中节、末节的桡侧缘着力，从两侧太阳穴起向后沿耳上后方做弧形摩动至枕骨两侧，反复数次（图3－29）。作用同扫散法。

6. 勒法。

勒法，又称理法。以屈曲的中指、食指夹住指（或趾）后，向指端滑勒，各指（或趾）均勒一遍（图3－30）。

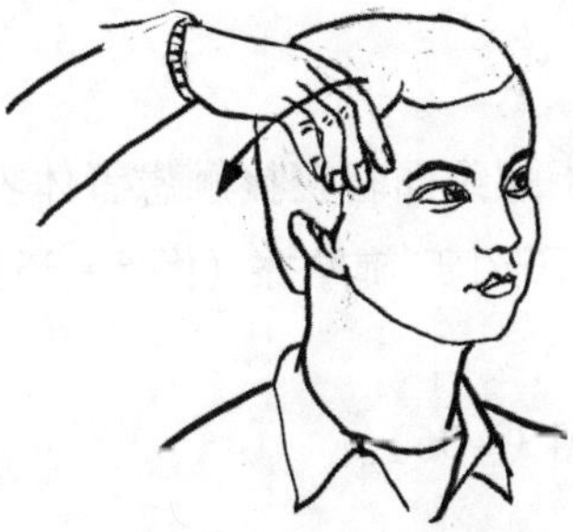

图3－29　钩法

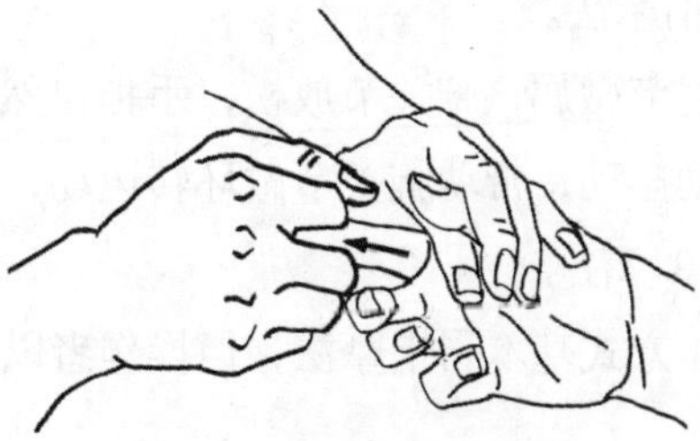

图3－30　勒法

7. 捋法、顺法。

以掌推法在四肢伸侧自近端推向远端，称捋法（图3－31）；肢屈侧自远端推向近端称顺法（图3－32）。

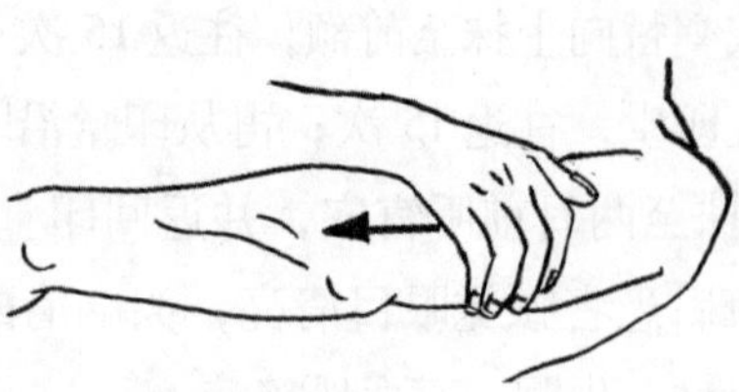

图 3－31　捋法

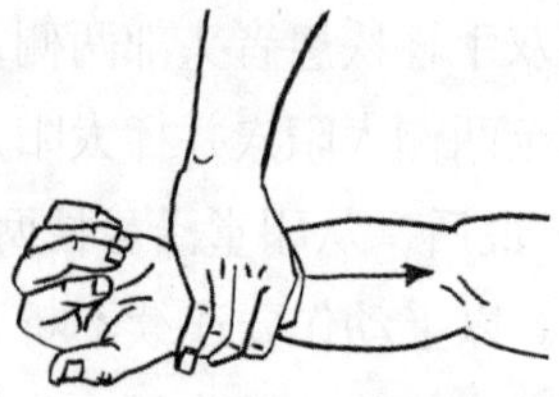

图 3－32　顺法

8. 拂法、刮法。

以四指螺纹面轻快地单方向掠擦皮肤的手法称拂法（图 3－33）。它与指直推法相近。以指螺纹面较重地单方向掠擦皮肤的手法，或以匙缘、铜钱边缘掠擦皮肤至皮下瘀血的手法，均称刮法（图 3－34）。

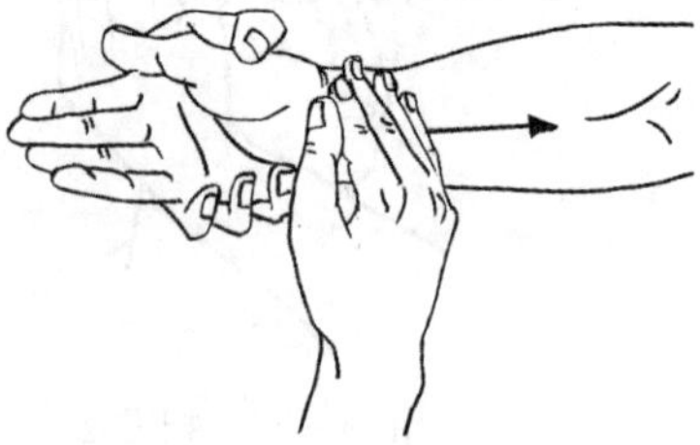

图 3－33　拂法

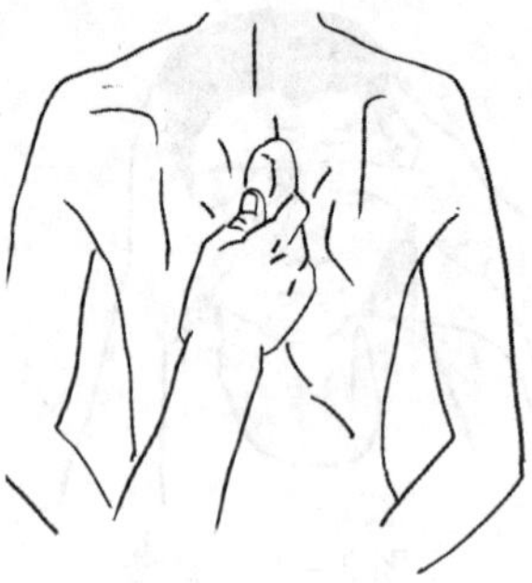

图 3－34　刮法

3.3.3　摩揉类手法

所谓摩揉类手法是指操作者以指、掌或身体其他部位接触患者体表，在保持一定垂直压力下做环旋运动的一类手法。

3.3.3.1　代表手法：摩法

摩为抚摩之意。摩法有两种操作方式，用食、中、无名指指面抚摩称指摩法，用手掌面抚摩称掌摩法。

1. 指摩法。

肘关节微屈，腕关节放松，手指自然伸直，以食、中、无名指螺纹面轻轻接触患者体表，以前臂主动摆动，带动腕关节做环转运动，使操作者指面在患者体表产生环旋摩擦（图 3－35）。

2. 掌摩法。

操作方式基本同指摩法，但操作者以掌面与患者体表接触（图 3－36）。

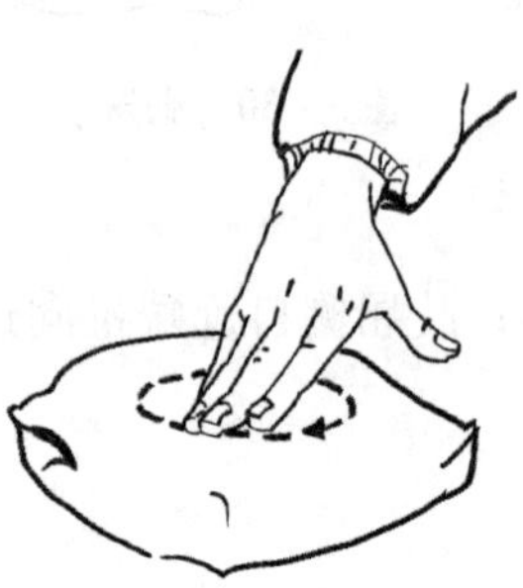

图 3－35　指摩法

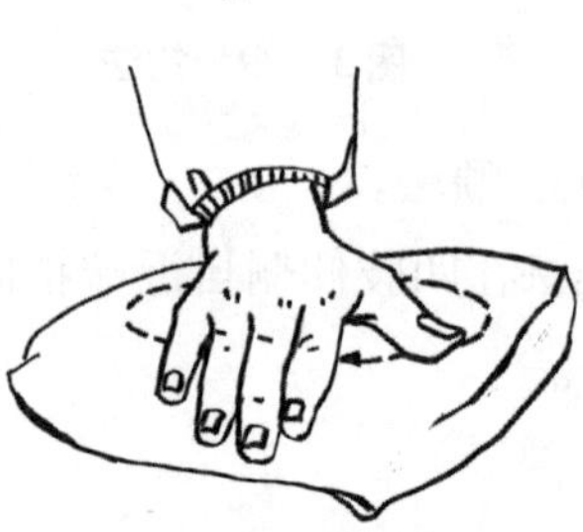

图 3－36　掌摩法

摩法操作时，动作宜轻柔，压力不要太大，顺时针方向与逆时针方向环摩均可，每分钟操作频率为 100～120 次。摩法刺激舒适缓和，适用于胸腹与胁肋部操作，也可在其他部位的损伤肿痛处操作。具有宽胸理气、疏肝和中、消积导滞和活血散瘀的作用，治疗胸胁胀闷、脘腹疼痛、消化不良、泄泻、便秘及外伤肿胀等症。古代应用摩法时常在施术皮肤涂以药膏，以加强手法的治疗作用，称之为膏摩。

3.3.3.2　摩法的衍化

1. 揉法。

在摩法操作的基础上，增加向下的垂直压力，减小环旋运动的幅度，使操作者指、掌黏附于患者体表，皮肤保持相对不动，而带动皮下浅层组织在深层组织界面上环转揉动，称为揉法。故《保赤推拿法》说：“揉者，医以指按儿经穴，不离其处而环转之也。”《厘正按摩要术》称：“揉法以手宛转回环，宜轻宜缓，绕于其上也，是从摩法生出者。”

揉法有指腹揉、掌根揉、大鱼际揉、拇指桡侧揉 4 种操作方式。

（1）指腹揉：以食指、中指、无名指指腹揉动，操作方法与指摩法相仿（图 3－37）。

（2）掌根揉：操作者腕关节略背屈，手指自然屈曲，以掌根部着力于患者体表做环旋揉动。操作方法与掌摩法相似（图 3－38）。

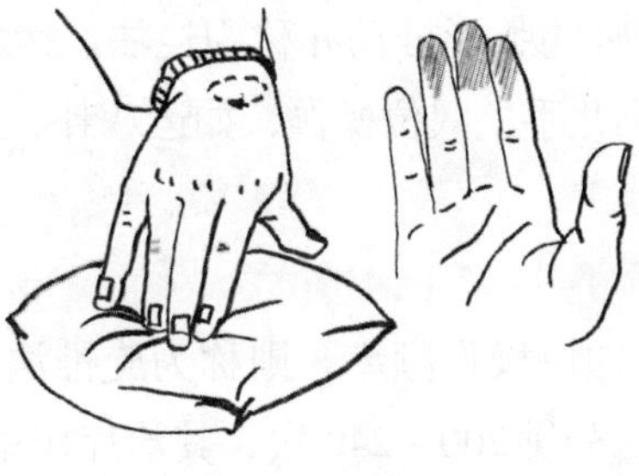

图 3－37　**指腹揉**

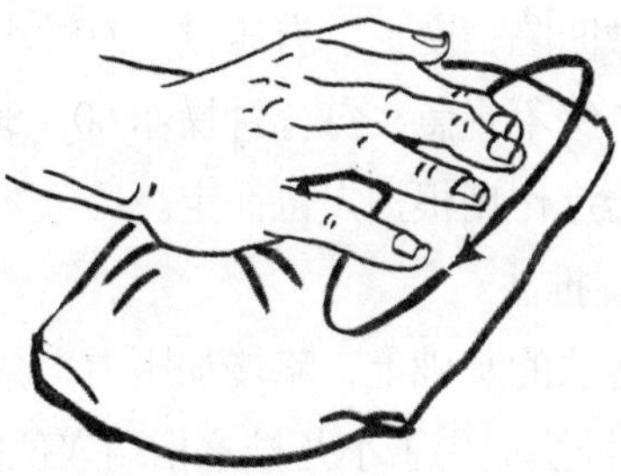

图 3－38　**掌根揉**

（3）大鱼际揉：肘关节屈曲 120°，腕关节放松，肘腕大致在同一水平线上；手尺侧缘在前，桡侧缘在后，以手掌大鱼际部位接触患者体表（图 3－39）；然后前臂做主动摆动，带动腕关节、第一腕掌关节环转运动，使大鱼际附着于皮肤，皮下组织在深层组织界面上环旋揉动（图 3－40，3－41）。

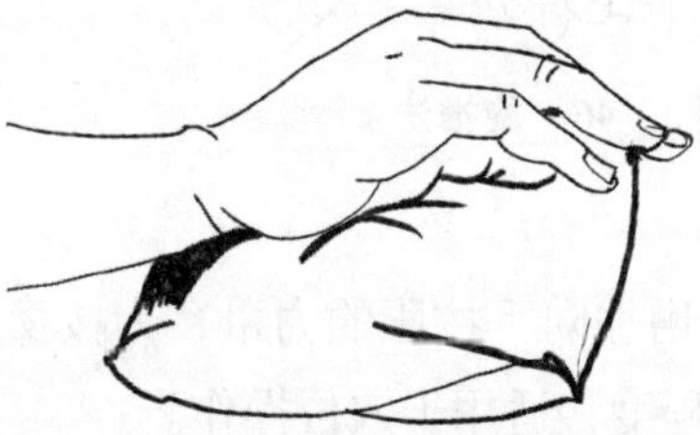

图 3－39　**大鱼际揉（前视）**

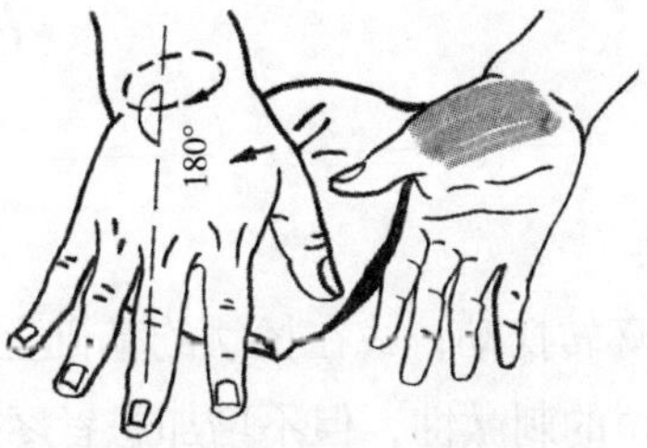

图 3－40　**大鱼际揉（前摆）**

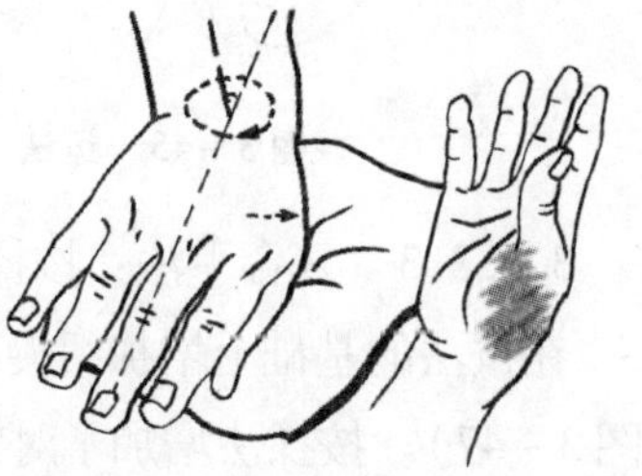

图 3－41　**大鱼际揉（后摆）**

（4）拇指桡侧揉：操作方式与大鱼际揉相仿，操作者以拇指桡侧缘接触患者体表揉动（图 3－42，3－44，3－44）。

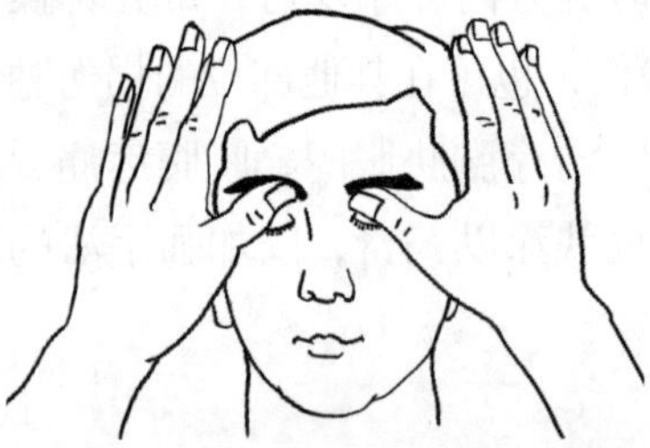

图 3－42　拇指桡侧揉

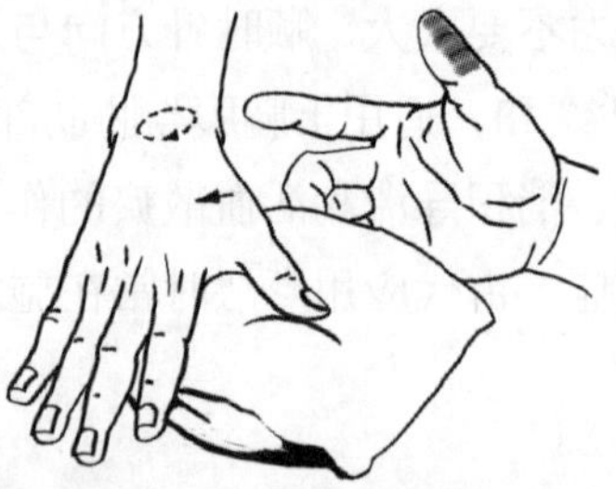

图 3－43　拇指桡侧揉（前摆）

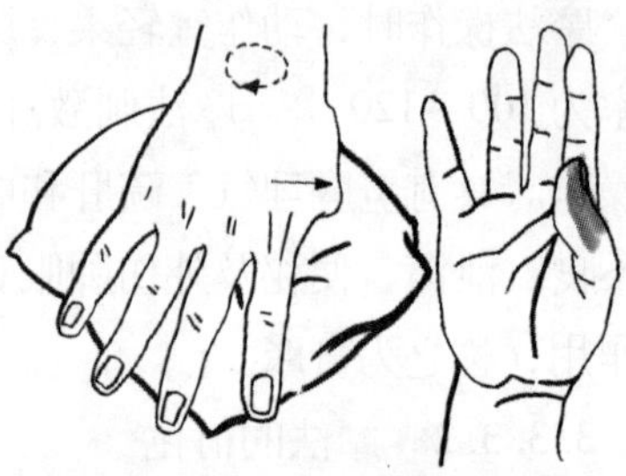

图 3－44　拇指桡侧揉（后摆）

揉法操作宜轻快柔和，压力不可过大，摆动频率为每分钟 120～160 次。揉法刺激轻柔缓和，其适用范围较广。指腹揉多用于小儿推拿，掌揉法常用于脘腹、胁肋、腰背等大面积平坦部位，大鱼际揉适用于头面部、胸胁部操作，拇指外侧揉适用于眼眶周围、肋间隙操作。具有宽胸理气、健脾和胃、活血化瘀、舒筋解痉、消肿定痛的作用，常用于治疗胸闷胁痛、脘腹胀满、泄泻、便秘、头痛眩晕、神衰失眠、口眼㖞斜、外伤肿痛等症。

2. 运法。

在指摩法的基础上，减轻向下的压力，使拇指或中指端轻触小儿穴位皮肤，然后做缓慢的环旋摩擦运动，称运法（图 3－45）。运法操作时，患者皮肤不变形，仅引起触觉；而摩按操作时，皮肤轻微凹陷、变形、有压觉。有时小儿推拿中把压力很轻的弧形推动亦称为运法。运法宜轻不宜重，宜缓不宜急，每分钟操作 60～80 次。运法适用于小儿手上穴位操作，如运八卦、运水入土等，其治疗作用根据穴位而定。

3. 旋推法。

在运法的基础上，略增加压力，减小环转运动幅度，加快操作频率，则称为旋推法（图 3－46）。旋推法适用于小儿推拿指端穴位操作，操作频率为每分钟 200～240 次，其治疗作用偏于补。

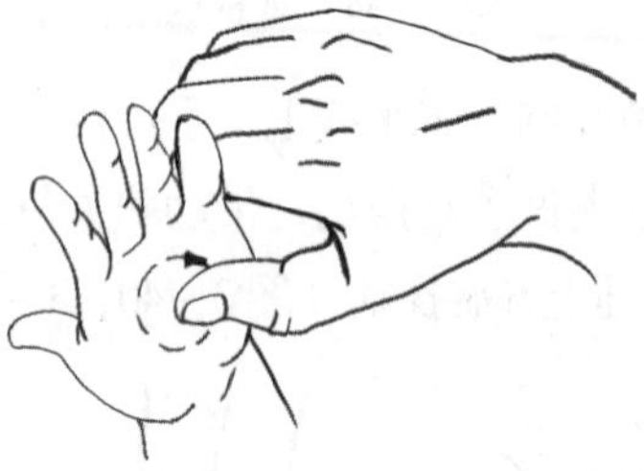

图 3－45　运法

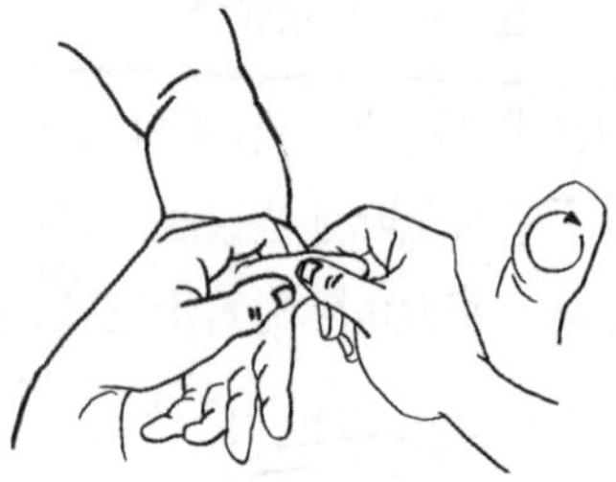

图 3－46　旋推法

3.3.3.3　复合手法：按揉法

在按法的基础上增加缓慢的环转揉动，或在揉法的基础上，增加向下按压的力量，为按揉法（图 3－47）。按揉法增加了对穴位的刺激性，但不增加患者疼痛程度，适用于穴位操作。

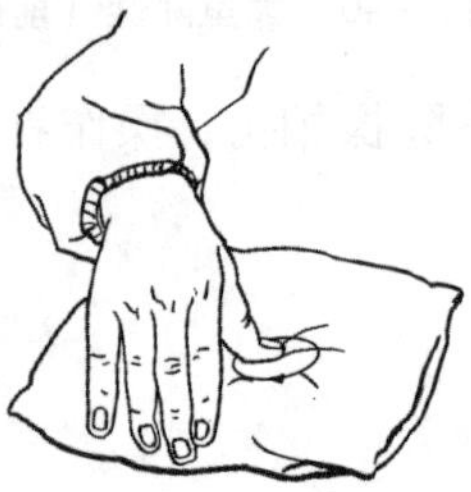

图 3－47　按揉法

[附] 摩揉法的操作练习

初学推拿手法者，在做摩法、揉法练习时，常觉动作生硬欠灵活。究其原因，一是未找到正确的操作方式，二是腕关节缺乏柔韧性。建议学习者做以下练习动作：

（1）两手十指交叉，然后做腕部扭转动作。每次练习1～2分钟，以增加腕关节柔韧性（图3－48）。

（2）腕关节放松，然后以前臂摆动，带动腕关节做侧向摆腕动作（图3－49）。这种侧向摆腕的前臂运动方式，就是摩揉法的前臂运动方式。只不过侧向摆腕时，手是游离的，其运动幅度大于腕部；当摩揉法操作指掌黏附于某一点后，腕部形成运动中心，自然就协调地摆动起来了。仔细体会一下侧向摆腕的前臂运动方式，然后按这一运动方式练习摩、揉法，将很快能掌握其操作方式。

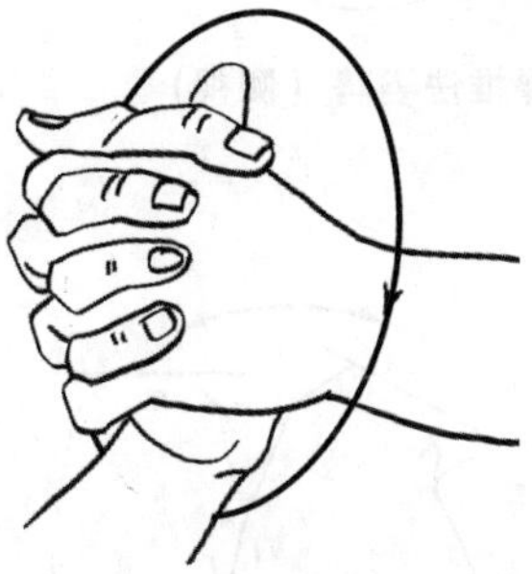

图3－48 扭腕练习

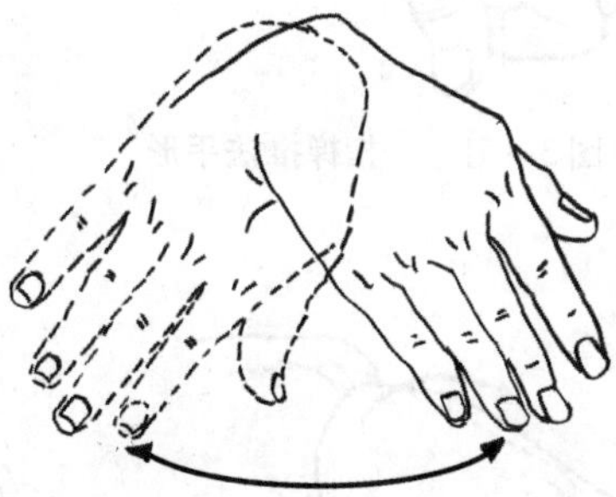

图3－49 摆腕练习

3.3.4 推擦类手法

所谓推擦类手法，是指以操作者的指端、手背与患者体表形成曲面接触，然后前臂主动摆动，带动腕关节（或拇指小关节）做屈伸运动，使接触部位来回滚动的一类操作。推擦类手法是中医推拿手法的特色和精华。

3.3.4.1 代表手法：一指禅推法

练习一指禅推法前，必须摆正姿势。端坐，含胸拔背；肩关节放松，肩胛骨自然下垂；上臂肌肉放松，肘部屈曲下垂，略低于腕部；腕关节放松，垂屈；四指自然屈曲，握成虚拳；拇指伸直，指端自然着力于一点，指掌侧遮盖拳眼，指间关节纹正好与食指桡侧缘相贴（图3－50，3－51，3－52）。

然后，操作者自我检查一下上肢除腕关节外，是否已经完全放松（初学者腕关节处可能有紧张感）。如感到某处僵硬不舒服，应随时调整之。只有在完全放松的基础上，才能做到动作灵活，操作持久，蓄力于掌，发力于指，刚柔相济，力透溪谷。否则，可能把动作练僵而不易纠正。

上肢完全放松后，再练习动作。先将肘关节略伸，前臂前摆旋后，腕部前移，带动拇指外展、伸直，虎口张开，以螺纹面接触米袋（图3－53）；随后，肘关节略屈，前臂回摆旋前，腕部后移，带动拇指内收、屈曲（也可不屈曲），以指端近指甲处接触米袋（图3－54）。把上述动作连续起来操作，不使其有瞬间停顿，就成为一指禅推法操作。操作中还应注意，前摆时前臂尺侧低于桡侧，回摆至极限时，前臂背面持平（图3－55）。

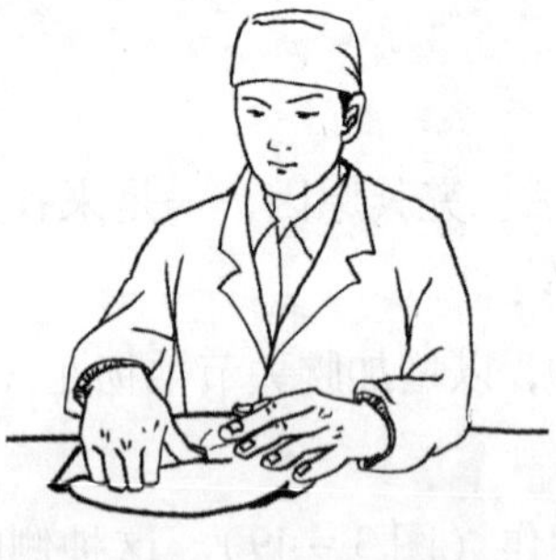

图3-50　一指禅推法姿势（前视）

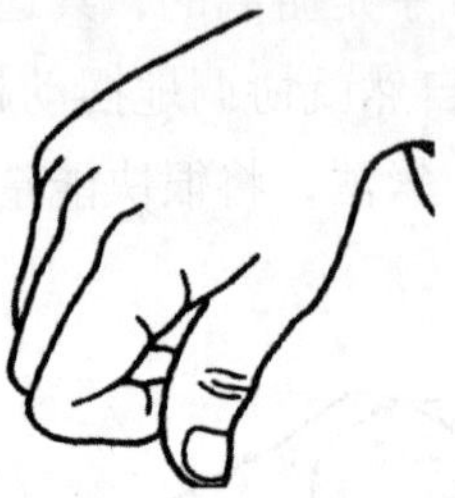

图3-51　一指禅推法手形

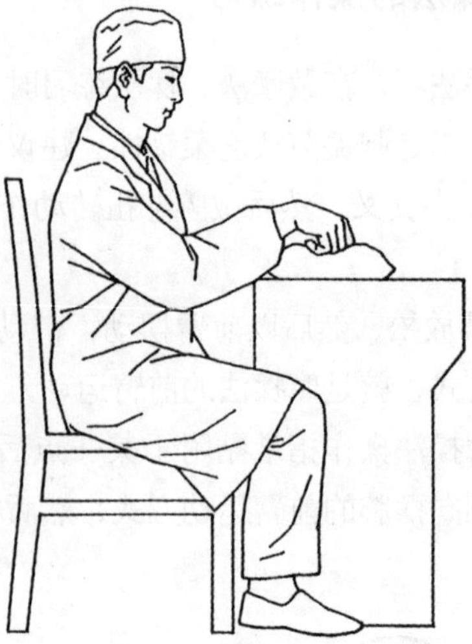

图3-52　一指禅推法姿势（侧视）

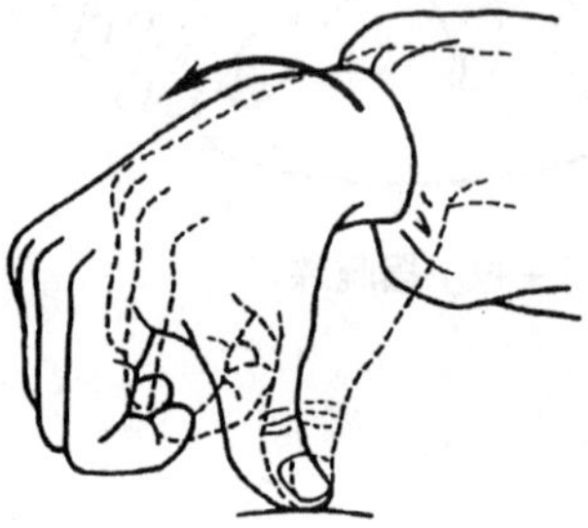

图3-53　一指禅推法前摆

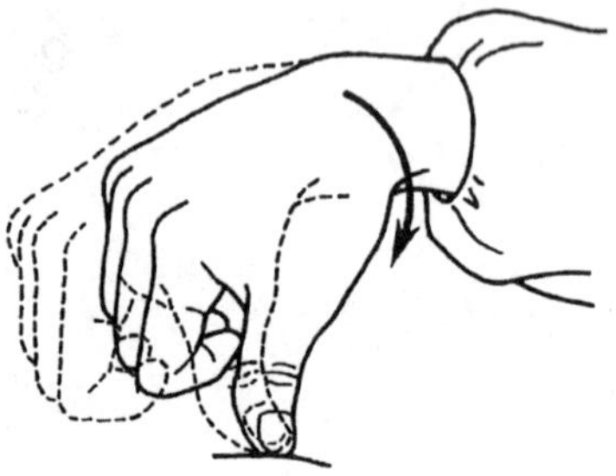

图3-54　一指禅推法回摆

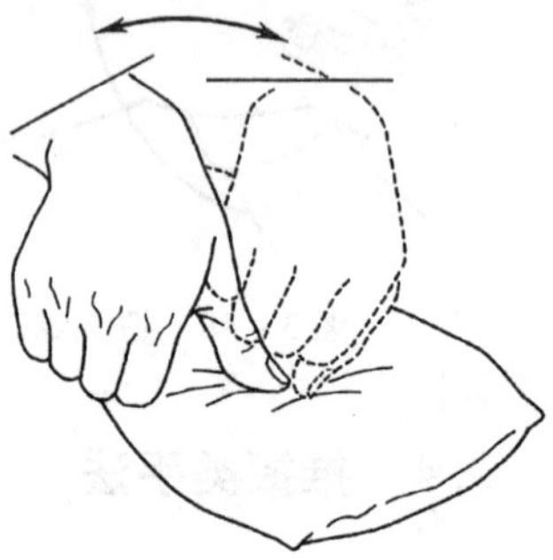

图3-55　前臂旋转幅度

一指禅推法操作时，要求动作协调灵活，压力均匀柔和，不可时轻时重、时快时慢。一指禅推法初练时，要求拇指指端吸定于一点，不能随着前后摆动而滑移。然后在吸定的基础上，再练习拇指沿一定路线移动的控制能力，要求其在操作过程中，能使指端随心所欲地沿着一定的路线（通常为经络路线）往返移动，做到紧推慢移。此外，操作时拇指端不可有意识地向下按压，操作频率为每分钟140～160次。

一指禅推法接触面小而柔软，对经络穴位发挥持续不断、柔和有力的刺激，适用于全身穴位、经络路线的操作。有舒筋通络、行气活血、调节内脏功能的作用，尤适宜于内科、妇科、儿科疾病的治疗，对头痛、失眠、口眼㖞斜、泄泻、便秘、月经不调有较好的治疗作用。

3.3.4.2　一指禅推法的衍化

由于人体各部位结构的不同，一指禅推法的这种标准操作方式在人体实际操作中，有时会感到困难。因此一指禅推拿流派在实际操作中，根据人体各部位结构的特点，创造了许多变法。常用的有：

1. 偏锋推。

在头面、胸胁部操作时，垂腕握拳方式可能造成手指与体表的撞击。故一指禅推法在头面部操作时，腕关节略屈曲，手指伸直，以拇指偏锋处着力于一定部位，做前后推动（图3-56）。实际上偏锋推的操作方与拇指桡侧揉法相近。头面部偏锋推的移动路线是有规律的。

2. 蝴蝶双飞。

风池穴为推拿治疗要穴。临床上以一指禅推法刺激风池穴时，通常以双手拇指操作，被形象地称为蝴蝶双飞（图3－56）。

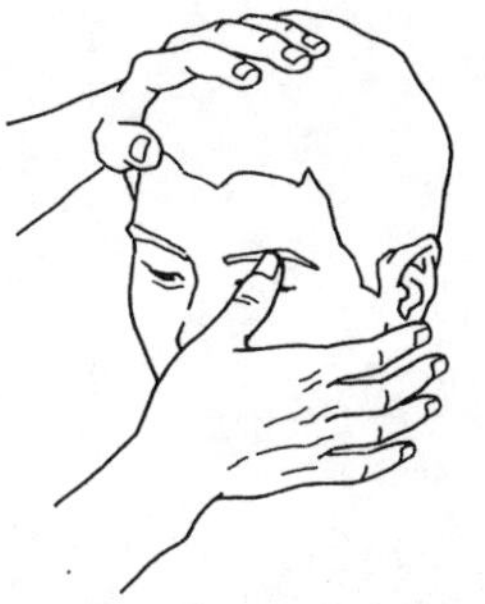

图3－56　偏锋推

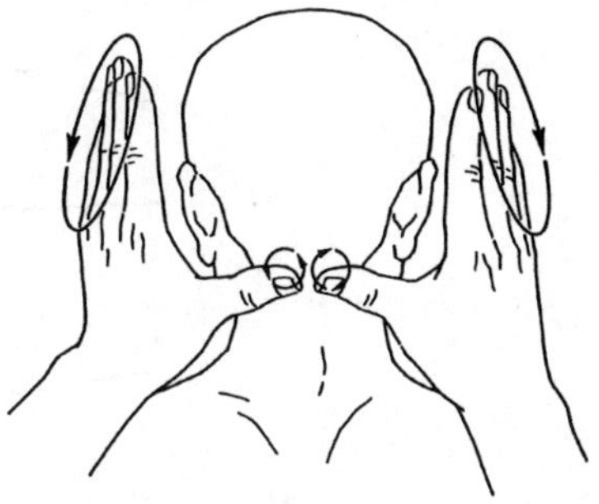

图3－57　蝴蝶双飞

3. 屈指推。

一指禅推法在项部操作时，不容易吸定。另外，颈椎病患者项肌强硬，压力较轻时，力量难以深透。将拇指屈曲，以拇指指间关节与指甲盖为着力面做一指禅推，称为屈指推（图3－58，3－59）。屈指推压力大，刺激强，吸定性好，适合于项枕部、关节骨缝处操作。

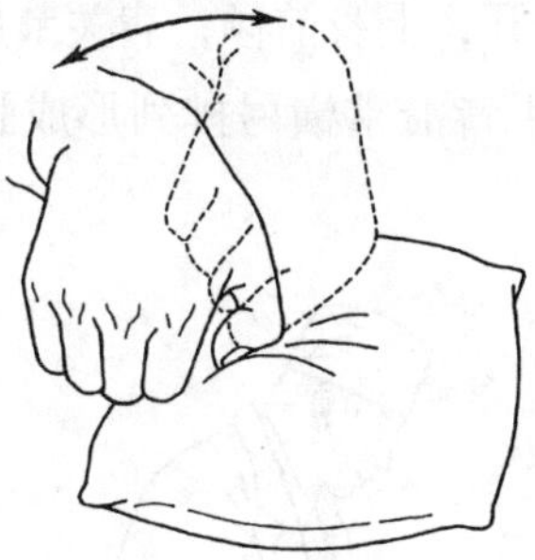

图3－58　屈指推

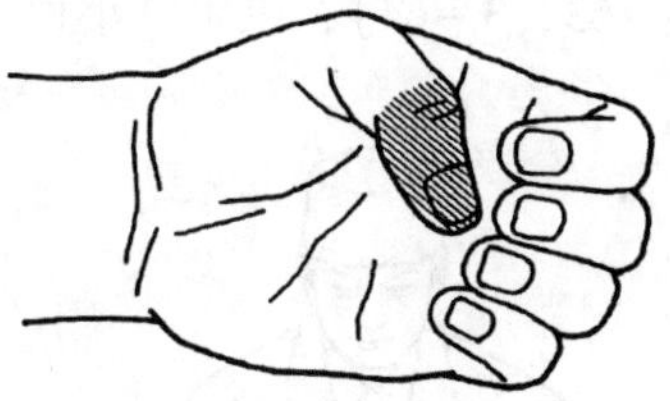

图3－59　屈指推接触面

4. 双手交叉扶持推。

四指伸直，虎口张开，以双手拇指指腹着力于患者颈椎对侧缘，四指则扶持于颈外侧，稳定操作，然后双手一起摆动，沿颈椎两侧推移。该法稳定性好，工作效率也高（图3－60）。

5. 单手扶持推。

在四肢关节处操作时，一般用单手扶持推（图3－61）。

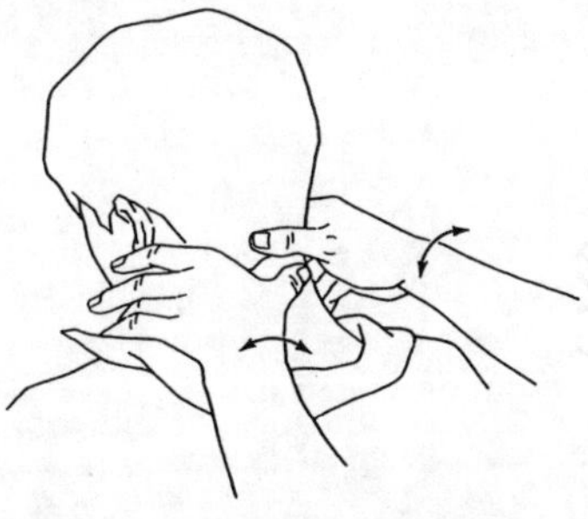

图3－60　双手交叉扶持推

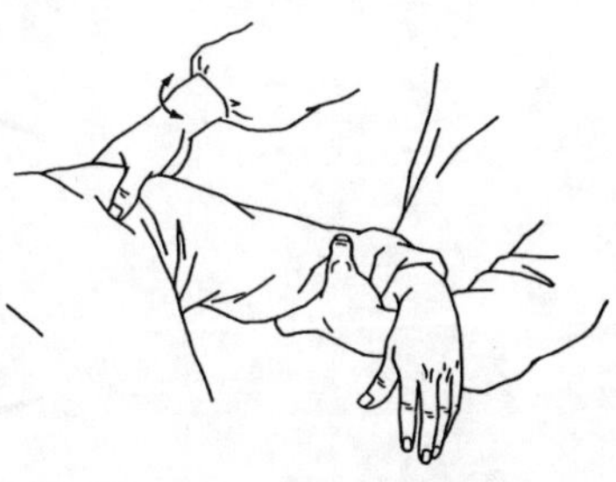

图3－61　单手扶持推

6. 推摩法。

推摩法是一指禅推法和摩法的复合操作，以拇指吸定于某穴，其余四指指腹在另外腹壁处做环旋摩动。推摩法适用于腹部（图3-62）。

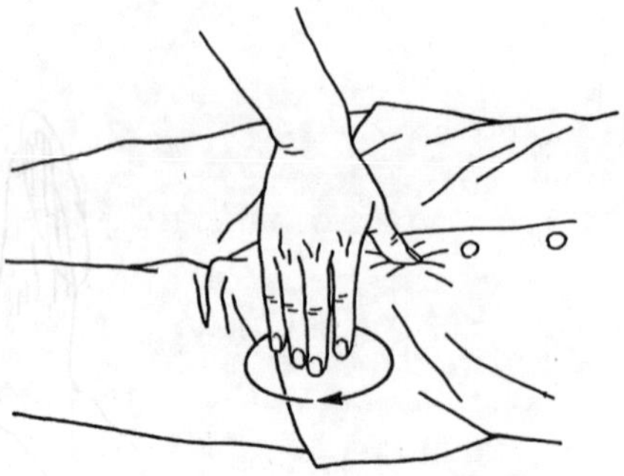

图3-62 推摩法

7. 缠法。

加快一指禅推法操作频率，使之每分钟超过200次，则称为缠法。缠法一般以偏锋着力，前后摆动的幅度亦较小，波动缓和而频率高。缠法对外科疮疡初起及外伤肿痛处有较好的消散作用。

3.3.4.3 代表手法：㨰法

㨰法操作练习前，应摆正姿势。操作者站立，两脚略前后分开，上身前倾；肩关节放松，肘关节屈曲呈140°，肘部距胸前壁为一拳左右；手指自然弯曲，手背沿掌横弓排列形成弧面（图3-62，3-63，3-64），以手掌小鱼际缘接触患者体表。

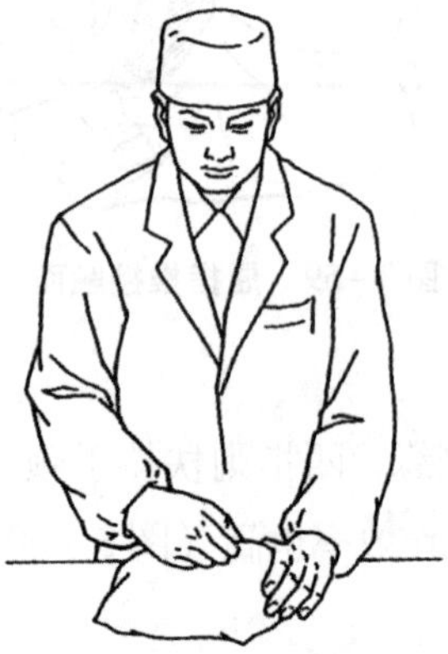

图3-63 㨰法姿势（前视）

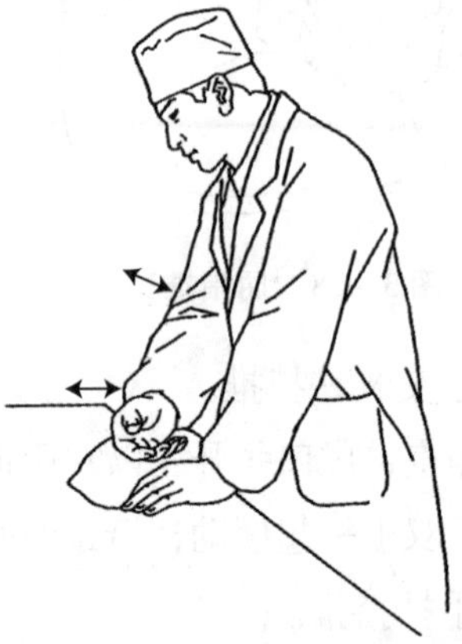

图3-64 㨰法姿势（侧视）

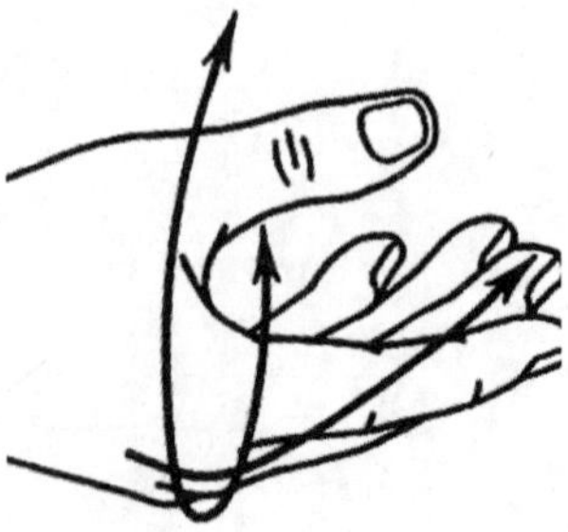

图3-65 手背弧面

在姿势正确的基础上，练习㨰法动作。先将肘关节略伸，前臂前摆旋后，腕关节逐渐掌屈前移，带动手背弧面向前方滚动，直至第二、三掌骨间隙接触患者体表（图3－66，3－67），紧接着，前臂后摆旋前，腕关节逐渐背伸后移，使手背弧面向后方滚动，直至以手尺侧缘接触体表（图3－68）。将上述操作连续起来，不使间断、停顿，就形成了轻重交替、持续不断的压力波动刺激（图3－69）。为了便于读者理解㨰法动作形式，以图3－70的机械模型说明。

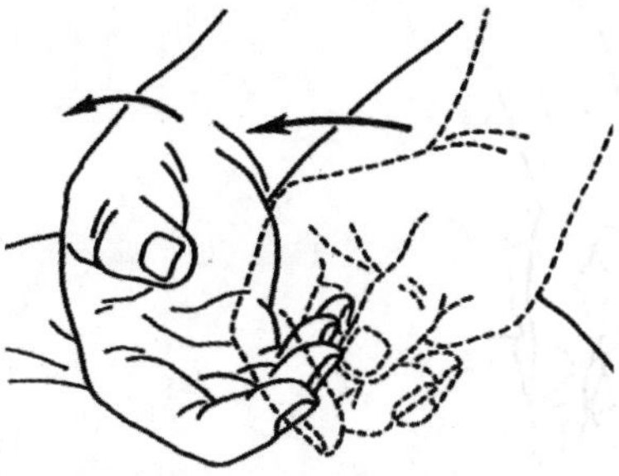

图3－66　前㨰运动

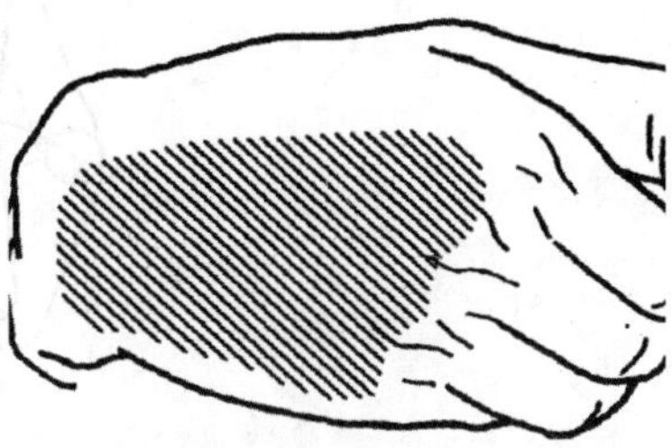

图3－67　前㨰时的接触面

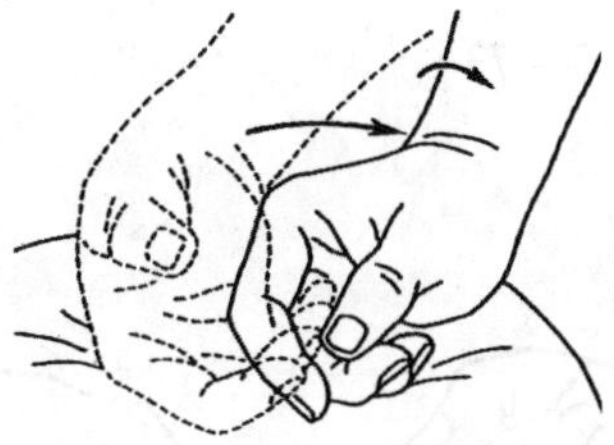

图3－68　㨰法回㨰时的接触面

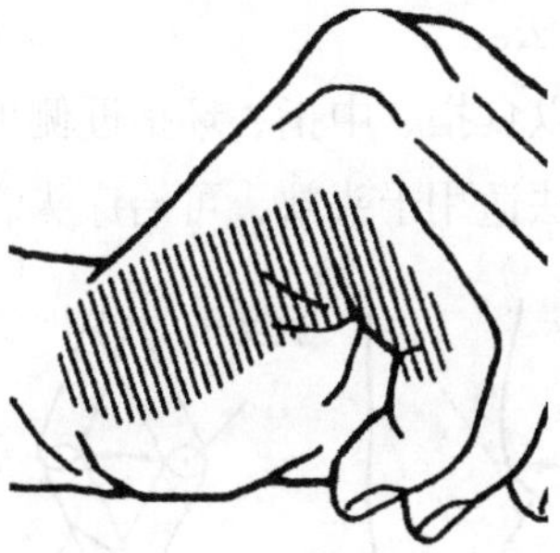

图3－69　㨰法回㨰运动

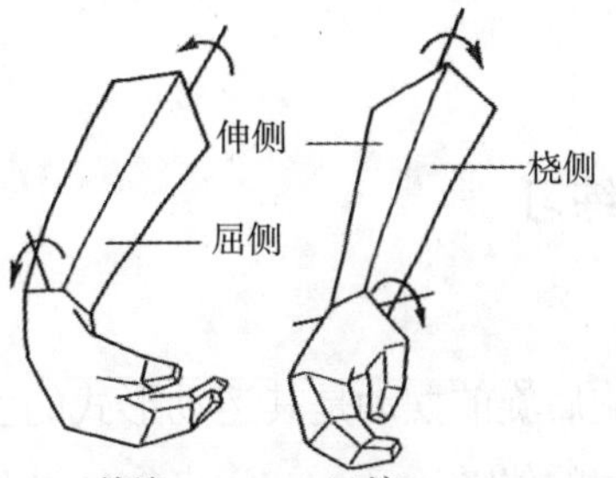

图3－70　㨰法操作机械模型

㨰法操作中，操作者手背弧面在患者体表形成滚动运动，若二者之间产生相对滑移（拖动）或手背相对体表而空转，都是不对的。㨰法操作过程中，要控制好腕关节的屈伸运动，不使腕关节出现折刀样的突变动作而造成跳动感。㨰法操作时也不可有意识地向下用力顶压，压力、频率、摆动幅度要均匀一致，动作协调而有节律性。

㨰法的压力大，接触面积也大，刺激刚柔相济，适用于颈项、肩背、腰臀、四肢大关节等肌肉丰厚部位。具有舒筋通络、滑利关节、增强肌肉韧带活动能力、促进血液循环及消除疲劳的作用，对软组织损伤、运动系统与神经系统疾病具有独特的疗效。

3.3.4.4 㨰法的衍化

1. 掌指关节㨰法。

㨰法以手背弧面与患者接触，刺激较为柔和舒适。在㨰法的推广应用过程中，一些操作者认为以掌指关节骨突形成接触，用腕关节单纯伸屈运动代替腕关节屈伸与前臂旋转的复合运动，能获得更大压力和刺激强度。图3－71为掌指关节㨰法，适用于对腰背肌僵硬、感觉迟钝者的治疗。

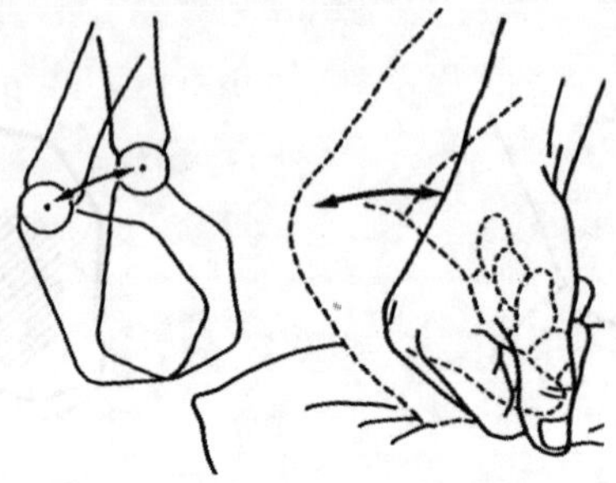

图3－71 掌指关节㨰法

2. 㨰法。

㨰法以食指、中指、环指近侧指间关节骨突形成接触，通过腕关节屈伸运动使指间关节前后滚动。㨰法适用于头部，可治疗头痛、失眠等症（图3－72，3－73）。

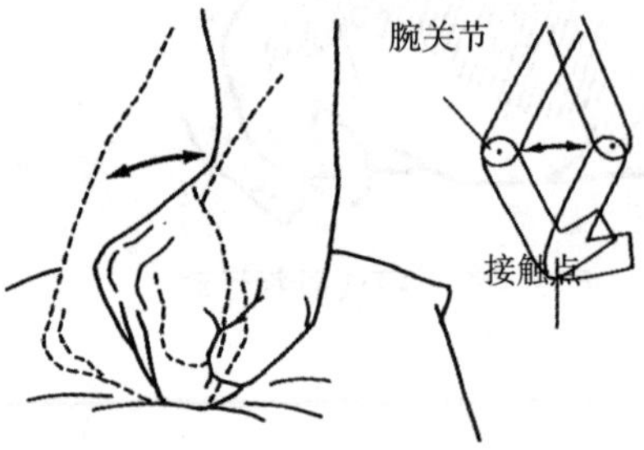

图3－72 㨰法

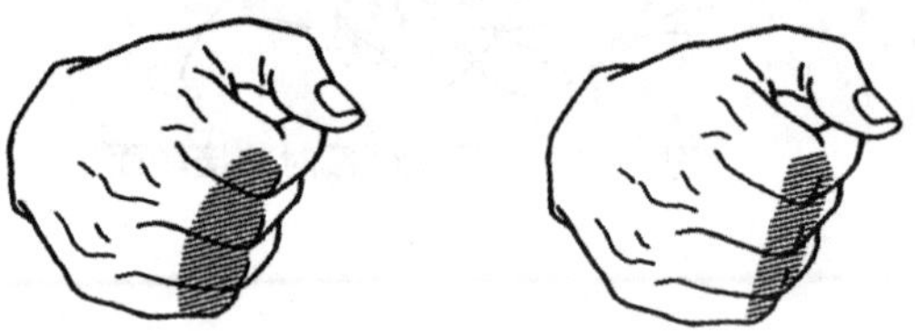

图3－73 㨰法接触面

［附］一指禅推法与㨰法练习

1. 一指禅推法练习。

一指禅推法操作中，前臂的旋后旋前摆动是其运动形式的主要方面，而拇指的运动则是由前臂摆动、腕部空间位置变化而引起的伴随运动。初学者往往过分重视拇指运动，甚至有意识地屈伸拇指，不但会引起大鱼际酸痛，而且易把手法练僵。因此，初学者在学习一指禅推法过程中，建议分两个阶段走。第一阶段，操作者主要练习正确的前臂摆动运动，不考虑拇指伴随摆动。可令操作者拇指与食指相贴，虎口闭拢，练习前臂摆动（图3－74）。第二阶段，在前臂摆动协调、熟练的基础上，再将虎口放松，使拇指与食指在前臂摆动过程中自然出现开合动作。

2. 㨰法练习。

㨰法操作中，腕关节的屈伸运动是其运动形式的主要方面。在初学者操作错误中，以腕关节屈伸运动不够占大多数，而前臂旋转运动大多存在。因此在学习㨰法过程中，笔者也建议分两步走。第一步，先练习腕关节屈伸运动，可令操作者一手轻握另一手的手指，使其位置相对固定；然后将腕关节前摆，掌屈至极限位，再使腕关节后摆，背伸至40°左右；连续以上操作，勿中断。

此阶段并不形成滚动，而是手小鱼际缘的摩擦滑动（图 3－75）。第二步，在腕关节屈伸摆动熟练、协调的基础上，解除对手指的固定，注意使手背接触部位随前后摆动不断改变，将摩擦运动改为滚动，就自然形成了腕屈伸与前臂旋转的复合。

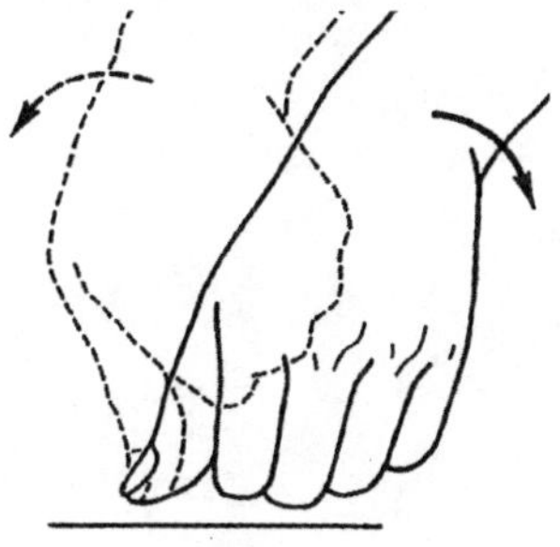

图 3－74　一指禅推法第一阶段学习

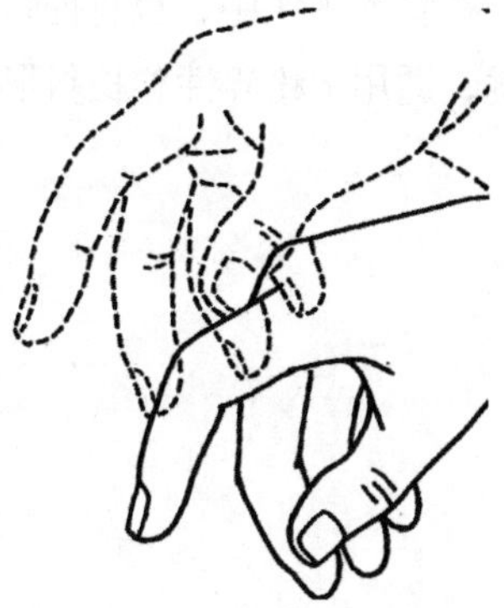

图 3－75　㨰法第一阶段练习

3.3.5　捏拿类手法

所谓捏拿类手法是指以操作者的指、掌从皮肤对称的位置向深部挤压的一类操作。

3.3.5.1　代表手法：捏法

以拇指与其他手指相对，将患者皮肤及少量皮下组织捏起，称捏法。捏法常用于小儿脊柱两侧操作，有两种操作方式。

1. 拇食指捏。

患儿俯卧，使背部肌肉松弛。操作者将两手食指屈曲，以食指中节背面紧触脊柱两侧皮肤，拇指前按皮肤后向后捏起，随捏随提，两手交替向前推进，自龟尾至大椎处（图 3－76，3－77）。

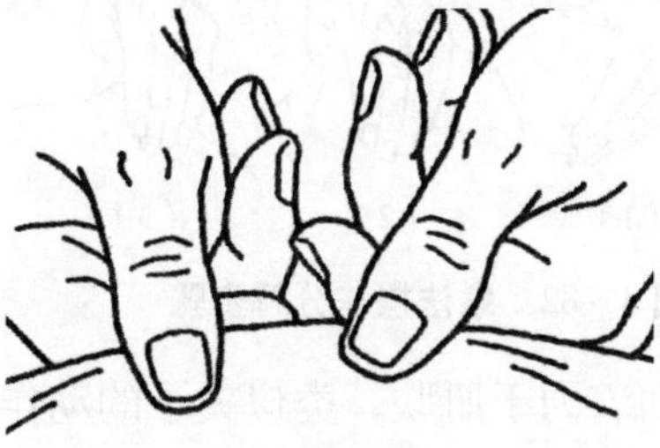

图 3－76　拇食指捏

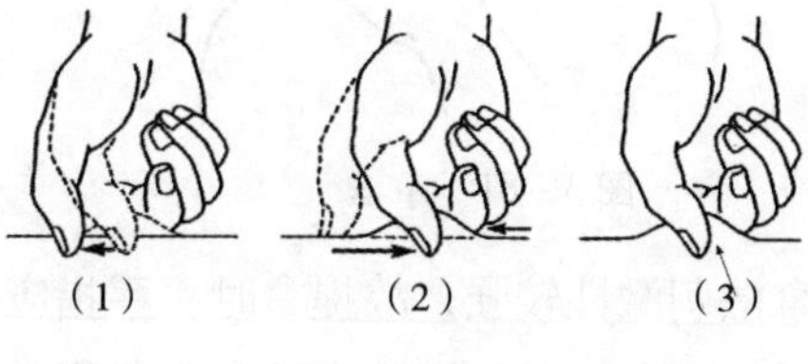

图 3－77　拇食指捏操作分解步骤

2. 拇食中指捏。

患儿体位同上。操作者将两手拇指桡侧偏锋紧触脊柱两侧皮肤，食中指前按皮肤后相对捏起。随捏随提，两手交替前进（图 3－78，3－79）。

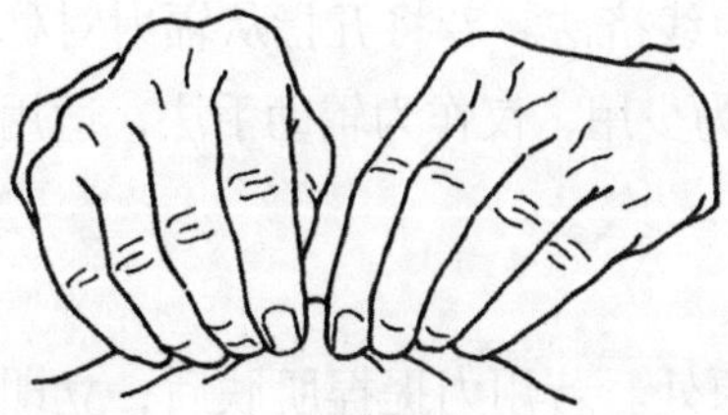

图 3－78　拇食中指捏

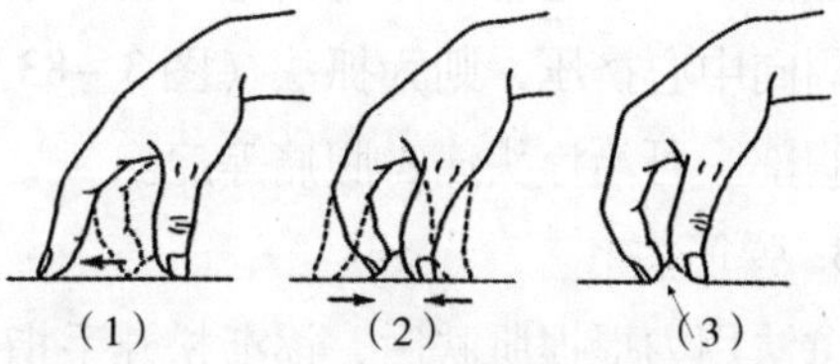

图 3－79　拇食中指捏操作分解步骤

捏脊法临床应用范围较广，在小儿推拿中尤为常用。一般认为捏脊法偏于补益，具有调和阴阳、健脾和胃、增强人体抗病能力的作用，常用于治疗小儿疳积、消化不良、腹泻呕吐、体弱多病等病症，也可治疗成人消化道疾患、月经不调、痛经、失眠等症。

此外，在骨科手法中，也有捏骨法（图3－80），是指操作者以两手掌相对挤压，使骨折碎片向纵轴线靠拢，适用于粉碎性和长斜形骨折、长螺旋形骨折的整复对位。是为同名异法，应分清。

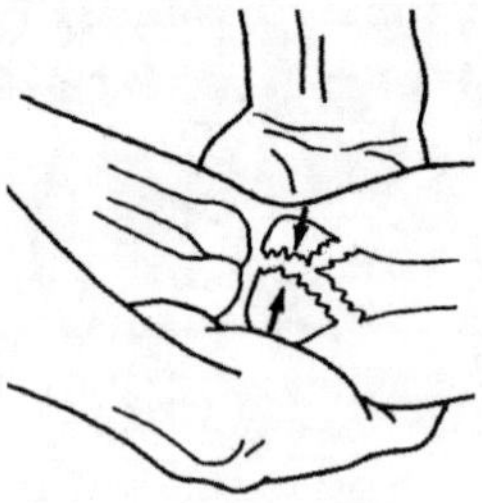

图3－80　捏骨法

3.3.5.2　捏法的衍化

1. 拿法。

拿法与捏法操作非常相似，在命名上也随个人的习惯称呼之，概念不十分清楚。一般而言，捏法是指捏拿皮肤及少量皮下组织的操作。在捏法的基础上，增加捏拿组织的体积和力量，将肌肉连同皮肤、皮下组织一起捏起上提，再让肌肤逐渐从手指间滑出，则为拿法（图3－81，3－82）。

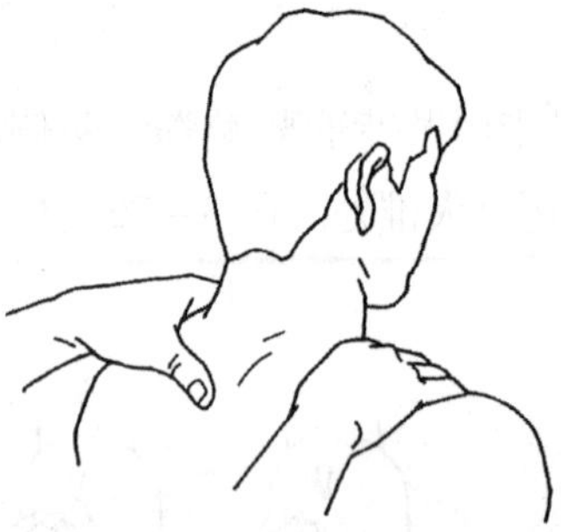

图3－81　拿法

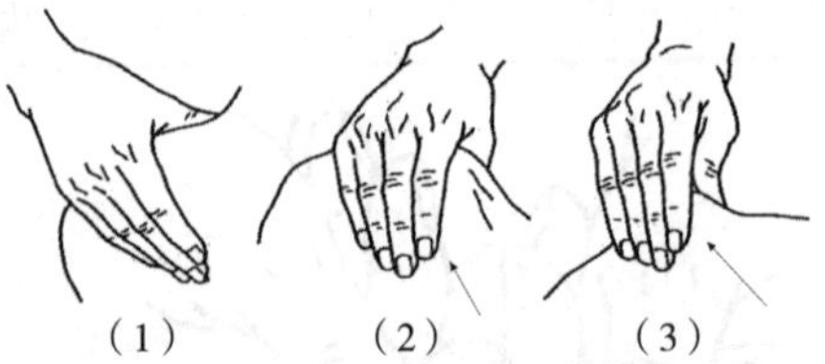

图3－82　拿法操作分解步骤

拿法刺激性较强，故提拿时，手指应伸直，以平坦的指面着力于肌肤，类似夹子的动作。不可将手指屈曲，以尖锐的指端着力，形成钳子样的动作，以免患者感觉不舒适。

拿法操作时，腕部放松，捏拿动作连绵不断，用力由轻到重，由重到轻。拿法适用于颈项、肩部和四肢肌肉丰厚处，具有疏通经络、放松肌肉、解表发汗、止痛活血的作用，可用于治疗头痛项强、关节痹痛、肌肉酸胀、感冒等症。

2. 抓法。

捏法、拿法是将拇指与其他手指从轴对称位置自两侧向中线挤法。若将五指从辐射对称位置自四周向中心挤压，则为抓法（图3－83）。抓法在临床上较为少用，仅作为辅助手法，适用于头部、腹部。可治疗头痛、腹痛等症。

3. 弹筋法。

拿法用力提捏肌肤后，逐渐松开手指，让肌肤慢慢滑回原处。若用力提捏肌肤后，立即松开手指，使紧张的肌肤迅速弹回原处，则称为弹筋法（图3－84）。弹筋法有剥离粘连、解除肌肉痉挛的作用，适用于肌腹、肌腱部位。

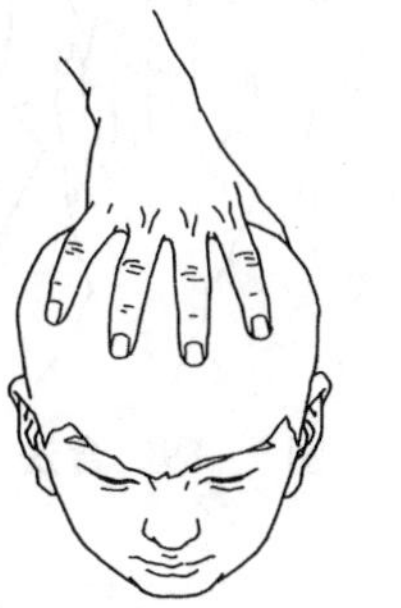

图 3－83　抓法

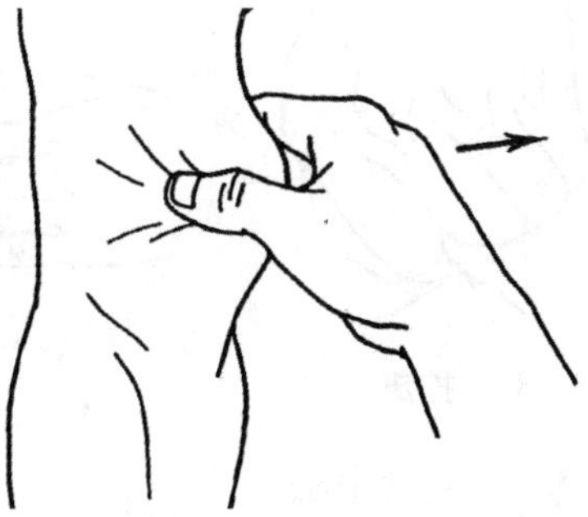

图 3－84　弹筋法

4. 挤法。

捏法挤压皮肤、皮下组织的力量很轻，一般以不引起痛苦为限，且捏挤的部位不断移动。若拇、食二指相对挤捏的力量很重，且重复在同一部位操作，直至皮下血管破裂，出现瘀血，则称为挤法，又称为挤痧（图 3－85）。

5. 扯法。

在挤法的基础上再增加上提皮肤的操作，直至皮下瘀血，则称扯法，或称扯痧（图 3－86）。

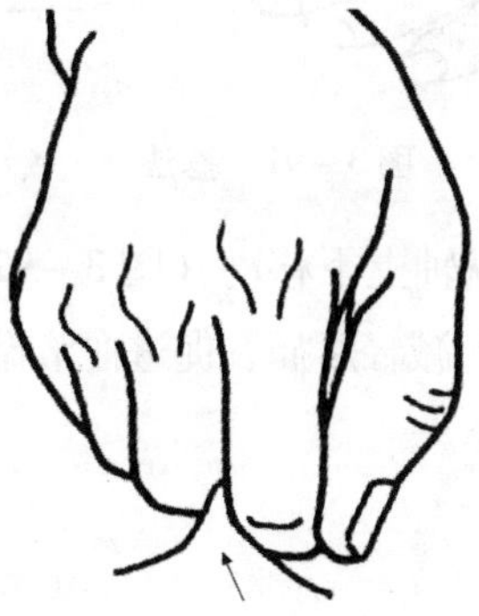

图 3－85　挤法

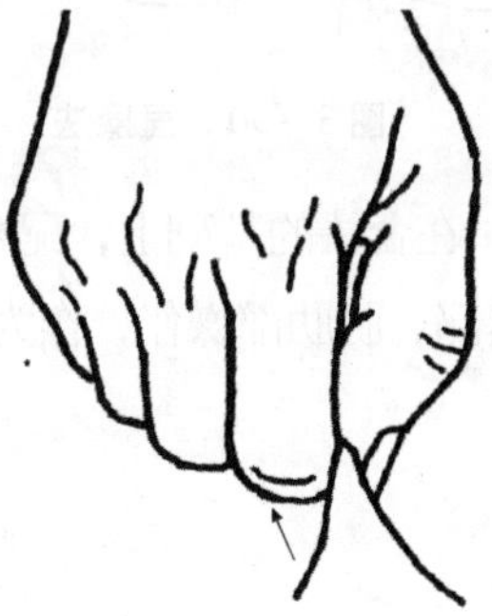

图 3－86　扯法

6. 拧法。

拧法，又称扭法。以弯曲的食、中指近侧指间关节处捏起皮肤后，左右扭转，使皮下瘀血，亦称拧痧、扭痧（图 3－87）。挤、扯、拧、扭法都是民间治疗痧证的一些手法，常在额面部、鼻梁、颈项部、胸部、脊椎两侧、肘窝、腘窝处操作，具有开通气机、发散病邪、开窍醒神的作用，对许多内科急症都有很好的疗效。

7. 挪法。

手掌平置于腹部，然后如握拳状将腹壁抓紧提起片刻，再松开手掌稍向前移，再抓提腹壁，不断地前移，直至整个腹部操作一遍（图 3－88）。本法刺激强烈，常用于小儿蛔虫性肠梗阻、肠粘连等症的治疗。

8. 合法。

两手掌对置关节对称位置，同时向关节纵轴相对挤压合拢，称合法或归合法。合法为理筋手法，常用于关节软组织损伤，如下尺桡关节分离者的治疗（图 3－89）。

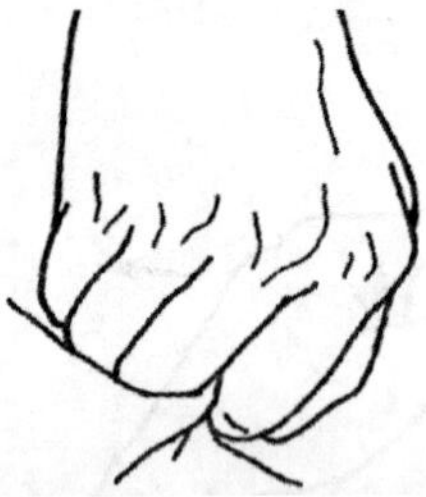

图 3－87　拧法

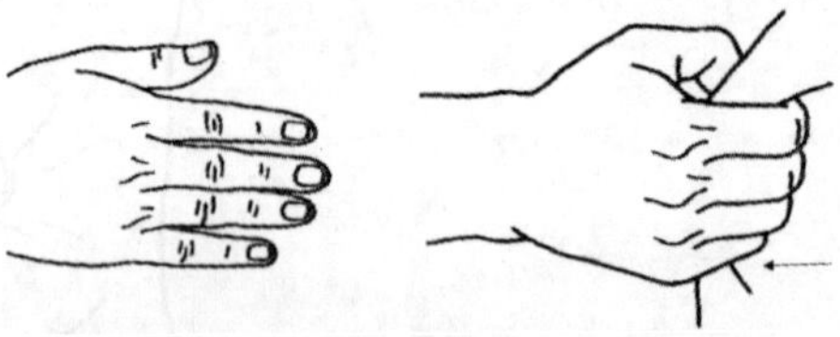

图 3－88　挪法

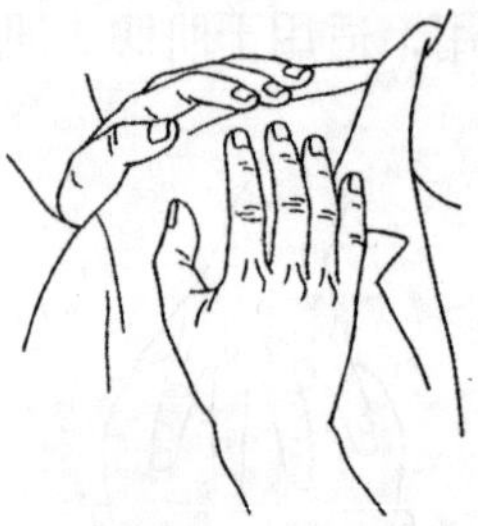

图 3－89　合法

3.3.5.3　复合手法

1. 捏揉法，又叫拿揉法。在揉法、拿法基础上，配合手指的揉捻动作（图 3－90）。

2. 捻法：在捏手指、足趾时，配合揉捻动作和指间关节、掌指关节的扭转运动（图 3－90）。捻法用于治疗指、趾疼痛，指间关节扭伤。

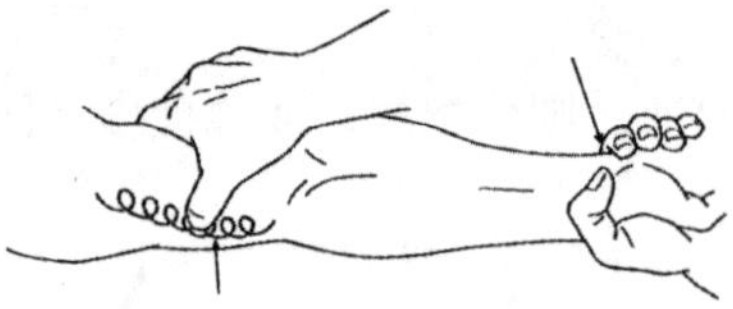

图 3－90　捏揉法

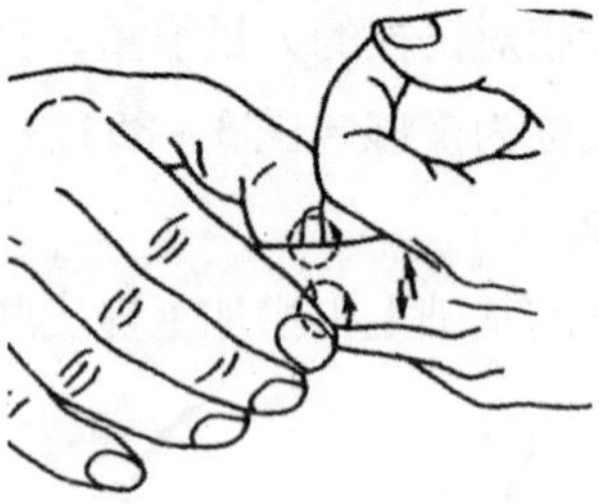

图 3－91　捻法

3. 搓法：在合法的基础上，配合手掌环转揉动，并沿肢体纵轴上下移动（图 3－92）。搓法常用于四肢、腰部、胁肋部操作，作为结束手法使用，有放松肌肉、减轻疼痛、促进血液循环的作用。

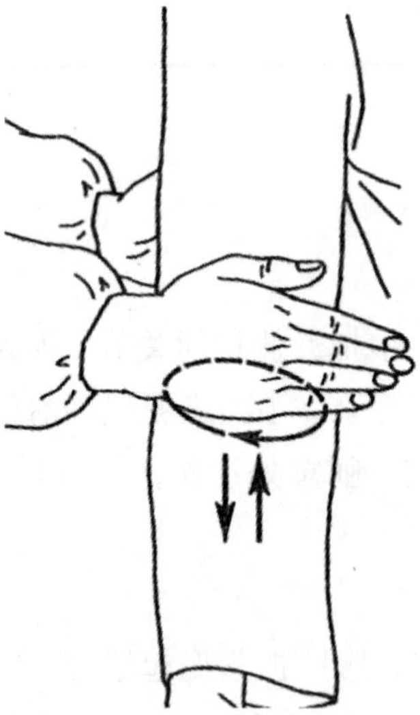

图 3－92　搓法

3.3.6　振动类手法

所谓振动类手法是指以指、掌轻触患者体表后，通过肌肉快速、小幅度运动产生较高频率的震颤，并将震颤波动传递给患者肌肤的一类操作。

3.3.6.1　代表手法：振法

振法根据操作者接触部位的不同而分为掌振法和指振法两种，但其姿势、操作方式基本相似。操作者肩关节外展30°左右，肘关节屈曲约140°。

1. 指振法。

垂腕，手指自然伸直，以食、中两指指端轻触患者一定穴位（图3－93）。

2. 掌振法。

腕关节略背伸，手指自然伸直，以手掌面轻按于患者体表某部位（图3－94）。

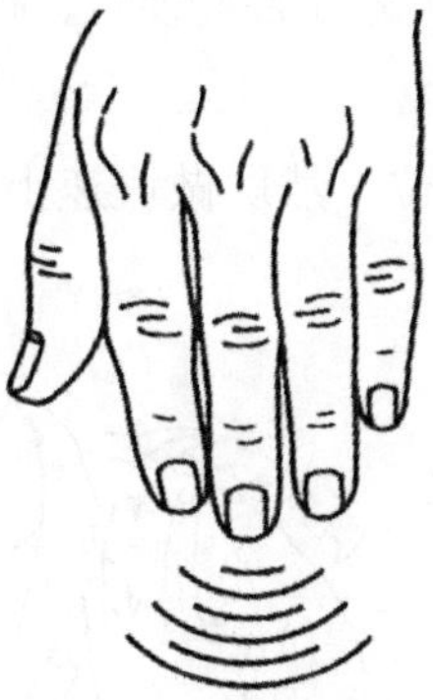

图3－93　指振法

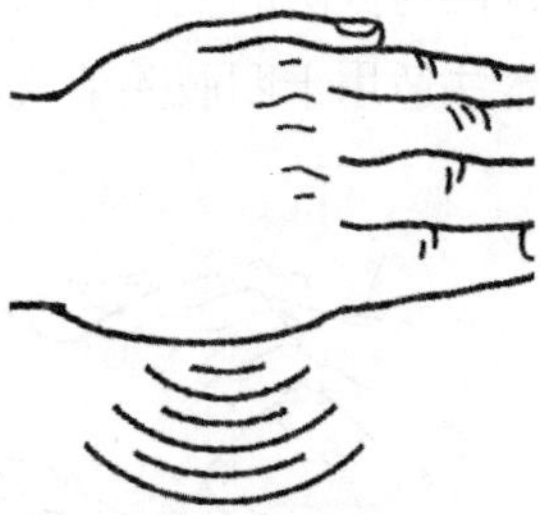

图3－94　掌振法

然后，操作者可用两种不同的运动方式产生高频振动。第一种为痉挛性肌震颤方式，前臂和手部肌强烈地做静止性收缩，产生振颤动作，振动频率可达每分钟600～800次。本法容易学习，但由于肌肉持续痉挛，影响本身血液循环，易疲劳。第二种为交替性肌收缩振动，操作者肌肉放松，前臂屈肌和伸肌做快速交替性收缩，但不产生明显的手部运动，而是产生细微振动，振动频率一般为每分钟300～400次。本法掌握困难，但由于肌肉交替地收缩、舒张，血液循环不受影响，不易疲劳。

振法操作的能量消耗较大，应保持自然呼吸，切忌憋气，以免影响操作者自身健康。也可在操作时将意念集中于操作部位上，即所谓“运气推拿”。本法可使局部产生温热舒适感，多用于脘腹胀痛、消化不良、中气下陷等症的辅助治疗，具有健脾消积、调节胃肠蠕动的疗效。

3.3.6.2　振法的衍化：摆法

振法所产生的振动是上下波动，若改变振动的方向，使波动向周围传导，则称为摆法。摆法操作时，以手尺侧缘置患者体表，腕关节放松，然后做快速小幅度的摆腕动作，带动体表组织产生高频振动（图3－95）。摆法适用于胸腹、腰背和四肢部位，具有放松肌肉、调和脾胃、促进血液循环、缓急止痛的作用，可用于治疗消化不良、肌肉痉挛、局部肿痛等症。

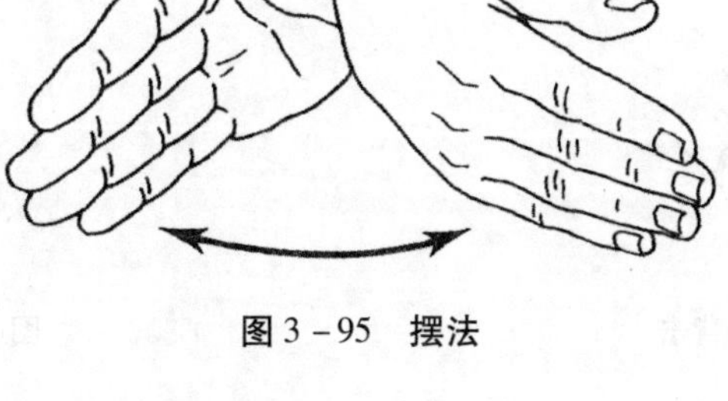

图3－95　摆法

3.3.6.3　复合手法

1. 提颤法。

本法为捏拿与振动的复合手法。手指分开呈半屈状态，以拇指与食指、中指轻轻捏提肌肤后，腕、指做快速颤抖动作，两手交替操作（图3－96）。提颤法具有放松肌肉、活血化瘀、止痛、分离粘连的作用，适用于颈项、四肢及腹部。

2. 荡法。

在提颤法的基础上，增大左右上下颤动的运动幅度，降低颤抖频率，则称为荡法（图3－97）。本法仅用于腹部，具有消积利气、分离粘连的作用，可用于治疗小儿蛔虫性肠梗阻、肠粘连等症。

3. 对掌振法。

本法为合法与振法的复合手法。两手掌分置于关节的对称部位，然后做快速上下（或左右）振颤动作。本法适用于四肢关节（图3－98）。

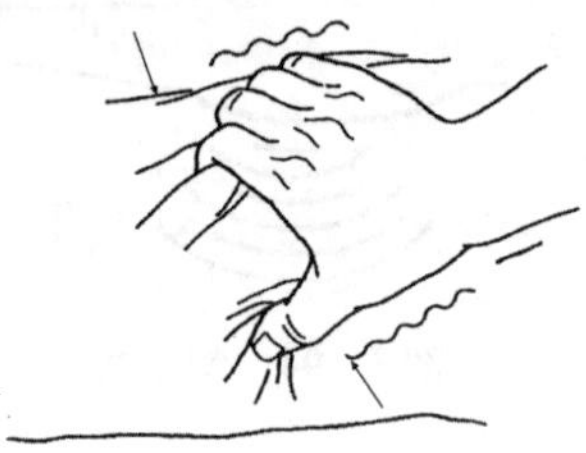

图3－96　提颤法

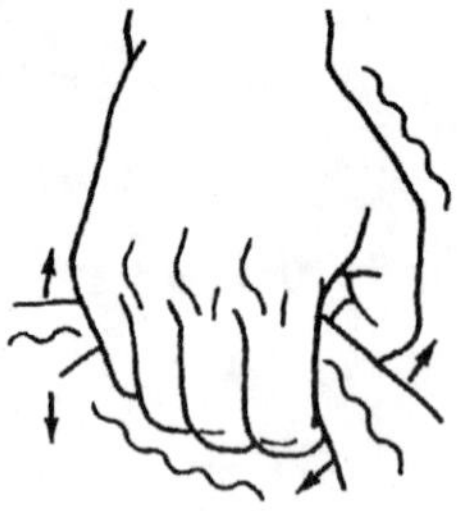

图3－97　荡法

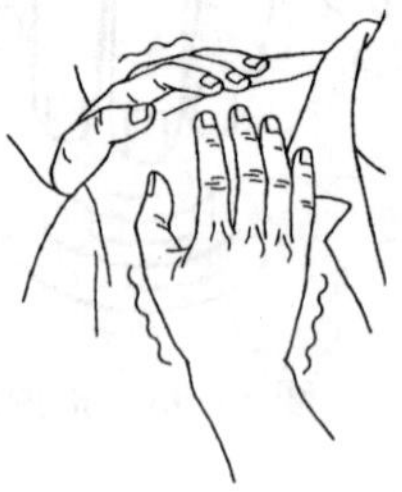

图3－98　对掌振法

3.3.7　叩击类手法

所谓叩击类手法是指以指、掌、拳或器具对患者体表进行有节律的、间断的击打的一类操作。

3.3.7.1　代表手法：击法

以较重的力量单次或多次击打某一体表部位，使击打力量作用到肌肉、骨骼等深部组织，称击法。击法可用拳、掌，也可用特制的棒（桑枝棒），故击法有以下不同操作方式：

1. 拳背击。

手握空拳，腕关节伸直，以肘部发力，使拳背有节律地反复击打某一部位；或边击打，边移动作用部位（图3－99）。拳背击适用于肩背部。

2. 捶击。

手握空拳，腕关节放松，以肘部发力，将两拳尺侧缘交替捶击某一部位，捶击法用力一般要比拳背击法轻（图3－100）。捶击法适用于肩背、四肢部位。

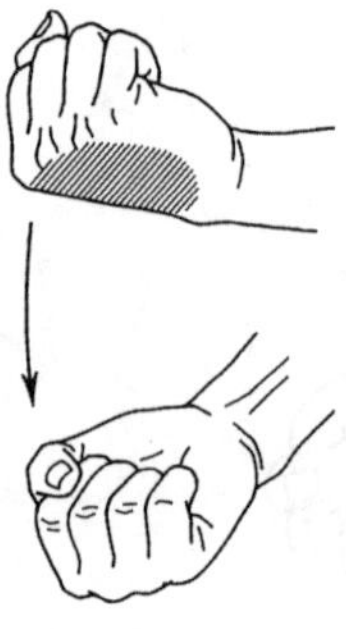

图3－99　拳背击

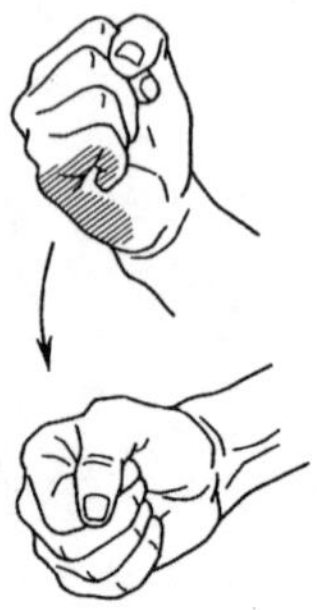

图3－100　捶击

3. 掌根击。

手指微屈，腕关节背伸至极限位，然后以肩关节发力，将掌根部反复击打某一部位；或边击打，边移动击打部位（图 3－101）。掌根击适用于臀部及大腿肌肉丰厚处。

4. 掌侧击。

手指伸直，腕关节放松，然后以腕关节发力，用手掌尺侧缘反复击打某一部位（图 3－102）。本法形如刀劈，故又称劈法，用于肩背、四肢关节及指（趾）缝处。

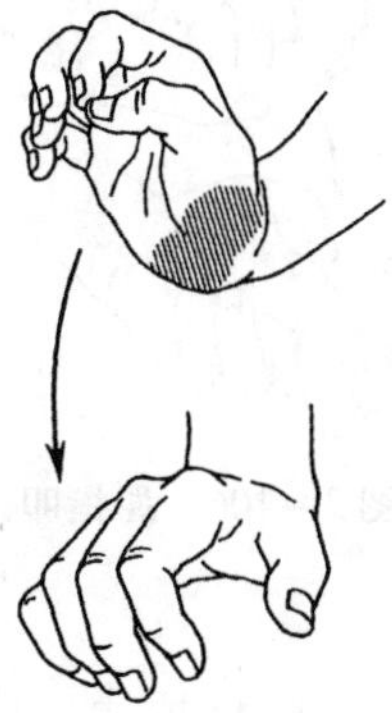

图 3－101　掌根击

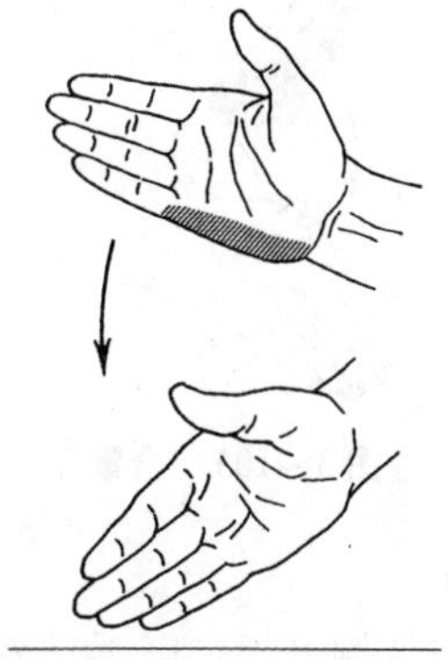

图 3－102　掌侧击

5. 棒击。

手握桑枝棒（略有弹性）的一端，腕关节放松，然后视需要，以肘关节发力（力量较轻）或肩关节发力（力量较大），用棒身连续在某一部位击打 3～5 下（图 3－103），再移动击打部位。棒击时，力量要由轻而重，适可而止；击打的方向应与肌肉、骨骼平行，棒身接触部位应尽可能大，不要用棒尖打，也不要打出头棒（图 3－104）。

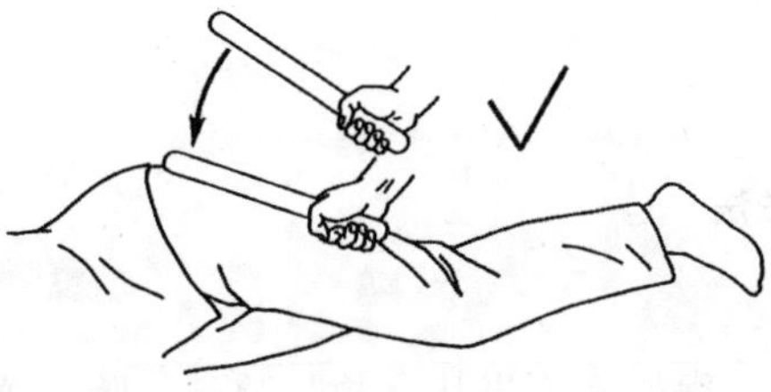

图 3－103　棒击（正确）

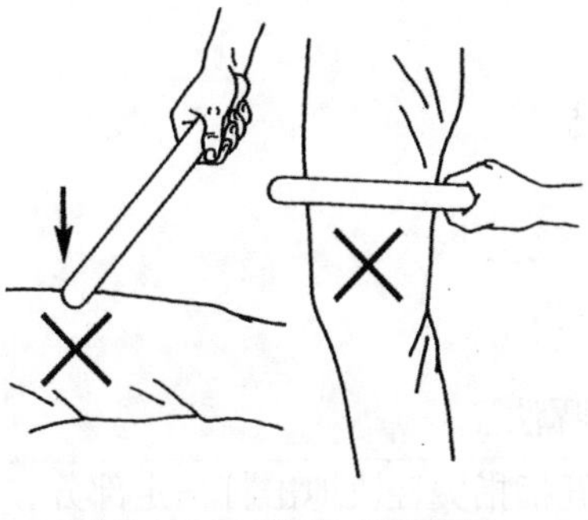

图 3－104　棒击（不正确）

击法力量较大，击打过程中不能有拖拉现象；击打过程要短促，一触即弹起，避免造成组织损伤。击法的操作频率为每分钟 45～80 次。

击法适用于肌肉丰厚处。具有开窍醒神、活血和通络的作用。治疗头目眩晕、肢体顽麻等症，也可用于体育比赛前运动员精神状态的调整。

3.3.7.2　击法的衍化

1. 叩法。

在击法的基础上减轻击打力量，使其作用传达于皮下组织、肌肉；并加快击打频率，使之达到每分钟 80～100 次，则称为叩法。有以下操作变化：

（1）合掌叩：两手手指伸直、并拢、相合，然后以掌尺侧缘快速击打某一部位（图 3－105）。

合掌叩适用于肩背、胸胁部位。

（2）屈指叩：手指半屈曲，以食指、中指近侧指间关节背面轻快地叩击某一部位（图3－106）。屈指叩适用于小儿推拿。

叩法操作轻快，具有舒松筋脉、促进血液循环、消除疲劳、镇静安神的作用，常用于精神紧张、失眠的治疗及体育比赛后的恢复。

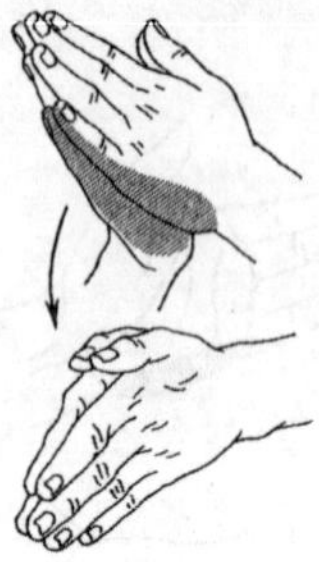

图3－105　合掌叩

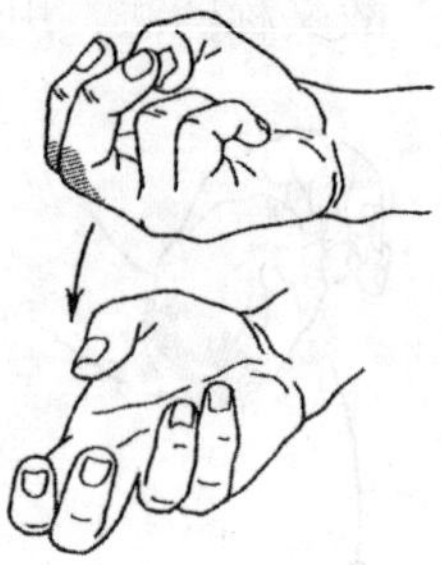

图3－106　屈指叩

2. 拍法。

掌根击与掌侧击都是以手掌着实地击打，若以虚掌轻快地击打，则称拍法。其法为：五指并拢，掌心凹陷成虚掌，腕关节放松；然后以腕关节力量，轻快地击打体表（图3－107）。拍法常用于肩背、腰骶及四肢关节处，且有舒松筋脉、促进血液循环的作用。

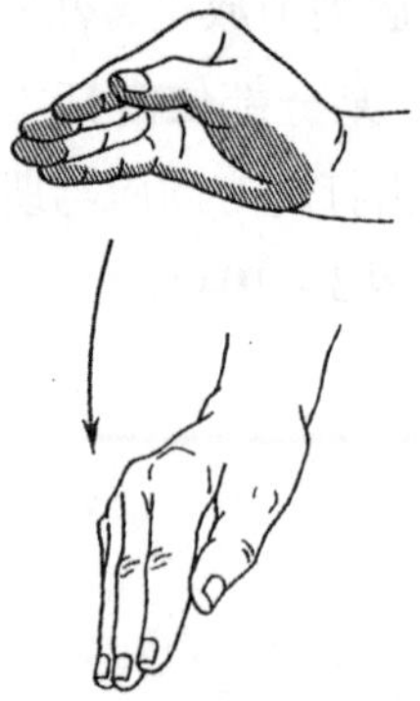

图3－107　拍法

3. 啄法。

以五指指尖轻快地击打一定部分，两手交替操作，犹如鸡啄米状，故称啄法。啄法操作既可手指分开如爪状（图3－108），也可互相聚拢成梅花状（图3－109）。啄法适用于头面部，有安神醒脑的作用，用于头痛、失眠的治疗。

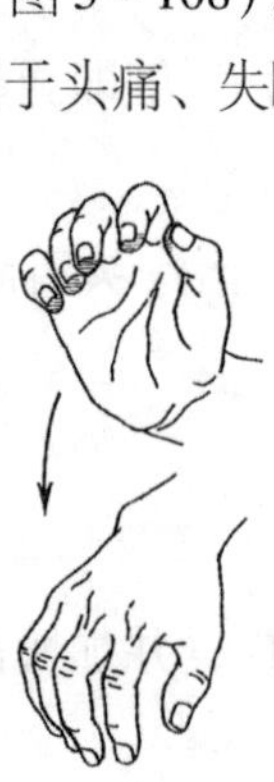

图3－108　啄法（爪状）

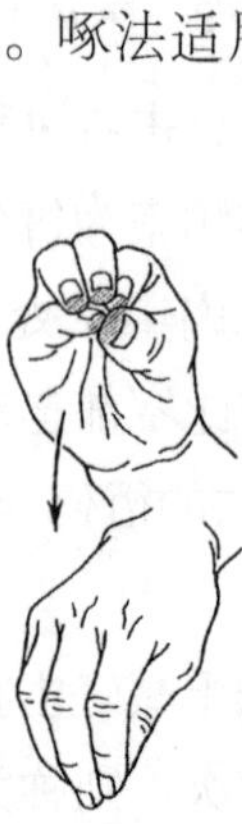

图3－109　啄法（梅花状）

4. 弹法。

啄法以腕关节力量击打，弹法则是用伸指肌的弹力进行击打。弹法既可用食指指腹抵住中指指甲（图3－110），也可用拇指指腹抵住中指指甲（图3－111），然后中指迅速弹出，以指尖击打某一穴位。弹法适用于头面部，作用同啄法。

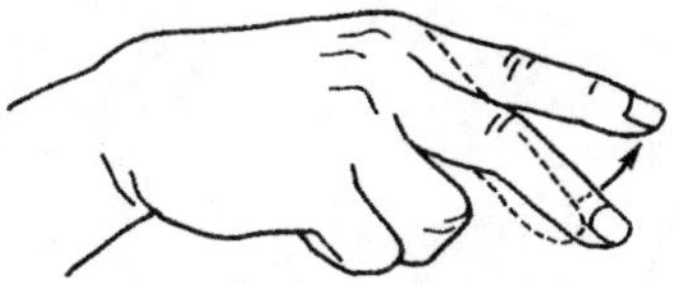

图3－110　弹法（食指指腹）

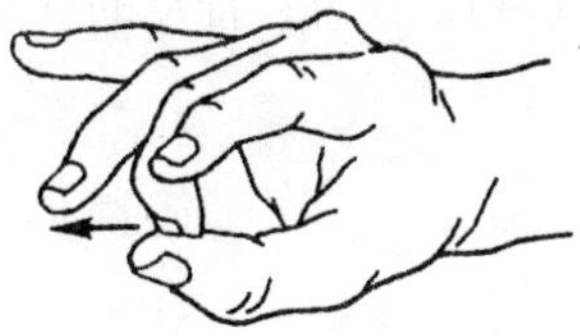

图3－111　弹法（拇指指腹）

拍法、啄法、弹法的操作频率为每分钟100～120次。

3.3.8　环摇类手法

所谓环摇类手法是指由操作者对病变关节做缓和回旋的环旋摇动的一类操作（图3－112），属松动性手法范畴。

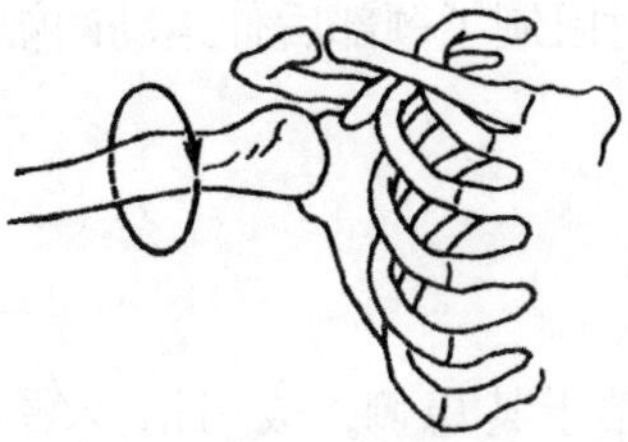

图3－112　环摇类手法模式图

环摇类手法操作时，通常以一手稳定被摇关节近端的肢体，另一手握住被摇关节的远端肢体，根据被摇关节的生理、病理活动范围，以稳妥缓和的力，带动关节做环转运动。关节运动的幅度，应由小到大，逐渐增强，可超过关节病理限制位，但一般不超过其生理限制范围。严禁粗暴动作和违反正常生理活动的运动。

3.3.8.1　摇颈

1. 坐位摇颈。

患者坐位，颈项放松，略前屈。操作者一手扶住其顶枕部，另一手托住下颏，双手协同将头摇转，顺时针与逆时针方向各5～7次（图3－113）。注意，环摇时不可将头过度后伸。

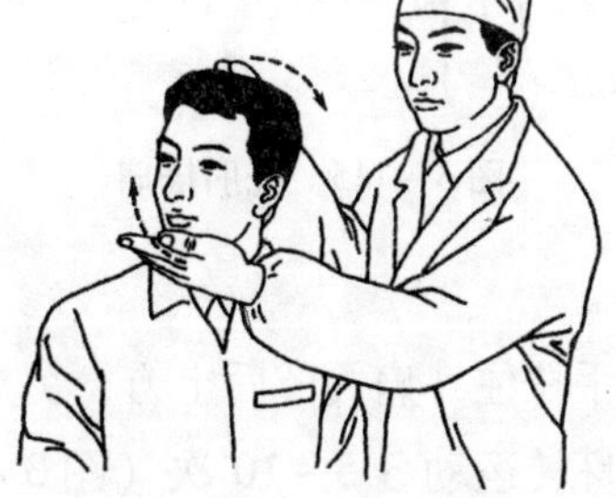

图3－113　坐位摇颈

2. 仰卧位摇颈。

患者仰卧，操作者站于其头端，先以右前臂伸侧托起患者枕部，右手则抓住患者左肩部，虎口朝向外侧；左手扶住患者头顶；然后利用右前臂的摆动，带动患者头颈做顺时针方向环转摇动3～5周。再交换一下左右手，以左前臂托起患者枕部，右手扶患者头顶，做逆时针方向环摇3～5周（图3－114）。注意，摇动的动作不能太快，幅度不可过大，以免引起患者眩晕。

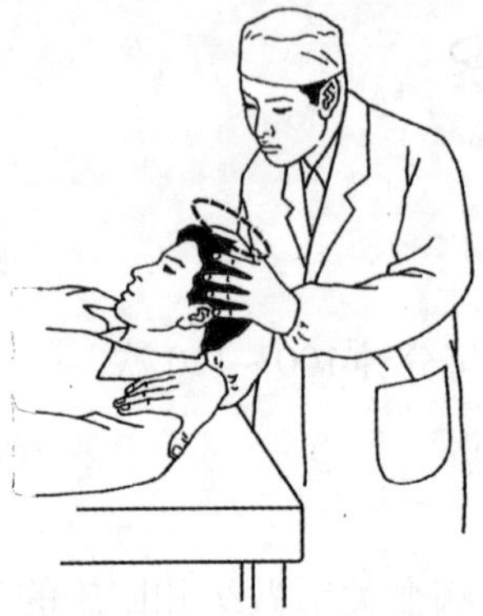

图3－114　仰卧位摇颈

仰卧位摇颈法操作较稳定，同时限制了颈部后伸运动的幅度，较为安全。适用于颈项疼痛僵硬、活动不利者的治疗。

3.3.8.2　摇肩

1. 托肘摇肩。

患者坐位，肩部放松。操作者站于其患侧，成弓箭步站立；一手按于肩关节后方，稳定肩部，另一手托起患者屈曲之肘关节，并使患者前臂搁置于自己前臂之上；然后带动患者肩关节做顺时针方向与逆时针方向环转运动各5～10次（图3－115）。本法操作时，按肩部之手可配合刺激肩部穴位，以减轻环转肩部可能引起的疼痛。本法适用于肩关节疼痛、抬举不利、关节运动障碍较严重者的治疗。

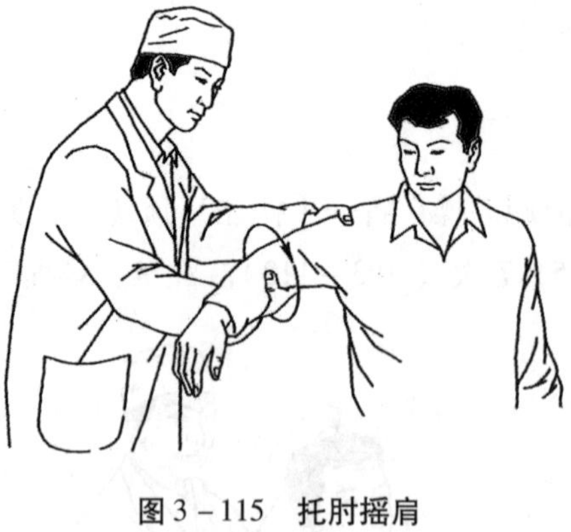

图3－115　托肘摇肩

2. 握手摇肩。

患者体位同上。操作者亦以一手扶住其肩关节后上方，另一手握住其手掌，然后带动患者肩关节做顺时针方向与逆时针方向的环转运动各5～10次（图3－116）。本法操作时，扶肩关节之手可配合刺激肩部穴位，以减轻运动疼痛。适应范围同上。

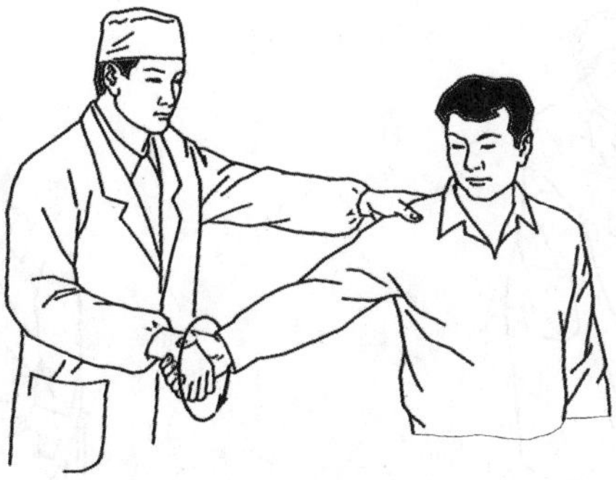

图3－116 握手摇肩

3. 抡摇肩关节。

以左肩关节为例，患者坐位，肩关节放松，自然下垂。操作者以丁字步站于其侧后方，以右手松握其腕背，左手手掌夹住其腕掌侧，慢慢向上举起（图3－117），当上举到60°～120°范围时，托腕之左手反掌握住患者腕部，握腕之右手顺势向下滑移至肩关节上方按住；两手协调用力，右手按肩关节下压，左手握腕部上拉，使肩关节伸展，并继续将肩关节向上转动（图3－118）；当环转至240°～300°范围时，按肩之右手顺势滑移至腕部并握住，握腕之左手手指松开，以手掌夹住患者腕掌侧，连续操作3～5次后，再做自前向后环摇（图3－119）。操作者站于其侧前方，以左手松握其腕背，右手掌面夹住其腕掌侧，慢慢向前上方举起（图3－120）；当上举到60°～120°范围时，托腕之右手翻掌握住患者腕部，握腕之左手顺势向下滑移至肩部按住；两手协调用力，左手按肩关节下压，右手握腕部上拉，使肩关节伸展，并继续将肩关节向后转动（图3－121）；当环摇至240°～300°范围时，握肩之左手顺势滑回腕部并握住患者手腕，握腕之右手手指松开，以掌面夹住患者腕掌侧，并继续向前下环转（图3－122）。连续操作3～5次。本法适用于肩关节疼痛、关节活动功能障碍较轻者，或经过推拿治疗，肩关节活动功能明显改善者的治疗。

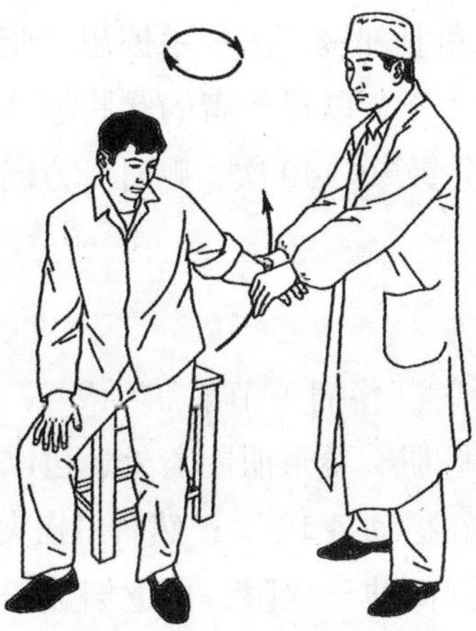

图3－117 抡摇肩关节（1）

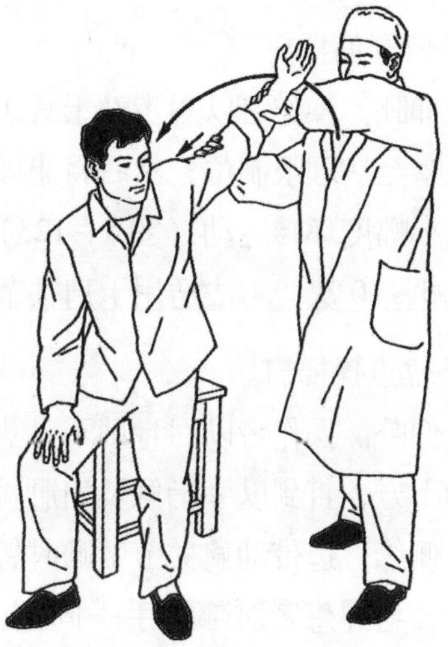

图3－118 抡摇肩关节（2）

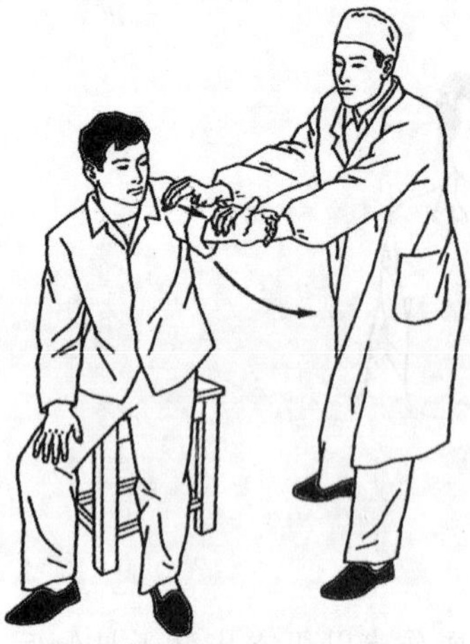

图 3－119　抡摇肩关节（3）

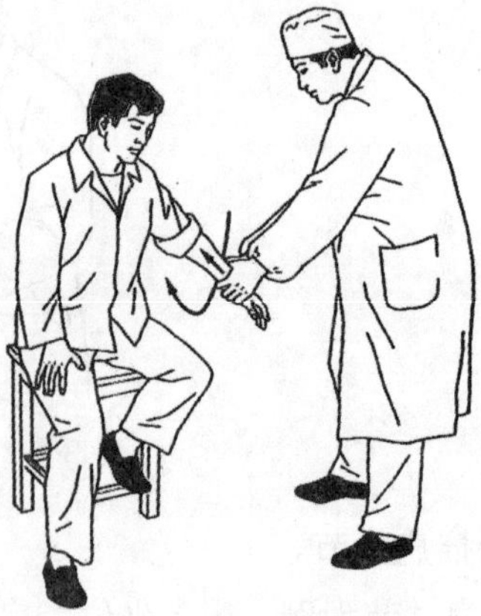

图 3－120　抡摇肩关节（4）

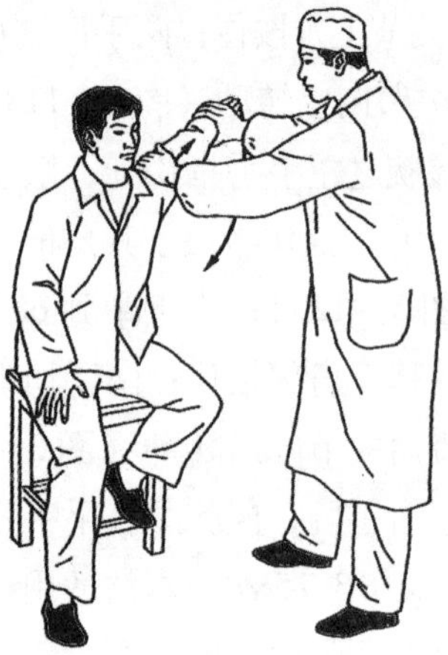

图 3－121　抡摇肩关节（5）

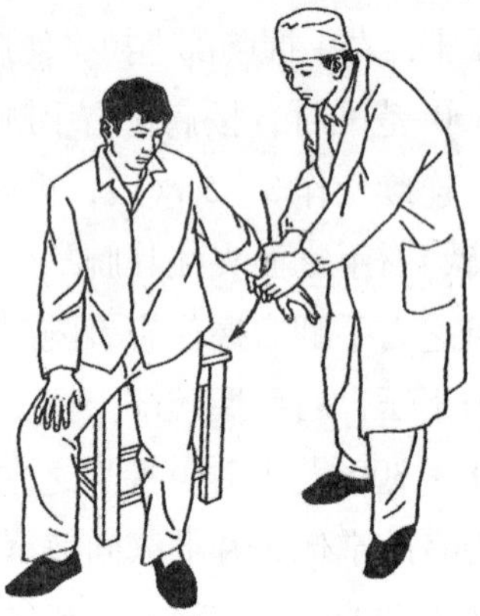

图 3－122　抡摇肩关节（6）

4. 卧位展筋摇肩。

患者仰卧。操作者以弓步站于其患侧，一手按住患者三角肌部位，另一手握患者腕部，将患肢伸直上举至病理限制位；然后将患肢在维持轻度纵向牵引力下，以操作者的腰胯运动带动患者肩关节做小幅度环转运动（图 3－123）。环转速度掌握在每分钟 30～40 次，顺时针方向、逆时针方向各做 5～10 次。本法适用于肩关节周围炎粘连期的治疗。

5. 卧位点揉摇肩。

患者仰卧。操作者以弓步站于其患侧，用一手握住患者肘部将肩关节前屈至 90°，另一手伸入肩胛骨下方，直到以手指触及肩胛骨内侧缘斜方肌、提肩胛肌、菱形肌附着处；边以指端点揉肩胛骨内侧缘，边带动肩关节做顺时针方向和逆时针方向环转摇动各 10 次；然后用指尖扣住肩胛骨内侧缘，与握患者肘部之手一同用力，将整个肩部向外侧拉伸至极限，再逐渐放松（图 3－124）。本法适用于肩周炎粘连期的治疗。

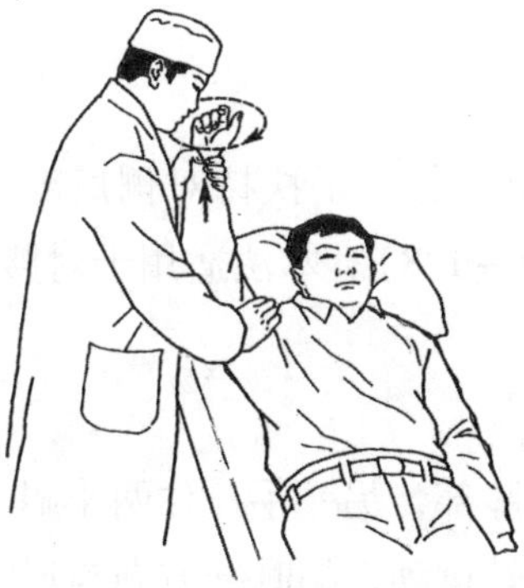

图 3－123　卧位展筋摇肩

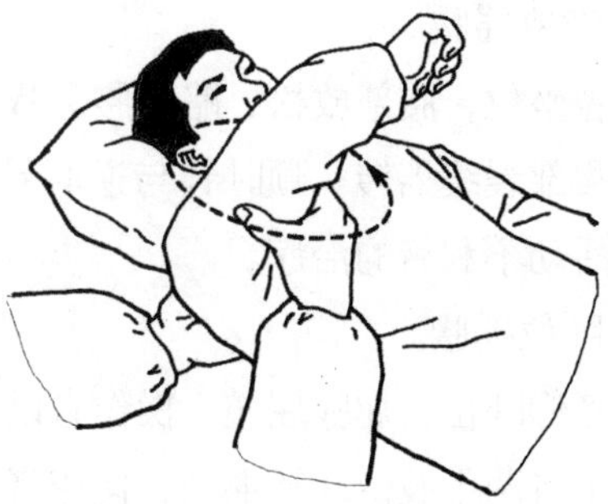

图 3－124　卧位点揉摇肩

3.3.8.3　摇肘

患者仰卧。操作者以弓步站于其患侧，一手抓住其肘部，另一手抓住其腕部，做相对拔伸；然后在伸肘、轻度拔伸状态下利用操作者的躯体运动，带动肘关节做小幅度环转运动，顺时针、逆时针方向各 10 次；再在屈肘、轻度拔伸状态下，带动肘关节做环转运动（图 3－125）。本法适用于对肘关节疼痛、活动受限者的治疗。

3.3.8.4　摇腕

患者坐位或仰卧位。操作者以一手握住患者前臂下端，另一手五指与患者手指相叉，做相对拔伸；然后在伸腕、轻度拔伸状态下带动腕关节做小幅度环转运动，顺时针与逆时针方向各 5 次。再在屈腕、轻度拔伸状态下带动腕关节做小幅度环转运动（图 3－126）。本法适用于对腕关节疼痛无力、活动有障碍者的治疗。

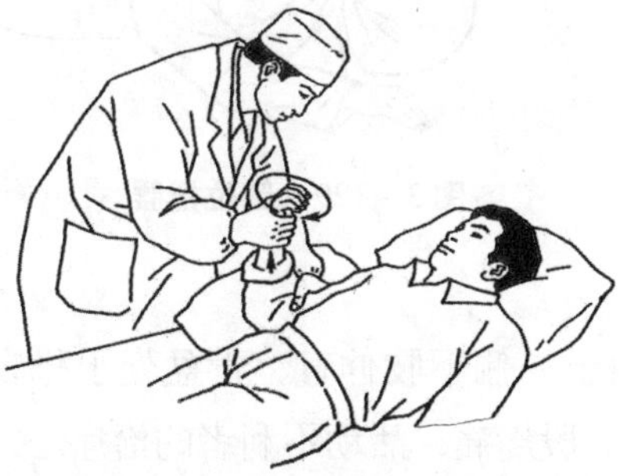

图 3－125　摇肘

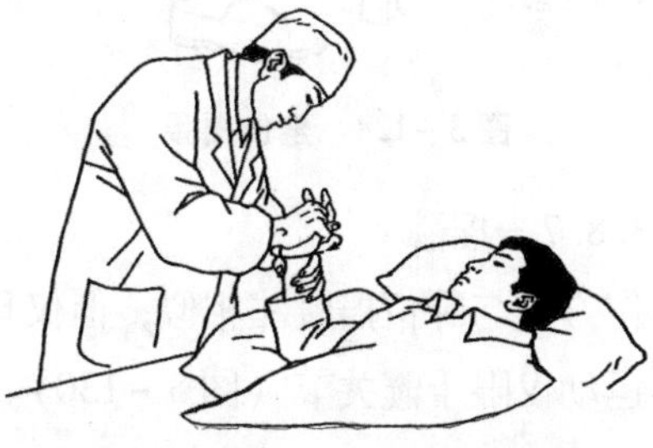

图 3－126　摇腕

3.3.8.5　摇指

患者坐位。操作者以一手握住患者手掌，另一手屈曲的食指和中指夹住患者手指，做相对拔伸；然后在维持拔伸状态下环摇掌指、指间关节（图 3－127）。本法适用于对指间、掌指关节疼痛肿胀、活动有障碍者的治疗。

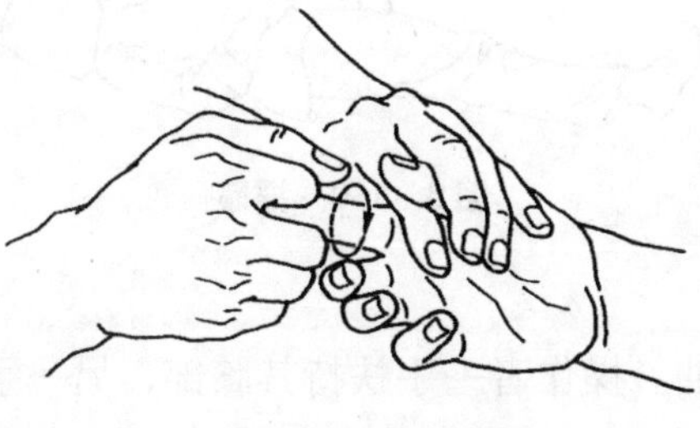

图 3－127　摇指

3.3.8.6　摇腰

1. 坐位摇腰。

患者坐位，腰部放松，略弯腰。操作者一手按住患者腰部，另一手扶持对侧肩部，两手协调，使腰部缓缓摇转。顺时针与逆时针方向各5～10次（图3－128）。本法适用于对腰背酸痛、僵硬、活动不利者的治疗。

2. 卧位摇腰。

患者仰卧位，屈膝屈髋。操作者以一手按于患者并拢之两膝部，另一手托住两小腿下端；然后带动患者两下肢做环转摇动，使患者骨盆与腰椎间亦产生环转运动，顺时针方向与逆时针方向各摇5～10次（图3－129）。本法适应证同上。

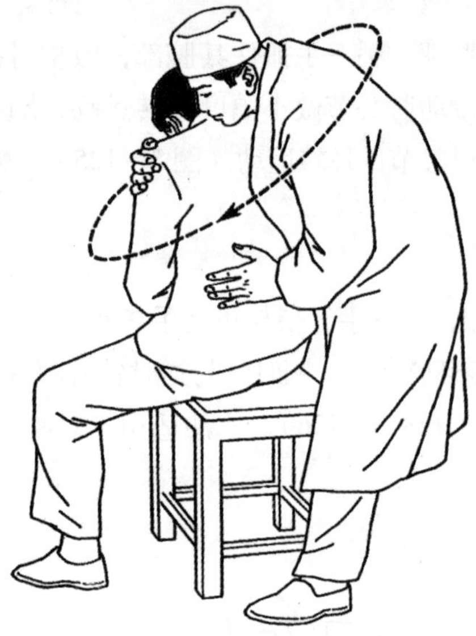

图3－128　坐位摇腰

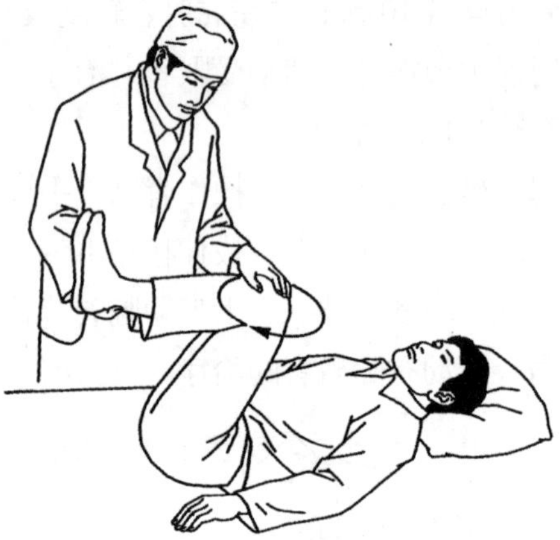

图3－129　卧位摇腰

3.3.8.7　摇髋

操作方式与卧位摇腰法相似，但仅环摇一侧下肢。由于一侧下肢伸直，骨盆处于稳定状态，故环转运动仅限于髋关节（图3－130）。本法适用于对髋、股疼痛，活动不利者的治疗。

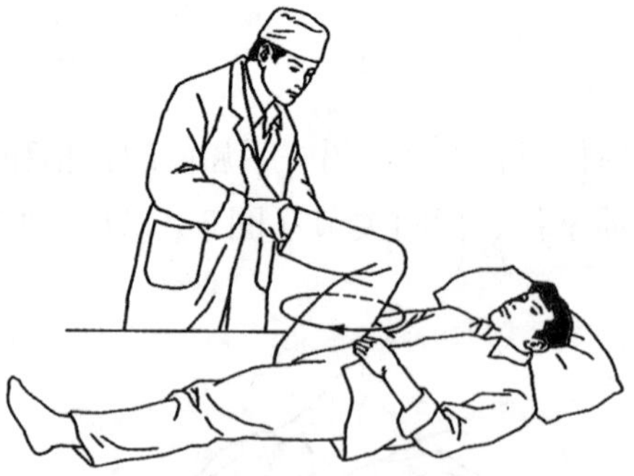

图3－130　摇髋

3.3.8.8　摇膝

患者仰卧位，膝关节半屈曲。操作者一手扶持其膝部，另一手握住其小腿下端；两手协调，使膝关节环转摇动，并边摇边慢慢将膝关节伸直，顺时针与逆时针方向各5～10次（图3－131）。

本法适用于对膝关节半月板处于破裂交锁状态者的治疗。

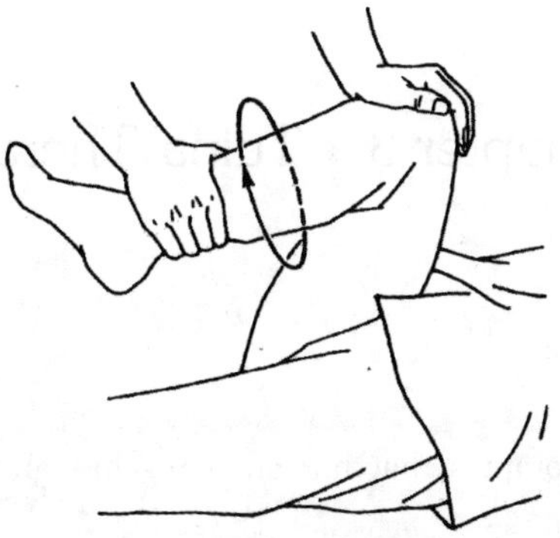

图 3－131　摇膝

3.3.8.9　摇踝

患者仰卧位，下肢伸直。操作者一手托起其足跟，另一手握住其足前部，做纵向拔伸片刻；然后在维持轻度拔伸力下带动踝关节环转摇动（图 3－132）。本法适用于对踝关节扭伤、活动不利者的治疗。

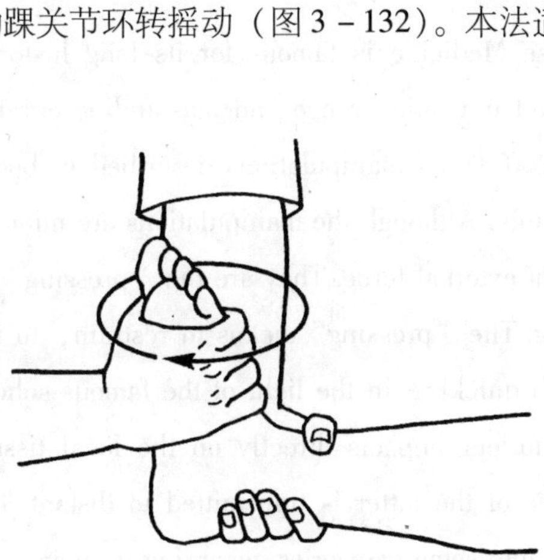

图 3－132　摇踝

Chapter 3 Tuina Therapy

Tuina is one of the oldest therapies that human being has grasped. Manipulation is the essential procedure of Tuina therapy.

3.1 Classification of the Manipulations

Tuina of Traditional Chinese Medicine is famous for its long history, numerous schools, plentiful manipulations, high skills, broad indication range and outstanding curative effects. According to present statistics, there are more than 200 Tuina manipulations described in books in China. And there are still more manipulations prevailed in folk. Although the manipulations are numerous, they can be classed into 2 phyla on the basis of the action of external force. They are the "pressing" and the "rectifying" written in the ancient classic book *Nei Jing*. The "pressing" means to restrain, to press skin and muscle while the "rectifying" means to move limb quickly, in the light of the famous scholar Wang Bing who lived in the Tang Dynasty. The force of the former impacts directly on the local tissues which are contacted by the manipulator's hand, but the force of the latter is transmitted to distant joints, muscles, tendons and so on. Each phylum can be divided into some categories according to their motion features. And each category contains several elementary manipulations. Even more, on the basis of their touch parts and motion changes, each elementary manipulation is sub-divided into some varieties. If the manipulations are classified according to their main effects, they can be divided into stimulating manipulations, rectifying manipulations and mobilizing manipulations. The essence of Tuina manipulations is external force. The force of the manipulations can either directly correct the subluxation or disalignments of the joints, cause the soft tissues to be deformed and the adhesion separated so as to redress the pathological status and cure disease. More important is that, the force of the manipulations, as a stimulating factor, activates adjusting function of the channel system to making rehabilitation.

The essence of Tuina manipulations is external force. The force of the manipulations can either directly correct the subluxation or disalignments of the joints, cause the soft tissues to be deformed and the adhesion separated so as to redress the pathological status and cure disease. More important it that, the force of the manipulations, as a stimulate factor, activates adjusting function of the channel system to make rehabilitation.

Relationships between various manipulations as Fig. 3－1：

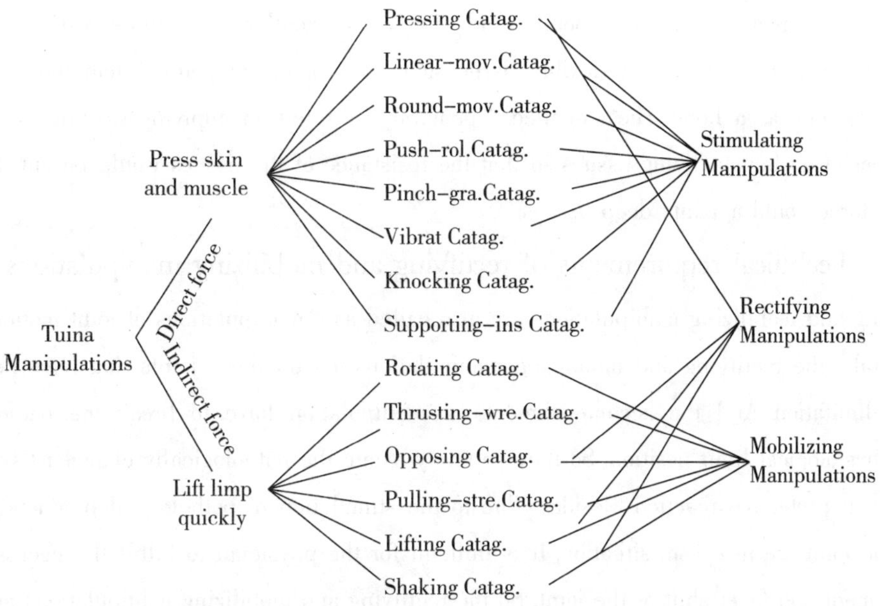

Fig. 3 – 1 Relationships between various manipulations

3.2 Technical Requirements of Tuina Manipulations

3.2.1 Technical requirement of stimulating manipulations

Most manipulations of the "Pressing skin and muscle" belong to the stimulating manipulation. The stimulating manipulations don't directly rely on their force to remove illness and make recovery. But they act on the channel system and then through its medium to promote the intrinsic adjusting and self – curing functions of the life to prevent or to heal disease. So the stimulating manipulations must tally with endurable, forceful, regular, gentle and penetrable technical requirements.

The so-called "endurable" means that the manipulations must be correctly handled for a long time according to specific rules. Thus the quantity of stimulation of the manipulation will accumulate to a critical point, which is big enough to push forward the adjusting function of the channel system, so as to improve pathological status. For example, "Pushing Sanguan" and "Retreating Liufu" in the Pediatric Tuina clinic must be manipulated for more than half an hour, only then can it exert a remarkable effect of diaphoresis or antifebrile on some serious infant patients. The so-called "forceful" means that the manipulations must keep in suitable force. In a given range, the quantity of manipulation force is directly proportion to the stimulating intensity to the channel system. But if it is over the limit, the force can injure the tissues or become an over-limitation suppressive massage to weaken the function of channel. The quantity of manipulation force is also not fixed. It must be adjusted according to the acting parts, the pathological features, and the patient's constitutions so on. To apply a suitable force on the basis of clinical conditions can be held only through a long-time practice. The so-called "regular" means that the motion of manipulations must have rhythm. The velocity can't be sometimes fast, and sometimes slow. The force can't be sometimes heavy, and sometimes light. The so-called "gentle" refers to the patterns of delivering force. The force, which is varied smoothly and slowly, is gentler than those varied violently and quickly. The touch styles with a soft flexible tissue such as a palm are gentler than those with a hard, inflexible tissue such as a bone. The so-called "penetrable" refers to applying skillful manipulations to reduce the tension of human living tissues so that the resistance of the tissues would be cut down and the manipulation force could act into deep tissues.

3. 2. 2 Technical requirements of rectifying and mobilizing manipulations

Rectifying and mobilizing manipulations are also called as "manipulations of joint motion".

In general, the rectifying and mobilizing manipulations act on those joints that have been suffering from motion limitation. And the accomplishments of manipulation have to break the pathological limit position or physiological limit position. So they certainly excite the pathologically changed tissues and give rise to pain and protective reaction. Beside, due to the stimulation of pathological products, the motion muscles of the joint are in spasm situation. It is difficult for the physician to fulfill the necessary range of passive movement and facet shift of the joint. So the rectifying and mobilizing manipulations must abide by the following requirements:

3. 2. 2. 1 Suitable posture

Before the rectifying and mobilizing manipulations are given, the patient must be put in suitable posture on the basis of human anatomy and biomechanics principles. In this way, the muscles will be relaxed, and the interval of joint will be broadened so as to make the manipulations less resisted and easy accomplished. For example, when an upper thoracic vertebral subluxation is reset, it is necessary to put a soft pad under the patient's chest and make the neck slightly flex down so that the cervical and the thoracic spine are in the same arc. If one wants to correct a lumbar vertebral subluxation, it is better to adjust the right rotation range of the spine and suitable flexion degree of hip. Thus the twisting center of the spine is just located at subluxation segment and the manipulation is easily accomplished.

3. 2. 2. 2 Smoothly, lightly, slightly, and briefly controlled

The manipulative course is usually divided into 2 phases. First, the joint is moved to a limited situation smoothly and slowly. Second, a light, ingenious, controlled and sudden thrusting is done to expand the range of joint motion. As soon as the thrusting is done, one must stop it and the joint regain its neutral status.

3. 2. 2. 3 Correct direction of exerting force

During the manipulative process, one must consider those things such as the shape of joint facet, the instantaneous center of joint motion and the direction at which the two joint surfaces will move along, in order to hold the correct force direction of manipulation. Otherwise, it is impossible to achieve the goal of the manipulation. For instance, there are posterior subluxation and anterior subluxation at sacroiliac joint. For the former, one should thrust the posterior superior iliac spine in the anterior lateral and inferior direction, and the lower end of sacrum in the superior direction at the same time. But for the latter, it is suitable to thrust the ischium directed anterior laterior and superior, and the upper end of sacrum directed anterior inferior in the same time. If the direction is controlled wrong, it is very difficult to restore the subluxation.

3.3　Commonly Used Techniques

3.3.1　Categories of pressing manipulations

The category of pressing manipulations refer to those actions in which the manipulator puts his palm, finger or other parts of the body on the patient's body surface and delivers force at the vertical direction to the body surface.

3.3.1.1　Principal techniques of pressing manipulations:

The pressings in which the manipulator presses on the patient's body with thumb tip or thumb pulp is called pressing with the thumb, while those with palm heel is called pressing with the palm. They may be done with a single hand, or with two overlapped hands in coordination to strengthen the pressing force.

1. Pressing with the thumb.

The operator extends the thumb with his four fingers flexed naturally and the index finger leaned against the thumb to enhance its strength; the manipulator extends the thumb and puts it at a point. Then applies forearm's power to press downward gradually. The force is varied from slight to heavy until the stimulation fully penetrates into the deep tissues; then reduce the strength gradually. This process is repeated for several times (Fig. 3-2). If you want to strengthen the pressing force, you can overlap the other thumb on the interphalangeal joint of the thumb to press down coordinately (Fig. 3-3).

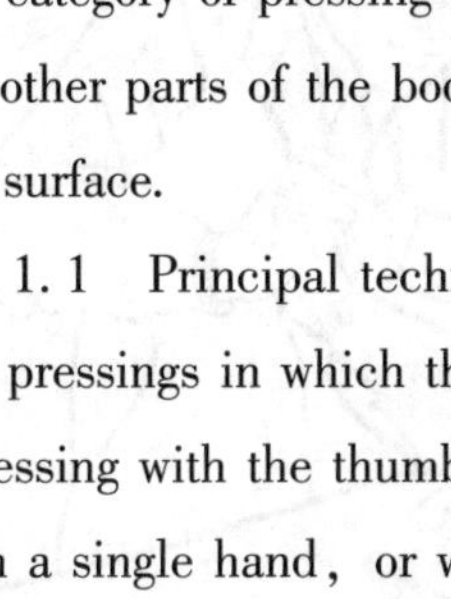

Fig. 3-2　Pressing with a thumb

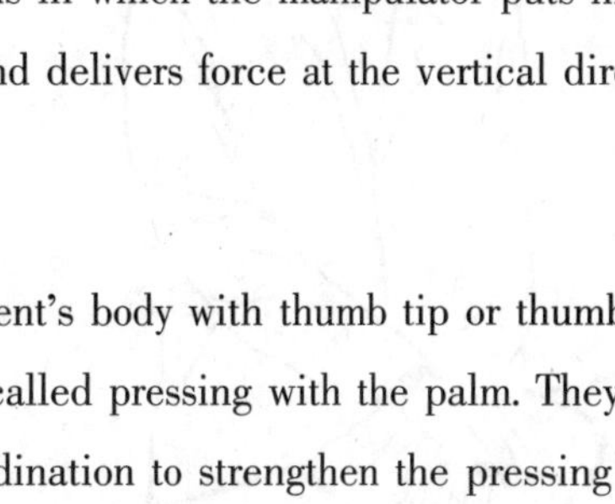

Fig. 3-3　Pressing with overlapped thumbs

The contact area of pressing with the thumb is small and concentrated. Its stimulating intensity can be controlled easily. So it is adopted for acting on all the acupoints, reflecting points and trigger points. It has strong analgesic effect and is often used to treat pain syndromes.

2. Pressing with the palms.

Two-hand pressing is more often seen than single-hand manner. During the manipulation, the manipulator extends the fingers and the wrist naturally, and puts the hand heel on the patient's body and overlaps the other hand on it. The force generated by the shoulder or the trunk is transmitted to the pressing areas along the straightening upper limbs. The pressing force is increased until the stimulation is fully and deeply penetrated; then it is reduced gradually. The above action is repeated for several times (Fig. 3-4).

The force of pressing with the palm is strong and its contact area is also big. It is suitable for acting on the back, buttocks, the thigh, the shank and the shoulder. It has a good effect to relax convulsive muscles and is usually applied to cure acute and chronic lumbar-leg pains and scapulohumeral periarthritis.

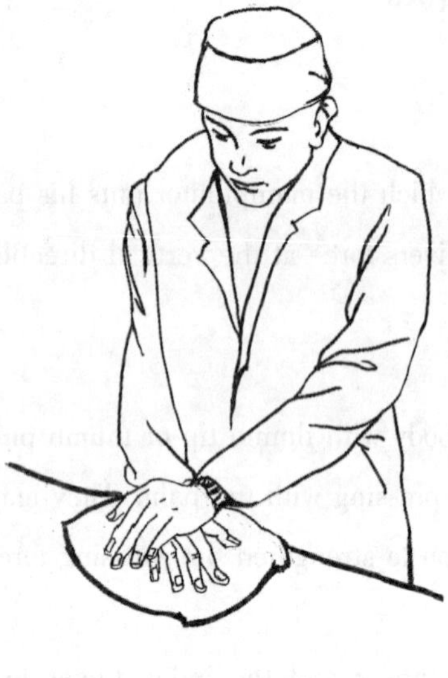

Fig. 3 – 4 **Pressing with palms**

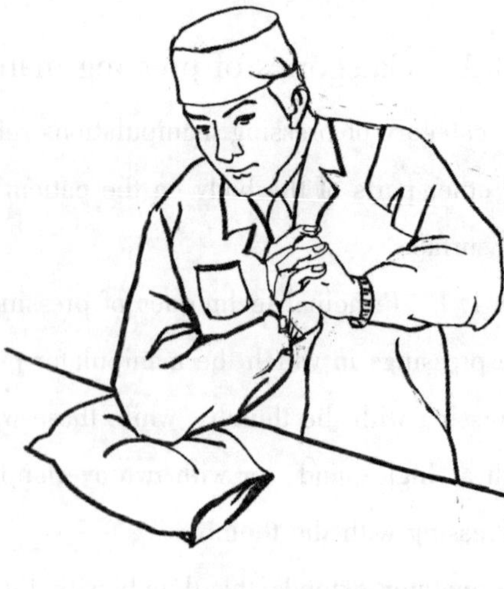

Fig. 3 – 5 **Compressing with the elbow**

3. 3. 1. 2 Evolution of pressings

1. Compressing with the elbow.

In Chinese, pressing refers to the motion pattern of manipulation while compressing refers to the effect caused by the manipulation. So the pressing and the compressing are often lumped together in Tuina books. If you want to strictly distinguish them, the "pressing" is inclined to motion, while the "compressing" is inclined to static. The duration time of the pressing is shorter than that of the compressing. The force and the stimulation intensity of the former are also slighter than those of the compressing. The manipulation in which the elbow is used to compress is used to being named as compressing with elbow. When you exercise compressing with elbow, you should flex the elbow joint, put the elbow tip on patient's body, and then deliver force from shoulder and trunk muscles to compress downward. Because its stimulation is fairly intense, it is only used on the low back and buttocks on which the muscles are well developed to cure persistent lumbar-leg pains and lumbar stiff.

2. Pointing.

If you want to get a stronger stimulation than pressing with the thumb, you may reduce the touching area and the manipulation becomes pointing. There are four manipulative manners in pointing. First, pointing with middle finger is manipulated as follows: First, extend thumb, index finger and middle finger naturally; put the thumb against the palm side of the middle finger and the index finger against the back side to strengthen the middle finger; then the manipulator delivers power from the wrist, elbow, or shoulder joint to point and press acupoints with the tip of the middle finger. When the stimulation penetrates into the deep tissue, lift the middle finger (Fig. 3 – 6). Second, pointing with the "sword fingers" can be done as follows: Stretch the index and the middle fingers to form so-called "sword fingers"; then the manipulator imitates the pattern of the pointing with the middle finger to deliver the power from the wrist, the elbow, or the shoulder to point and press acupoints with the tip of the fingers (Fig. 3 – 7). Third, pointing with the interphalangeal joint of the thumb, is manipulated as: make a hollow fist; then the manipulator points and presses acupoints with the bone bulge on back side of the interphalangeal joint of a flexed thumb (Fig. 3 – 8). Fourth, pointing with the interphalangeal joint of the index finger, may be done in this way. Make a hollow fist; support the index finger nail with the palm side of the thumb; then the manipulator points and presses acupoints with the bone bulge on the back side of the proximal interphalangeal joint of the flexed index finger (Fig. 3 –9).

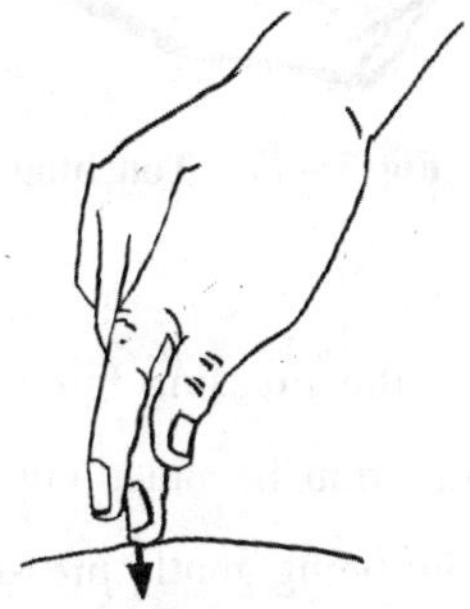

Fig. 3 –6 Pointing with the middle finger

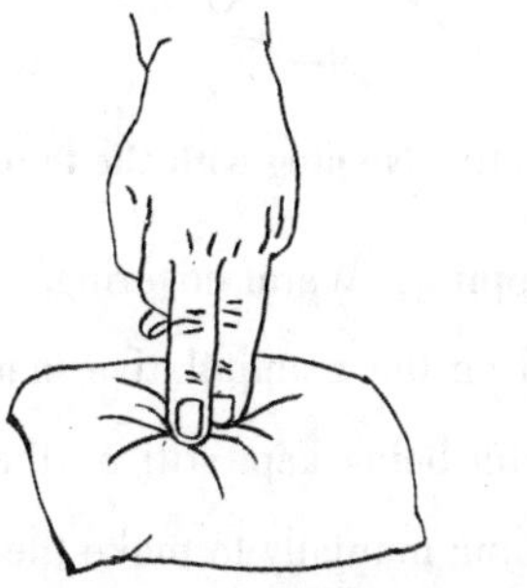

Fig. 3 –7 Pointing with the "sword fingers"

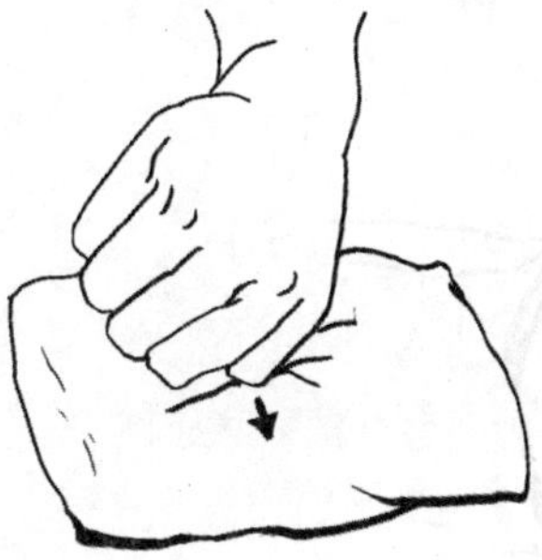

Fig. 3 –8 Pointing with interphalangealjoint of the thumb

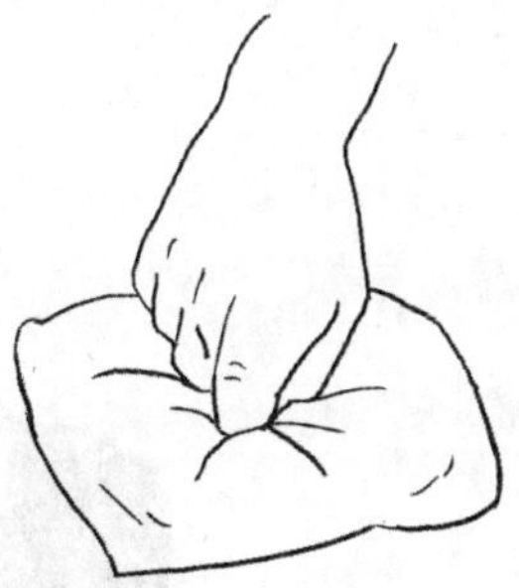

Fig. 3 –9 Pointing with interphalangealjoint of the index finger

The stimulation force of pointing is stronger than that of pressing, but its duration is shorter than that of the latter. Pointing is adapted for acting on the points which situate in bone cracks and joint interval or the treatment severe pain and paralysis. But for common patients, pressing is more frequently used.

3. Nipping with the thumbnail.

If you want to reduce the touching area of pressing and make the stimulation stronger and sharper, you may employ the thumbnail to press acupoints and the manipulation is called nipping with the thumbnail, or scratching or cutting (Fig. 3 – 10). The nipping with the thumbnail has a strong stimulus, and it is often manipulated on the first-aid acupoints such as Shuigou, Suliao, Neiguan, Zhongchong and Laolong etc. Since it may resuscitate one's life and dispel epileptic attack, it is used for curing coma, convulsion and shock. In order to relieve acute pain caused by the nipping with the thumbnail, you may use the kneading manipulation at the nipping area after it.

4. Touching.

Based on the manipulative manner of pressing with the fingers, one reduces pressing force and keeps the fingerprint in still on acupoints. The manipulation is called touching (Fig. 3 – 11). The touching is usually used to seek the accurate location of the acupoints and for convenience of "getting Qi".

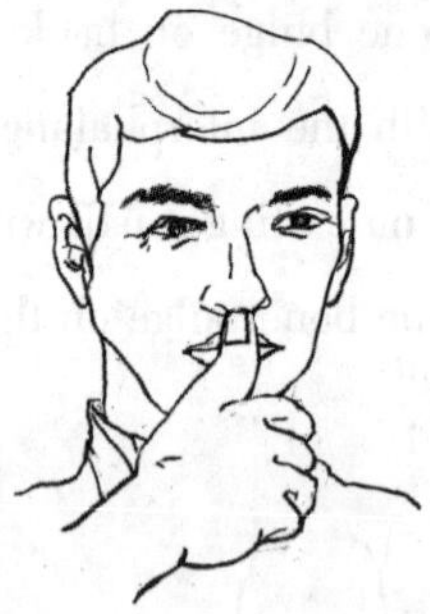

Fig. 3 - 10 **Nipping with the thumbnail**

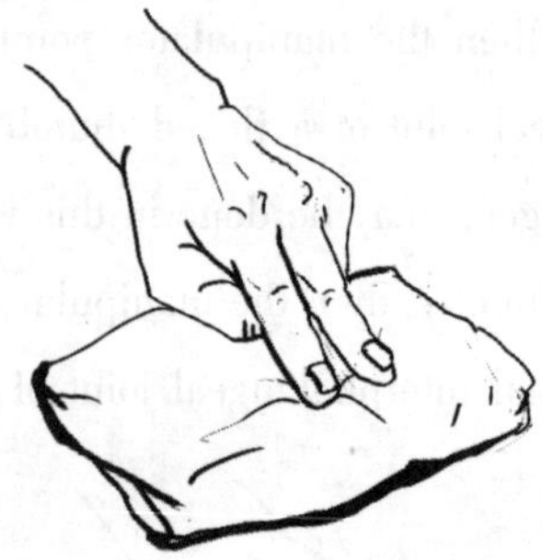

Fig. 3 - 11 **Touching**

5. Cupping, Warm covering.

Based on the manipulative manner of the pressing with the palm, the pressing force being reduced and the palm being kept still on the chest or the abdomen, the manipulation becomes cupping. With two palms rubbing mutually to make the palm warm, and then the warm palm being gently pressed on the body and kept in still, it is named as warm covering (Fig. 3 - 12). But in present clinic application of Tuina, they have not been distinguished strictly and both are called pressing with the palm.

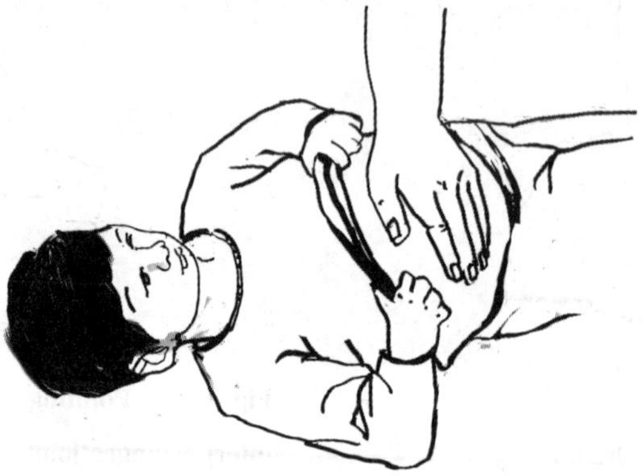

Fig. 3 - 12 **Cupping, Warm covering**

3.3.2 Category of linear-moving manipulations

Manipulations of linear - moving category are referred to those actions in which the manipulator puts his fingers, palm or other body parts on patient's body surface and moves straightly or cursively while keeping a constant pressing force.

3.3.2.1 principal techniques of linear-moving

1. Linear-pushing with the thumb.

The physician stretches all fingers, with the thumb being put behind and the rest four fingers in front of the acting point. Then through nimble moving, in which the thumb and the other fingers are gathered and separated, the thumb is pushed forward with the frequency of 200 to 240 times per minute (Fig. 3 - 13).

2. Linear - pushing with the "sword-fingers".

With the index and the middle fingers being stretched to form "sword-fingers", the physician touches the patient's skin with print regions of the two fingers, and moves the forearm forth and back quickly so as to cause the fingers to skate forward on the skin nimbly and then return back (Fig. 3 - 14).

The frequency of manipulation is 200 to 240 times a minute. Linear-pushing is the lightest manipulation in pushing. It is required that the patient's skin be not changed in form during manipulation and in color after manipulation. Before the pushing is being done, it is necessary to have the fingers soaked with clear water or ginger sauce to keep the skin in moist condition. Linear-pushing is employed in pediatric Tuina such as "pushing Sanguan", and "Retreating Liufu" etc. Their effects rely on which point is acted and what direction is moved along.

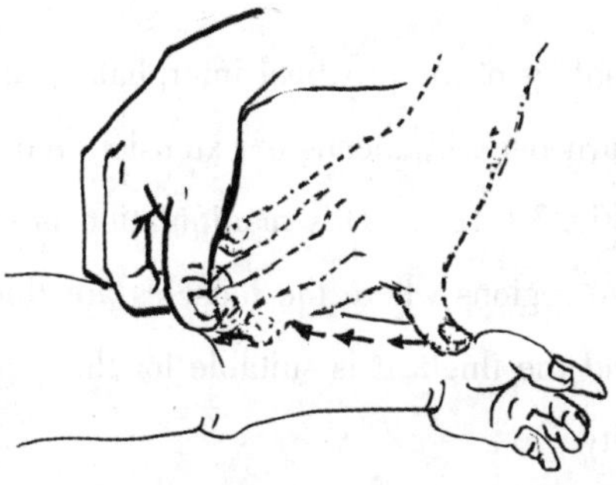

Fig. 3 - 13 Linear-pushing with the thumb

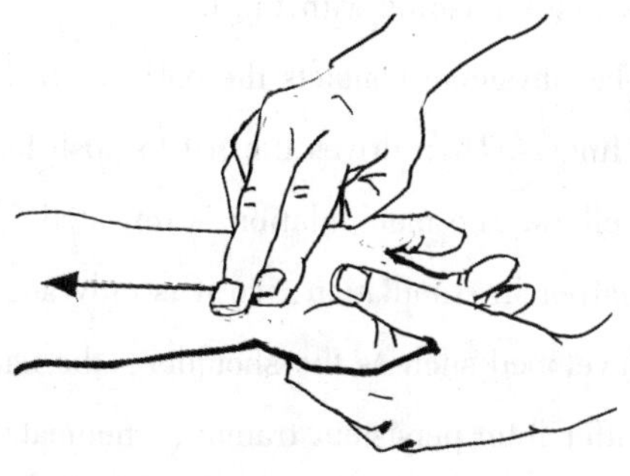

Fig. 3 - 14 Linear-pushing with the "sword - fingers"

3. Flat-pushing with the thumb.

The physician contacts the patient's body with the print region of the thumb that is strengthened and supported by the rest opened finger. Then drives the thumb to push forward slowly and steadily along muscles or channels by means of extending and flexing of elbow. The manipulation is repeated 5 to 15 times (Fig. 3 - 15). The pressing force of flat pushing is heavier than that of the linear pushing. It is suitable for manipulation on shoulder, back, chest, abdomen, lumbar, buttock and limb. Dredging blocked channel, vivifying Qi and blood, setting tendon in order, and relieving pain are its common functions. It is often applied to cure shoulder and back pain, stuffed thorax and abdomen, muscle spasm, inflexible joint and so on.

4. Flat-pushing with the palm.

The physician contacts the patient's body with his palm heel, with his fingers being stretched. Then drives the palm to push forward slowly and steadily along channel route by means of extension and flexion movement of the elbow. The manipulation is repeated 5 to 15 times (Fig. 3 - 16). This pushing is gentler than the flat pushing with thumb. It is adapted to manipulation on those flat body regions such as back, chest, abdomen and thigh for promoting blood circulation, relieving spasm, comforting thorax, and regularizing Qi. It is usually used to heal back pain and stuffed thorax and abdomen.

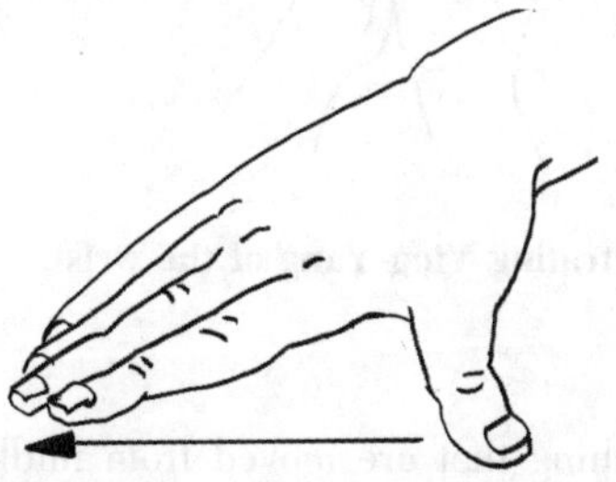

Fig. 3 - 15 Flat-Pushing with the thumb

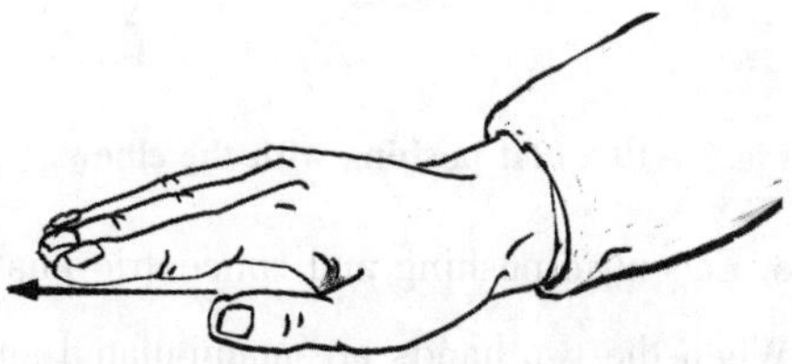

Fig. 3 - 16 Flat-pushing with the palm

5. Planing-pushing.

The physician holds the patient's limb gently with one hand. Then drives the palm to push forward along the longitudinal axis of the limb by means of extension and flexion of the elbow. This manipulation is repeated 5 to 10 times (Fig. 3 – 17). The stimulation of planing-pushing is gentle and suitable for manipulation on the limbs. It has functions such as relaxing muscle and sinew, promoting blood circulation, relieving swelling and relieving pain. It is usually used to treat soft tissue injuries of limbs, arthritis and arthralgia.

6. Flat – pushing with the fist.

The physician contacts the patient's body with a fist bone bulges of the proximal interphalangeal joints of the fingers. Then drives the fist to push forward and then return back by means of extension and flexion of the elbow. The manipulation is repeated for 5 to 10 times (Fig. 3 – 18). This manipulation is stronger and sharper in stimulation, so it is only adapted to act on those regions where the muscles are thick and well developed such as the shoulder, the back, the buttock and the thigh. It is suitable for those patients who suffer from persistent trauma, rheumatalgia and insensitivity.

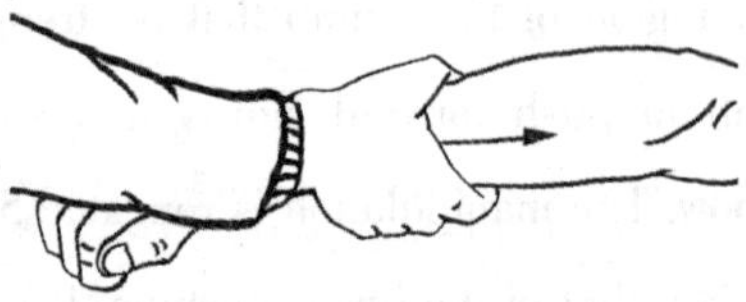

Fig. 3 – 17 Planing-pushing

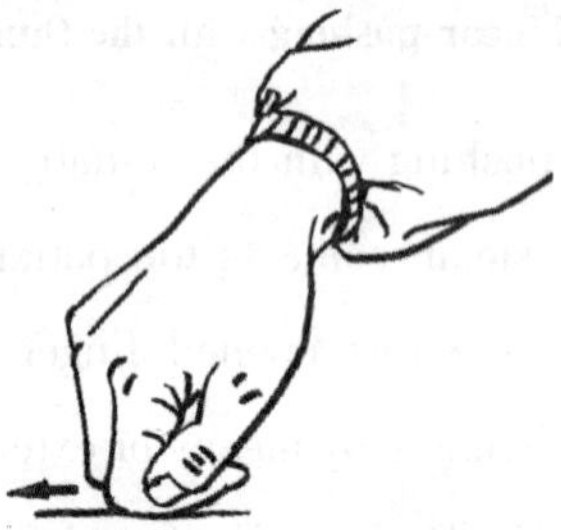

Fig. 3 – 18 Flat-pushing with the fist

7. Flat – pushing with the elbow.

The physician contacts the patient's body with a flexed elbow, and then drives the elbow to push forward and return back by means of extension and flexion of the shoulder. The manipulation is repeated 5 to 10 times (Fig. 3 – 19). Its stimulation is the strongest in all pushing, so it is only used to those who have very strong physiques. The adapted range is like the flat-pushing with fist.

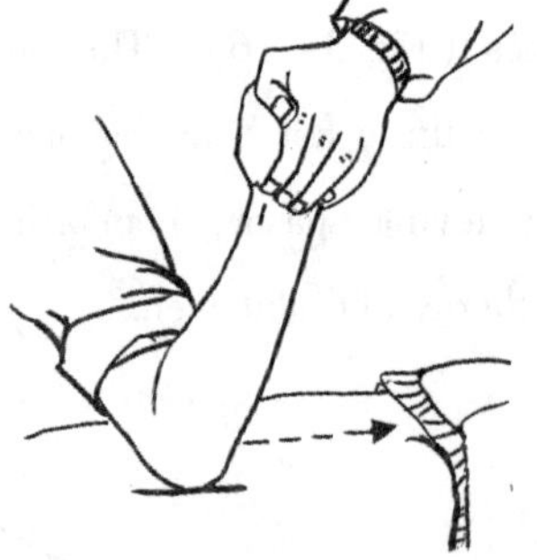

Fig. 3 – 19 Flat-pushing with the elbow

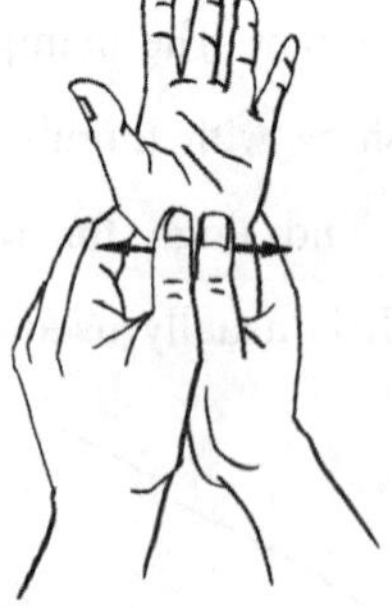

Fig. 3 – 20 Eccentrating Ying-Yang of the wrist

8. Eccentric-pushing and concentric-pushing.

When the two hands are manipulated simultaneously, those pushing that are moved from midline to two lateral sides are named as eccentric-pushing, while those from two lateral sides to the midline are named as concentric-pushing. The eccentric – pushing and concentric-pushing have different names as they are applied on different parts of the body, such as centrifugal yin-yang of the wrist (or concentrating yin-yang of the wrist) (Fig. 3 – 20), eccentrating the Tanzhong (Fig. 3 – 21), adapted to pediatric Tuina, "八" shaped eccentric-pushing (Fig. 3 – 22), adapted to back pain etc.

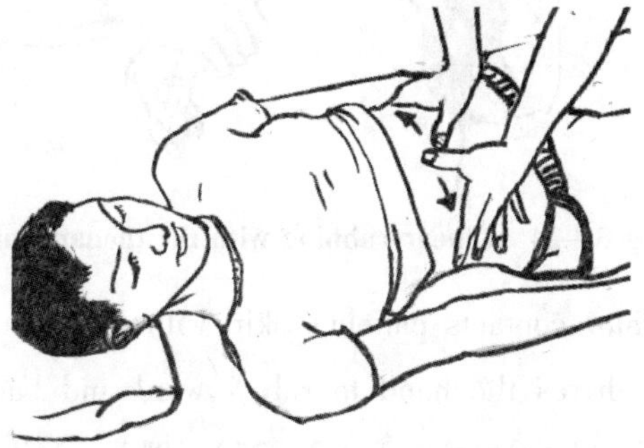

Fig. 3 – 21 Eccentrating the Tanzhong

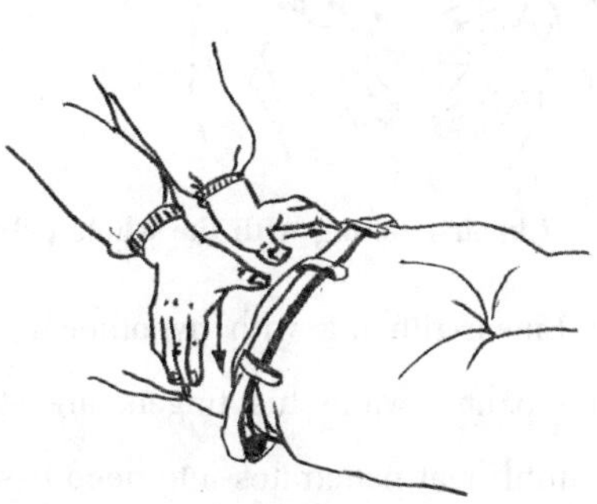

Fig. 3 – 22 "八" shaped eccentric-pushing

3. 3. 2. 2 Evolution of pushing

1. Linear-rubbing.

The aim of pushing is to promote Qi and blood circulation in channels and vessels. So the pushing is one-way forcible moving. The goal of Linear-rubbing is to transform the friction produced between the palm and the skin as well as the superficial and the deep tissues into heat energy. So the linear-rubbing must move forcibly forth and back. The pressing force of the linear-rubbing can't be too strong. It is suitable that no wrinkles appear on skin when the linear-rubbing is being done. The moving velocity of linear-rubbing is quicker than that of flat pushing and its frequency is about 100 to 120 times per minute.

(1) linear-rubbing with the whole palm: It is similar to flat pushing with palm, but its pressing force is slighter than that of the latter. The manipulator contacts the selected areas of the patient's body with the whole palm. Then drives the palm to rub the skin forth and back straightly until heat penetrates into deep tissues (Fig. 3 – 23). This manipulation is adapted to manipulation on shoulder, back, chest and abdomen. Those effects such as warming channels, dredging vessels, comforting thorax, settling Qi disorder, regulating digestive function and building up health are distinguishing. It is often employed in treating the illnesses of respiratory system and digestive system as well as poor health condition.

(2) Linear rubbing with the thenar eminence: The manipulator closes and slightly flexes all fingers to make a vacuous palm, and puts the thenar eminence and the base of the palm on skin. Then drives the hand to rub forth and back straightly until heat penetrates into the deep tissues of the manipulated area (Fig. 3 – 24). This manipulation is more steadily manipulated on limbs. It has functions such as promoting blood circulation, dredging blocked channels and vessels, relieving swelling and relieving pain etc. Those troubles such as injuries of the soft tissues on limbs, swollen joints and persistent rheumatalgia are all adapted.

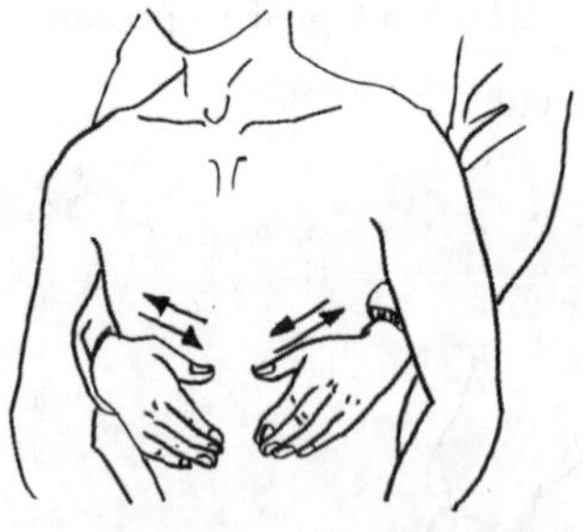

Fig. 3 – 23 **Linear-rubbing with the whole palm**

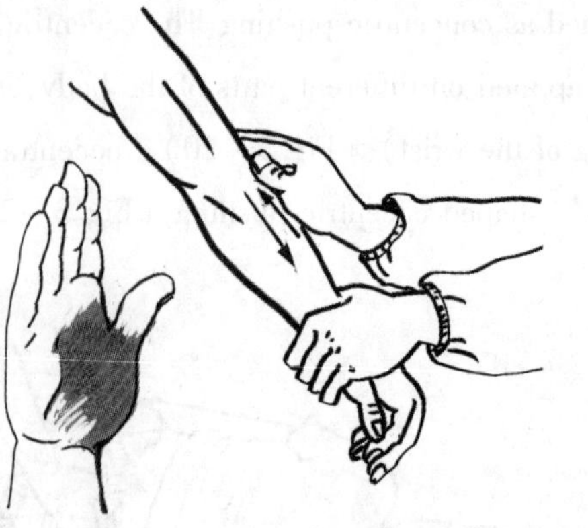

Fig. 3 – 24 **Linear-rubbing with the thenar eminence**

(3) Linear-rubbing with hypothenar: The manipulator contacts patient's skin with the hypothenar side of the palm, while his fingers are stretched. Then drives the hand to rub forward and backward straightly until heat penetrates into deep tissues of the manipulated area (Fig. 3 – 25). This manipulation has strong warm effect and is adapted to manipulation on back, sacrum and lower abdominal regions. Warming channels, eliminating cold evil, reinforcing kidney, building up health, promoting blood circulation and dispelling wind evil are all its distinguished functions. It is often applied to the treatments of back pain, muscle and tendon spasms, cold and pain in the lower abdomen, and weak condition etc. When the linear-rubbing is manipulated, one should smear some grease on skin in order to protect skin as well as promote heat penetrating. After linear-rubbing, there may be slight injury on skin, therefore the linear-rubbing must be used at the end of manipulations so as to avoid abrasion of skin.

2. Plucking.

Also named as catapult plucking. When the pushing and linear-rubbing are being done, the pressing force is lighter while the moving range is longer, so there is friction between hand and skin. When the plucking is being done, the press force is heavier while the moving range is shorter, and the thumb fixes on the skin and moves at a very short range to make each layer of deep tissue move relatively (Fig. 3 – 26). This manipulation stimulus is strong and it is usually applied to trigger point to treat the adherence and contraction of soft tissue. It can peel off adherence, relax muscle and sinew and relieve spasm.

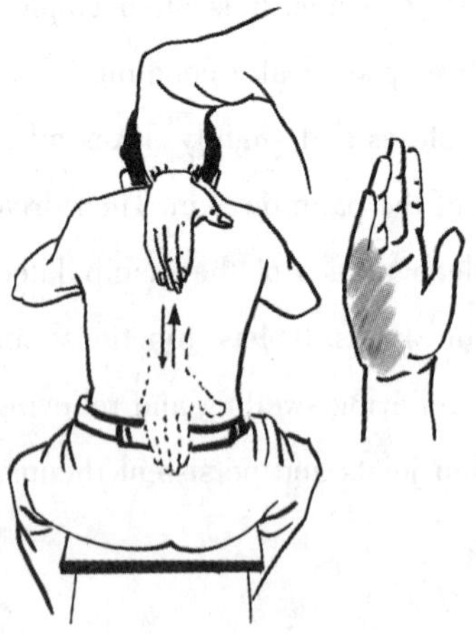

Fig. 3 – 25 **Linear-rubbing with the hypothenar**

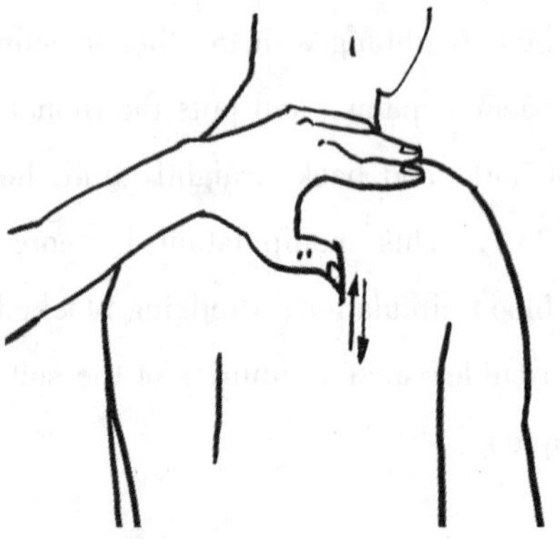

Fig. 3 – 26 **Plucking**

3. Wiping.

Wiping is referred to those flat-pushing with the thumb or with the palm on the face and head following a fixed program. This program is as follows: The physician stands in front of the patient, with his hands being put on both side of the patient's temporal regions, and moves the thumbs in turn for 15 times by wiping from the point Yintang to the point Shenting, and then from the point Yintang to the point Taiyang, from the point Jingming to the point Taiyang along the upper and lower borders of the eyesockets and from Yintang through Jingming, the lateral sides of the nose, the low rims of the cheek bones to Tinggong. All the wiping routes are repeated for 15 times (Fig. 3 –27). The above actions must be done continuously and not be broken. After wiping, the patient immediately refreshes seeing and thinking. Because wiping on the face and head may dispel the wind evil, clear seeing, calm mind and reduce blood pressure etc. Those illnesses such as cold, headache, insomnia, hypertension show good responses to it.

4. Sweeping.

The doctor gently supports patient's head with one hand and contacts the patient's temporal region with the radial side of the thumb and the tips of four fingers of the other hand. Then moves the hand along an arc route from the temporal region (along the Gall Bladder Channel route) to occipital region (Fig. 3 – 28). This manipulation possesses effects of inhibiting Liver Yang, dispelling the wind evil and relieving pain. Therefore those illnesses such as headache, dizziness, hypertension show good responses to it.

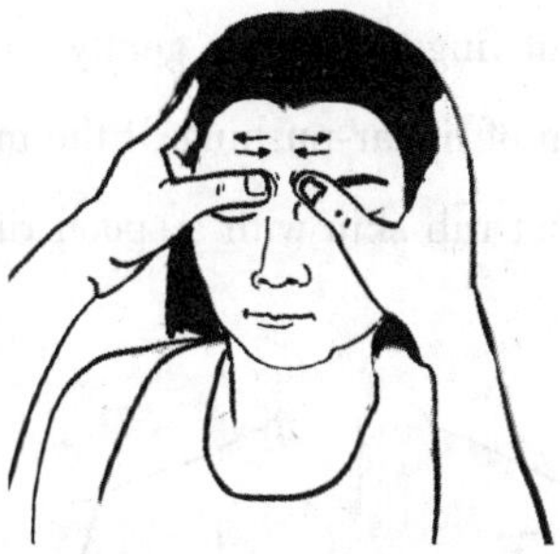

Fig. 3 –27 **Wiping**

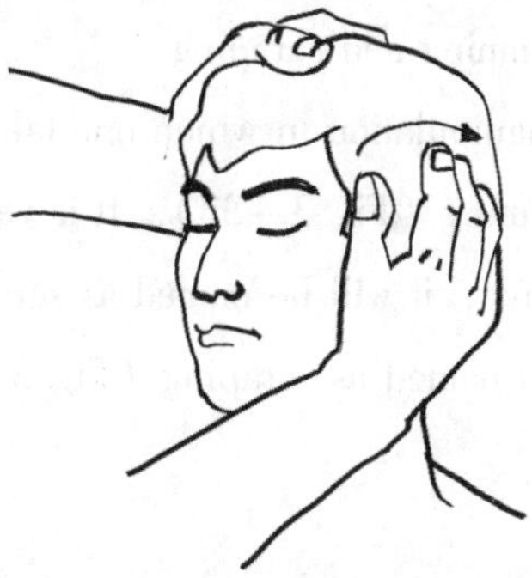

Fig. 3 –28 **Sweeping**

5. Canceling.

It is like the sweeping. The doctor stands behind the patient. With his two thumbs being put on the lateral sides of the occipital bone, his radial sides of the index fingers that are slightly flexed as a "hook" and the rest fingers are put on the temporal regions. Then drives the fingers to rub on the temporal regions along an arc route from the point Taiyang to the occipital bone. The manipulation is repeated for several times (Fig. 3 –29). Its effects are similar to those of the sweeping.

6. Tweezering.

It is also named for stripping or arranging. The doctor clamps patient's finger between flexed index finger and middle finger (or toe), then slips out of the finger tip. Each finger (or toe) is manipulated a time (Fig. 3 –30).

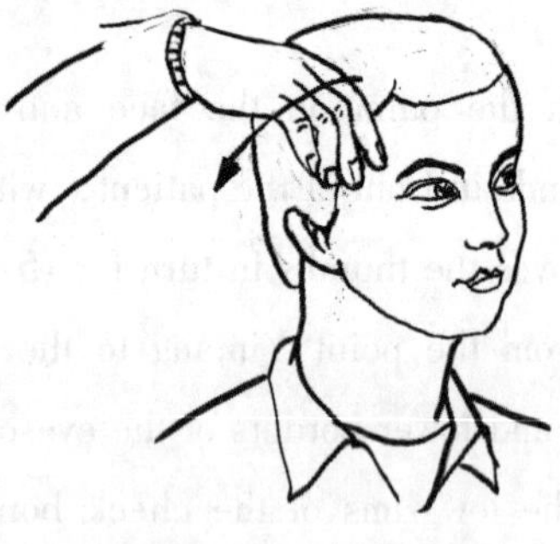

Fig. 3 – 29 **Canceling**

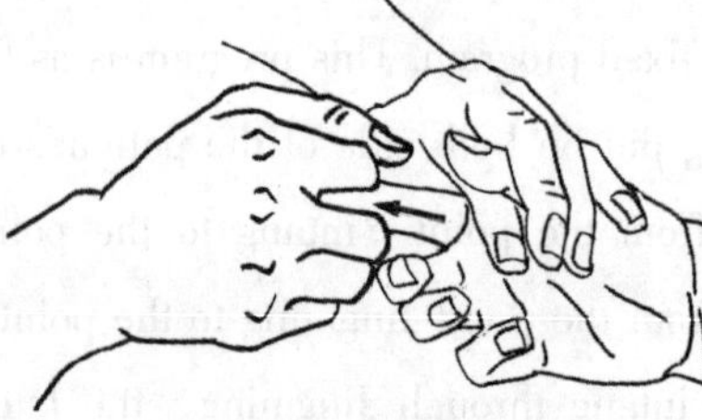

Fig. 3 – 30 **Tweezering**

7. Stripping and conforming

When manipulated on the limbs, pushing with palm moving from the proximal to the distal on the extensional side is named as stripping (Fig. 3 – 31), while from the distal to the proximal on the flexion side is named as conforming (Fig. 3 – 32).

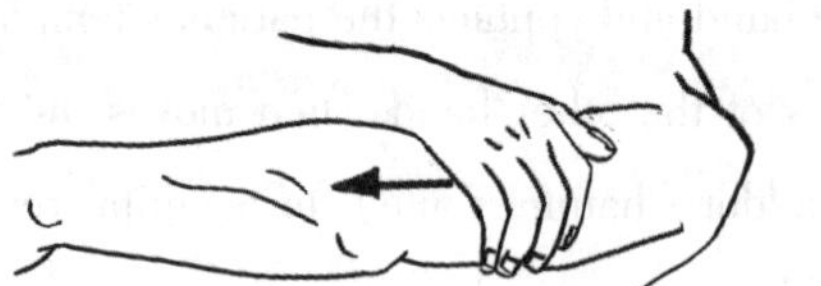

Fig. 3 – 31 **Stripping**

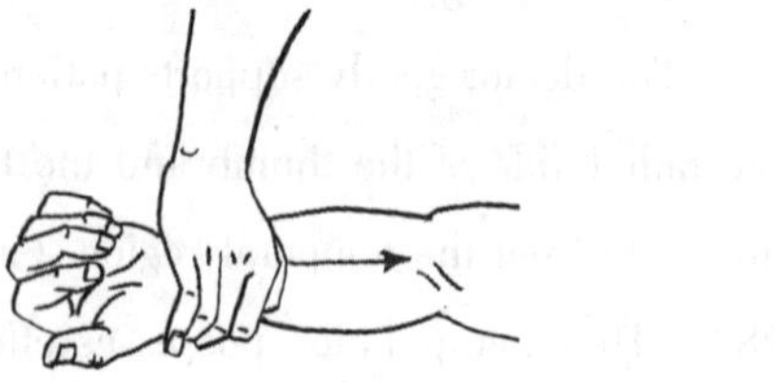

Fig. 3 – 32 **Conforming**

8. Skimming and scraping

The manipulation in which one takes the print regions of the four fingers to skim gently on the skin is called skimming (Fig. 3 – 33). It is very similar to the manipulation of linear-pushing. If the manipulative force is heavy, it will be named as scraping. Those manipulations that rub skin with a spoon rim or a coin rim are also named as scraping (Fig. 3 – 34).

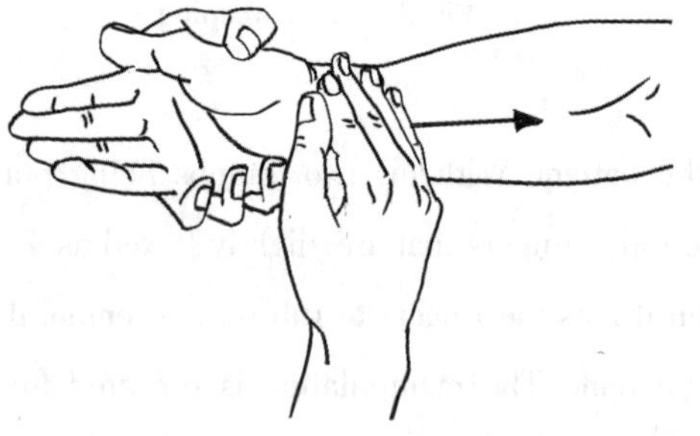

Fig. 3 – 33 **Skimming**

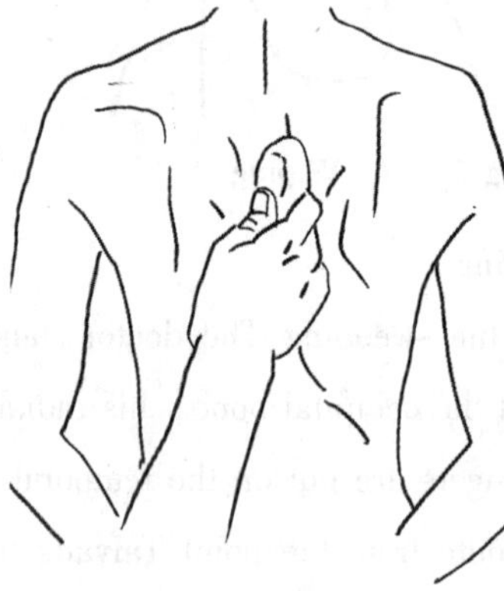

Fig. 3 – 34 **Scraping**

3.3.3 Category of circular-moving manipulations

Circular-moving manipulations refer to those actions during which the manipulator puts his fingers, palms or other parts of body on the patient's body and moves them circularly while keeping in constant pressing force.

3. 3. 3. 1 Principal techniques of circular – moving manipulations: circular-rubbing

Rubbing means to stroke. There are two main manipulative manners in circular-rubbing. The manipulative manner in which the print regions of the index, middle and ring fingers are put on the patient's body is named as circular-rubbing with the fingers; while the whole palm is put on body, it is named as circular-rubbing with the palm.

1. Circular – rubbing with the fingers.

With his elbow flexed slightly, the wrist and fingers extended naturally, the manipulator puts the print regions of the fingers on the patient's body surface, then swings the forearm actively to rotate the wrist joint and cause the fingerprints to rub on the body surface passively in circular form (Fig. 3 – 35).

2. Circular – rubbing with the palm.

The manipulative pattern is similar to circular-rubbing with the fingers. But the manipulator touches patient's skin with whole palm (Fig. 3 – 36).

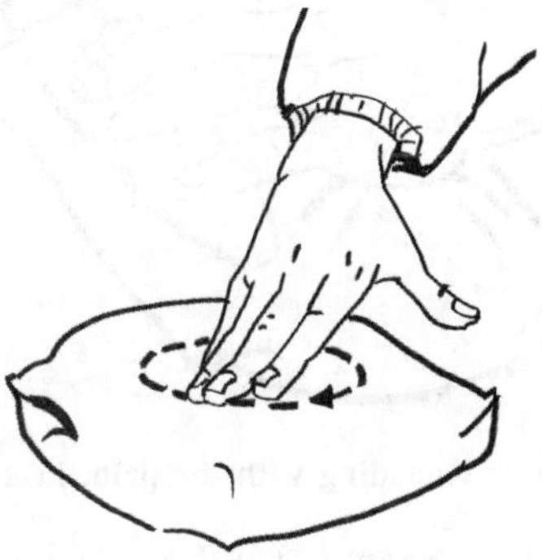

Fig. 3 – 35 Circular – rubbing with the fingers

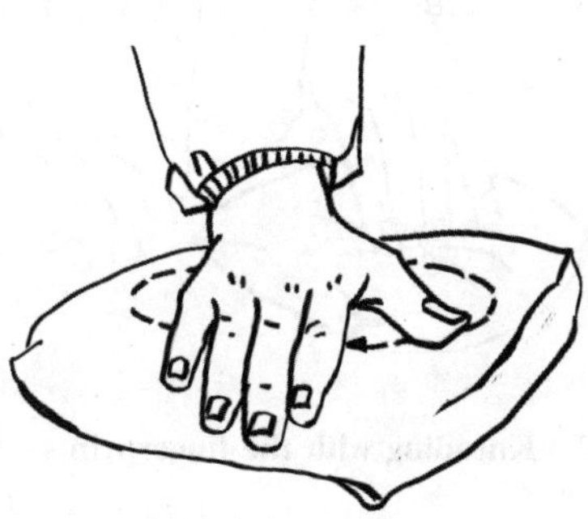

Fig. 3 – 36 Circular – rubbing with the palm

When applying circular-rubbings, the motion should be gentle; the force should not be too heavy, and both rubbings in clockwise and anti-clockwise are feasible. The manipulative frequency is about 100 to 120 times per minute. The stimulation of circular-rubbing is comfortable and mild. It is suitable for manipulation on the thorax, the abdomen, the rib regions as well as other parts where the soft tissues is injured and swollen. It has the effects of comforting thorax, regulating Qi, smoothing liver, regulating digestive function and promoting blood circulation. So the circular-rubbing is used to treat stuffed thorax and rib regions, stomach and abdomen pain, indigestion, diarrhea, constipation, sprain or contusion of soft tissue. In ancient times, the doctor often applied some herb paste on skin to enhance the curative effects of manipulation when the circular-rubbing was done. This is named as paste circular-rubbing.

3. 3. 3. 2 Evolution of circular-rubbing

1. Kneading.

Based on the action of circular-robbing, if the vertical pressing force is increased and the range of circular moving is reduced, the manipulator's hand will adhere to the patient's skin and keep in relatively fixed location, but drive the shallow subcutaneous tissue to knead on the deep tissue circularly. The manipulation becomes kneading. So the ancient book, *Bao Chi Tui Na Fa* said: "The kneading is referred to the manipulation in which the doctor puts his fingers to press baby's acupoints and rotates on the skin circularly without leaving his fingers from the acupoints." The book *Li Zheng An Mo Yao Shu* states that, "Kneading means to revolve, to circle on the skin with hand. It should be light and mild. It is developed from the circular-rubbing."

There are as many as 4 different manipulative patterns in kneading. They are kneading with the fingerprints, kneading with the palm heel, kneading with the thenar, and kneading with radial side of the thumb etc.

(1) kneading with the fingerprints: It is referred to kneading on patient's skin with the print regions of the index, middle and ring fingers. The manipulative manner is similar to circular-rubbing with fingers (Fig. 3 – 37).

(2) kneading with the palm heel: The manipulator extends his wrist joint slightly, flexes his fingers naturally, and puts his palm heel on the patient's skin to knead circularly. The action manner is very similar to circular-rubbing with the palm (Fig. 3 – 38).

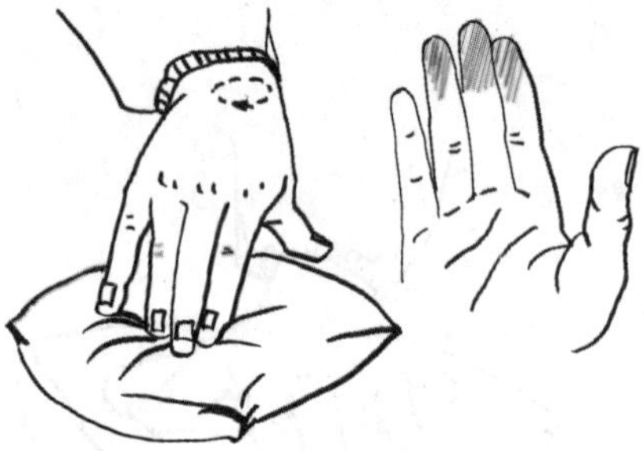

Fig. 3 – 37 Kneading with the fingerprints

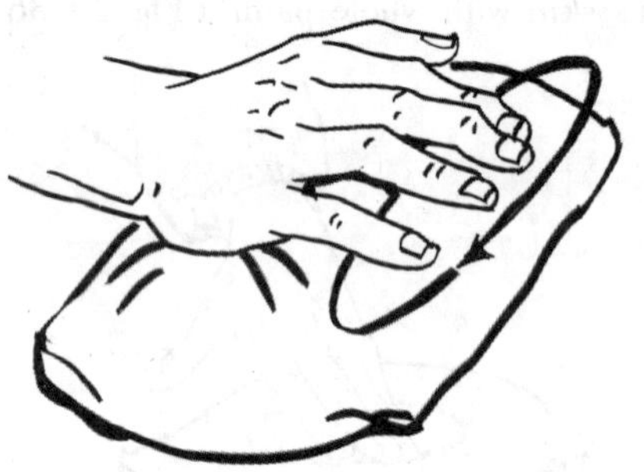

Fig. 3 – 38 Kneading with the palm heel

(3) kneading with the thenar: With the elbow joint flexed about 120° and the wrist joint relaxed, the manipulator keeps the two joints at the same level and the ulnar side of the hand in anterior while the radial side in posterior. Then puts the thenar eminence on the patient's skin (Fig. 3 – 39), and swings the forearm actively to drive the wrist joint and the first metacarpophalangeal joint to turn around. In this way, the thenar eminence and the skin and the subcutaneous tissues is moved together on the interface of the deep tissue (Fig. 3 – 40, 3 – 41).

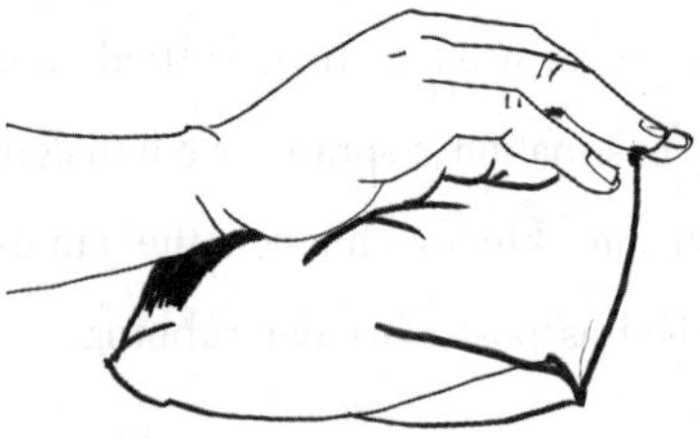

Fig. 3 – 39 Front view of kneading with the thenar

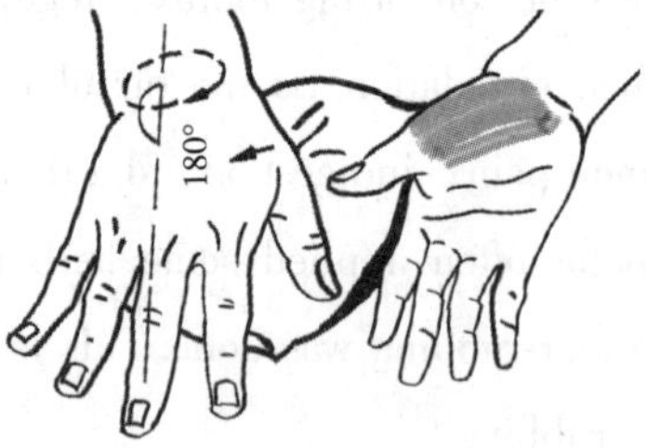

Fig. 3 – 40 Anterior swinging of kneading with the thenar

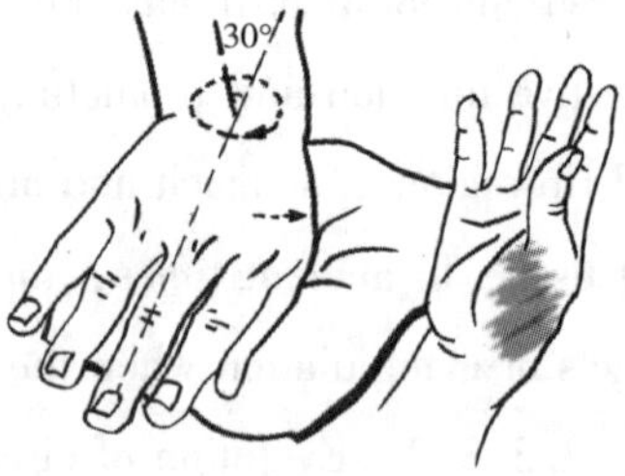

Fig. 3 – 41 Posterior swinging of kneading with the thenar

(4) kneading with the radial side of the thumb: The manipulative manner is similar to kneading with the thenar. But the manipulator touches patient's skin with his radial side of the thumb to knead (Fig. 3 – 42, 3 – 43, 3 – 44).

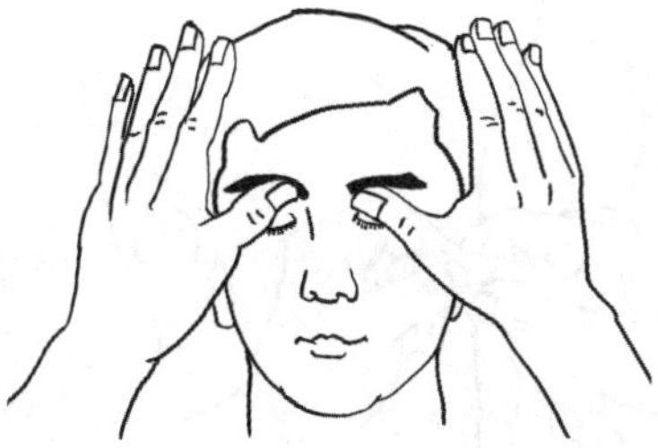

Fig. 3 – 42 Kneading with the radial side of the thumb

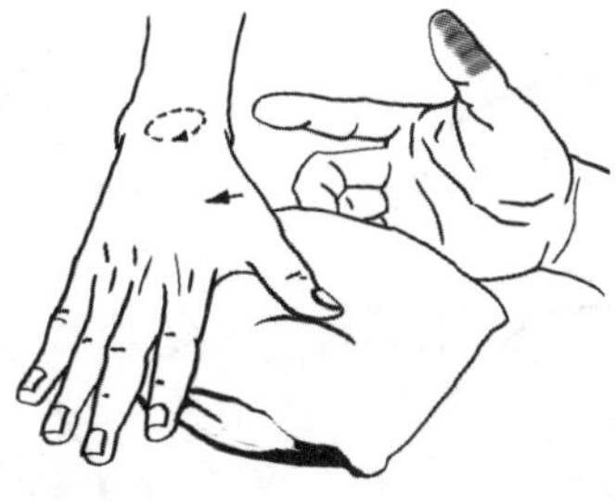

Fig. 3 – 43 Anterior swinging of kneading with the radial side of the thumb

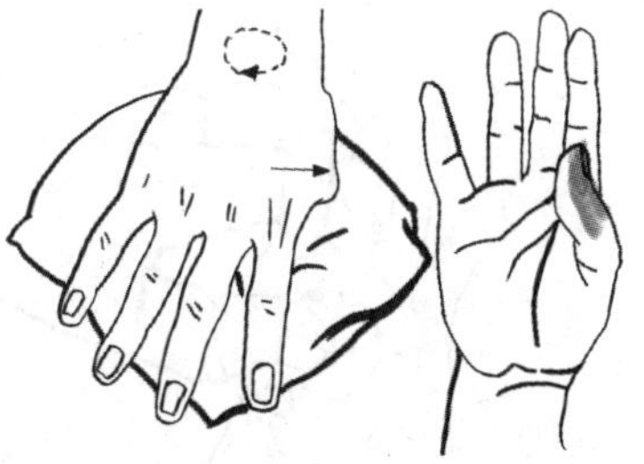

Fig. 3 – 44 Posterior swinging of kneading with the radial side of the thumb

The kneading manipulation should be slight, quick and gentle, but not be heavy. Its frequency is about 120 to 160 times per minute.

The stimulation of kneading is gentle and mild. Its adapting range is very broad. The kneading with finger prints is mainly applied to pediatric Tuina. The kneading with palm heel is often used for manipulating on those body parts whose surfaces are flat, such as abdomen, rib region and back. The kneading with thenar is frequently employed for manipulation on head, face, thorax and rib regions. And the kneading with radial side of the thumb is used for manipulating on eyehole and intercostal space. The manipulation have those effects such as conforming thorax, regularizing Qi, tonifying the spleen and harmonizing the stomach, promoting blood circulation to eliminate homeostasis, relaxing muscles and tendons, removing swelling and relieving pain etc. Those illness such as thoracic and hypochondriac pain, fullness in stomach and abdomen, diarrhea, constipation, headache, dizziness, insomnia due to neurasthenia, facial paralysis, injury of soft tissues etc. are all its indications.

2. Transporting.

Based on the action of circular-rubbing, if the pressing force is decreased, the tip of the thumb or the middle finger gently touches the skin of baby, and the rubbing is moved very slowly, the manipulation is changed into transporting (Fig. 3 – 45). During transporting manipulation, the baby's skin is not out of shape and only the tactile sensation is felt. But during circular-rubbing, the skin is slightly pressed and the pressures sensation is caused. Sometimes the arch-shaped pushing whose force is very light is also called transporting in pediatric Tuina. Transporting should be slight and mild, but not heavy and rapid. It should be manipulated 60 to 80 times per minute. Transporting is adapted to manipulating on the acupoints of baby's hand, such as transporting Eight Diagrams, transporting Water to Earth. The curative effects are determined by what points are acted.

3. Circular-pushing.

Based on the action of transporting, if the pressing force is increased and the range of circular moving is reduced, the manipulation is called circular-pushing (Fig. 3 – 46). Circular pushing is suitable for acting on the acupoints on baby's fingers. The frequency is 200 to 240 times per minute. Its curative effects are inclined to tonifying.

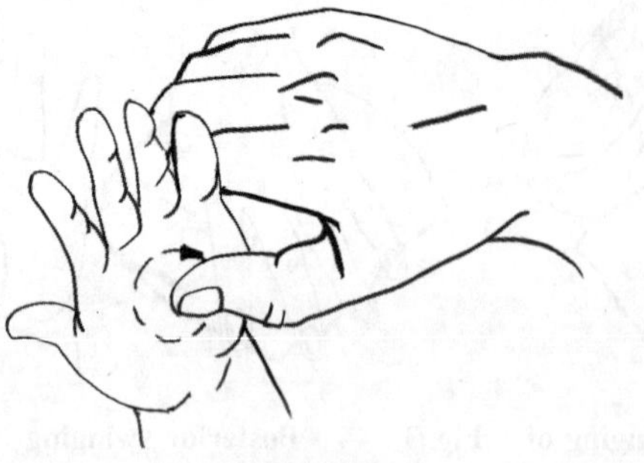

Fig. 3 – 45 **Transporting**

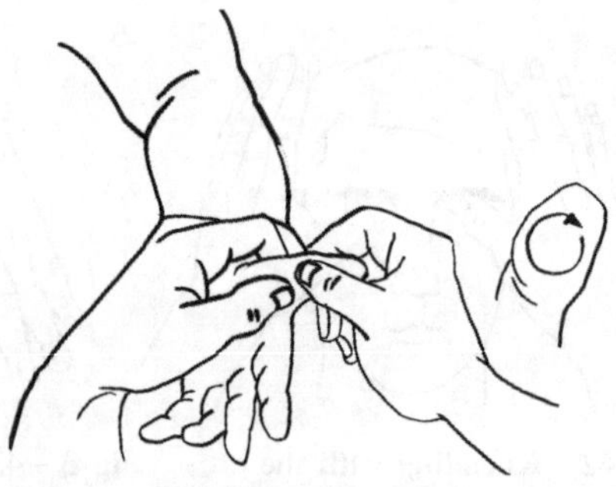

Fig3 – 46 **Circular-pushing**

3. 3. 3. 3 Compound manipulation: pressing – kneading

Based on the pressing manipulation and adding slow circular motion, or based on the kneading manipulation and increasing the pressing force, the manipulation becomes pressing – kneading. The pressing-kneading (Fig. 3 – 47) increases stimulation to the acupoints, but doesn't raise pain level. It is suitable for manipulation on acupoints.

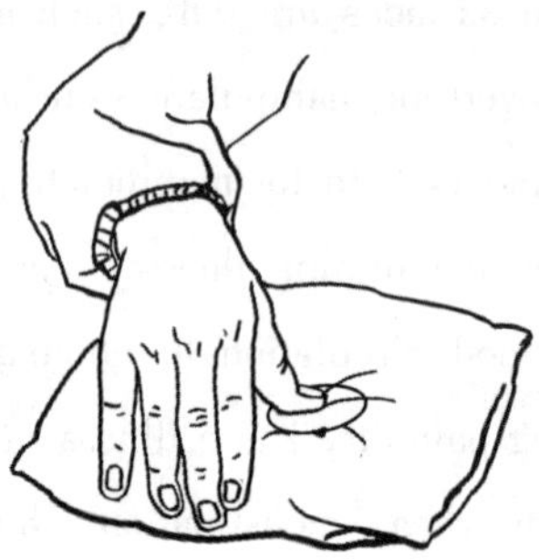

Fig. 3 – 47 **Pressing-kneading**

[Appendix] Manipulation exercise of circular-rubbing and kneading

When one drills circular rubbing or kneading, the beginner will often feel the action being stiff and rough. What is the matter? First, one has not found out the right manipulative manner. Second, his wrist joint lacks pliability and toughness. It is suggested that the learner adopt the following drills:

(1) Turning the wrist round with crossing the ten fingers for 1 to 2 minutes each time to increase the pliability and toughness of the wrist joint (Fig. 3 – 48).

(2) With relaxing of the wrist joint, swinging the forearm actively to make the wrist joint swung from side to side (Fig. 3 – 49), in which the motion manner of the forearm is just the motion manners of the circular-rubbing and the kneading of doing the exercise, but the hand is free and its motion range is broader than that of the wrist. During circular-rubbing and kneading, since the hand is adhered to a point, the wrist becomes motion center and swings naturally and coordinately. Considering how the forearm acts during swinging wrist side to side, then drilling circular-rubbing and kneading according to this manner, one will quickly familiarize the right manipulative manner.

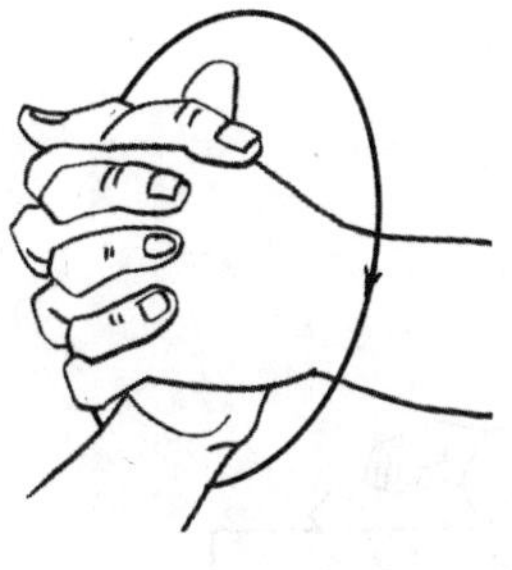

Fig. 3 – 48 **Exercise of turning wrists around**

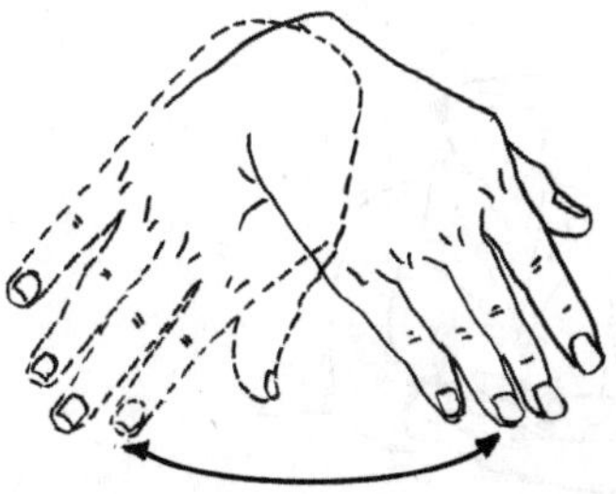

Fig. 3 – 49 **Exercise of swinging wrist**

3.3.4 Category of pushing-rolling manipulations

Category of pushing-rolling manipulation refers to those actions during which the manipulator makes his finger tip or hand back camber shapes to touch the patient's body surface; then his forearm swings actively to drive the wrist joint (or joints of thumb) to extend and flex and makes the contact part roll forward and backward. These manipulations are the characters and the creams of the Tuina of TCM.

3.3.4.1 Principal techniques of pushing-rolling: dhyana-thumb-pushing

Before drilling the Dhyana-thumb-pushing, it is necessary to rectify postures as follows. The manipulator sits upright with the thoracic and lumbar spine being flexed slightly, the shoulder and the arm relaxed, the scapula bone descended naturally, the elbow flexed and descended lower than the wrist, the wrist flexed fully, and the fingers flexed naturally to make an empty fist. Then he should put the thumb tip, which is extended naturally, on a point. Thus the palm side of the thumb just covers the "fist eye" and its transverse crease of the interphalangeal joint keeps close to index finger (Fig. 3 – 50, 3 – 51, 3 – 52).

Then, the manipulator makes sure that the upper limb is relaxed except for the wrist (The beginner probably has the tight feeling on the wrist region). If somewhere is felt stiff and uncomfortable, one must correct it at any time. Only being completely relaxed, will one be possible to achieve moving nimbly, manipulating durably, delivering force from the palm to the thumb, combining stiffness and flexibility, penetrating into muscles and tendons. Otherwise, the action will become rigid and hard to correct again.

After the upper limb is completely relaxed, one can drill the manipulation. At first, the elbow joint is extended slightly; the forearm is supinated and swung forward, and the wrist region moves forward. Thus the thumb is driven straight; the thumb-index web of the hand is opened, and the thumb print touches the exercise bag (Fig. 3 – 53). Then, the elbow joint is flexed slightly, the forearm pronated and swung backward, and the wrist moved backward. In this way, the thumb is driven to adduct and flex (It is not allowed to flex either); the first web is closed, and the thumb tip touched the exercise bag (Fig. 3 – 54). By combining these actions, the right manipulative manner of dhyana-thumb-pushing is gotten. It should be noted that, the ulnar side of the forearm is lower than the radial side during the forward swinging, but at the same level when the wrist swings backward to its limit (Fig. 3 – 55).

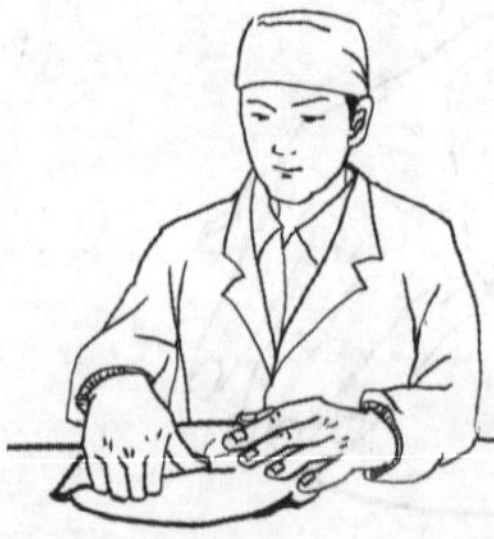

Fig. 3 – 50 **Posture of Dhyana – thumb – pushing (Frontal view)**

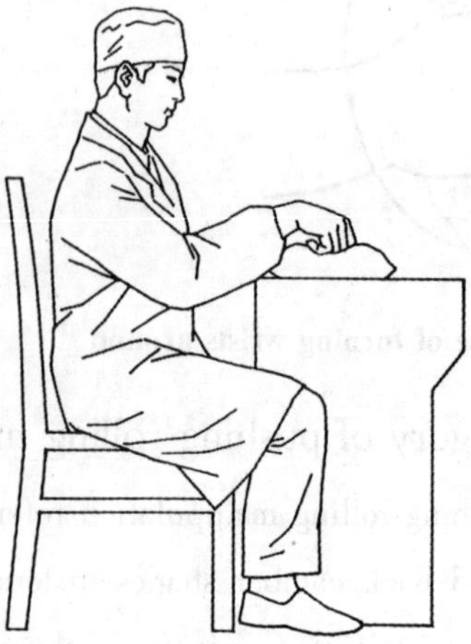

Fig. 3 – 51 **Posture of Dhyana – thumb – pushing (Lateral view)**

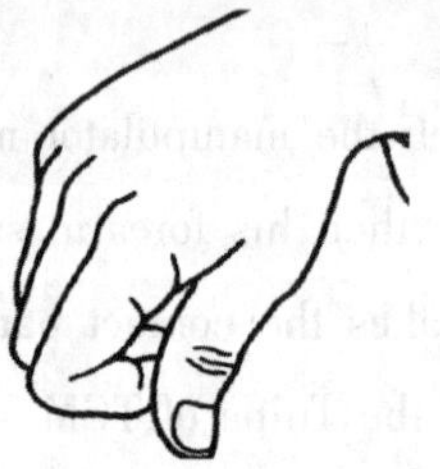

Fig. 3 – 52 **Hand shape of Dhyana – thumb – pushing**

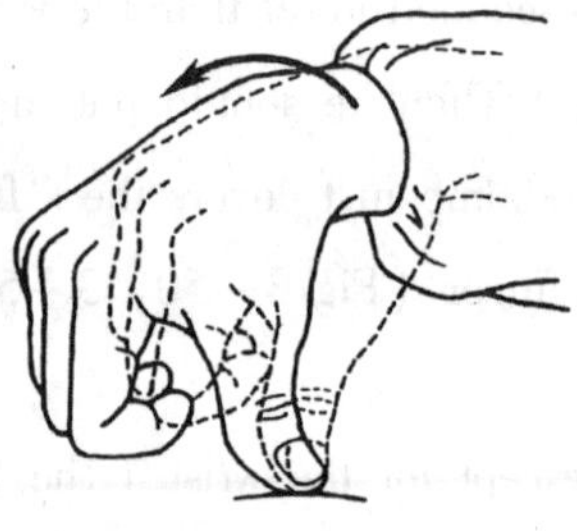

Fig. 3 – 53 **Forward swinging of Dhyana-thumb-pushing**

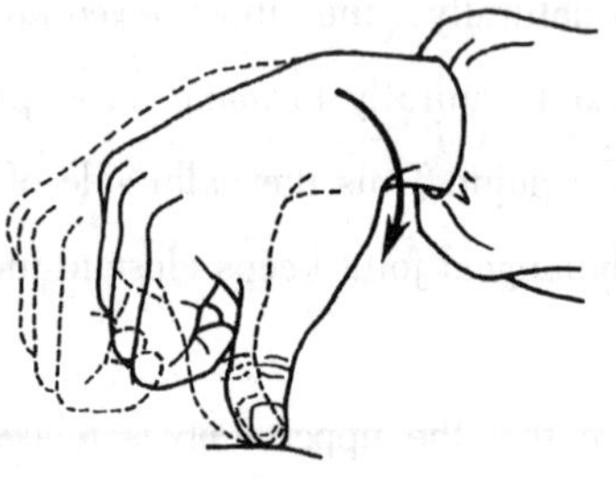

Fig. 3 – 54 **Back swinging of Dhyana-thumb-pushing**

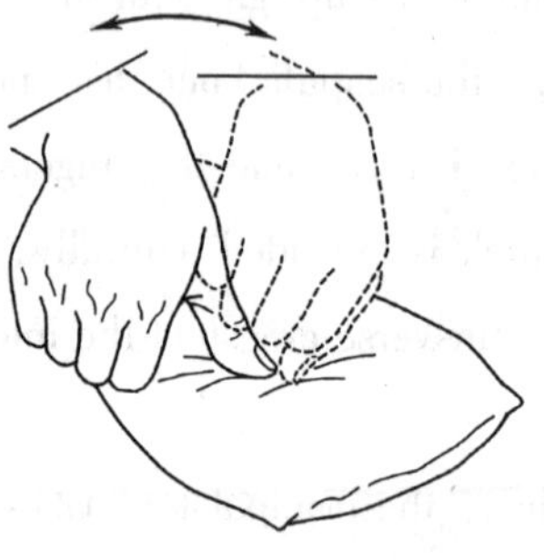

Fig. 3 – 55 **Illustration of the forearm rotation**

The manipulation of the dhyana-thumb-pushing requires that the action be harmonious and nimble, the pressing force be uniform and gentle. Sometimes light and sometimes heavy as well as sometimes quick and sometimes slow are not allowed. When you start drilling the manipulation, you ought to keep the thumb tip on one point, but not to make it slide during swinging of the wrist and the forearm. When you control the above requirements, you can learn to control your thumb tip along some specially selected lines (usually a channel route) to and fro. Follow your inclinations during manipulation. Besides, it is not permitted to press down deliberately and too forcefully. Its frequency is about 140 to 160 times per minute.

The contact area of the dhyana-thumb-pushing is small and soft. It can stimulate the channels and acupoints continuously, gently and forcefully. All the acupoints and the channel routes are adapted to be acted by this manipulation. It can relax muscles and tendons, dredge blocked channels and collaterals, promote Qi and blood circulation, adjust the functions of viscera. It is especially suitable for treating the diseases of internal medicine, gynecology and pediatrics. Those illnesses such as headache, insomnia, facial paralysis, diarrhea, constipation and irregular menstruation, show good responses to this manipulation.

3. 3. 4. 2 Evolution of dhyana-thumb-pushing

The above mentioned standard manipulative manner of dhyana-thumb-pushing sometimes is difficult to do in clinic due to the construction differences in different parts of the human body surface. So the Dhyana-thumb-pushing school of Tuina has created several variations. The frequently used are as follows:

1. Thumb-pushing with the side tip.

When the standard manipulative manner is applied on the head, face or thorax regions, the manner in which the manipulator flexes his wrist and holds his fist may make the fingers bump against the body surface. So if one manipulate on these regions with Dhyana-thumb-pushing, he should flex the wrist joint slightly, extend the fingers and put the radial side tip of the thumb on a point to swing forward and backward (Fig. 3 - 56). In fact, this manipulative manner and the kneading with the radial side of thumb are fairly alike. The moving route of thumb pushing with the side tip on head and face is fixed.

2. Couple flying butterflies.

Fengchi is an important acupoint in clinic of Tuina therapy. Generally, if manipulated on the neck, one should use two hands to do thumb-pushing with tips so as to stimulate the bilateral acupoints Fengchi at the same time. Therefore, it is vividly named as couple flying butterflies (Fig. 3 -57).

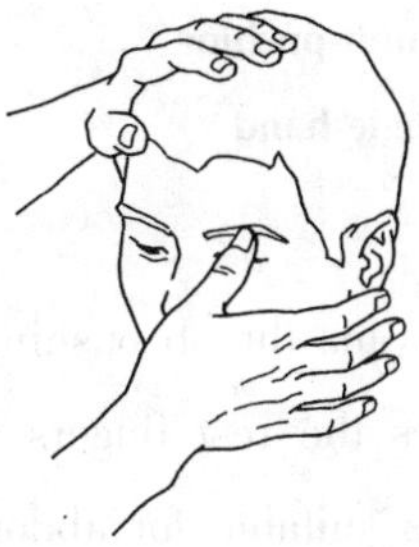

Fig. 3 - 56 Thumb-pushing with the side tip

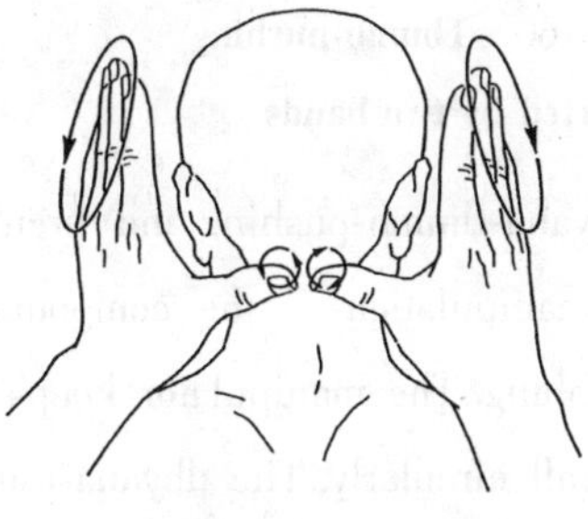

Fig. 3 - 57 Couple flying butterflies

3. Pushing with flexed thumb.

It is not easy to keep the thumb tip at a point when the Dhyana-thumb-pushing is done on the nape region. Moreover, since the nape muscles of the cervical spondylopathy sufferers are rigid, the manipulation force is hardly to penetrate into the deep tissues. The manipulative manner that the back side of the interphalangeal joint of flexed thumb is taken for touching area to do Dhyana-thumb-pushing is referred as pushing with flexed thumb (Fig. 3 - 58, 3 - 59). Its pressure is higher, its stimulation is stronger, and its stability is better. So the pushing with flexed thumb is adapted to manipulation on the nape-occipital region and the interval of bones and joins.

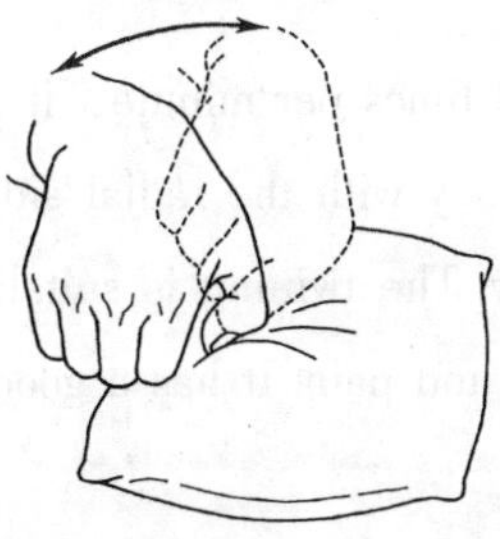

Fig. 3 - 58 Pushing with flexed thumb

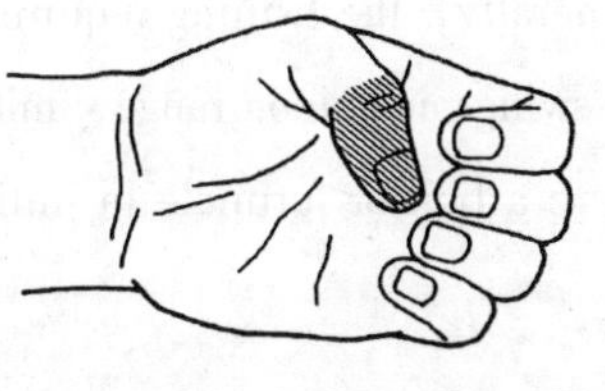

Fig. 3 - 59 Touching surface of pushing with flexed thumb

4. Thumb-pushing supported by two hands.

With extended fingers and opened first web, the manipulator puts two crossed thumbs on the two opposite sides of the patient's cervical spine and the rest fingers on the homolateral sides of the neck to stabilize the hands. Then swings two hands and moves the thumbs along the cervical spine in the meantime. The manipulation has good stability and high efficiency (Fig. 3 – 60).

5. Thumb-pushing supported by single hand.

When it is manipulated on joints of limbs, one generally used manner is the thumb – pushing supported by single hand (Fig. 3 – 61).

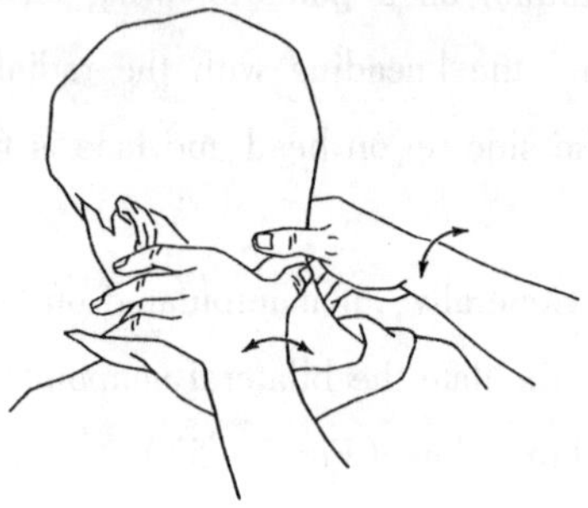

Fig. 3 – 60 Thumb-pushing supported by two hands

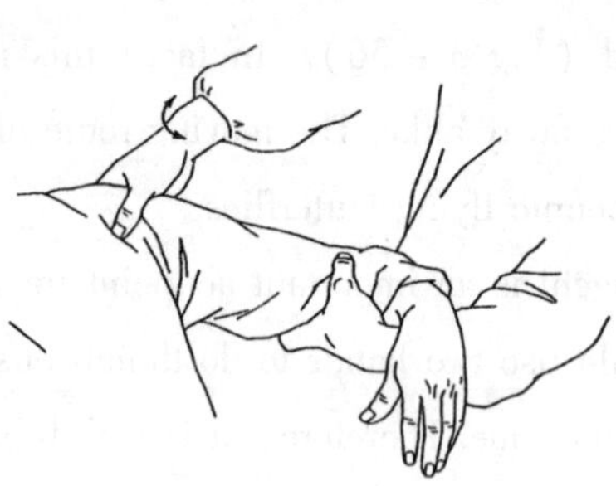

Fig. 3 – 61 Thumb-pushing supported by single hand

6. Dhyana-thumb-pushing and circular-rubbing.

This manipulation is the compound manipulation combining the Dhyana-thumb-pushing with the circular-rubbing. The manipulator keeps the thumb at acupoints and makes the rest fingers rub on the abdomen wall circularly. The dhyana-thumb-pushing and circular-rubbing is suitable for abdomen region (Fig. 3 – 62).

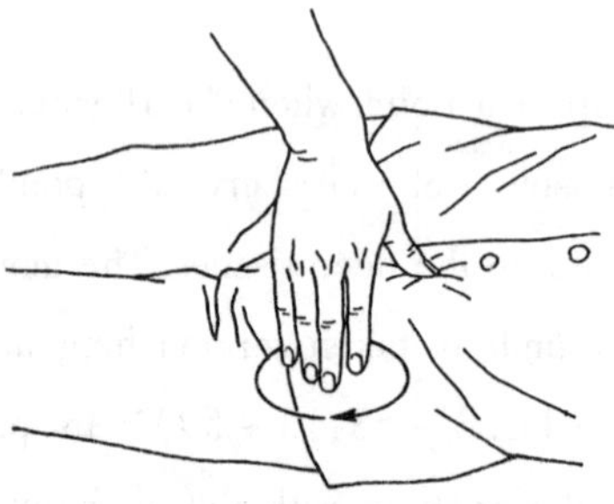

Fig. 3 – 62 Dhyana-thumb-pushing and Circular-rubbing

7. Twining.

If the manipulative frequency of dhyana-thumb-pushing is over 200 times per minute, it is named as twining. Generally, the twining requires that the manipulator touches body with the radial side tip of the thumb and swings in minor range, mitigative wave and high frequency. The twining is suitable for local regions where a boil or furuncle in initiating stage or the swollen injury and pain. It has a good dispersing effect.

3.3.4.3 Principal technique of pushing-rolling manipulation: rolling

Before drilling the rolling, you ought to hold the right posture as follows. The manipulator stands with two feet separated and the upper trunk inclined anteriorly. Relaxes his shoulders, flexes his elbow joint to about 140°, keeps his elbow a fist away from the anterior wall of the thorax, flexes his fingers naturally, and makes the hand back cambered shape along the transverse metacarpal arch (Fig. 3-63, 3-64, 3-65). Then puts the ulnar side of the palm on the patient's body.

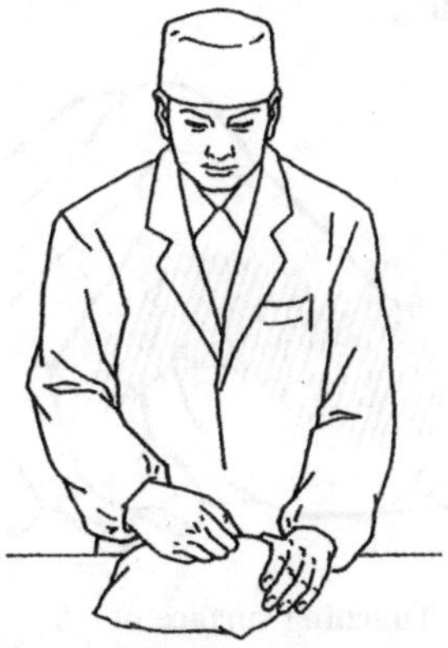

Fig. 3-63 Posture of rolling (Frontal view)

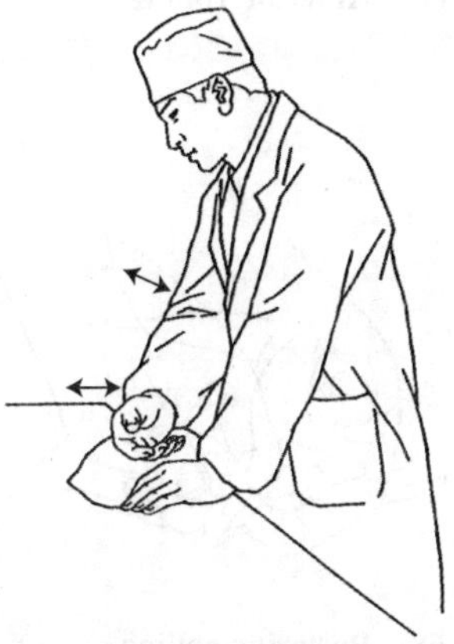

Fig. 3-64 Posture of rolling (Lateral view)

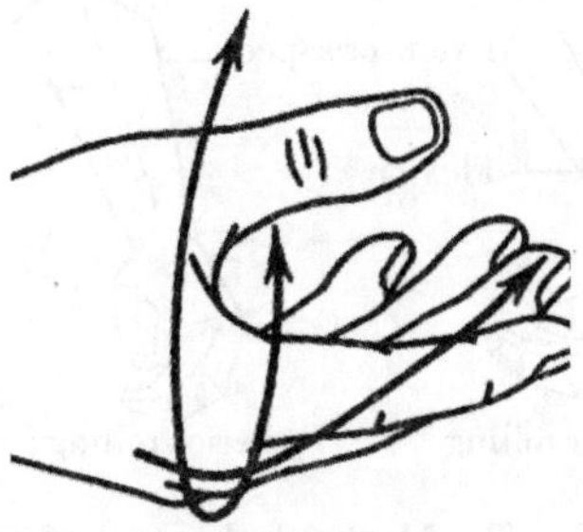

Fig. 3-65 Camber of hand back

When the posture is correct, one may drill the rolling manipulation. At first, the elbow joint is slightly extended, the forearm is swung anteriorly and supinated, and the wrist joint is relaxed and moved forward gradually. Thus the arch surface of hand back is driven to roll ahead until the interval between the second and the third metacarpal bone touches the body surface (Fig. 3-66, 3-67). Immediately, the elbow is flexed slightly, the forearm is swung posterior and pronated, the wrist is extended and moved backward and the hand back is rolled to back until the hypothenar side of the hand touches the body surface (Fig. 3-68). When the above actions are linked without breaking, the manipulation becomes a lasted stimulation with slight and heavy strength alternately (Fig. 3-69). In order to help readers to understand the manipulative manner of the rolling, one mechanical model is provided in Fig. 3-70.

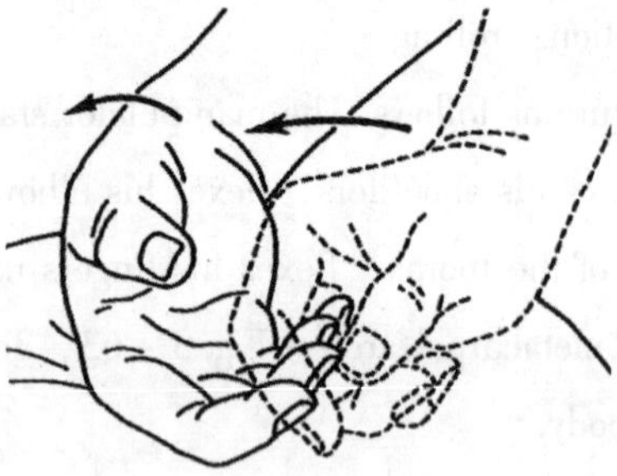

Fig. 3 – 66 **Anterior rolling**

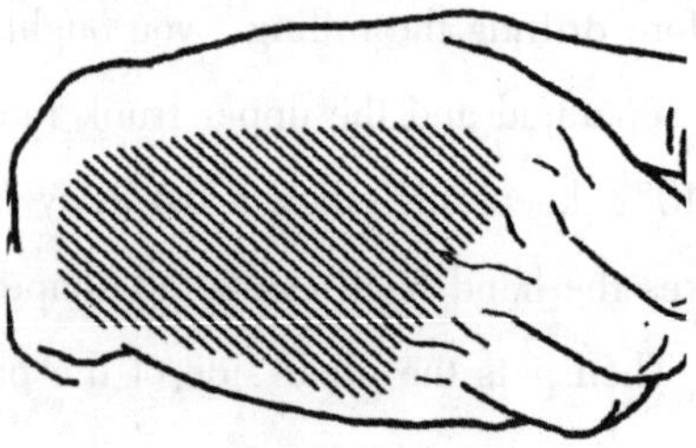

Fig. 3 – 67 **Touching surface of anterior rolling**

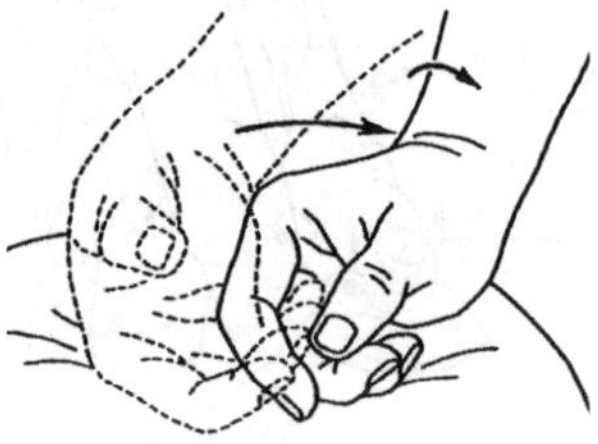

Fig. 3 – 68 **Posterior rolling**

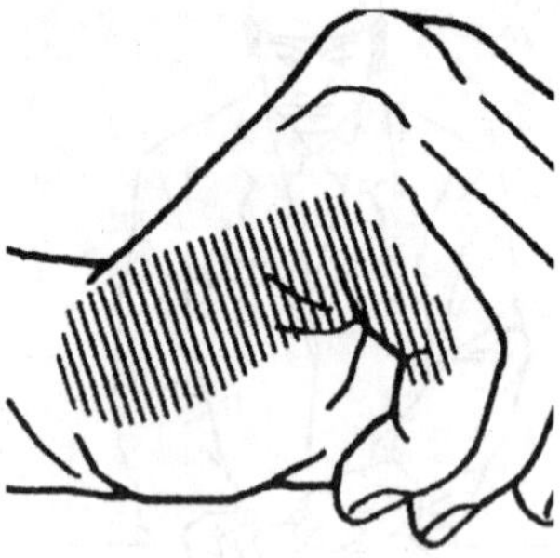

Fig. 3 – 69 **Touching surface of posterior rolling**

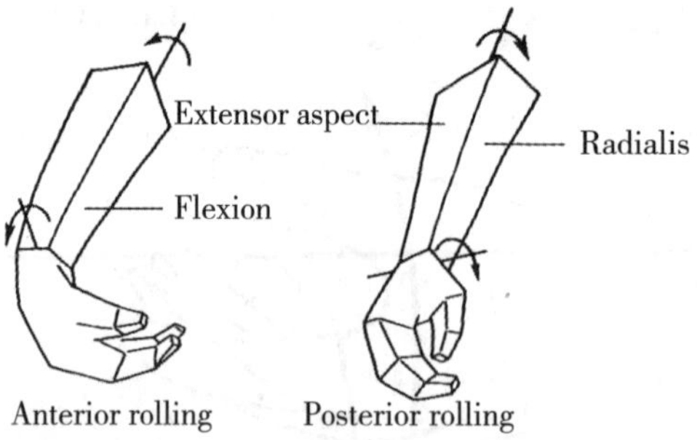

Fig. 3 – 70 **Mechanical model of rolling**

During rolling, the back of the manipulator's hand is rolled on the patient's body. If the two touching aspects slide relatively or the back of hand turns without touching, it is not right. During rolling manipulation, one must control the flexion-extensional movement of the wrist to keep the patient from feeling jumping sensation caused by sudden movement of the wrist as a folding knife. It is also not allowed to press down consciously. The pressing force, frequency and the swinging range ought to be uniform. The action must be harmonious and rhythmical.

The rolling has strong pressing force and large touching area. Its stimulation is both forceful and mild. It is suitable for manipulating on neck, shoulder, back, waist, buttocks and the major joints of limbs where the muscles are well developed. Rolling can relax the muscles and tendons, dredge blocked channels, lubricate joints, enhance the motive ability of the muscle and the ligaments, promote the blood circulation and remove fatigue. It has unique curative effects on healing the injury of soft tissues, the diseases of the kinetic system and the nervous system.

3.3.4.4 Evolution of rolling

1. Rolling with the metacarpo-phalangeal joints.

During rolling, the manipulator touches the body surface with the cambered surface of the back of hand, so its stimulation is relatively mild and comfortable to the patient. In the spreading and applying course of the rolling, it was thought that if the bone bulges of the metacarpo-phalangeal joints are taken to touch body surface and use the simple flexion-extension movement of the wrist instead of the compound movements of the flexion-extension of the wrist and the rotation of forearm, stronger force and stimulation could be achieved. The rolling with the metacarpo-phalangeal joints is adapted to cure those who suffer from stiff muscles and insensibility on back. Fig. 3 – 71 is the illustration of rolling with the metacarpo-phalangeal joints.

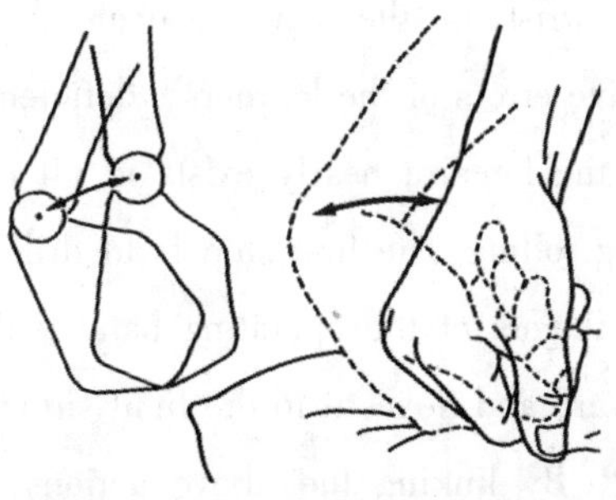

Fig. 3 – 71 Rolling with the metacarpo-phalangeal joints

2. Rolling with the proximal interphalangeal joints.

In this rolling, the proximal interphalangeal joints of the index, middle and ring fingers are used to touch body surface with the flexion-extension of the wrist joint to make the joints roll forward and backward. Rolling with the proximal interphalangeal joints is adapted to manipulate on head for curing headache, insomnia etc. Fig. 3 – 72 shows rolling with the proximal interphalangeal joints and the Fig. 3 – 73 shows its touching surface.

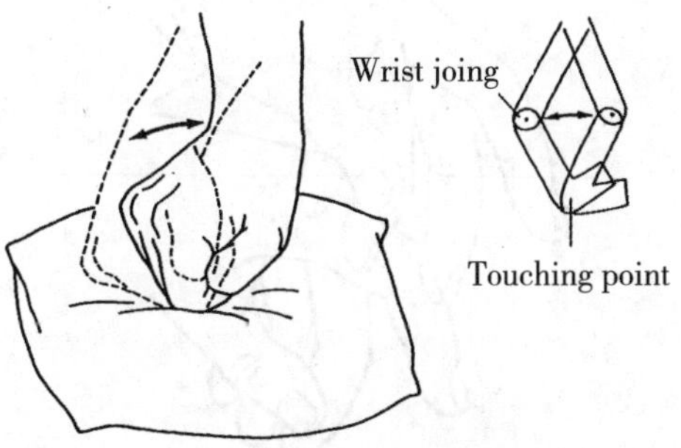

Fig. 3 – 72 Rolling with the proximal interphalangeal joints

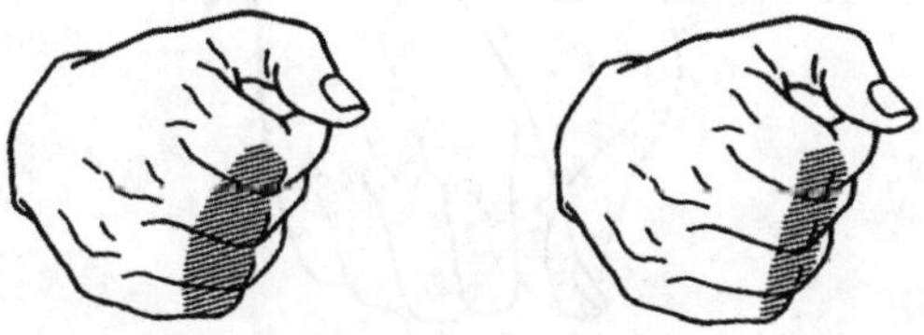

Fig. 3 – 73 Touching surface of rolling with the proximal interphalangeal joints

[Appendix] The drilling of dhyana-thumb-pushing and rolling

1. Drill of dhyana-thumb-pushing.

During the manipulative procedure of the Dhyana-thumb-pushing, the pronation and supination are the main aspects of its action manner. While the motion of the thumb is the accompanied motion caused by the wrist location variation in space due to swinging of the forearm. The learners usually pay too much attention to the motion of the thumb, and even more, they flex and extend the thumb consciously. Thus not only does the big thenar eminance feel painful and sore, but also the manipulation becomes inflexible. Because of these, the writer suggests learners to take two steps in the drill process of the dhyana-thumb-pushing. In the first step, the learners mainly drill correct swinging motion of the forearm and do not consider the passive motion of the thumb. One may close the first web of the hand, keep the thumb against the index finger, and then swing the forearm to and fro simply (Fig. 3 – 74). The second step is that, on the basis of harmonious and skilled swinging of the forearm, the manipulator relaxes the first web to make the thumb and the index finger opened and closed during the swinging process of the forearm.

2. Drill of rolling.

The flexion-extension of the wrist is the main aspect of the motion pattern in the rolling manipulation. Among the manipulative errors of the learners, deficiency of flexion-extension of the wrist is the commonest and the rotation of the forearm nearly exists in all cases. So the writer also suggests the learner to take two steps in learning rolling. The first step is to drill the flexion-extension of the wrist as follows. The manipulator holds the fingers of the operating hand with his other hand to fix it in certain location, then swings the wrist forward and flexes it to the limit situation, and then makes the wrist swing backward and extend to about 40°. By linking the above actions without breaking, the drill process becomes smoother and faster. In fact, during first step, the manipulative manner isn't the rolling movement but rubbing and slipping under the hypothenar side of the hand (Fig. 3 – 75). In the second step, after achieving harmonious and skilled flexion-extension swing of the wrist, the manipulator removes the fixation of the fingers and makes the touching part of the back of hand be changed constantly. Thus the rubbing movement is replaced with rolling, and the profound movements of the flexion-extension of the wrist and the rotation of the forearm is naturally formed.

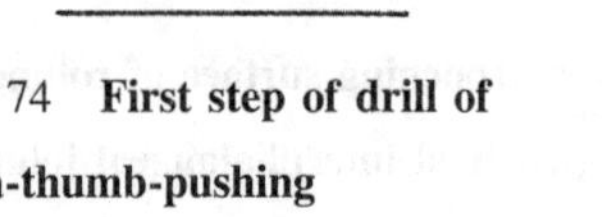

Fig. 3 – 74 First step of drill of Dhyana-thumb-pushing

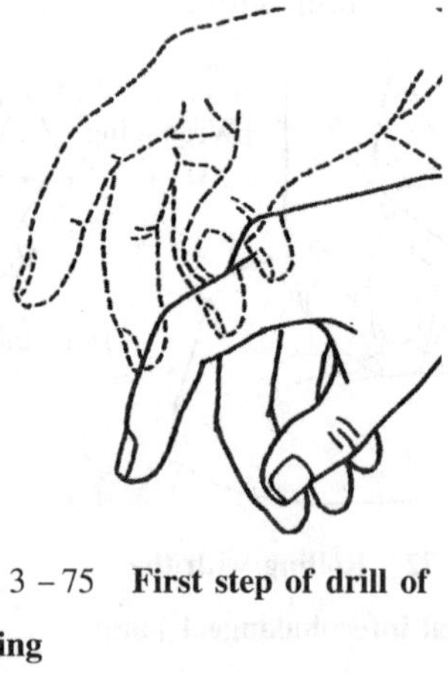

Fig. 3 – 75 First step of drill of rolling

3.3.5 Category of pinching-grasping manipulations

Category of pinching-grasping refers to those actions in which the manipulator squeezes body tissues from two opposite sides with his fingers or palms.

3.3.5.1 Principal techniques of pinching

The manipulation that the manipulator holds the patient's skin and some subcutaneous tissues and pulls them up with the thumb and other fingers oppositely is called pinching. The pinching is often applied on two sides of infant's spine. There are two different manipulative manners.

1. Pinching with the thumb and index finger.

The suffered infant lies prostrately to make the back muscles relaxed. The manipulator touches the paraspinal skin of the infant with the backside of the middle section of the index finger, which is flexed. Then moves the thumb forward to presses skin and pinches the skin between the thumb and the index finger. As the skin is pinched, the manipulator pulls it up and then lets it off. This action is done alternately by two hands from the point Guiwei to the point Dazhui (Fig. 3-76, 3-77).

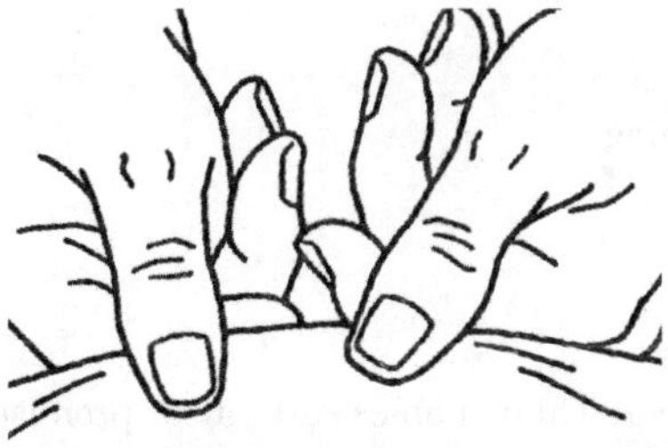

Fig. 3-76 Pinching with the thumb and the index finger

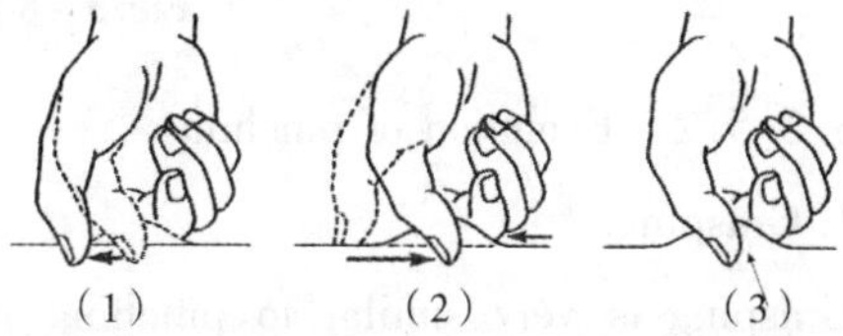

Fig. 3-77 Decomposed steps of pinching with the thumb and index finger

2. Pinching with the thumb, the index and middle fingers.

The infant's posture is the same as the above. With the thumb putting behind to touch the paraspinal skin, and the index and middle fingers moving forward to press the skin, the manipulator pinches the skin between the thumb and the two fingers. Then pulls it up and then lets it off. The two hands move forward alternately (Fig. 3-78, 3-79).

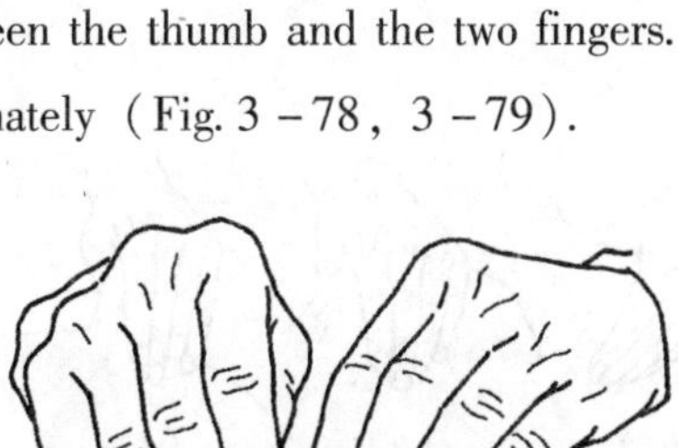

Fig. 3-78 Pinching with the thumb, the index and middle fingers

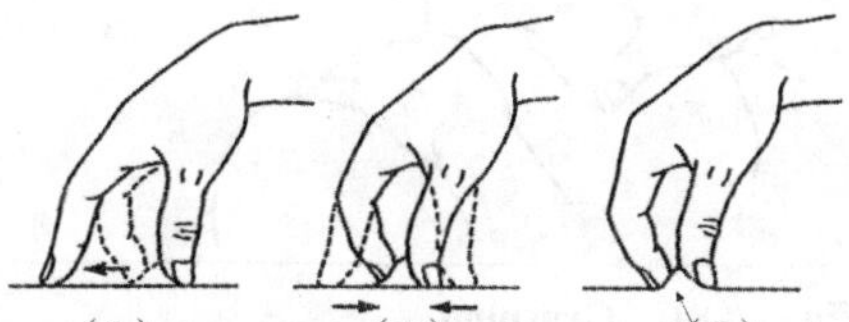

Fig. 3-79 Decomposed steps of pinching with the thumb and index and middle fingers

The clinical applying range of pinching spine is very broad, and it is especially frequently used in pediatric Tuina. It is generally believed that the functions of pinching spine incline to nourishing and invigorating. It can balance yin and yang, reinforce the spleen and normalize the stomach and strengthen the body resistance. It is used for curing malnutrition and food stagnation in children, indigestion, diarrhea, vomiting and poor health condition. It is also used for curing adult's diseases, such as digestive tract disorders, irregular menstruation, dysmenorrhoea, and insomnia etc.

Besides, there is pinching in orthopedic manipulations as well (Fig. 3-80). It is referred to that the manipulator squeezes the limb with his palms oppositely to make the pieces of broken bone close up to the longitudinal axis. It is suitable for correcting fracture such as comminuted fracture, long oblique fracture and long spiral fracture. The two pinching are different in manipulation but the same in name. Therefore, they should be distinguished.

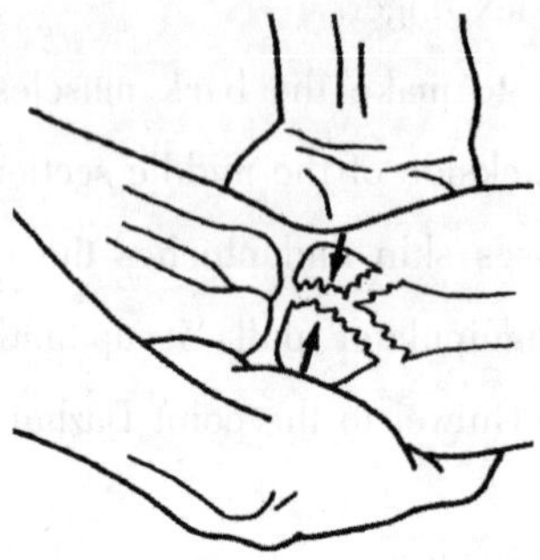

Fig. 3 – 80 Pinching of bone setting

3.3.5.2 Evolution of pinching

1. Grasping.

Grasping is very similar to pinching in manipulative manner. Their names are also promiscuous together due to writers' habits in various books because the concepts of them are not very clear. In general, pinching refers to the manipulation that only the skin and a little subcutaneous tissue are held. While grasping refers to the manipulation that not only the skin and the subcutaneous tissue are held, but the muscles as well, and then the muscles are slipped out of the fingers (Fig. 3 – 81, 3 – 82).

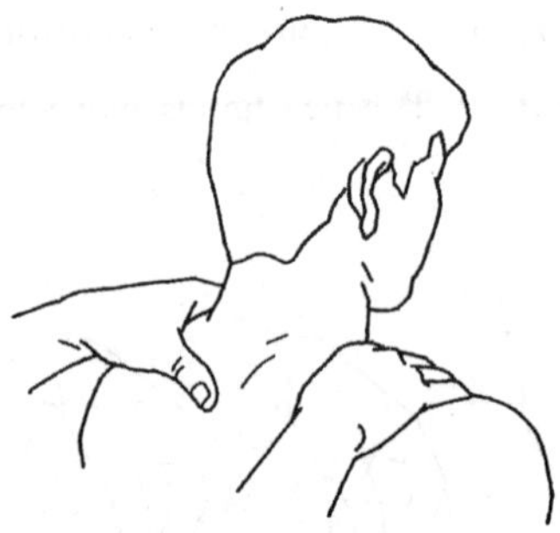

Fig. 3 – 81 Grasping

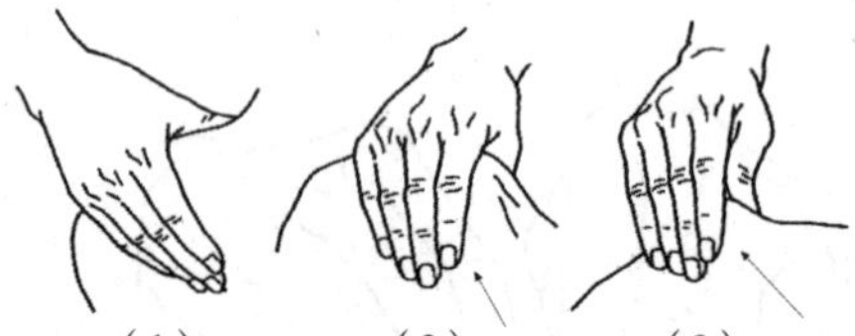

(1) (2) (3)

Fig. 3 – 82 Decomposed steps of grasping

The stimulation of grasping is relatively stronger. So you ought to straighten the fingers and put the flat finger-print regions on the skin. This action is like the action of a clip. You mustn't flex your fingers and put the sharp fingertips on the skin to cause pincer like action. Thus the patient can avoid uncomfortable sensation.

During the grasping manipulation, the wrist is relaxed; the pinching-grasping action is uninterrupted; the power is changed from mild to strong and then from strong to weak. Grasping is adapted on the neck, shoulder and limb regions where the muscles are developed. It has the abilities to dredge blocked channel and collateral, relax the muscle, relieve superficial syndrome by means of diaphoresis, relieve pain and invigorate the blood circulation. Those illnesses such as headache, stiff neck, arthrilgia, muscle sore, cold etc. can be treated by grasping.

2. Seizing.

Both in pinching and grasping, the manipulator compresses the tissues from both sides to the middle line with thumb and other fingers. If one compresses from several points to the central point with fingers, this manipulation is called seizing (Fig. 3 – 83). Seizing is a supplementary manipulation and is not so frequently used as pinching and grasping in clinic. It is suitable for manipulation on head, abdominal regions to cure headache and abdominal pain.

3. Plucking tendon.

In grasping manipulation, after the skin and muscles are held and pulled, the fingers are gradually loosened to let the skin and muscles go back to the original situation. If the fingers are loosened immediately to make the strained skin and muscles jump to original situation swiftly after the skin and muscles are held and pulled, the manipulation is called plucking tendon (Fig. 3 – 84). The plucking tendon is able to peel off adherence and relieve muscle convulsion and it is suitable for manipulation on muscles and tendons.

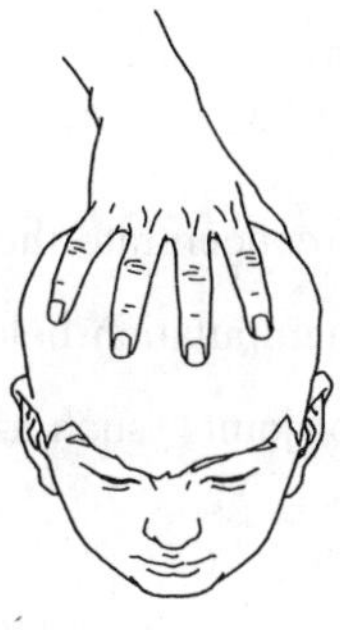

Fig. 3 – 83 Seizing

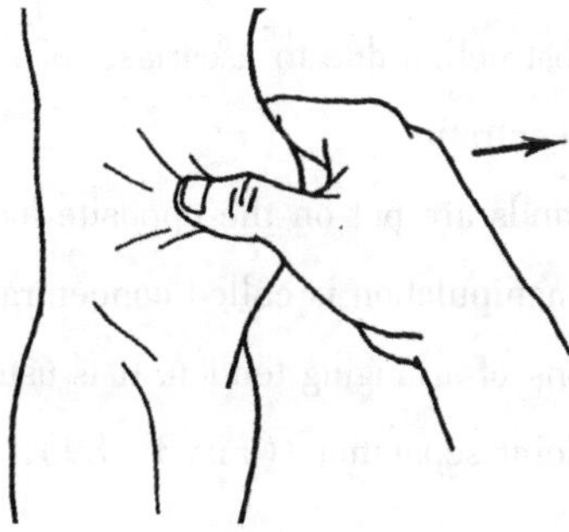

Fig. 3 – 84 Plucking tendon

4. Squeezing.

The force of pinching is very mild. Generally, the force is controlled not to cause pain, and the pinched points are changed continuously. If the compressing force of the thumb and index finger is stronger, and the action is repeated at the same site until the subcutaneous vessels are broken and some petechiae appear, the manipulation is named squeezing, or squeezing "Sha" (Fig. 3 – 85).

5. Tearing.

On the basis of the squeezing manipulation, if one proceeds to do the action of pulling until some petechiae appear under the subcutaneous tissues, the manipulation is named tearing or tearing "Sha" (Fig. 3 – 86).

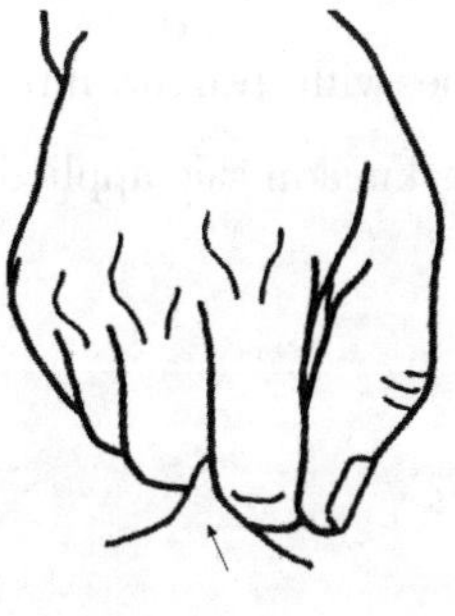

Fig. 3 – 85 Squeezing

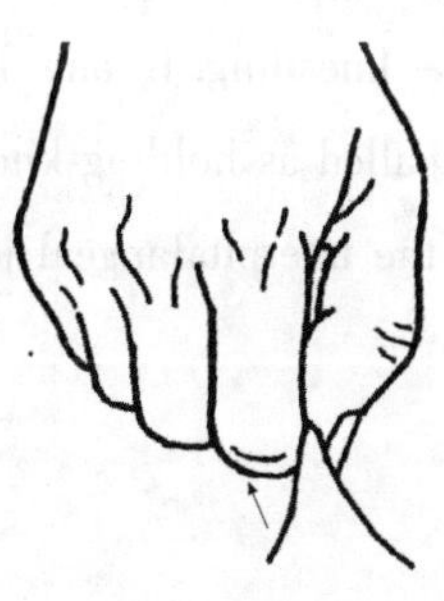

Fig. 3 – 86 Tearing

6. Twisting.

It is also called turning. In twisting, the manipulator pinches the skin with flexed proximal interphalanaeal joints of the index and middle fingers, then twists the skin rightward and leftward to make some petechiae appear within the subcutaneous tissue. It is also named twisting "Sha" or turning "Sha" (Fig. 3 – 87). Squeezing, tearing, twisting, and turning are all the folk methods used for "Sha" in early stage. They are often adapted on the forehead, bridge of the nose, neck and nape, chest, paraspinal region, and hollow of the elbow, and hollow of the knee. They have the effects of ventilating Qi, dispersing ill evil and regaining consciousness. And a lot of internal emergencies show good responses to them.

7. Shifting.

Putting the hand on the abdomen, the manipulator holds the abdomen as holding fists and pulls it up, then loosens the hand and moves forward a bit and repeat the above actions until the whole abdomen has been acted thoroughly (Fig. 3 – 88). This manipulation stimulation is strong and is applied to treat intestinal obstruction due to ascariasis of the children and the intestinal adhesion.

8. Concentrating.

Two hands are put on the opposite locations of a joint to squeeze it so as to concentrate the separated joint. This manipulation is called concentrating or concentrating reduction. This manipulation belongs to the manipulations of arranging tendon. It is usually applied to cure soft tissue injury of joint, such as the distal radioulnar joint separation (Fig. 3 – 89).

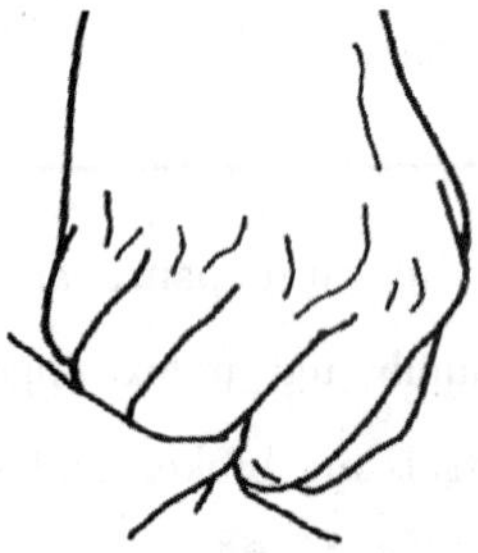

Fig. 3 – 87 Twisting (Turning)

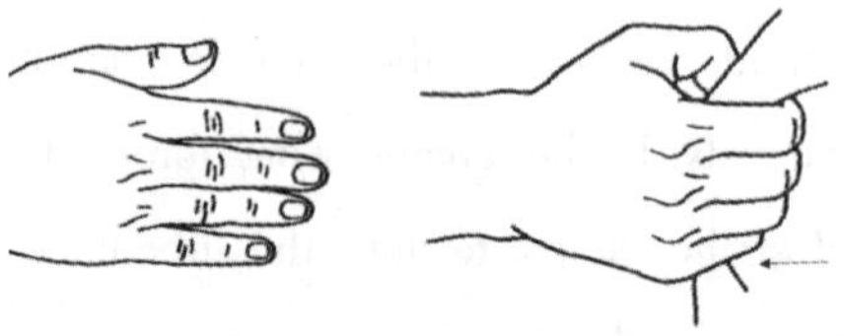

Fig. 3 – 88 Shifting

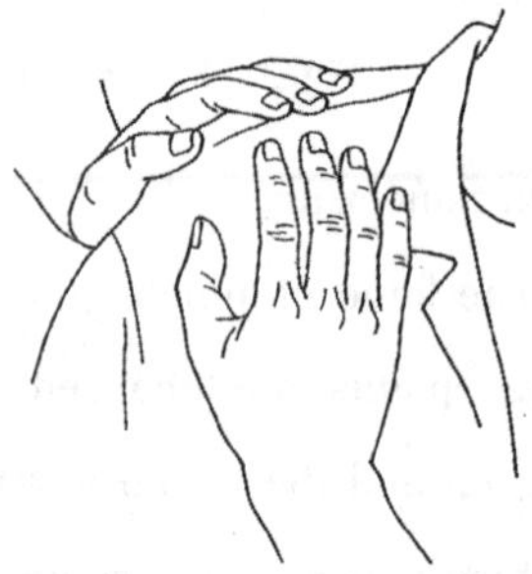

Fig. 3 – 89 Concentrating

3.3.5.3 Compound-manipulations

1. Pinching-kneading, also named grasping-kneading. On the basis of pinching or grasping manipulation and coordinating with kneading and twisting action, the manipulation becomes pinching-kneading or grasping-kneading (Fig. 3 – 90).

2. Holding – kneading. If one kneads and rotates a finger or toe with two or three fingers, the manipulation is called as holding-kneading (Fig. 3 – 91). The holding-kneading is applied to cure finger or toe pain and the interphalangeal joint sprain.

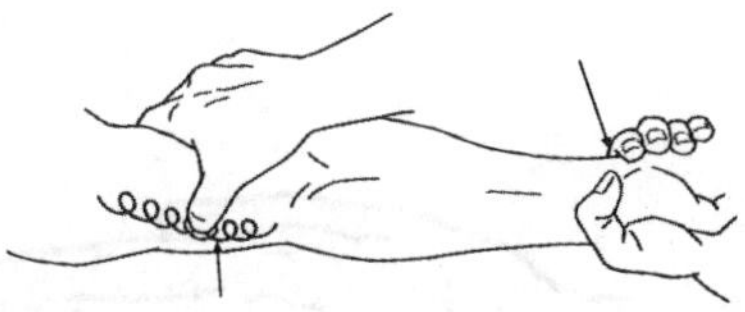

Fig. 3 – 90 **Pinching-kneading**

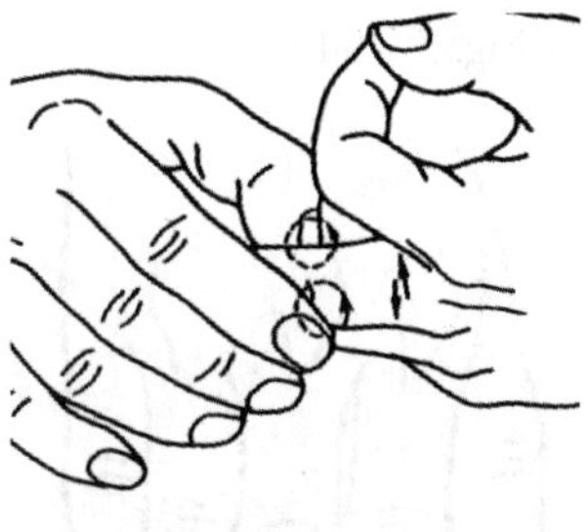

Fig. 3 – 91 **Holding-kneading**

3. Rubbing with two palms. Rubbing with two palms refers to concentrating manipulation coordinated with circular rubbing and shifting the palms along axis of the limb (Fig. 3 – 92). It is often used on the limbs, back and rib regions as an ending manipulation. It can relax muscles, relieve pain and promote the blood circulation.

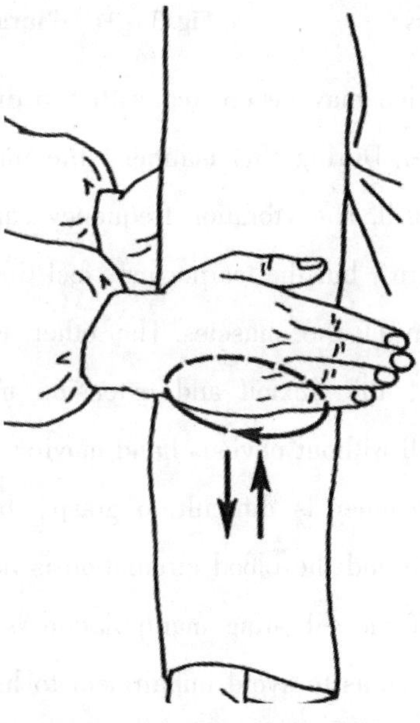

Fig. 3 – 92 **Rubbing with two palms**

3.3.6 Category of vibrating manipulations

The so-called "Category of Vibrating manipulations" mean those actions that the fingers or palms are put on the patient's body slightly, and then some higher frequency vibration produced by speedy and fine muscle motion of the manipulator is transmitted to the patient's tissues.

3.3.6.1 Principal techniques of vibrating manipulations: vibrating

The vibrating manipulations are divided into two manipulative manners, vibrating with palm and vibrating with fingers, according to the touching parts. But, their postures, manipulative manners are very similar. The manipulator abducts his shoulder about 30° and flexes his elbow about 140°.

1. Vibrating with the fingers.

The manipulator flexes the wrist, extends the fingers naturally and puts the tip of the index and middle finger at a point of the patient's body gently (Fig. 3 – 93).

2. Vibrating with the palm.

The manipulator extends the wrist and the fingers naturally and puts the palm on a part of the patient's body gently (Fig. 3 –94).

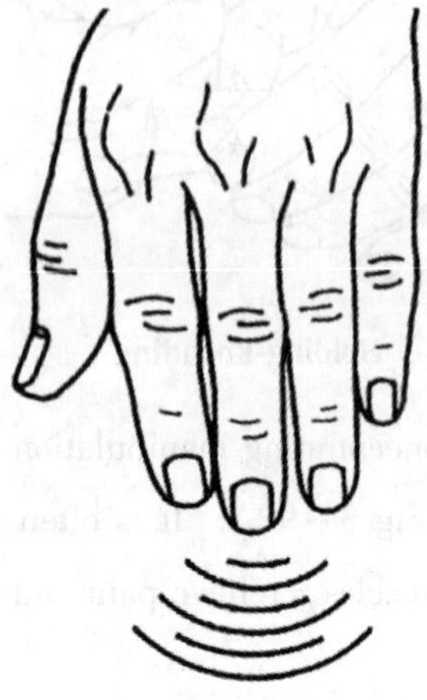

Fig. 3 –93 **Vibrating with the fingers**

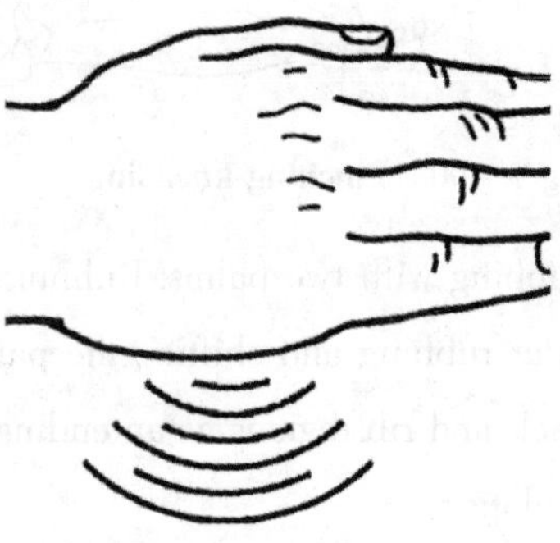

Fig. 3 –94 **Vibrating with the palm**

Then the higher frequency vibration may be created with two different manners of muscle motion. A sort of them is the convulsive manner. During this manner, the muscles of the arm are kept in static contraction intensely to bring about thrill. The vibration frequency can reach as high as 600 to 800 times per minute. This manner is easy to learn, but the learner may feel tired because of the muscles contraction that may block the blood circulation of the muscles. The other is alternative contraction manner of muscle. In this manipulative manner, the flexion and extension muscles make speedy contraction or dilatation in turn to engender fine thrill without obvious hand moving. The vibration frequency is about 300 to 400 times per minute. The later manner is difficult to grasp, but more durable, since the muscle contracting and relaxing are alternative and the blood circulation is not obviously affected.

Since the energy consumption of the vibrating manipulation is high, one should maintain natural breath and avoid holding respiration, so as to avoid impairment to his health. That the manipulator keeps his mind on the acted part of the patient is also allowed in vibrating manipulation. Thus it is so called "Tuina of Transferring Qi". Vibrating manipulation can cause the local tissues to feel warm and comfortable. It is usually applied to the supplementary manipulation for fullness and pain in epigastric and abdominal regions, indigestion and descended Qi in middle Jiao. It has functions such as invigorating the spleen, removing stagnant food, regulating the gastrointestinal peristalsis etc.

3.3.6.2 Evolution of vibrating: waving

The vibration of the vibrating manipulation is oscillated up and down. If the direction of vibration is changed to surrounding area transversely, the manipulation is called waving. When waving is done, the ulnar side of the hand is put on the patient's body with his wrist joint relaxed. Then the manipulator makes speedy and minor ringed movement of flexion and extension of wrist to cause the superficial tissues of the patient's body to generate high frequency vibration (Fig. 3 –95). Waving is manipulated on the chest, abdomen and limb regions. It has the effects of relaxing the muscles, regulating the digestive function, promoting blood circulation, alleviating spasm and relieving pain. It is often used to cure indigestion, muscle convulsion and swelling pain on local tissue.

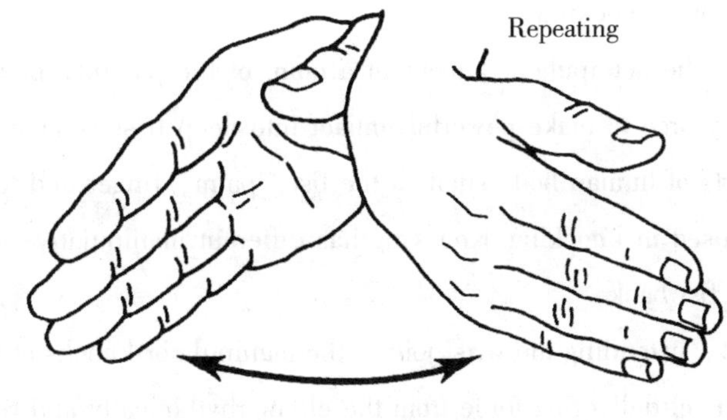

Fig. 3 – 95 Waving

3. 3. 6. 3 Compound manipulations

1. Lifting-trembling.

This manipulation is a compound manipulation combining grasping with vibrating. With opening the fingers to form semiflexion condition, the manipulator holds the patient's skin and muscles gently with the thumb, the index and middle fingers, and then makes the wrist and the fingers tremble quickly. This manipulation can be done with the two hands one by one (Fig. 3 – 96). This manipulation has the functions of relaxing muscles, promoting blood circulation and removing blood stasis, relieving pain, separating adhesion and so on. It is suitable for manipulation on the neck, limbs and abdominal regions.

2. Swinging.

Based on the lifting-trembling manipulation, the so-called swinging requires the manipulator to increase the movement range of trembling but reducing the frequency (Fig. 3 – 97). The manipulation is only used on the abdomen. It has the effects to remove stagnant food, smooth Qi, and separate adhesion. It is adapted to treat ascarid ileus of children and intestinal adhesion etc.

3. Concentrating-vibrating.

This manipulation is the compound manipulation combining concentrating with vibrating. Two palms are put on the symmetrical sides of the joint and then tremble and vibrate up and down (or left and right) quickly. This manipulation is suitable for manipulating on the joints of the limbs (Fig. 3 – 98).

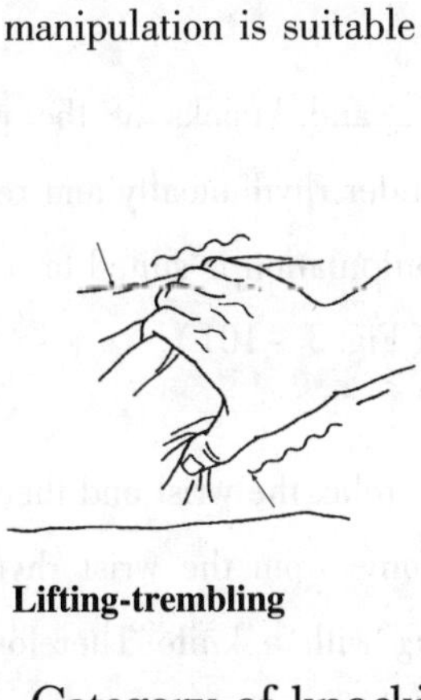

Fig. 3 – 96 Lifting-trembling

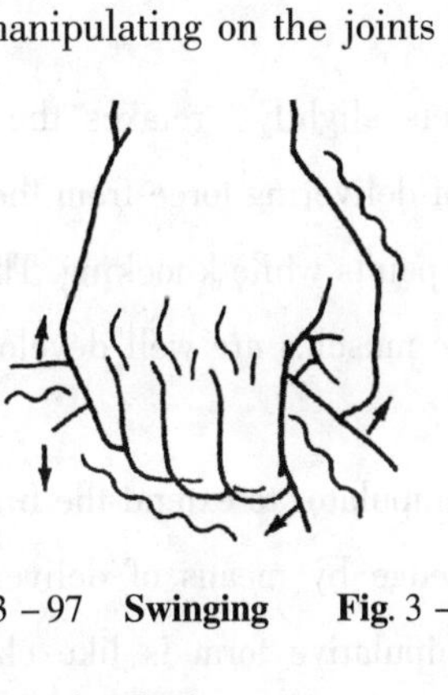

Fig. 3 – 97 Swinging

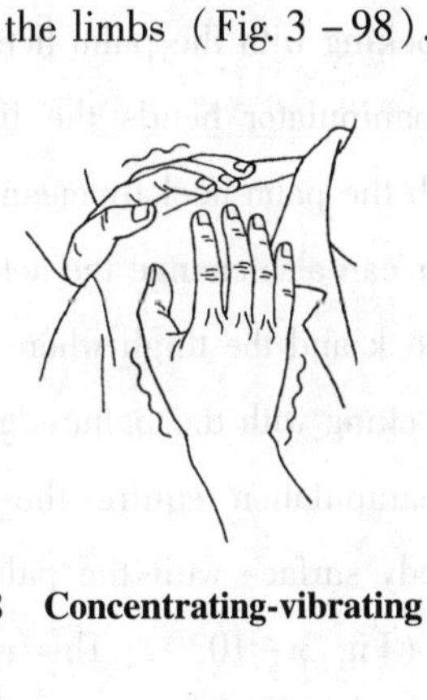

Fig. 3 – 98 Concentrating-vibrating

3. 3. 7 Category of knocking manipulations

Categories of knocking manipulation mean those actions during which the manipulator knocks the patient's body rhythmically and disconnectedly with one's finger, palm, fist or tools.

3. 3. 7. 1　Manipulation: knocking

The manipulation that the manipulator knocks at a point of the patient's body for one time or several times with relatively strong force to make powerful impact into deep tissues such as muscles, bone etc. is called knocking. Some parts of human body such as the fist, palm, finger and tools such as a stick made of mulberry twigs can be used in knocking. Knocking has different manipulative manners as below.

1. Knocking with the fist back.

Holding an empty fist, extending the wrist joint, the manipulator knocks at the patient's body surface with the fist back by means of delivering force from the elbow rhythmically and repeatedly. Or changes the acted points while knocking (Fig. 3 - 99). This manipulation is adapted to the shoulder and back regions.

2. Thumping.

Thumping requires the manipulator to hold two empty fists, relax the wrists, then knock at a point with the ulnar sides of the fists in turn by means of delivering force from the elbow. The force of thumping is generally lighter than that of knocking with the fist back. Thumping is usually applied on the shoulder, back and limb regions (Fig. 3 - 100).

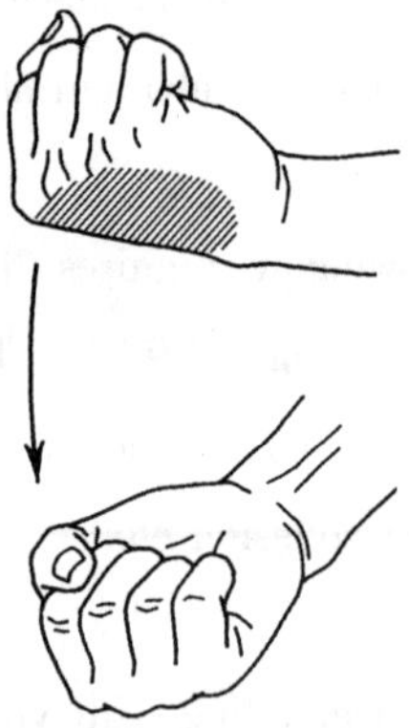

Fig. 3 - 99　**Knocking with the fist back**

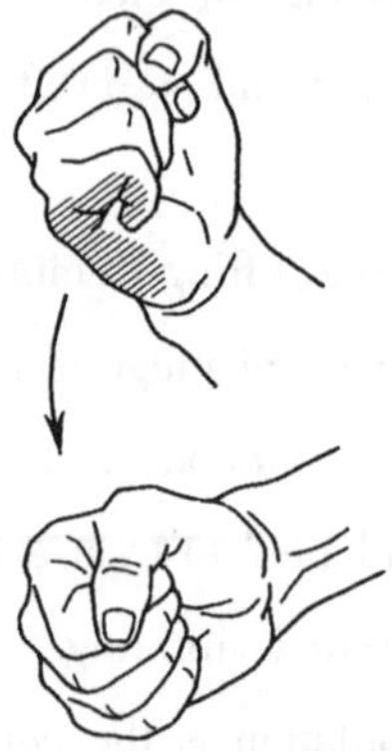

Fig. 3 - 100　**Thumping**

3. Knocking with the palm heel.

The manipulator bends the fingers slightly, relaxes the wrist, and knocks at the patient's body surface with the palm heel by means of delivering force from the shoulder rhythmically and repeatedly. The manipulator can also change the acted points while knocking. This manipulation is suited to be manipulated on the buttock and the thigh where the muscles are well developed (Fig. 3 - 101).

4. Knocking with the palm edge.

The manipulation requires the manipulator to extend the fingers, relax the wrist and then knock at the patient's body surface with the palm edge by means of delivering force from the wrist rhythmically and repeatedly (Fig. 3 - 102). This manipulative form is like chopping with a knife. Therefore, it is also named chopping. This manipulation is suitable for the shoulder, back, joints of the limbs and the cracks between fingers (or toes).

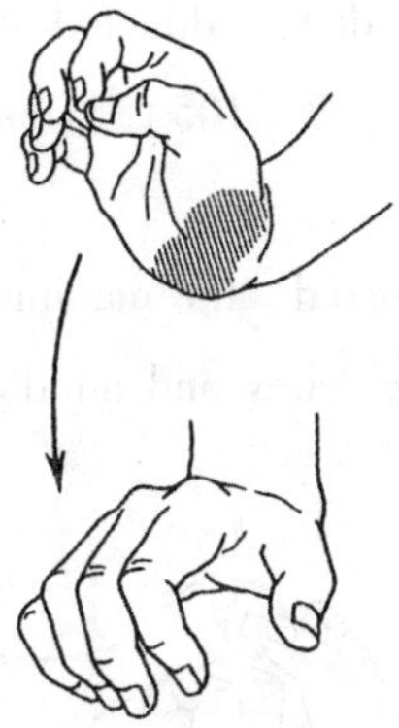

Fig. 3 – 101 Knocking with the palm heel

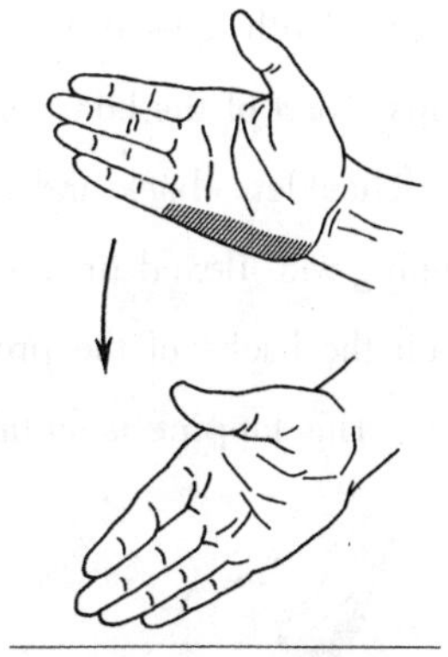

Fig. 3 – 102 Knocking with the palm edge

5. Knocking with the stick.

During this manipulation, the manipulator holds one end of a stick made of mulberry twigs (which is slightly elastic), relaxes the wrist and then knocks at the patient's body surface with the stick by means of delivering force from the elbow (it is slighter), or from the shoulder (it is stronger), rhythmically and repeatedly for 3 to 5 times, according to clinical condition (Fig. 3 – 103). Then move the impacting point while knocking. The force should be changed from light to strong but not too heavy. The stick axis should be parallel to the muscles and bones. The touching part of stick should be as large as possible. It isn't allowed to knock with the stick tip or to make the stick tip out of the patient's body (Fig. 3 – 104).

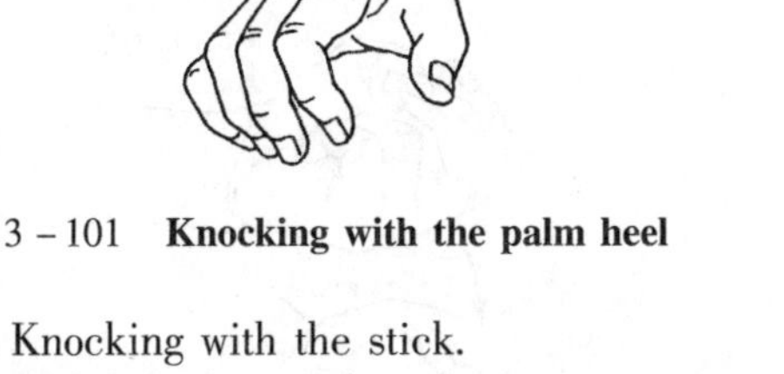

Fig. 3 – 103 Knocking with the stick (proper)

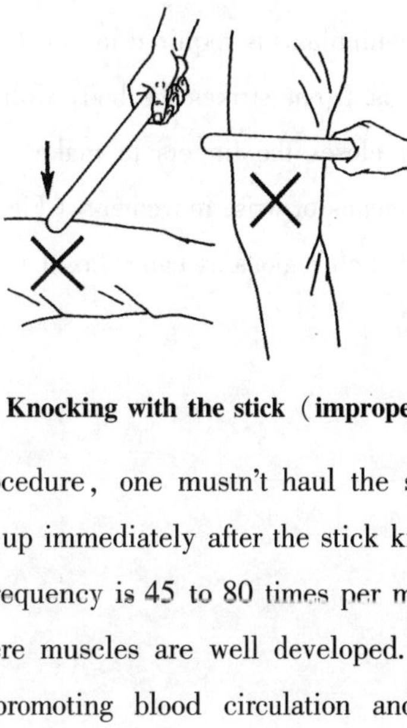

Fig. 3 – 104 Knocking with the stick (improper)

The force of knocking is strong. During the knocking procedure, one mustn't haul the stick while knocking. The knocking procedure should be brief, and spring up immediately after the stick knocking on the body so as to avoid injury of the tissue. The manipulation frequency is 45 to 80 times per minute.

Knocking is suitable for manipulation on those parts where muscles are well developed. It has the functions of refreshing the mind, restoring consciousness, promoting blood circulation and dredging channels. It is often used to treat dizziness and persistent numb limbs. It is also used to regularize the sportsman's spiritual condition before games.

3.3.7.2 Evolution of knocking

1. Tapping.

Based on the knocking manipulation, if the force is reduced to make its effect arrive only at the subcutaneous tissues and the muscles, and the frequency increase up to 80 to 100 times per minute, the manipulation is called tapping. Variations of tapping are as follows.

(1) Tapping with closed palms: With his fingers being extended, adducted and closed, the manipulator taps a part of the body with the ulnar sides of the palms (Fig. 3 – 105). This manipulation is suitable for the shoulder, back and thoracic regions.

(2) Tapping with flexed fingers: With his fingers being semi – flexed, the manipulator taps a part of the body with the backs of the proximal interphalangeal joints of the index and middle fingers briskly (Fig. 3 – 106). This tapping is suitable for pediatric Tuina.

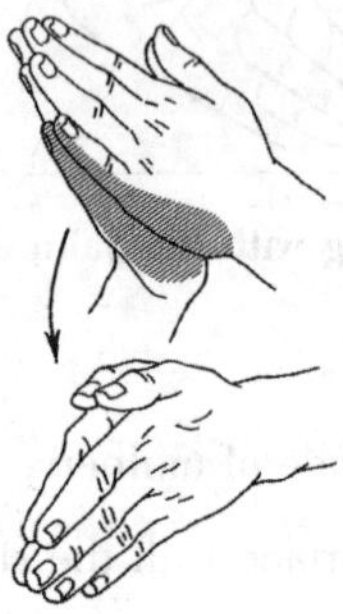

Fig. 3 – 105 Tapping with closed palms

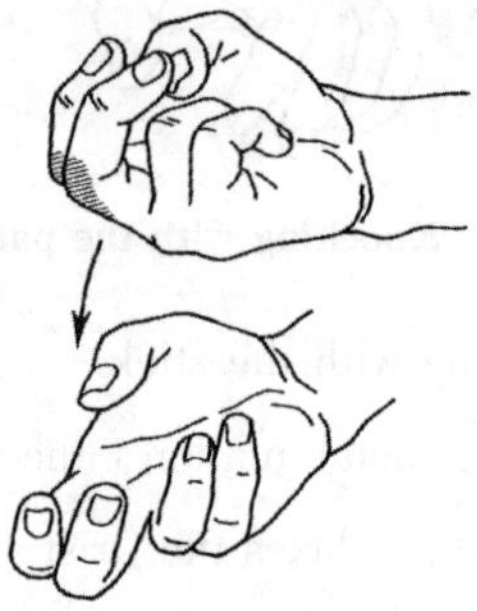

Fig. 3 – 106 Tapping with flexed fingers

Tapping is brisk in manipulating. It possesses the effects of relaxing muscles and tendons, promoting blood circulation, relieving tiredness, tranquilizing the mind and allaying excitement, and is applied to treat stress and insomnia, as well as restore energy after sport games.

2. Patting.

The manipulator is required to knock the body solidly both in knocking with palm heel and palm edge manipulations. If one strikes the body with a hollow palm briskly, the manipulation is called patting. The manipulator closes the fingers to make a hollow palm, and then knocks at the patient's body surface briskly by means of wrist movement (Fig. 3 – 107). Patting is usually applied on the shoulder, back, sacrum and limb regions. It can relax the muscles and tendons, promote the blood circulation.

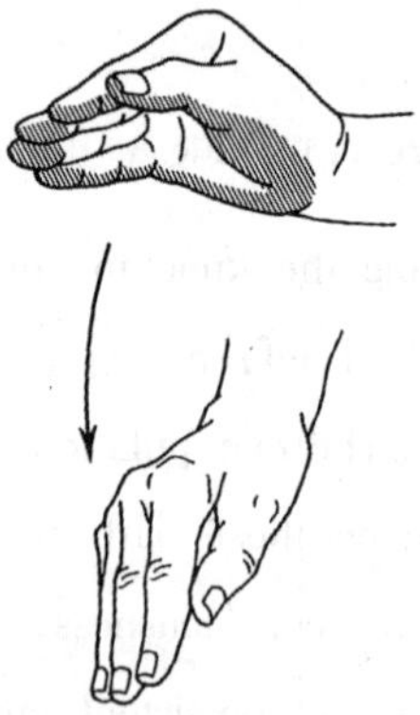

Fig. 3 – 107 Patting

3. Pecking.

The manipulator takes the fingers tips of two hands to knock at the body briskly and alternatively. Because this manipulation is like the pecking movement of a chicken, it is called pecking. In manipulation, the fingers tips are opened as a bird talon (Fig. 3 – 108) or closed as a plum flower (Fig. 3 – 109). Pecking is suited for manipulating on the head and face. It possesses the effects of tranquilizing the mind, restoring consciousness and is applied to treat headache and insomnia.

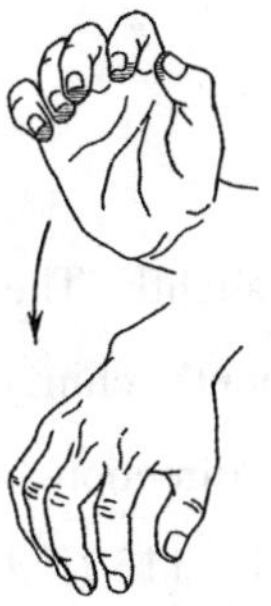

Fig. 3 – 108 **Pecking**

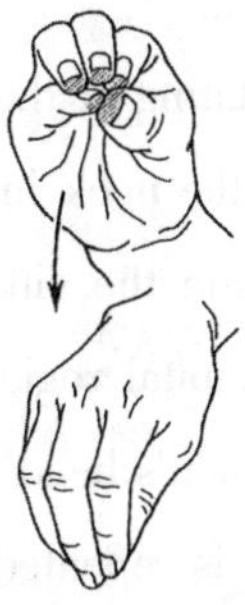

Fig. 3 – 109 **Pecking**

4. Flicking.

The power of the wrist is used in pecking manipulation, while the elastic force of the extensor of the fingers is delivered in flicking manipulation. That the print region of the index finger contracts on the middle finger nail (Fig. 3 – 110) and that the thumb print contracts on the middle fingernail are both allowed (Fig. 3 – 111). Then the middle finger pops swiftly to knock at a point with the fingertip. Flicking is suited for manipulation on the head and face. Its functions are like those of pecking.

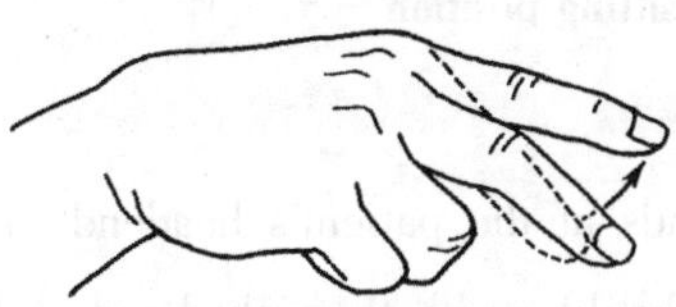

Fig. 3 – 110 **Flicking**

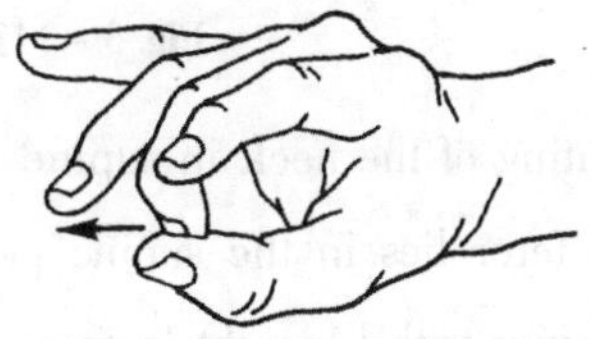

Fig. 3 – 111 **Flicking**

The frequency of patting, pecking and flicking are 100 to 120 times per minute.

3.3.8 Category of the rotating manipulations

The so-called "category of the rotating manipulation" means those actions that the manipulator makes the patient's suffered joints to be rotated slowly and mildly. It belongs to mobilizing manipulation (Fig. 3 – 112).

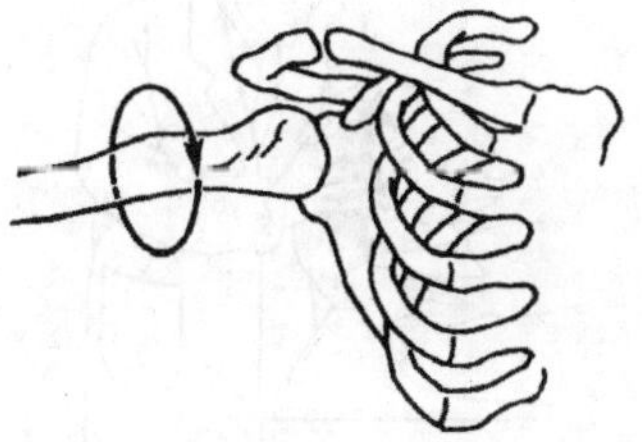

Fig. 3 – 112 **Model of Category of Rotating Manipulation**

When rotating manipulations are being done, the manipulator usually takes one hand to stabilize the proximal part of the joint and the other hand to hold the distal part. Then he holds the joint to rotate with steady and gentle force. The motion breadths should be restricted according to the physiological and pathological motion range. The rotation range should be varied from narrower to broader and increased gradually. It is allowed to exceed the pathological limit, but it mustn't be allowed to exceed the physiological limit. Both violent actions and those actions that transgress the physiological motion manner are strictly forbidden.

3.3.8.1 Rotating of the Neck

1. Rotating of the neck in sitting position.

The sufferer is in the sitting position, relaxes and flexes his neck slightly. The physician holds the patient's parieto-occipital region with one of his hands and supports patient's chin with the other hand, then rotates the patient's head and neck at the clockwise and anticlockwise directions with placid force. The above manipulation is repeated for 5 to 7 times in each direction (Fig. 3 – 113). One should be aware that it isn't allowed to overextend the head during rotation.

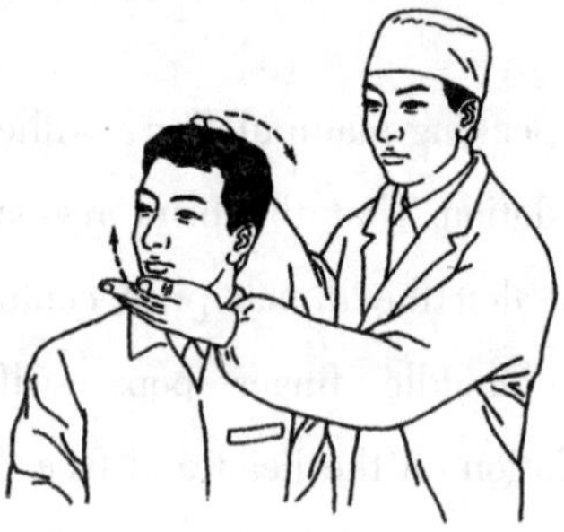

Fig. 3 – 113 Rotating of the neck in sitting position

2. Rotating of the neck in supine position.

The sufferer lies in the supine position. The physician stands at the patient's headend, supports the patient's occiput with his right forearm and grasps patient's left shoulder with the right hand, while holding the patient's head top with the left hand. Then inducts the patient's head and neck to rotate at the clockwise direction with placid force. Then exchanges the role of left and right hand to do the same rotating, at the anticlockwise direction. The above rotation is repeated for 3 to 5 times in each direction (Fig. 3 – 114). One should pay attention to that it isn't allowed to overextend the head during rotation, so as to avoid dizziness.

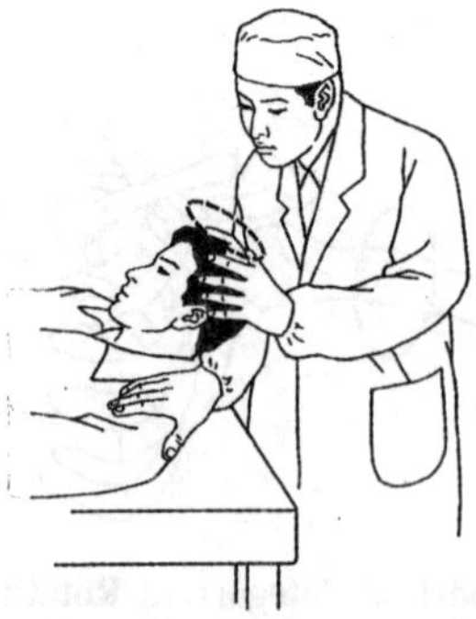

Fig. 3 – 114 Rotating of the neck in supine position

The rotating of neck in supine position is relatively steady, and it's safer to restrict the range of extension in the meantime. These manipulations are adapted to heal pain and stiff in neck and inconvenient motion of the neck.

3.3.8.2 Rotating of the shoulder

1. Rotating of the shoulder while supporting the elbow.

The patient is in the sitting position with relaxed shoulders. While standing on the suffered side in the posture of bow step, the physician puts one hand on the posterior side of the shoulder to stabilize it, supports the flexed elbow and the forearm with his other hand and forearm. Then holds the shoulder joint to rotate annularly at the clockwise and anti-clockwise direction for 5 to 10 circles each direction (Fig. 3 - 115). During this manipulation, the hand that put on the shoulder may cooperate to stimulate the acupoints on the shoulder region, so as to relieve pain caused by rotation motion. The manipulation is suitable for those serious patients who have the troubles of shoulder pain, inconvenient movement of the shoulder.

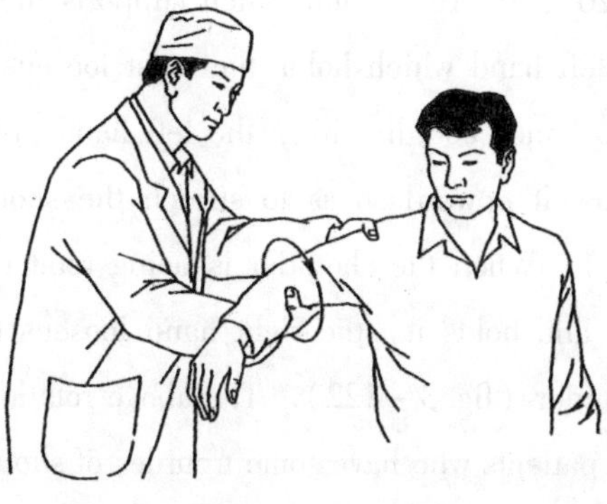

Fig. 3 - 115 Rotating of the shoulder while supporting the elbow

2. Rotating of the shoulder while holding the hand.

The patient's position is the same as the above. The physician puts one hand on the posterior superior part of the shoulder and holds the patient's hand with the other hand. Then holds the patient's shoulder to rotate at both clockwise and anti-clockwise direction for 5 to 10 circles (Fig. 3 - 116). During this manipulation, the hand that puts on the shoulder may cooperate to stimulate the acupoints so as to relieve pain caused by motion. The scope of application is the same as the above one.

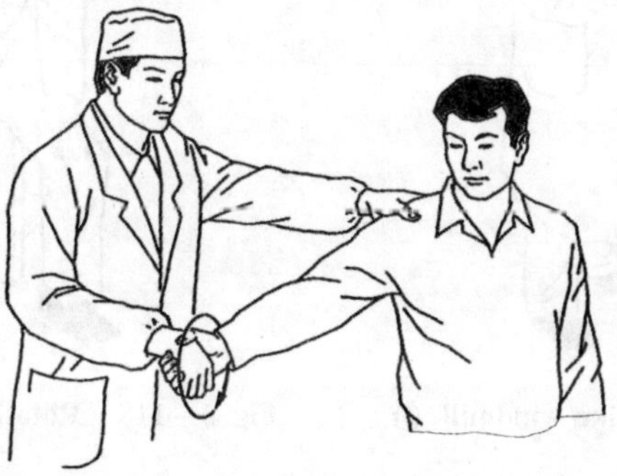

Fig. 3 - 116 Rotating of the shoulder while holding the hand

3. Rotating of the shoulder like windmill.

Take the left shoulder for example. The patient is in the sitting position with his shoulder relaxed. The physician stands on the postero-laterior side with T step, loosely holds the wrist back with the right hand and clips the palm side of the wrist with the left palm. Then lifts the arm slowly (Fig. 3 - 117). When the arm suffered should is being lifted for 60° to 120°, the left hand which supports patient's wrist turns the palm and holds the wrist to continue lifting the arm up while the right hand moves along the arm to the superior side of the shoulder. With two hands cooperating continually, the left hand drives the arm up and the right hand presses the shoulder down to stretch the shoulder and continue rotating (Fig. 3 – 118). When the shoulder is being rotated for 240° to 300°, the right hand which presses on the shoulder moves to the wrist and holds it while the left hand which holds the wrist loosens the fingers and clips the wrist. And then the two hands continue rotating shoulder downward. After repeating rotation for 3 to 5 times, rotates the shoulder again anteriorly to posteriorly (Fig. 3 – 119). The physician stands on the anterio – lateral side of the patient, loosely holds the wrist back with left hand, supports the palm side of the wrist with the right palm to lift the arm slowly, anteriorly and superiorly (Fig. 3 – 120). When the arm is being rotated for 60° to 120°, the right hand which supports the wrist turns to hold the palm and continues to hold the wrist; the left hand which holds the wrist loosens the fingers to move up along the arm to the shoulder. With the two hands coordinating, the left hand presses the shoulder down while the right hand holds the wrist to draw it upward so as to stretch the shoulder. Then continues rotating the shoulder backward (Fig. 3 – 121). When the shoulder is being rotated for 240° to 300°, the left hand moves along the arm to the wrist and holds it, the right hand loosens the fingers and supports the palm side of the wrist to rotate the shoulder (fig. 3 – 122). The above rotation is repeated for 3 to 5 times. This manipulation is suitable for those patients who have some troubles of shoulder pain, inconvenient motion of the shoulder or those patients whose motion function of the shoulder has been improved after Tuina therapy.

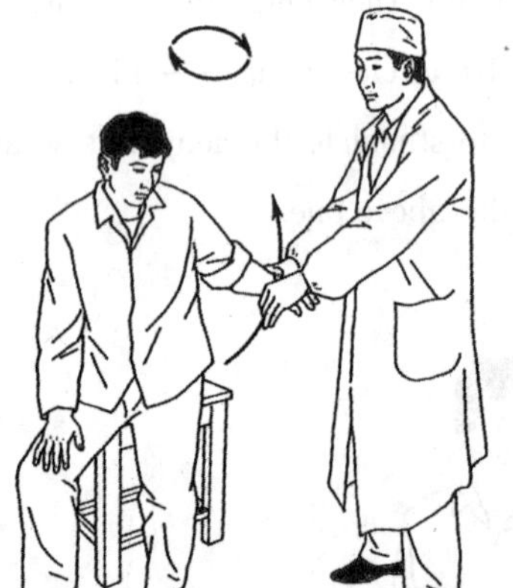

Fig. 3 – 117 Rotating of shoulder like windmill (1)

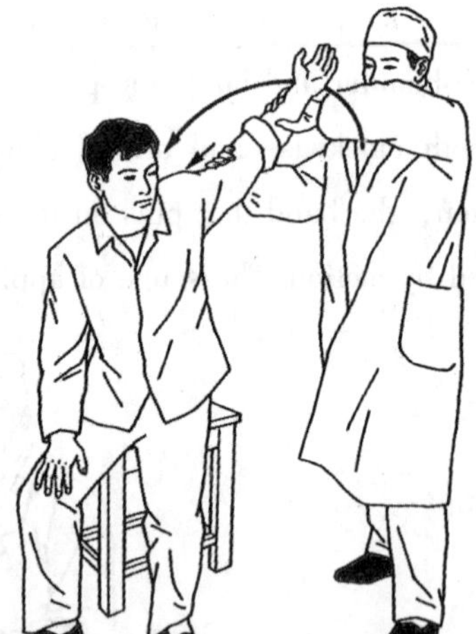

Fig. 3 – 118 Rotating of shoulder like windmill (2)

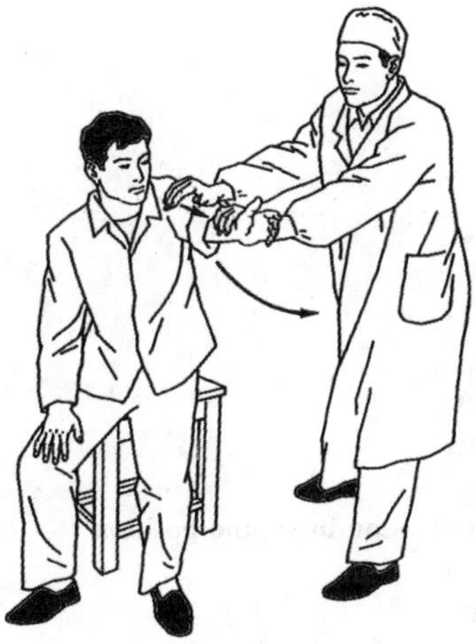

Fig. 3 – 119 **Rotating of shoulder like windmill** (3)

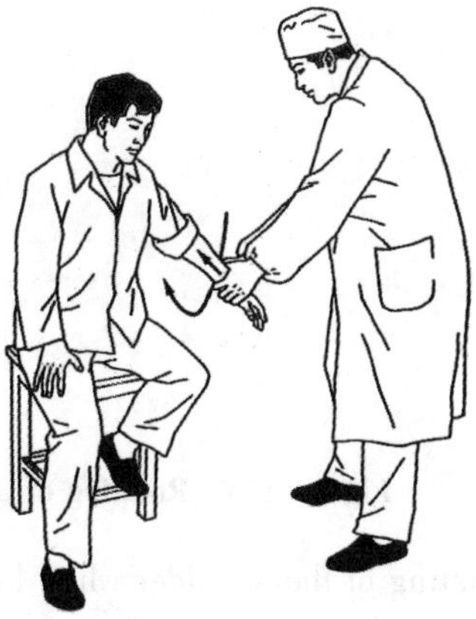

Fig. 3 – 120 **Rotating of shoulder like windmill** (4)

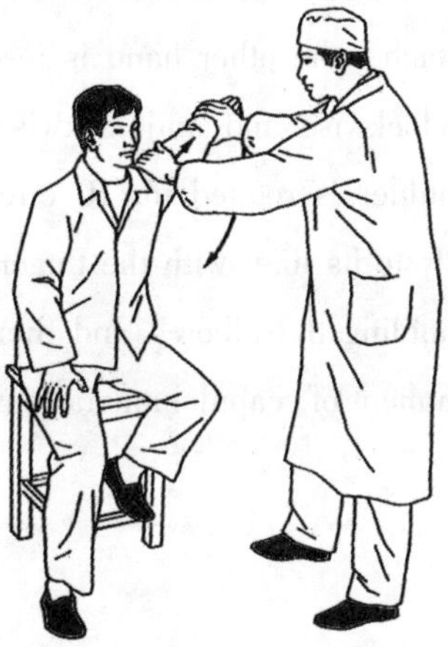

Fig. 3 – 121 **Rotating of shoulder like windmill** (5)

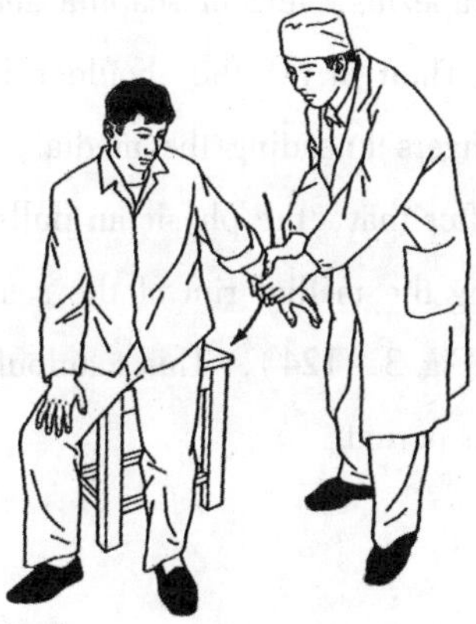

Fig. 3 – 122 **Rotating of shoulder like windmill** (6)

4. Rotating of the shoulder for stretching the tendon in supine position.

The sufferer is in the supine position. The physician stands on the suffered side with bow step, and contacts the patient's deltoid with one hand and holds the wrist with the other hand. Then stretches and lifts the arm upward to the pathological limit position, then drives the shoulder to be rotated in narrow range with the physician's lumbar and hip motion while the arm is being kept in slight traction (Fig. 3 – 123). The speed of rotation is about 30 to 40 times per minute. The rotation is repeated for 5 to 10 circles at both clockwise and anticlockwise direction. This manipulation is adapted to cure the scapulohumeral periarthritis in the adhesion period.

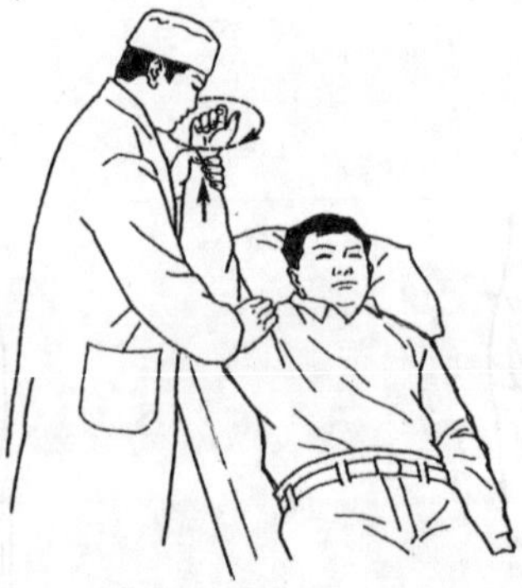

Fig. 3 – 123 Rotating of the shoulder for stretching the tendon in supine position

5. Rotating of the shoulder while kneading in supine position.

The patient is in the supine position. The physician stands on the suffered side in the posture of forward lunge, holds the patient's elbow to flex 90° with one hand, touches the medial rim of the scapula where the trapezius, levator scapula and rhomboid muscles are attach, the other hand is inserted under the scapula. Then drives the shoulder joint to be rotated at the clockwise and anticlockwise direction, while the fingers kneading the medial rim of the scapula. The shoulder is rotated for 10 circles at each direction. After that, the physician pulls the whole shoulder laterally to its limit with the finger tips of one hand hooking the medial rim of the scapula and the other hand holding the elbow, and then loosens it gradually (Fig. 3 – 124). This manipulation is suitable for the treatment of scapulohumeral periarthritis in the adhesion period.

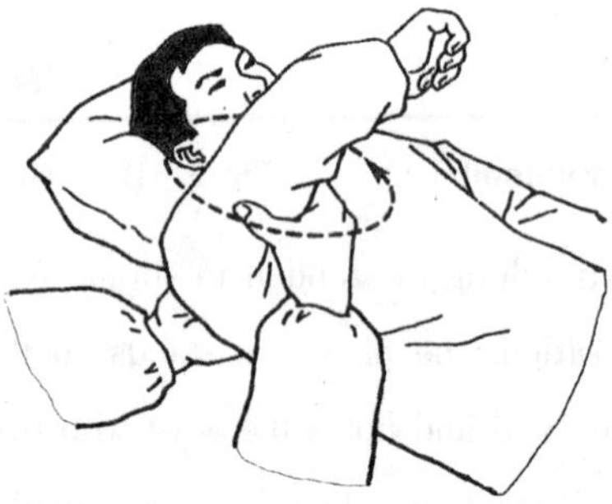

Fig. 3 – 124 Rotating of the shoulder while kneading in supine position

3.3.8.3 Rotating of the elbow

The patient is in the supine position. The physician stands on the suffered side in the posture of forward lunge, and holds the patient's elbow with one hand and the wrist with the other to pull the elbow oppositely. Then inducts the elbow to be rotated in a narrow range with his trunk motion, while the suffered elbow is being in the extension and slight traction. The rotation is repeated for 10 times at both clockwise and anticlockwise direction. And then drives the elbow to do rotation in flexion and slight traction (Fig. 3 – 125). This manipulation is suitable for the treatment of elbow pain with movement disorder.

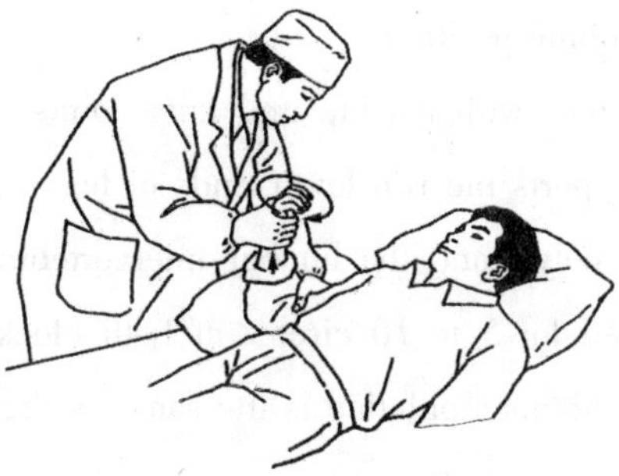

Fig. 3 – 125 Rotating of the elbow

3.3.8.4 Rotating of the wrist

The patient is in the sitting position or supine position. The physician holds the lower end of the forearm with one hand and crosses his own fingers with the fingers of the patient to pull the wrist oppositely. Then inducts the wrist to be rotated in a narrow range, while the suffered wrist is kept in extension and slight traction condition. The rotation is repeated for 5 times at both clockwise and anticlockwise direction. And then drives the wrist to be rotated in flexion and slight traction condition (Fig. 3 – 126). This manipulation is suitable for the treatment of wrist pain with movement disorder.

3.3.8.5 Rotating of the finger

The patient is in the sitting position. The physician holds the suffered palm with one hand and clips the suffered finger with the index and middle fingers of the other hand to pull the metacarpopha-langeal joint or the interphalangeal joint oppositely. Then keeps the joint in traction and rotates the joint in a narrow range (Fig. 3 – 127). This manipulation is suitable for the treatment of pain, swolling and movement disorder in the metacarpopha-langeal joint or the interphalangeal joint.

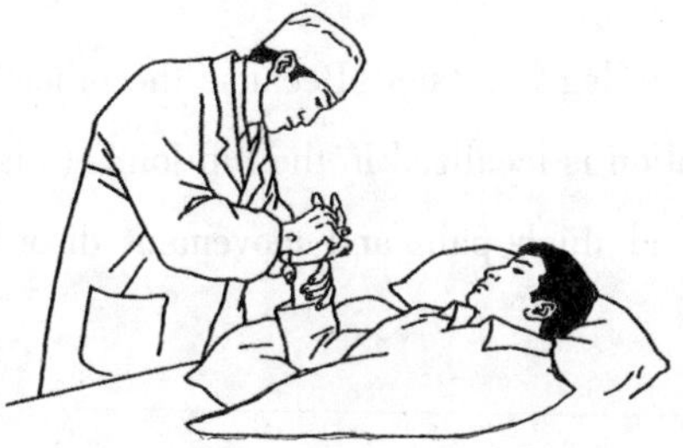

Fig. 3 – 126 Rotating of the wrist

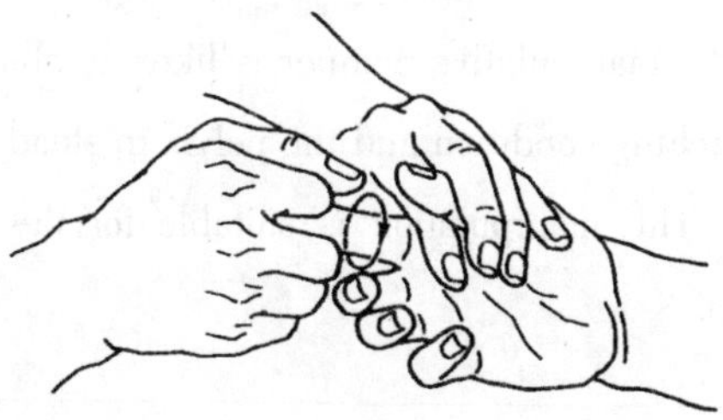

Fig. 3 – 127 Rotating of the finger

3.3.8.6 Rotating of the lumbus

1. Rotating of the lumbus in sitting position.

The patient is in the sitting position, relaxes his lumbar muscles and flexes the lumbar slightly. The physician contacts the suffered side of the waist with one hand and supports the opposite shoulder with the other hand to rotate the lumbar slowly and coordinately. The rotation is repeated for 5 to 10 circles at both clockwise and anti – clockwise directions (Fig. 3 – 128). This manipulation is suitable for the treatment of lower back pain, stiff lower back, and movement disorder in lower back.

2. Rotating of the lumbus in supine position.

The patient is in supine position, with his hip and knee joints flexed. The physician holds the two closed knees with one hand and supports the two lower ends of legs with the other hand. Then drives the two legs to be rotated, so that the pelvis and the lumbar intervertebral discs are also rotated slowly and coordinately. The rotation is repeated for 5 to 10 circles at both clockwise and anti-clockwise directions (Fig. 3 - 129). The indication of this manipulation is the same as the above one.

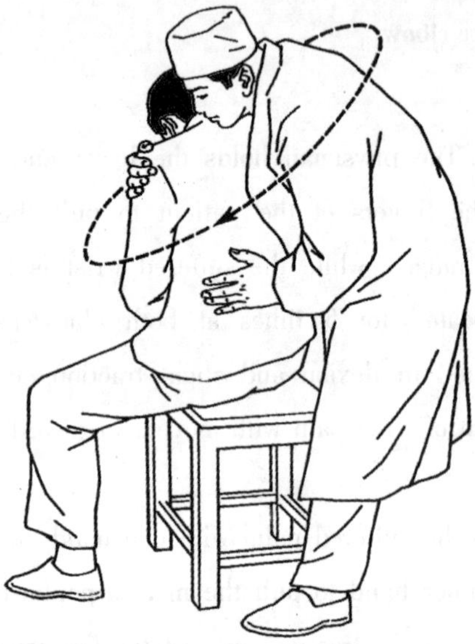

Fig. 3 - 128 Rotating of the lumbus in sitting position

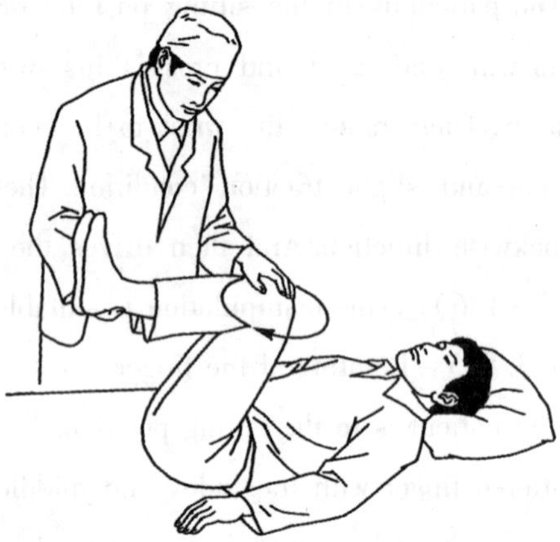

Fig. 3 - 129 Rotating of the lumbus in supine position

3.3.8.7 Rotating of the hip

The manipulative manner is like the above one, but only one leg is rotated. Because the other leg is in stretching condition and the pelvis in steady position, the rotation is localized in the hip joint (Fig. 3 - 130). This manipulation is suitable for the treatment of hip and thigh pain and movement disorder of the hip.

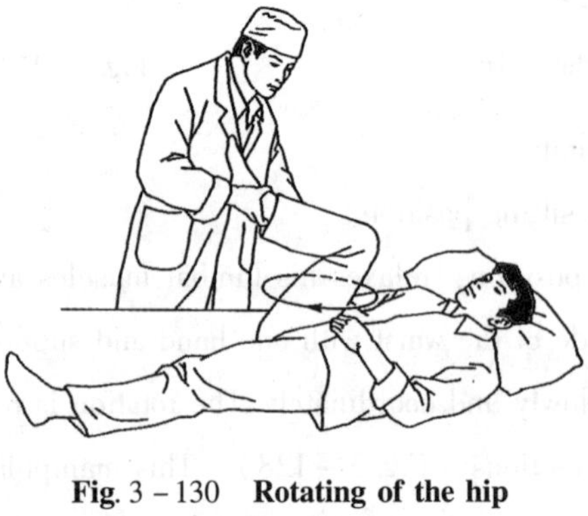

Fig. 3 - 130 Rotating of the hip

3.3.8.8 Rotating of the knee

The patient is in supine position, with his knee joints semi-flexed. The physician supports the knee with one hand and holds the end of leg with the other hand. Then drives the leg to be rotated slowly and coordinately, and then extends the knee while rotating. The rotation is repeated for 5 to 10 circles at both clockwise and anti – clockwise directions (Fig. 3 – 131). This manipulation is suitable for the treatment of meniscus injury in lock condition.

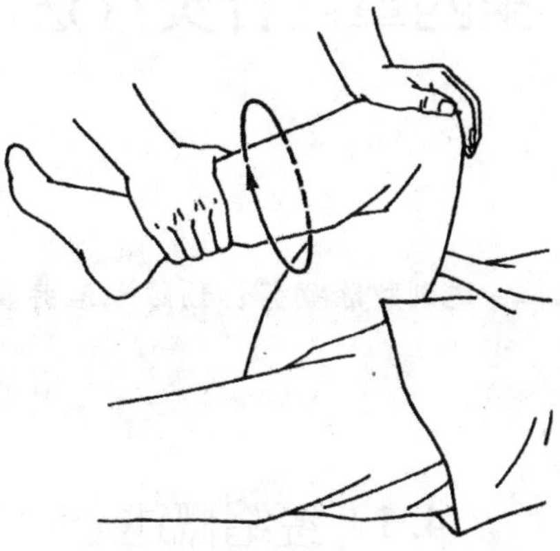

Fig. 3 – 131 Rotating of the knee

3.3.8.9 Rotating of the ankle

The patient is in supine position, with his leg stretched. The physician supports the heel with one hand and holds the forefoot with the other hand. Then hauls the ankle joint for a while. And then drives the ankle joint to be rotated while keeping slight traction (Fig. 3 – 132). This manipulation is suitable for the treatment of sprain of the ankle, as well as inconvenient motion of the ankle.

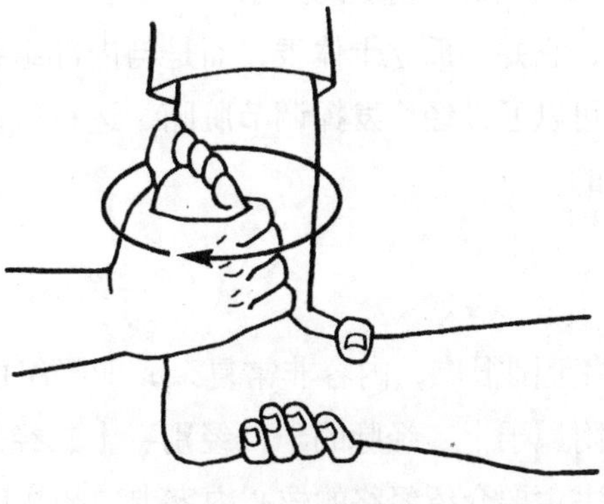

Fig. 3 – 132 Rotating of the ankle

第四章 针灸疗法

针灸主要是通过刺激经络和穴位，达到解除疲劳、预防或治疗疾病的目的。针灸利用针刺或艾灸进行刺激。

4.1 经络概述

经络学说是针灸学的理论基石。经络是人体联络脏腑、运行气血的通路。经络分为经脉和络脉，“经”有路径的含义，经脉贯穿上下、沟通内外，直行而分布较深部，是经络系统的主干；“络”有网络的含义，络脉是纵横交错的分支，较经脉细小。经络对内属于脏腑，对外联络四肢，沟通于内脏与体表之间，把人体的五脏六腑、四肢百骸、五官九窍、皮肉筋脉等组织器官联结成一个有机的整体，使人体各部分的功能活动保持相对的协调和平衡。经络学说几千年来一直指导着中医临床，尤其与针灸、推拿、气功有密切的关系。

穴位是经络线上的特定点，它并不孤立于体表，而是与内部组织、器官有一定联系的一些特定部位。刺激一定的穴位，就可以通过经络发挥调节脏腑、运行气血的功能，激发机体内在的抗病能力，以达到防治疾病的目的。

4.1.1 经络的组成

《黄帝内经》所论述的经络范围很广，内容非常复杂，即经络由经脉和络脉组成，经脉又包括十二经脉和奇经八脉，以及附属于十二经脉的十二经别、十二经筋、十二皮部等；络脉则包括十五络脉、浮络、孙络等。本书主要介绍经络的核心内容十二经脉和奇经八脉。

4.1.2 十二经脉和奇经八脉

4.1.2.1 十二经脉

十二经脉是手太阴肺经、手厥阴心包经、手少阴心经、手阳明大肠经、手少阳三焦经、手太阳小肠经、足太阴脾经、足厥阴肝经、足少阴肾经、足阳明胃经、足少阳胆经、足太阳膀胱经的总称，一侧共十二条，左右对称。

十二经脉的体表分布：阴经分布于四肢内侧面和胸腹部，阳经分布于四肢外侧面及头面躯干。其中手三阴经和足三阴经在四肢内侧面的排列是：太阴在前缘，厥阴居中，少阴在后缘；手三阳经和足三阳经在四肢外侧面的排列是：阳明在前缘，少阳居中，太阳在后缘。如表4－1及图4－1所示。

手太阴肺经（简称肺经）与手阳明大肠经（简称大肠经），分别循行于上肢内侧前缘和上肢外侧前缘，内外对应，相互联络，称为“表里经”；手厥阴心包经与手少阳三焦经，手少阴心经与手太阳小肠经，足太阳脾经与足阳明胃经，足厥阴肝经与是少阳胆经，是少阴肾经与是太阳膀胱经，均为表里经。表里经之间的对应关系，使之在治疗疾病中有密切的联系。当十二经脉发生病变时，会出现各经特有的一些病症，如手太阳肺经发病有咳嗽、哮喘、胸痛等呼吸系统症状及循经所过的前臂内侧前缘痛，治疗时可取手太阳肺经和手阳明大肠经的某些穴位；手厥阴心包经发病有心痛、心悸、失眠、喜笑不休等心血管和神志症状。

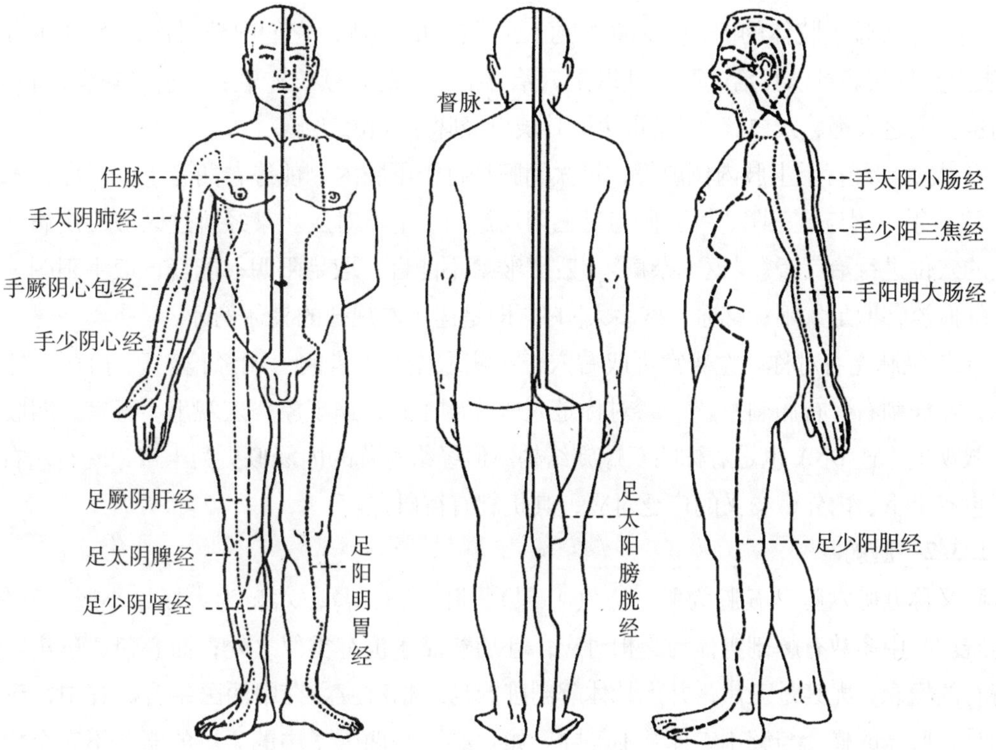

图 4－1

表 4－1　十二经脉分布表

阴经（属脏）	循行路径	阳经（属腑）	循行路径
手太阴肺经	胸，上肢内侧前缘	手阳明大肠经	头面，上肢外侧前缘
手厥阴心包经	胸，上肢内侧中间	手少阳三焦经	颈耳，上肢外侧中间
手少阴心经	胸，上肢内侧后缘	手太阳小肠经	肩中，上肢外侧后
足太阴脾经	腹，下肢内侧前缘	足阳明胃经	胸腹头面，下肢外侧前缘
足厥阴肝经	腹，下肢内侧中间	足少阳胆经	胁肋，下肢外侧中间
足少阴肾经	胸腹，下肢内侧后缘	足太阳膀胱经	后背，下肢外侧后缘

说明：在小腿下半部和足背部，足厥阴肝经在前缘、足太阴脾经在中间；至内踝上八寸处交叉之后，足太阴脾经在前缘、足厥阴肝经在中间。

4.1.2.2　奇经八脉

奇经八脉是任脉、督脉、冲脉、带脉、阴维脉、阳维脉、阴跷脉、阳跷脉的总称，是对十二经脉的补充。它与十二经脉不同，不直属某个脏腑，也无表里配合，因而称之为奇经。在奇经八脉中，任脉和督脉具有所属穴位，它们与同样具有所属穴位的十二经脉合称“十四经”（图 4－1）。十四经具有一定的循行路线、主治病症及所属穴位，是经络系统中最重要的部分，在临床上是针灸推拿取穴治病的基础。

4.1.3 经络学说的基本概念

4.1.3.1 阴阳

阴阳是中医学的重要概念之一，是传统中国文化对人体和疾病进行高度归纳的抽象分类，且在不同的分类中其内涵有所不同。在经络学说中，阴阳的精髓含义是“对称（对应）”。

1. 六条阴经位于肢体的内侧，六条阳经位于肢体的外侧，它们内外对应，术语称为“表里经”，表里经的疾病可以互治或两经共取配穴治疗。《灵枢·厥病》载：“腹胀胸满，心尤痛甚，胃心痛也。取之大都、太白。”即是胃病取其表里经脾经穴位之例。

2. 手太阴肺经行于上肢内侧前缘，足太阴脾经行于下肢内侧前缘，两者上下对应，术语称为“同名经”。手三阴与足三阴、手三阳与足三阳均是一一上下对应。某经所过区域的疾病常取其同名经上的穴位进行治疗。《灵枢·杂病》载：“喉痹不能言，取足阳明；能言，取手阳明……衄而不止，衃血流，取足太阳；衃血，取手太阳。”即是运用本规律的具体例证。

3. 十二经脉左右对称。左病常可取右穴，右病取左。《素问·调经论》王冰注：“巨刺者，刺经脉，左痛刺右，右痛刺左。”“缪对称是人体所存在的普遍现象，宏观上，五官、四肢、躯干对称；微观上，连DNA也是对称的双螺旋结构。但经络对称的内涵似更为丰富，既有左右的对称关系，也有上下、内外、交叉的广泛对应，其机制有待研究。”

4.1.3.2 脏腑

脏腑又称五脏六腑。五脏为肺、心（心包）、肝、脾、肾，六腑为大肠、小肠、三焦、胆、胃、膀胱。其中多数有解剖实体与之相对应，且功能描述也有类似之处；而心包、三焦则是中医学中特有的概念，尤其是三焦，并无具体解剖脏器与之相对应。在中西医结合研究中，应该特别注意的是，脏腑的概念与解剖实体并不等同。如“心”与西医学中的心脏的概念不完全相同，中医学中的“心”除包括心血管外，还包括精神、神经的范畴，具有大脑和脊髓的功能；“脾”并非我们所熟知的西医学中的免疫器官，而是与“胃”相对应，与消化功能关系密切、与某些泌尿系统疾病也有关的概念。在此，脏腑与其说是解剖所见的内脏，不如看作经络与疾病之间的桥梁更为贴切。在经络学说中，脏腑理论的精髓含义是“内脏与体表相关”的规律，其相关性已为神经解剖学、生理学实验所证实。今后的研究重点应该是如何从脏腑理论中，找出古人千年临床经验的线索，用现代的语言阐述其机制。

4.1.3.3 运行气血

“气”和“血”也是中医学的重要概念，在不同地方，内涵不同。经络学说中，“气”的概念首先来源于针刺感应，尤其是循经感传。针刺感应古称“得气”。

经络学说中“运行气血”的概念，有“传递刺激信息、加快血液循环”的含义。

4.2 穴位概述

4.2.1 穴位的分类

穴位又叫“腧穴”，分三大类。

1. 十四经穴，简称“经穴”，即分布在十二经脉和任脉、督脉上的穴位。有309对双穴，52个单穴，总计361穴。

2. 经外奇穴，简称“奇穴”，是指既有一定的穴名，又有明确的位置，但未被列入十四经系统的其他穴位。这些穴位历代都有所发现。

3. 阿是穴，又称“天应穴”，是指患病时，在身体上暂时出现的压痛点或反应点。这些穴位既无具体名称，也无固定位置。

4.2.2　穴位的治疗作用

1. 近治作用，指穴位能治疗所在部位及其邻近组织、器官的病症的作用。此为穴位作用的普遍规律。如睛明、四白，能治眼科疾病；中脘、下脘，能治胃炎等。

2. 远治作用，指某些穴位能治疗远离该穴区域部位的疾病的作用。如四肢肘膝以下部位的穴位，常能治疗头面、胸腹部疾病。如合谷治头面五官部疾病、足三里治消化系统疾病等。

3. 特殊作用，一般指穴位对机体的双相调节作用。如泄泻时，针刺天枢能止泻；便秘时，针刺天枢又能通便。心动过缓时，针刺内关能增快心率；心动过速时，针刺内关又能减缓心率。此外，某些穴位主治具有相对特异性，如大椎穴退热；至阴穴矫治胎位不正等，也属特殊作用范畴。

4.2.3　穴位的定位

4.2.3.1　体表标志法

体表标志法分为定型标志和动态标志。

1. 定型标志：以人体上有关的体表解剖标志作为定穴的依据。如头面部有五官、眉发等标志；背部有脊椎棘突和肩胛骨、肋骨、髂嵴等标志；胸腹部有乳头、胸骨、脐孔、耻骨联合等标志；四肢有关节、骨突等标志。以背部为例，常用的有：两肩胛冈平第三胸椎棘突；两肩胛下角平第七胸椎棘突；两髂嵴平第四腰椎棘突（图4－2）。

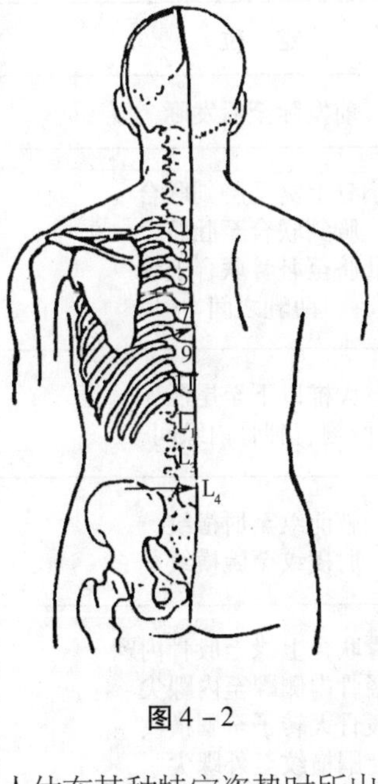

图4－2

2. 动态标志：姿势取穴法，是以人体在某种特定姿势时所出现的标志作为定穴的依据。如垂手中指尖所达的大腿侧面处取风市；两手虎口交叉，食指尖所达桡骨茎突凹陷处取列缺穴等（见图4－9）。

4.2.3.2　指量法

指量法即手指同身寸法，是以患者的手指为标准，进行测量定穴的方法。如果医生和病人的手大小相仿，也可以医生的手指为标准。临床常用的指量法有中指同身寸、拇指同身寸、横指同身寸3种。

1. 中指同身寸：以患者中指中节屈曲时内侧两端纹头之间作为1寸，用于四肢部定穴的直寸和背部取穴的横寸（图4－3）。

2. 拇指同身寸：以患者拇指关节的横度作为1寸，也适用于四肢部的直寸取穴（图4－4）。

3. 横指同身寸：将食、中、无名、小指等四指并拢，以中指中节横纹处为准，横量作为3寸（图4－5）。

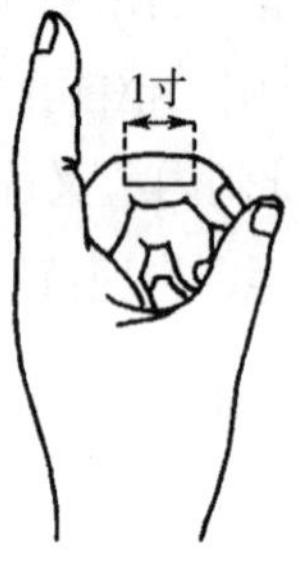

图4－3

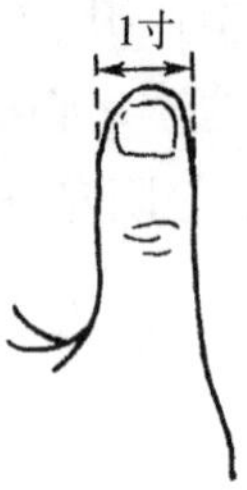

图4－4

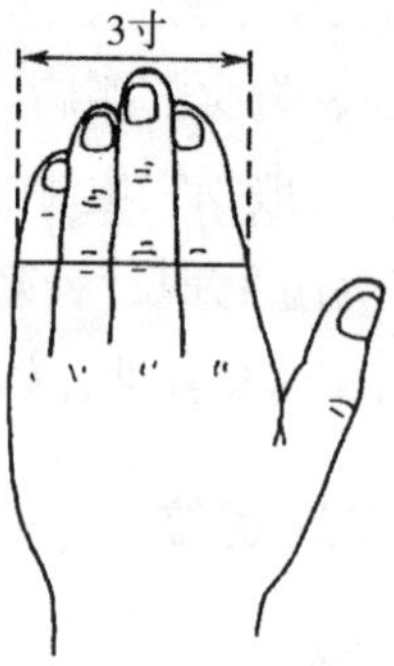

图4－5

4.2.3.3　折量寸法

折量寸法是将人体各部分分成若干等分以折量定穴的方法，每一等分为1寸。常用的分寸见表4－2和图4－6。

表4－2　常用折量寸表

身体部位	定　位	比　例
头部	前发际至后发际	12寸
胸腹部	胸骨上窝至胸剑联合 胸剑联合至肚脐 肚脐至耻骨联合上缘 两乳之间	9寸 8寸 5寸 8寸
背腰部	大椎以下至尾骶 两侧肩胛骨内缘间	21椎 6寸
上肢	腋前纹至肘横纹 肘横纹至腕横纹	9寸 12寸
下肢	耻骨联合上缘至股骨内踝 胫骨内侧踝至内踝尖 股骨大转子至腘横纹 腘横纹至外踝尖	18寸 13寸 19寸 16寸

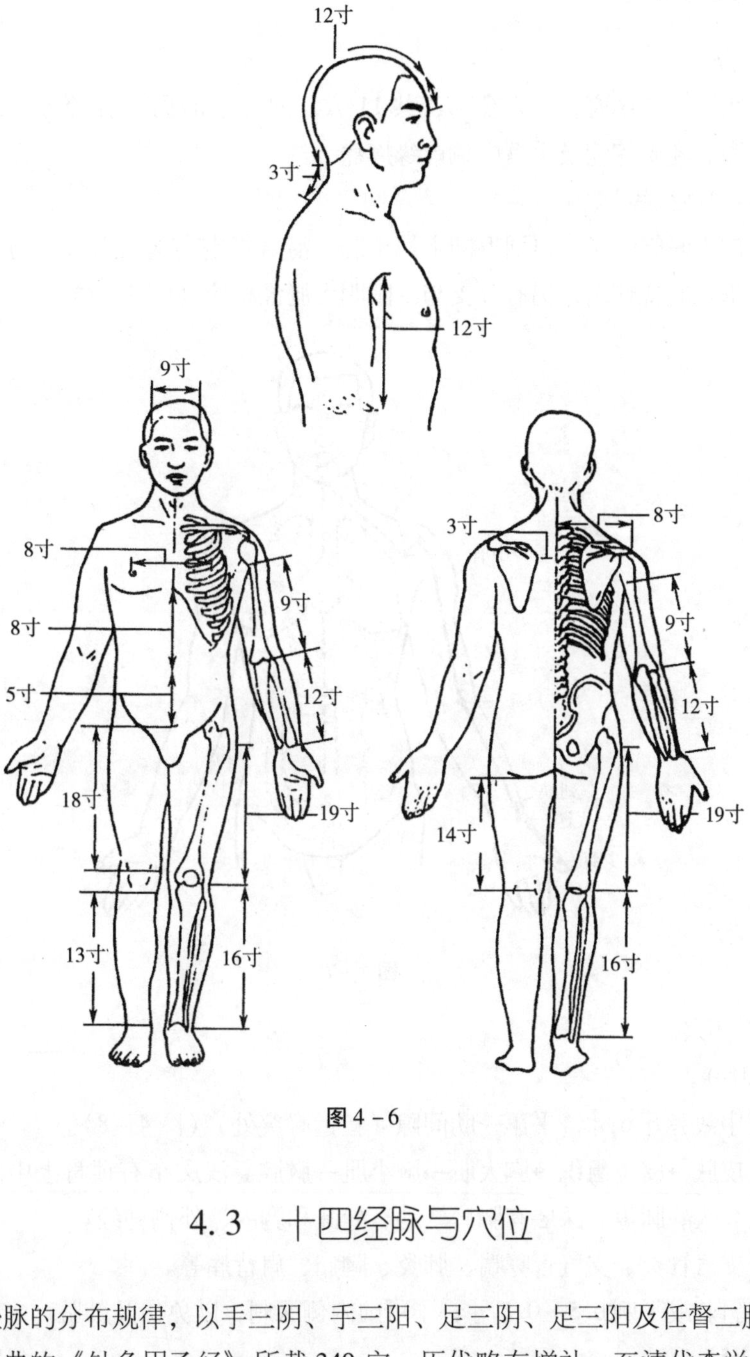

图4-6

4.3　十四经脉与穴位

本节按十四经脉的分布规律，以手三阴、手三阳、足三阴、足三阳及任督二脉的次序进行介绍。十四经穴从经典的《针灸甲乙经》所载349穴，历代略有增补，至清代李学川《针灸逢源》记载361穴，一直沿用至今。本书择要介绍其中的常用穴和次常用穴。穴位的定位、英文编号均按1991年实施的中国国家标准化方案执行。各穴的针灸操作方法，一般仅介绍毫针的常规进针深度及角度，穴位的推拿操作方法，多采用点按法、按揉法、一指禅推法等，本节各穴中仅对某些特殊用法加以说明。

4.3.1 手太阴肺经

4.3.1.1 概况

本经从胸至手，首穴中府，末穴少商，共11穴。穴位主治据《针灸大成》所载，治肺、喉症，还治疗心、眼、乳腺等症及手臂内侧前缘疼痛。

4.3.1.2 主要循行线

起于胃部，向下联络大肠；再回返向上属于肺，沿气管走向胸前臂外上方，经上肢掌侧面的桡侧缘，止于大拇指的桡侧端，另有分支与手阳明大肠经相接（图4-7）。

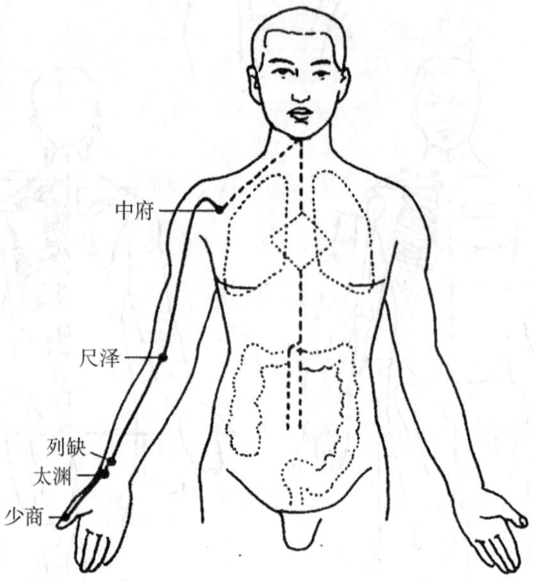

图4-7

4.3.1.3 常用穴位

1. 中府（LU1）。

定位：前正中线旁开6寸，平第一肋间隙（接近喙突处）（图4-8）。

层次解剖：皮肤→皮下组织→胸大肌→胸小肌→胸腔。浅层布有锁骨上中间神经、第一肋间神经的外侧皮支和头静脉等。深层有胸肩峰动、静脉和胸内、外侧神经。

主治举例：支气管炎、支气管哮喘、肺炎、胸痛、肩背痛等。

操作：向外斜刺或平刺0.5~0.8寸；不可向内侧深刺，以免伤及肺脏。

2. 尺泽（LU5）。

定位：肘横纹中，肱二头肌腱桡侧凹陷处（图4-8）。

层次解剖：皮肤→皮下组织→肱桡肌→桡神经→肱肌。浅层有头静脉、前臂外侧皮神经等。深层有桡神经，桡侧副动、静脉前支，桡侧返动、静脉等。

主治举例：支气管炎、支气管哮喘、胸膜炎、肘臂痛等。

操作：直刺0.5~1寸。

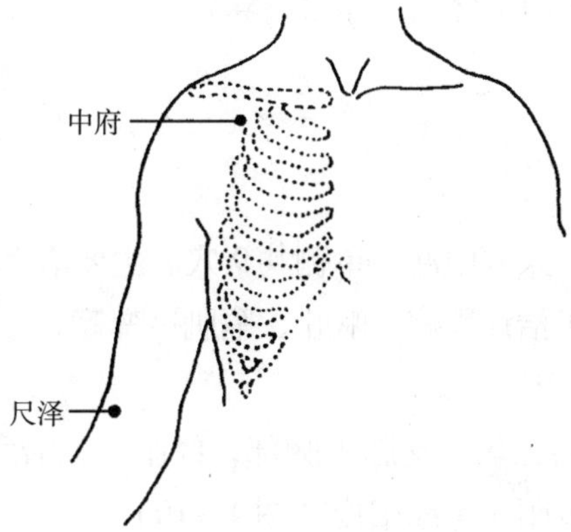

图4－8

3. 列缺（LU7）。

定位：桡骨茎突上方，腕横纹上1.5寸。简便取穴法可以两手虎口交叉，食指尖所指凹陷处（图4－9）。

层次解剖：皮肤→皮下组织→拇长展肌腱→肱桡肌腱→旋前方肌。浅层布有头静脉、前臂外侧皮神经和桡神经浅支。深层有桡动脉、静脉分支。

主治举例：感冒、支气管炎、哮喘、头痛、面神经麻痹、落枕、荨麻疹、手腕酸痛等。

操作：向肘斜刺0.5～1寸。

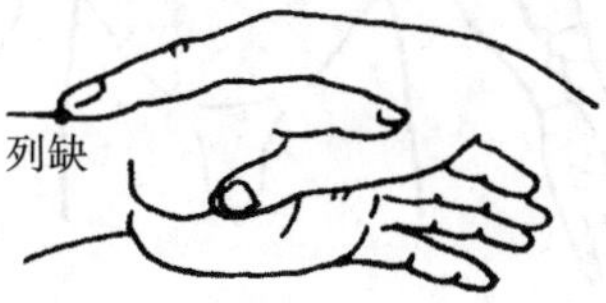

图4－9

4. 太渊（LU9）。

定位：腕横纹上，桡动脉外侧与拇长展肌腱之间凹陷处（图4－7）。

层次解剖：皮肤→皮下组织→桡侧腕屈肌腱与拇长展肌腱之间。浅层布有前臂外侧皮神经、桡神经浅支和桡动脉掌浅支等。深层有桡动、静脉。

主治举例：感冒、支气管炎、哮喘、心绞痛、肋间神经痛、无脉症、手腕酸痛等。

操作：直刺0.5寸，避开动脉。

5. 少商（LU11）。

定位：拇指桡侧，距指甲角约0.1寸（图4－7）。

层次解剖：皮肤→皮下组织→指甲根。有正中神经的指掌侧固有神经之指背支和拇主要动、静脉与第一掌背动、静脉分支所形成的动、静脉网。

主治举例：感冒发热、肺炎、腮腺炎、急性咽喉炎、急性扁桃体炎、昏迷、精神病等。

操作：向上斜刺0.1寸，急症重症可速刺出血。

4.3.1.4 次常用穴位

孔最（LU6）：腕横纹上7寸，尺泽与太渊连线上。

经渠（LU8）：腕横纹上1寸，桡骨茎突与桡动脉之间凹陷处。

鱼际（LU10）：约第一掌骨中点桡侧，赤白肉际处。

4.3.2 手厥阴心包经

4.3.2.1 概况

本经从胸至手，首穴天池，末穴中冲，单侧共9穴。主要治疗心血管病和神志病。如心绞痛、心律不齐、昏迷、无脉症。还可治疗胃病、呕吐、膈肌痉挛等。

4.3.2.2 主要循行线

起于胸中，属于心包，下络三焦。支脉出胸部，经腋窝，沿手臂掌侧面的中间进入手掌中，止于中指末端。另一分支与手少阳三焦经相接（图4－10）。

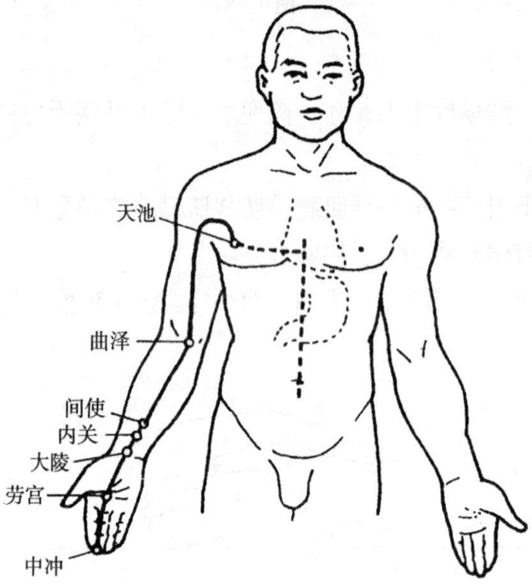

图4－10

4.3.2.3 常用穴位

1. 曲泽（PC3）。

定位：肘横纹中，肱二头肌腱尺侧缘（图4－11）。

层次解剖：皮肤→皮下组织→正中神经→肱肌。浅层有肘正中静脉，前臂内侧皮神经。深层有肱动、静脉，尺侧返动、静脉的掌侧支与尺侧下副动、静脉前支构成的动、静脉网，正中神经的本干。

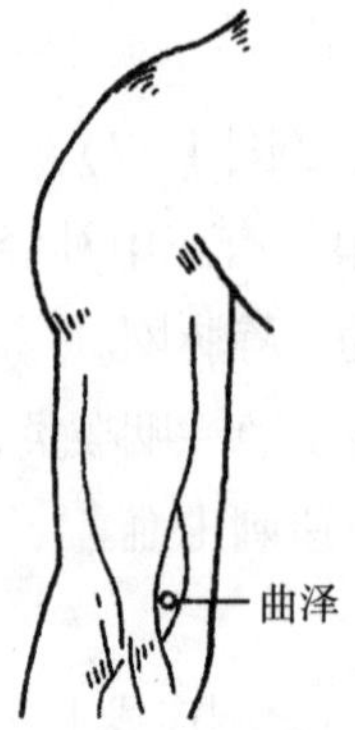

图4－11

主治举例：急性胃肠炎、支气管炎、中暑、高热、心绞痛、风湿性心脏病、小儿舞蹈病、肘关节内侧疼痛等。

操作：直刺0.5~1寸；急性吐泻，民间用三棱针点刺放血。

2. 内关（PC6）。

定位：腕横纹上2寸，掌长肌腱与桡侧腕屈肌腱之间（图4-10）。

层次解剖：皮肤→皮下组织→桡侧腕屈肌腱与掌长肌腱之间→指浅屈肌→指深屈肌→旋前方肌。浅层有前臂内侧皮神经，前臂外侧皮神经的分支和前臂正中静脉。深层在指浅屈肌、拇长屈肌和指深屈肌三者之间有正中神经和正中神经伴行动、静脉。在前臂骨间膜的前方有骨间前动、静脉和骨间前神经。

主治举例：心动过速或过缓、心绞痛、心肌炎、神经衰弱、胃炎、恶心呕吐、膈肌痉挛、急性胆囊炎、甲状腺功能亢进、血栓闭塞性脉管炎、血管性头痛等。

操作：直刺或向上斜刺0.5~1.2寸。

3. 大陵（PC7）。

定位：在腕掌横纹的中点处，掌长肌腱与桡侧腕屈肌腱之间（图4-10）。

层次解剖：皮肤→皮下组织→掌长肌腱与桡侧腕屈肌腱之间→拇长屈肌腱与指浅屈肌腱、指深屈肌腱之间→桡腕关节前方。浅层布有前臂内、外侧皮神经，正中神经掌支，腕掌侧静脉网。深层在掌长肌与桡侧腕屈肌之间的深面可能刺中正中神经。

主治举例：心动过速、心绞痛、心律不齐、胃炎、扁桃体炎、桡腕关节痛、精神病等。

操作：直刺0.3~0.5寸。

4.3.3 手少阴心经

4.3.3.1 概况

本经从胸至手，首穴极泉，末穴少冲，单侧共9穴。主治心血管及神经、精神病症，还可治疗穴位所在局部疾患。如心动过速或过缓、心绞痛、失眠、精神病、癫痫、癔症、手臂内侧后缘痛等。

4.3.3.2 主要循行线

起于心中，下行联络小肠。直行的经脉，从心上行抵肺部，再向下出腋窝，沿上肢掌侧面的尺侧缘下行，经四、五掌骨之间，止于手小指桡侧端（图4-12）。

4.3.3.3 常用穴位

1. 极泉（HT1）。

定位：在腋窝正中，腋动脉内侧（图4-13）。

层次解剖：皮肤→皮下组织→臂丛、腋动脉、腋静脉→背阔肌腱→大圆肌。浅层有肋间臂神经分布。深层有桡神经、尺神经、正中神经、前臂内侧皮神经、臂内侧皮神经、腋动脉、腋静脉等结构。

主治举例：肋间神经痛、上肢瘫痪、颈淋巴结核等。

操作：直刺0.5~0.8寸。

2. 少海（HT3）。

定位：屈肘，在肘横纹尺侧纹头凹陷者中（图4-13）。

层次解剖：皮肤→皮下组织→旋前圆肌→肱肌。浅层有前臂内侧皮神经，贵要静脉等分布。深层有正中神经，尺侧返动、静脉和尺侧下副动、静脉的吻合支。

主治举例：心绞痛、癫痫、精神病、尺神经麻痹、肋间神经痛、颈淋巴结核、手臂震颤、上肢麻木、肘关节痛等。

操作：直刺0.5~1.0寸。

3. 通里（HT5）。

定位：腕横纹上1寸，当尺侧腕屈肌腱桡侧（图4-12）。

层次解剖：皮肤→皮下组织→尺侧腕屈肌与指浅屈肌之间→指深屈肌→旋前方肌。浅层有前臂内侧皮神经，贵要静脉属支等分布。深层有尺动、静脉和尺神经分布。

主治举例：心动过缓、心绞痛、神经衰弱、癔症、扁桃体炎、失语、手腕痛等。

操作：直刺0.3~0.5寸。

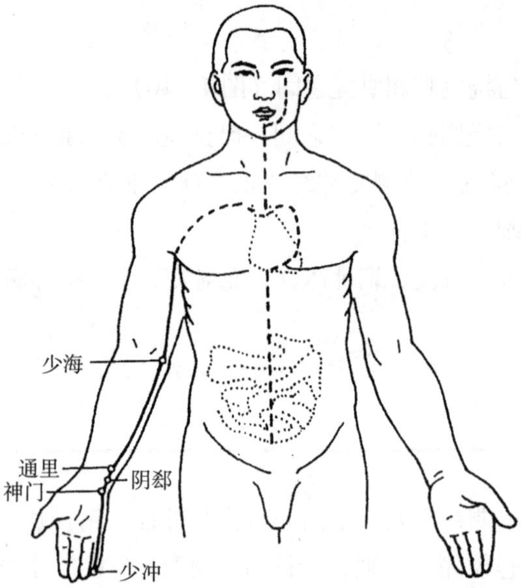

图4-12

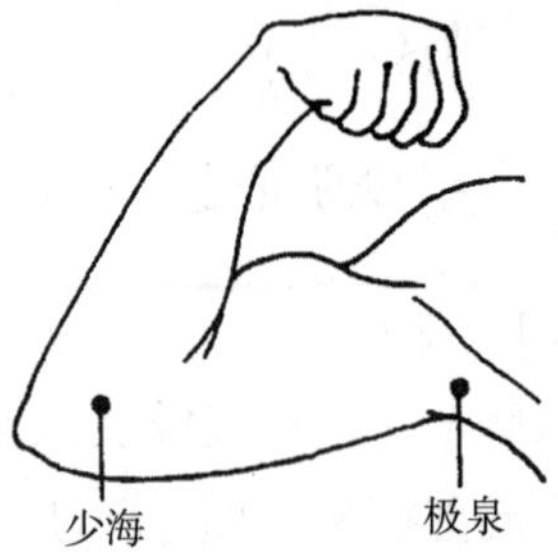

图4-13

4. 阴郄（HT6）。

定位：腕横纹上0.5寸，尺侧腕屈肌腱的桡侧缘（图4-12）。

层次解剖：皮肤→皮下组织→尺侧腕屈肌腱桡侧缘→尺神经。浅层有前臂内侧皮神经，贵要静脉属支等分布。深层有尺动、静脉。

主治举例：心动过速、心绞痛、心律不齐、胃出血、鼻出血、神经衰弱、低热等。

操作：直刺0.5寸。

5. 神门（HT7）。

定位：在腕横纹上，当尺侧腕屈肌腱桡侧（图4-12）。

层次解剖：皮肤→皮下组织→尺侧腕屈肌腱桡侧缘。浅层有前臂内侧皮神经，贵要静脉属支和尺神经掌支等分布。深层有尺动、静脉和尺神经分布。

主治举例：心动过速、心绞痛、心律不齐、失眠、神经衰弱、癔症、精神病等。

操作：直刺0.3~0.5寸。

6. 少冲（HT9）。

定位：小指桡侧，距指甲角约0.1寸（图4－12）。

层次解剖：皮肤→皮下组织→指甲根。布有尺神经的指掌固有神经指背支和指掌固有动、静脉指背支形成的动、静脉网。

主治举例：心绞痛、精神病、昏迷、发热等。

操作：毫针浅刺或点刺出血。

4.3.4　手阳明大肠经

4.3.4.1　概况

本经从手至头面，首穴商阳，末穴迎香，单侧共20穴。主要治疗头面、五官疾病和大肠有关的病症，以及经脉循行部位的病变，如头痛、三叉神经痛、面瘫、眼病、齿痛、鼻塞、咽喉炎、甲状腺肿、胃肠道疾病，上肢的疼痛、麻木、瘫痪。

4.3.4.2　主要循行线

起于食指桡侧端，经第一、二掌骨之间，沿腕臂背侧面的桡侧缘到达肩部，进入锁骨上窝，联络肺，属于大肠，其分支从锁骨上窝上行，经面颊，入下齿，回绕上唇，左侧的经脉向右，右侧的经脉向左，止于鼻翼两旁（图4－14）。

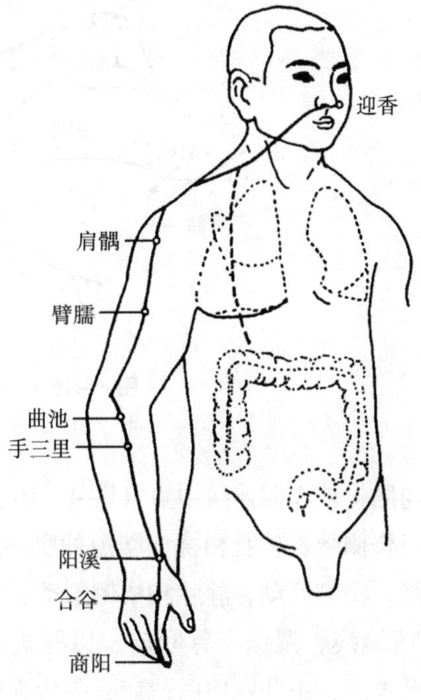

图4－14

4.3.4.3　常用穴位

1. 商阳（LI1）。

定位：食指桡侧端，距指甲角约0.1寸（图4－14）。

层次解剖：皮肤→皮下组织→指甲根。有正中神经的指掌侧固有神经之指背支和食指桡侧动、静脉与第一掌背动、静脉分支所形成的动、静脉网。

主治举例：发热、昏迷、急性咽喉炎及扁桃体炎、腮腺炎、口腔炎等。

操作：毫针浅刺或三棱针点刺。

2. 合谷（LI4）。

定位：手背第一、二掌骨之间，近第二掌骨中点的桡侧（图4－15）。

层次解剖：皮肤→皮下组织→第一骨间背侧肌→拇收肌。浅层布有桡神经浅支、手背静脉网的桡侧部和第一掌背动静脉的分支或属支。深层有尺神经深支的分支等结构。

主治举例：感冒、扁桃体炎、腮腺炎、头痛、面瘫、面肌抽搐、三叉神经痛、舌炎、牙龈炎、近视眼、高血压、中风后遗症、多发性神经炎、胃肠炎、阑尾炎、便秘、痛经、难产、荨麻疹等。

操作：直刺0.5～1寸。

3. 手三里（LI10）。

定位：肘横纹下2寸，当阳溪与曲池连线上（图4－16）。

层次解剖：皮肤→皮下组织→桡侧腕长伸肌→桡侧腕短伸肌→指伸肌的前方→旋后肌。浅层布有前臂外侧皮神经、前臂后皮神经等。深层由桡侧返动、静脉的分支或属支以及桡神经深支。

主治举例：腹痛、腹泻、牙痛、颈椎病、中风后遗症、咽喉炎、肘臂疼痛等。

操作：直刺0.8～1.5寸。

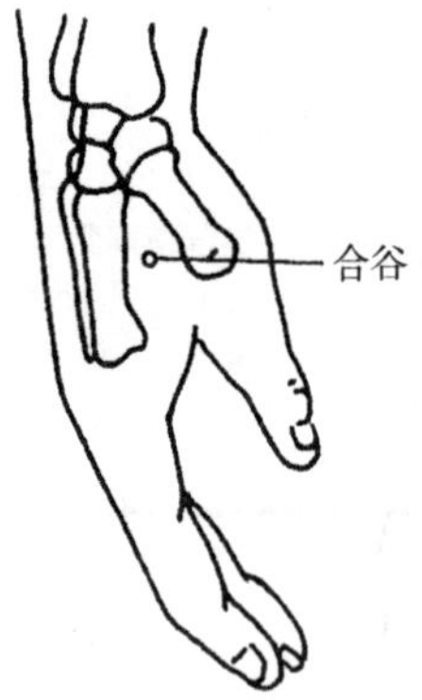

图4－15

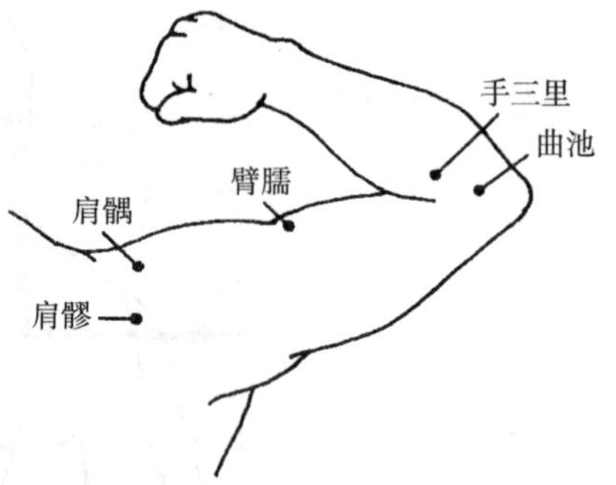

图4－16

4. 曲池（LI11）。

定位：屈肘，肘横纹外侧端与肱骨外上髁连线中点（图4－16）。

层次解剖：皮肤→皮下组织→桡侧腕长伸肌和桡侧腕短伸肌→肱桡肌。浅层布有头静脉的属支和前臂后皮神经。深层有桡神经，桡侧返动、静脉和桡侧副动、静脉间的吻合支。

主治举例：上肢疼痛、麻木或瘫痪、湿疹、荨麻疹、胃肠炎、感冒、扁桃体炎、疟疾、发热、高血压、神经衰弱、癫痫、精神病、小儿麻痹后遗症、甲状腺肿大等。

操作：直刺0.8～1.5寸。

5. 肩髃（LI15）。

定位：锁骨肩峰下缘，上臂平举时，肩部出现两个凹陷，前方的凹陷即为本穴（图4－16）。

层次解剖：皮肤→皮下组织→三角肌→三角肌下囊→冈上肌腱。浅层有锁骨上外侧神经、臂外侧上皮神经分布。深层有旋肱后动、静脉和腋神经的分支。

主治举例：上肢瘫痪、肩关节周围炎等。

操作：上臂平举时直刺1～1.5寸；如上臂不能平举时，向下斜刺。

6. 迎香（LI20）。

定位：鼻翼外缘中点旁，当鼻唇沟中（图4－17）。

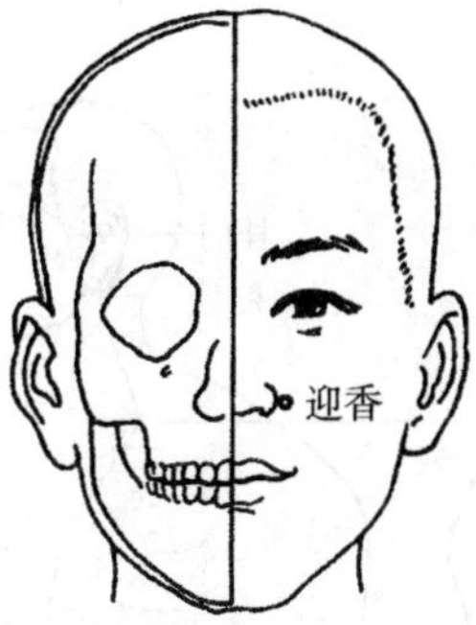

图4－17

层次解剖：皮肤→皮下组织→提上唇肌。浅层有上颌神经的眶下神经分支等结构。深层有上唇动、静脉和面神经颊支等分布。

主治举例：慢性鼻炎、面瘫、三叉神经痛等。

操作：向鼻根部斜刺0.5～1寸。

4.3.4.4　次常用穴

二间（LI2）：微握拳，在手食指本节前，桡侧凹陷处。

三间（LI3）：微握拳，在手食指本节后，桡侧凹陷处。

阳溪（LI5）：在腕背横纹桡侧，手拇指向上翘起时，拇长、短伸肌腱之间的凹陷中。

偏历（LI6）：腕横纹上3寸，阳溪与曲池连线上。

温溜（LI7）：腕横纹上5寸，阳溪与曲池连线上。

下廉（LI8）：肘横纹下4寸，阳溪与曲池连线上。

上廉（LI9）：肘横纹下3寸，阳溪与曲池连线上。

肘髎（LI12）：屈肘，曲池上方1寸，肱骨边缘处。

手五里（LI13）：曲池上方3寸，曲池与肩髃连线上。

巨骨（LI16）：锁骨肩峰端与肩胛冈之间凹陷处。

天鼎（LI17）：结喉旁，胸锁乳突肌后缘，扶突穴与缺盆连线中点。

扶突（LI18）：结喉旁，胸锁乳突肌的前、后缘之间。

4.3.5　手少阳三焦经

4.3.5.1　概况

本经从手至头，首穴关冲，末穴丝竹空，单侧共23穴。主要治疗耳、侧头部、胁肋部以及眼、咽喉部疾病，如耳鸣、耳聋、中耳炎、结膜炎、近视、咽喉炎，还可治疗发热、肩臂肘部外侧疼痛。

4.3.5.2　主要循行线

起于无名指端，沿上肢背侧面中间上行至肩，向前进入锁骨上窝，联络心包，属于三焦。一分支从胸中上行，循颈部到耳后，直上耳上角，由此屈而下行，绕颊部到眼眶下。另一分支与足少阳胆经相接（图4－18）。

4.3.5.3 常用穴位

1. 关冲（SJ1）。

定位：在手环指末节尺侧，距指甲角0.1寸（图4－18）。

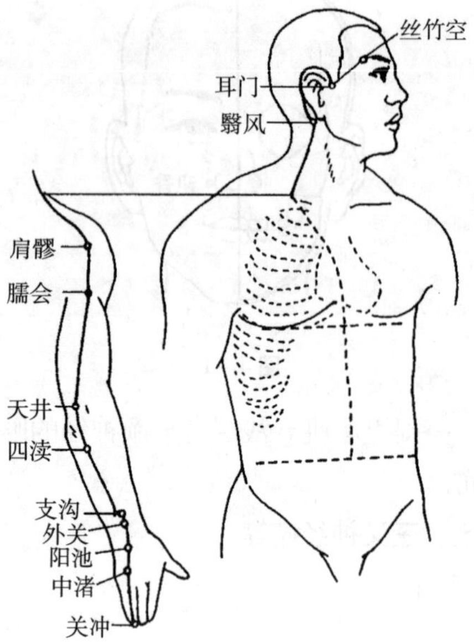

图4－18

层次解剖：皮肤→皮下组织→指甲根。皮下组织内有尺神经指掌侧固有神经的指背支的分支，指掌侧固有动、静脉指背支的动、静脉网。

主治举例：感冒、发热、角膜炎、急性咽喉炎、扁桃体炎、流行性腮腺炎、耳聋、昏迷、中暑等。

操作：浅刺0.1寸或三棱针点刺出血。

2. 中渚（SJ3）。

定位：手背第四、五掌指关节后凹陷中（图4－18）。

层次解剖：皮肤→皮下组织→第四掌骨肌背侧肌。浅层布有尺神经的指背神经，手背静脉网的尺侧部。深层有第四掌背动脉。

主治举例：耳聋、耳鸣、颞颌关节炎、落枕、肋间神经痛、小指麻木等。

操作：直刺或斜刺0.3~0.8寸。

3. 外关（SJ5）。

定位：腕背横纹上2寸，桡骨、尺骨之间（图4－18）。

层次解剖：皮肤→皮下组织→小指伸肌和指伸肌→拇长伸肌和食指伸肌。浅层布有前臂后皮神经，头静脉和贵要静脉的属支。深层有骨间后动、静脉和骨间后神经。

主治举例：感冒、发热、耳聋、耳鸣、偏头痛、肋间神经痛、高血压、上肢瘫痪、小儿麻痹后遗症、指腕关节痛等。

操作：直刺0.5~1寸。

参考：透内关、配养老治腕关节痛；配大陵、支沟治便秘。

4. 支沟（SJ6）。

定位：腕背横纹上3寸，尺骨与桡骨之间（图4－18）。

层次解剖：皮肤→皮下组织→小指伸肌→拇长伸肌→前臂骨间膜。浅层布有前臂后支皮神经，头静脉和贵要静脉的属支。深层有骨间后动、静脉和骨间后神经。

主治举例：耳鸣、耳聋、习惯性便秘、发热、肋间神经痛、手指震颤、肘臂痛痪等。

操作：直刺0.5～1寸。

5. 四渎（SJ9）。

定位：阳池与肘尖的连线上，肘尖下5寸，尺骨与桡骨之间（图4－18）。

层次解剖：皮肤→皮下组织→小指伸肌与尺侧腕伸肌→拇长展肌和拇长伸肌。浅层布有前臂后支皮神经，头静脉和贵要静脉的属支。深层有骨间后动、静脉和骨间后神经。

主治举例：颈椎病、耳聋（暴聋）、声音嘶哑、上肢瘫痪等。

操作：直刺0.5～1寸。

6. 肩髎（SJ14）。

定位：肩峰后下方，上臂平举时肩后凹陷处，当肩髃穴后1寸（图4－18）。

层次解剖：皮肤→皮下组织→三头肌→小圆肌→大圆肌→背阔肌腱。浅层布锁骨上外侧神经。深层有腋神经和旋肱后动、静脉。

主治举例：肩关节及上肢部外侧病症等。

操作：直刺或斜刺0.6～1.2寸。

7. 翳风（SJ17）。

定位：耳垂后方，下颌角与乳突之间（图4－18）。

层次解剖：皮肤→皮下组织→腮腺。浅层布有耳大神经和颈外静脉的属支，深层有颈外动脉的分支及耳后动脉，面神经。

主治举例：耳聋、耳鸣、中耳炎、腮腺炎、颞下颌关节炎、面瘫、偏头痛等。

操作：直刺0.8～1.2寸。

8. 耳门（SJ21）。

定位：耳屏上切迹前方，下颌关节后缘张口呈凹陷处（图4－18）。

层次解剖：皮肤→皮下组织→腮腺。布有耳颞神经，颞浅动、静脉耳前支，面神经颞支结构。

主治举例：耳聋、耳鸣、中耳炎、颞下颌关节炎、牙痛等。

操作：张口，直刺0.5～1寸。

9. 丝竹空（SJ23）。

定位：眉梢凹陷处（图4－18）。

层次解剖：皮肤→皮下组织→眼轮匝肌。布有眶上神经，颧面神经，面神经颞支和颧支，颞浅动、静脉的额支。

主治举例：偏头痛、眩晕、角膜炎、视神经萎缩、睑腺炎、近视眼、眼睑下垂、眼肌痉挛、牙痛、精神病等。

操作：平刺0.5～1寸。

4.3.5.4 次常用穴位

液门（SJ2）：在手背部第四、五指间，指蹼缘后方赤白肉际处。

阳池（SJ4）：指伸肌腱的尺侧缘凹陷处。

会宗（SJ7）：腕背横纹上3寸，支沟尺侧，尺骨的桡侧缘。

三阳络（SJ8）：腕背横纹上4寸，尺骨与桡骨之间。

天井（SJ10）：屈肘，肘尖直上1寸凹陷处。

臑会（SJ13）：肘尖与肩髎的连线上，肩髎下3寸，三角肌的后下缘。

4.3.6 手太阳小肠经

4.3.6.1 概况

本经从手至头，首穴少泽，末穴听宫，单侧共19穴。主治头、枕、项背、肩胛部疼痛，眼、耳及其他本经循行部位的病症。

4.3.6.2 主要循行线

起于小指尺侧端，沿上肢背侧面尺侧缘上达肩，绕肩胛部，交会于大椎，向下进入锁骨上窝，联络心，下属小肠。其一支脉从锁骨上窝上行，循颈部上达面颊至目外眦，再进入耳内。分支与足太阳膀胱经相接（图4－19）。

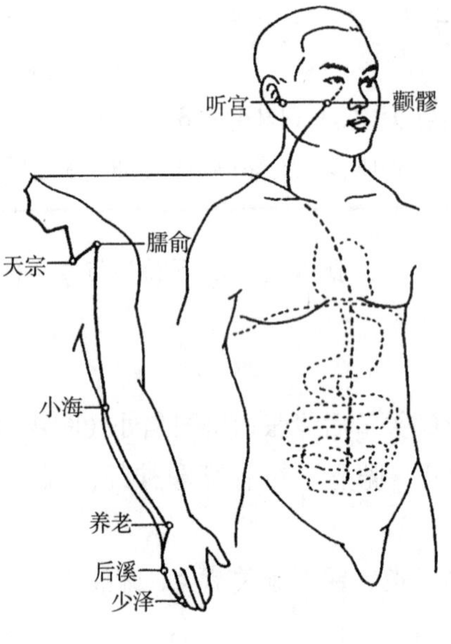

图4－19

4.3.6.3 常用穴位

1. 少泽（SI1）。

定位：小指尺侧，距指甲角约0.1寸（图4－19）。

层次解剖：皮肤→皮下组织→指甲根。有尺神经指掌侧固有神经的指背支和小指尺掌侧动、静脉指背支形成的动、静脉网。

主治举例：乳汁分泌不足、乳腺炎、昏迷、中暑、发热、指端麻木等。

操作：毫针浅刺或点刺出血。

2. 后溪（SI3）。

定位：第五掌指关节尺侧后方，赤白肉际凹陷中，握拳横纹尽处取之（图4-19）。

层次解剖：皮肤→皮下组织→小指展肌→小指短屈肌。浅层布有尺神经手背支、尺神经掌支和皮下浅静脉等。深层有小指尺掌侧固有动、静脉和指掌侧固有神经。

主治举例：神经性头痛、癫痫、落枕、耳聋、耳鸣、角膜炎、扁桃体炎、肩背痛、急性腰扭伤等。

操作：直刺0.6~1.5寸。

3. 养老（SI6）。

定位：掌心向胸，尺骨小头桡侧缘的骨缝中（图4-19）。

层次解剖：皮肤→皮下组织→尺侧腕伸肌腱。浅层布有前臂内侧皮神经，前臂后皮神经，尺神经手背支和贵要静脉的属支等。深层布有腕背动、静脉网等。

主治举例：视力减退、外眼炎症、肩背痛、急性腰扭伤等。

操作：掌心向胸时，向肘方向斜刺0.5~0.8寸。

4. 小海（SI8）。

定位：尺骨鹰嘴与肱骨内上髁之间凹陷处（图4-19）。

层次解剖：皮肤→皮下组织→尺神经沟。浅层有前臂内侧皮神经尺侧支，臂内侧皮神经，贵要静脉属支等结构。深层：在尺神经沟内有尺神经，尺神经的后外侧有尺侧上副动、静脉与尺动、静脉的尺侧返动、静脉后支吻合成的动、静脉网。

主治举例：尺神经痛、癫痫、神经衰弱、精神病、耳鸣、耳聋等。

操作：直刺0.5~1寸。

5. 天宗（SI11）。

定位：肩胛部，冈下窝中央凹陷处（图4-19）。

层次解剖：皮肤→皮下组织→斜方肌→冈上肌。浅层布有第四胸神经后支的皮支和伴行的动、静脉。深层布有肩胛上神经的分支和旋肩胛动、静脉的分支或属支。

主治举例：肩周炎、冈上肌肌腱炎、肩背肌筋膜炎、颈椎病、哮喘、乳腺炎等。

操作：直刺或斜刺0.8~1.2寸。

6. 听宫（SI19）。

定位：耳屏中点和下颌关节之间，张口凹陷处取穴（图4-19）。

层次解剖：皮肤→皮下组织→外耳道软骨。布有耳颞神经，颞浅动、静脉耳前支的分支或属支等结构。

主治举例：耳聋、耳鸣、中耳炎、颞下颌关节紊乱、聋哑等。

操作：直刺0.5~1寸。

4.3.6.4 次常用穴

前谷（SI2）：微握拳，当第五掌指关节前方，掌指横纹头赤白肉际。

腕骨（SI4）：第五掌骨基底与钩骨之间的凹陷处，赤白肉际。

阳谷（SI5）：尺骨茎突与三角骨之间的凹陷处。

支正（SI7）：腕背横纹上5寸，阳谷与小海的连线上。

肩贞（SI9）：在肩关节后下方，臂内收时，腋后纹头上1寸。

臑俞（SI10）：在肩部，腋后纹头直上，肩胛冈下缘凹陷中。

秉风（SI12）：冈上窝中央，天宗直上，举臂有凹陷处。

肩外俞（SI14）：第一胸椎棘突下，旁开3寸。

肩中俞（SI15）：第七颈椎棘突下，旁开2寸。

颧髎（SI18）：目外眦直下，颧骨下缘凹陷处。

4.3.7 足太阴脾经

4.3.7.1 概况

本经从足至腹，首穴隐白，末穴大包，单侧共21穴。主要治疗消化系统的病症，亦可治疗泌尿系统疾病，还可治疗与出血有关的病症及穴位所处局部的疾患。如消化不良、痢疾、肠炎、尿潴留、遗尿、崩漏、便血、膝痛等。

4.3.7.2 主要循行线

起于足大趾内侧端，沿足背内侧、内踝前面、胫骨内侧后方上行，在内踝上8寸处交会到足厥阴肝经的前面，经膝、股部内侧前缘进入腹部，属于脾，联络胃。分支与手少阴心经相接（图4-20）。

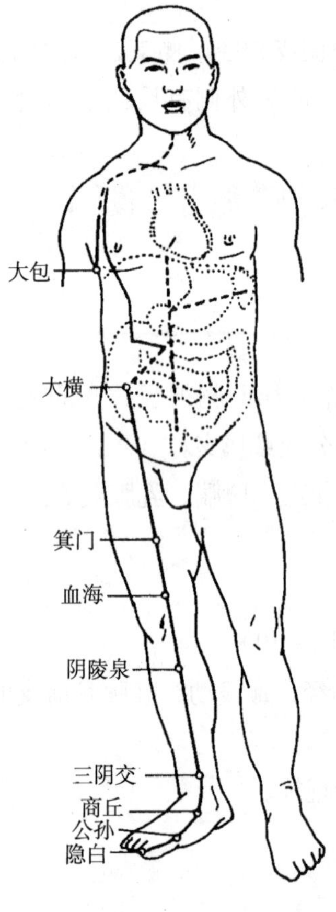

图4-20

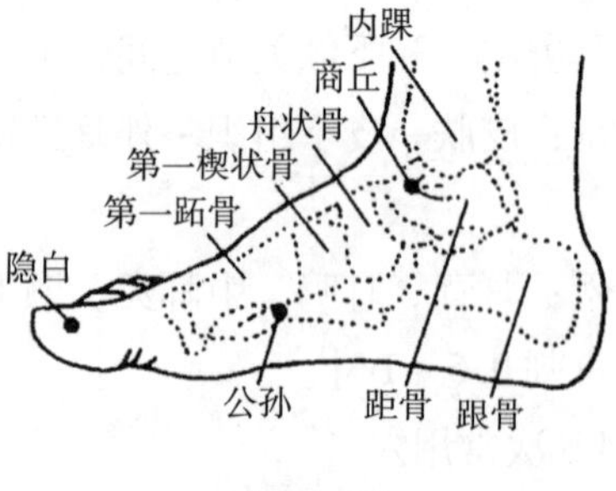

图4-21

4.3.7.3 常用穴位

1. 隐白（SP1）。

定位：足踇指内侧，距趾甲角0.1寸（图4-21）。

层次解剖：皮肤→皮下组织→甲根。布有足背内侧皮神经的分支，趾背神经和趾背动、静脉。

主治举例：消化不良、急慢性肠炎、上消化道出血、功能性子宫出血、月经不调（灸）、神经衰弱、精神病、昏迷、足趾痛等。

操作：毫针浅刺。

2. 公孙（SP4）。

定位：在足内侧缘，当第一跖骨基底的前下方（图4－21）。

层次解剖：皮肤→皮下组织→踇展肌→踇短屈肌→踇长屈肌腱。浅层布有隐神经的足内侧缘支，足背静脉弓的属支。深层有足底内侧动、静脉的分支或属支，足底内侧神经的分支。

主治举例：消化不良、神经性呕吐、急慢性胃炎、急慢性肠炎、腹水、踇囊炎、痛风等。

操作：直刺0.5～1寸。

3. 三阴交（SP6）。

定位：内踝尖上3寸，当胫骨的后缘（图4－22）。

层次解剖：皮肤→皮下组织→趾长屈肌→胫骨后肌→踇长屈肌。浅层布有隐神经的小腿内侧皮支，大隐静脉的属支。深层有胫神经和胫后动、静脉。

主治举例：腹痛、腹泻、月经不调、痛经、闭经、难产、遗尿、尿潴留、神经性皮炎、湿疹、荨麻疹、失眠、下肢瘫痪等。

操作：直刺0.5～1寸。

参考：①古籍记载本穴孕妇禁针。②为剖宫产、全子宫及附件切除术、卵巢囊肿摘除术、膀胱切开取石术等手术的针麻常用经穴。③另：有人认为高血压处于第一、二期，主要是小血管痉挛的阶段，应该选用三阴交、膈俞等与解除小血管痉挛有关的经穴。

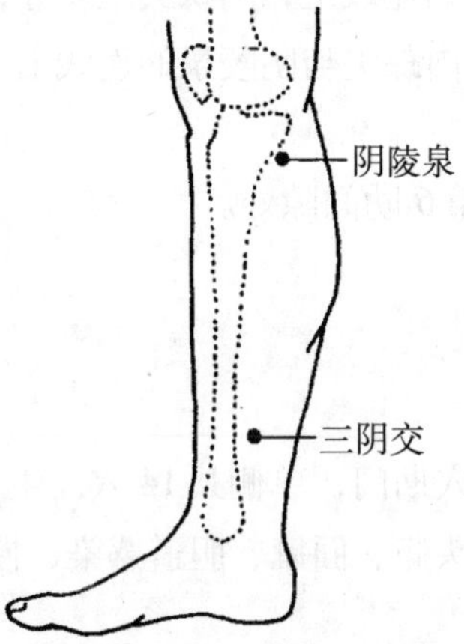

图4－22

4. 阴陵泉（SP9）。

定位：胫骨内侧髁下缘，胫骨内侧缘的凹陷处（图4－22）。

层次解剖：皮肤→皮下组织→半腱肌腱→腓肠肌内侧头。浅层布有隐神经的小腿内侧皮支，大隐静脉和膝降动脉分支。深层有膝下内侧动、静脉。

主治举例：腹痛、腹泻、水肿、尿潴留、尿路感染、遗尿、膝关节及周围软组织损伤等。

操作：直刺0.5～1寸。

参考：《千金翼方》，水肿不得卧，灸阴陵泉百壮。

5. 血海（SP10）。

定位：髌骨内上缘上2寸（图4－23）。

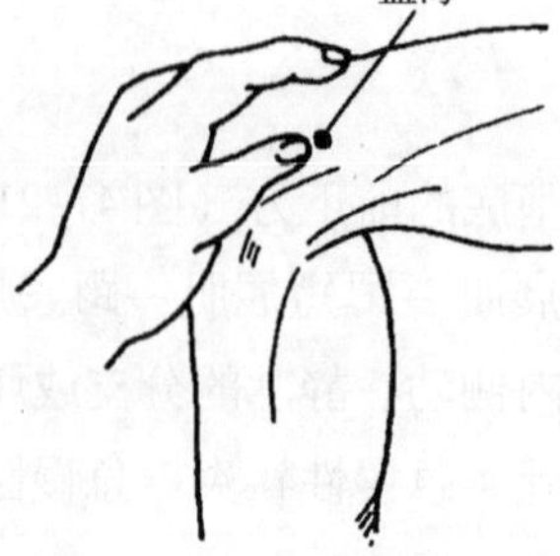

图4－23

层次解剖：皮肤→皮下组织→股内侧肌。浅层布有股神经前皮支，大隐静脉的属支。深层有股动、静脉的肌支和股神经肌支。

主治举例：月经过多、尿血、荨麻疹、湿疹、膝关节疼痛等。

操作：直刺0.5～1寸。

参考：配曲池、定喘、三阴交治荨麻疹。

4.3.7.4　次常用穴

大都（SP2）：第一跖趾关节前下方，赤白肉际凹陷处。

太白（SP3）：第一跖趾关节后下方，赤白肉际凹陷处。

商丘（SP5）：在足内踝前下方凹陷中，舟骨结节与内踝尖连线的中点处。

漏谷（SP7）：内踝尖与阴陵泉的连线上，内踝尖上6寸，胫骨内侧缘后方。

地机（SP8）：阴陵泉下3寸，内踝尖与阴陵泉的连线上。

大横（SP15）：肚脐旁开4寸。

大包（SP21）：腋中线上，当第6肋间隙处。

4.3.8　足厥阴肝经

4.3.8.1　概况

本经从足至腹，首穴大敦，末穴期门，单侧共14穴。主要治疗头顶、口唇、下腹部、前阴及肝胆、目病症，如痛经、睾丸炎、头痛、面瘫、胆道感染、慢性肝炎等疾病。

4.3.8.2　主要循行线

起于足大趾上，从足背经内踝前面，沿胫骨内侧上行，到踝上8寸处交叉到足太阴脾经的后面，再沿大腿内侧中间上行，环绕阴部，到达腹腔，夹胃属肝络胆，分布于胁肋。循喉咙后面上行，联系目，到头顶部。分支与手太阴肺经相接（图4－24）。

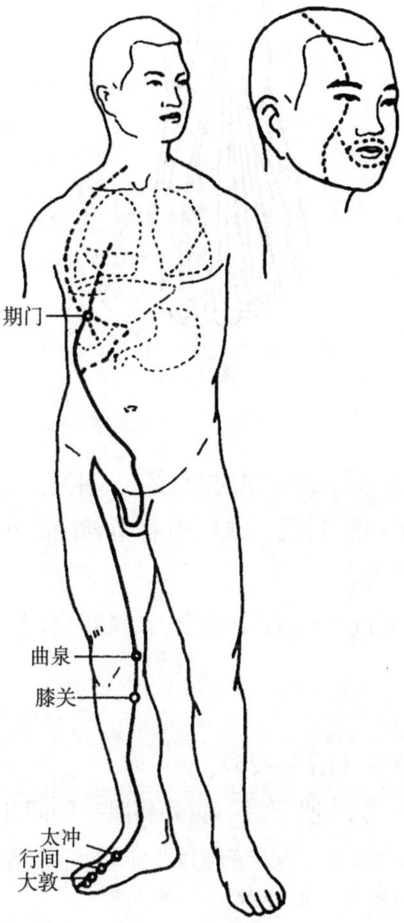

图4－24

4.3.8.3 常用穴位

1. 大敦（LR1）

定位：拇指外侧甲角旁约0.1寸（图4－25）。

层次解剖：皮肤→皮下组织→甲根。布有腓深神经的背外侧神经和趾背动、静脉等结构。

主治举例：疝气、精索神经痛、阴茎痛、功能性子宫出血、尿失禁、癫痫、昏迷等。

操作：毫针浅刺或三棱针点刺出血。

参考：据报道，对治疗急性附睾炎有显著效果，临床多配太冲、气海、归来、曲泉等穴使用。

2. 太冲（LR3）。

定位：足背第一、二跖骨结合部前的凹陷处（图4－25）。

层次解剖：皮肤→皮下组织→䟎长伸肌腱与趾长伸肌腱之间→䟎短伸肌腱的外侧→第一骨间背侧肌。浅层布有足背静脉网，足背内侧皮神经等。深层有腓深神经和第一趾背动、静脉。

主治举例：头痛、眩晕、高血压病、面瘫、面肌抽搐、䟎囊炎、痛风、精神病、癫痫等。

操作：直刺0.5～1寸。

参考：①对施行胆囊切除术和胆总管探查术的急性胆道疾病患者观察到，单刺太冲能使注射吗啡后胆道压力不仅停止上升，而且迅速下降。②针刺太冲缓解奥狄氏括约肌痉挛的作用大于足三里、阳陵泉。针刺委中、期门无改变。

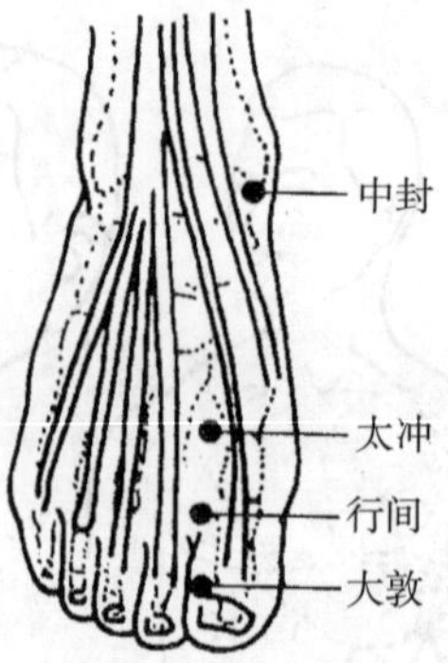

图 4－25

3. 膝关（LR7）。

定位：胫骨内侧髁的后下方，阴陵泉后1寸（图4－24）。

层次解剖：皮肤→皮下组织→腓肠肌。浅层布有隐神经的小腿内侧皮支，大隐静脉的属支。深层有腘动、静脉，胫神经等结构。

主治举例：膝关节内侧副韧带损伤、髌下滑囊炎、膝关节炎、急慢性咽喉炎等。

操作：直刺0.5～1寸。

4. 期门（LR14）。

定位：乳头直下第六肋间隙中（图4－26）。

层次解剖：皮肤→皮下组织→胸大肌下缘→腹外斜肌→肋间外肌→肋间内肌。浅层布有第六肋间神经的外侧皮支，胸腹壁静脉的属支。深层有第六肋间神经和第六肋间动、静脉的分支或属支。

主治举例：肋间神经痛、胆囊炎、肝炎等。

操作：斜刺，针0.3～0.5寸。

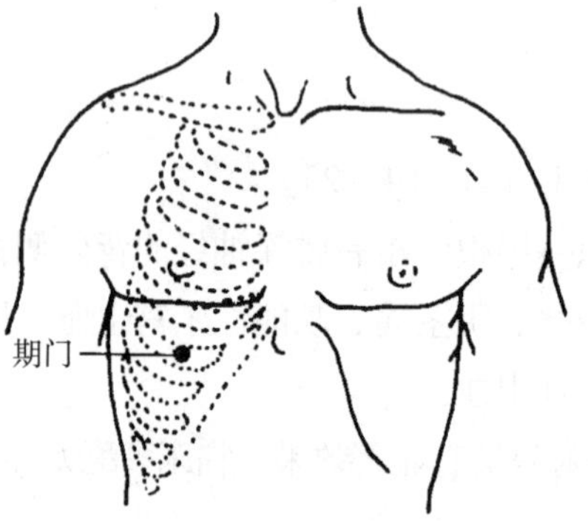

图 4－26

4.3.8.4 次常用穴

行间（LR2）：在足背第一、二趾间，趾蹼缘的后方赤白肉际处。

中封（LR4）：足内踝前，商丘与解溪连线之间，胫骨前肌腱的内侧凹陷处。

蠡沟（LR5）：足内踝尖上5寸，胫骨内侧面的中央。

中都（LR6）：在小腿内侧，足内踝尖上7寸，胫骨内侧面的中央。

曲泉（LR8）：屈膝，膝关节内侧面横纹内侧端，胫骨内侧髁的后缘，半膜肌止端的前缘凹陷处。

章门（LR13）：在侧腹部，第十一肋游离端的下方。

4.3.9　足少阴肾经

4.3.9.1　概况

本经从足至腹，首穴涌泉，末穴俞府，单侧共27穴。主要治疗泌尿、生殖系统的病症，以及由于“肾虚”引起的呼吸系统和神经系统疾病。如遗精、阳痿、早泄、浮肿、尿潴留、遗尿、喘咳、咽喉炎、失眠、耳鸣、耳聋、眩晕、腰痛等。

4.3.9.2　主要循行线

起于小趾下，斜走足心，沿内踝之后，转行足跟部，由下肢内侧后缘，上行脊柱，属肾络膀胱。直行经脉从肾上行肝，进入肺，沿喉咙到舌根部。分支与手厥阴心包经相接（图4－27）。

4.3.9.3　常用穴位

1. 涌泉（KI1）。

定位：约当足底（去趾）前1/3与后2/3交界处，卷足时呈凹陷（图4－28）。

层次解剖：皮肤→皮下组织→足底腱膜（跖腱膜）→第二趾足底总神经→第二蚓状肌。浅层布有足底内侧神经的分支。深层有第二趾足底总神经和第二趾足底总动、静脉。

主治举例：昏迷、头痛、眩晕、高血压、神经衰弱、失眠、小便不利等。

操作：直刺0.5～1寸。

参考：配关元、丰隆治虚劳咳嗽；配人中、十宣、足三里治晕厥、抽搐。

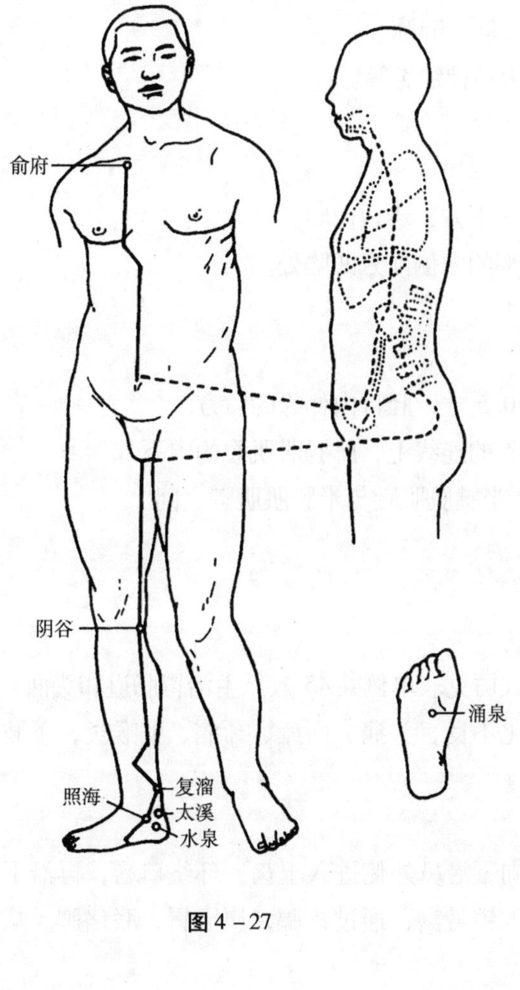

图4－27

图4－28

2. 太溪（KI3）。

定位：内踝与跟腱之间凹陷中，平内踝尖（图 4－29）。

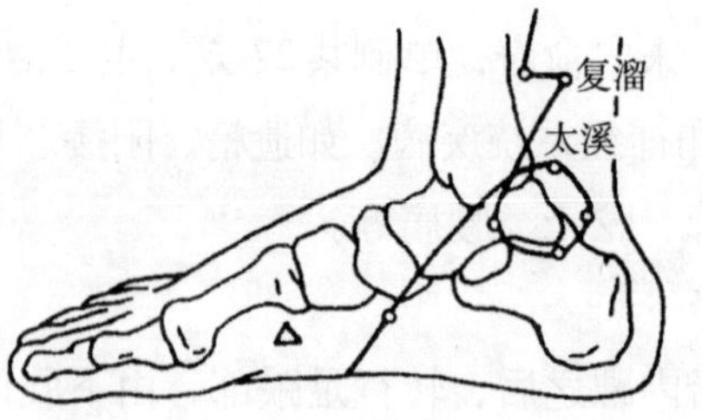

图 4－29

层次解剖：皮肤→皮下组织→胫骨后肌腱、趾长屈肌腱与跟腱、跖肌腱之间→踇长屈肌。浅层布有隐神经的小腿内侧皮支，大隐静脉的属支。深层有胫神经和胫后动、静脉。

主治举例：头痛、眩晕、耳鸣、视力减退、牙痛、慢性咽喉炎、足跟痛、遗精、阳痿、慢性前列腺炎、踝关节扭伤等。

操作：直刺 0.6～1 寸。

参考：配昆仑、申脉治足肿难行；配神门、三阴交治失眠、神经衰弱。

3. 复溜（KI7）。

定位：在小腿内侧，太溪直上 2 寸（图 4－29）。

层次解剖：皮肤→皮下组织→跖肌腱和跟腱前方→踇长屈肌。浅层布有隐神经的小腿内侧皮支，大隐静脉的属支。深层有胫神经和胫后动、静脉。

主治举例：慢性腰痛、肾炎、水肿、末梢神经炎等。

操作：直刺 0.5～1 寸。

4.3.9.4　次常用穴位

然谷（KI2）：在足内侧缘，足舟骨粗隆下方，赤白肉际。

大钟（KI4）：内踝后下方，跟腱附着部的内侧前方凹陷处。

水泉（KI5）：内踝后下方，太溪直下 1 寸。

照海（KI6）：内踝尖下方凹陷处。

交信（KI8）：太溪直上 2 寸，复溜前 0.5 寸，胫骨内侧缘的后方。

筑宾（KI9）：太溪上 5 寸，太溪与阴谷的连线上，腓肠肌肌腹的内下方。

阴谷（KI10）：在腘窝内侧，屈膝时，半腱肌肌腱与半膜肌肌腱之间。

4.3.10　足阳明胃经

4.3.10.1　概况

本经从头面走向下肢，首穴承泣，末穴厉兑。单侧共 45 穴。主治胃肠道和头面五官疾病以及经脉循行部位的病变。如胃炎、肠炎、消化不良、头痛、面瘫、牙痛、咽喉炎，下肢的瘫痪、麻木、疼痛等。

4.3.10.2　主要循行线

起于鼻旁，交会鼻根中及目内眦，又向下沿鼻外侧进入上齿，环绕口唇，再沿下颌角上行到前额。其下行的经脉，从下颌部下行，进入锁骨窝，通过横膈，属于胃，联络脾。从胃口分出的一条支脉，沿腹壁里面走到腹股沟部，与循行于体表的经脉相会合，行于大腿前面、胫骨外侧到足背部，止于第二趾外侧端。另有分支与足太阴脾经相接（图4－30）。

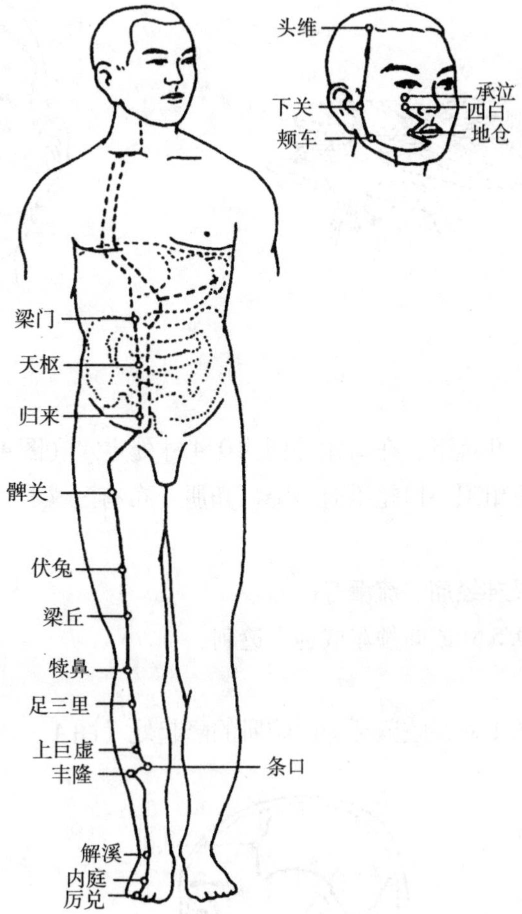

图4－30

4.3.10.3　常用穴位

1. 承泣（ST1）。

定位：目正视前方，瞳孔直下，在眶下缘与眼球之间取穴（图4－30）。

层次解剖：皮肤→皮下组织→眼轮匝肌→眶脂体→下斜肌。浅层布有眶下神经的分支、面神经的颧支。深层有动眼神经分支，眼动、静脉分支或属支等结构。

主治举例：角膜炎、急慢性结膜炎、斜视、白内障、青光眼、夜盲、视神经炎、视神经萎缩、近视、色盲、眼睑抽动、面瘫、面肌抽搐、眼睑下垂等。

操作：沿眶下缘直刺0.3～0.5寸，不作捻转（图4－31）。

2. 四白（ST2）。

定位：目正视前方，瞳孔直下，眶下孔凹陷处（图4－32）。

层次解剖：皮肤→皮下组织→眼轮匝肌、提上唇肌→眶下孔或上颌骨。浅层布有眶下神经的分支、面神经颧支。深层在眶下孔内有眶下动、静脉和神经穿出。

主治举例：面瘫、面肌抽搐、三叉神经痛、近视、角膜炎、结膜炎、眼睑下垂、青光眼、鼻炎、胆道蛔虫症等。

操作：直刺0.4～0.6寸，不宜灸。

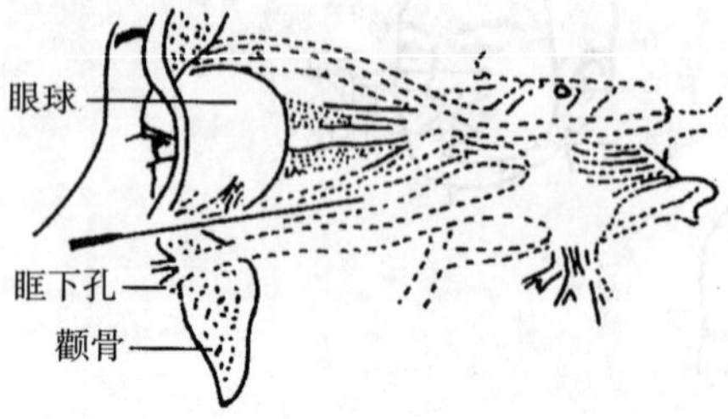

图4－31

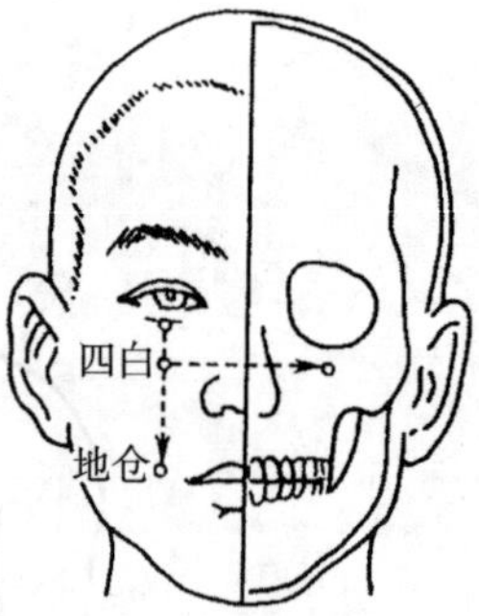

图4－32

3. 地仓（ST4）。

定位：目正视前方，瞳孔直下，在口角外侧约0.4寸处定穴（图4－32）。

层次解剖：皮肤→皮下组织→口轮匝肌→降口角肌。布有三叉神经颊支和眶下支，面动、静脉的分支或属支。

主治举例：面瘫、三叉神经痛、流涎等。

操作：斜刺或沿皮刺0.5寸或向颊车或迎香透刺。

4. 颊车（ST6）。

定位：下颌角前上方约1寸，咬紧牙齿时咬肌的隆起处（图4－33）。

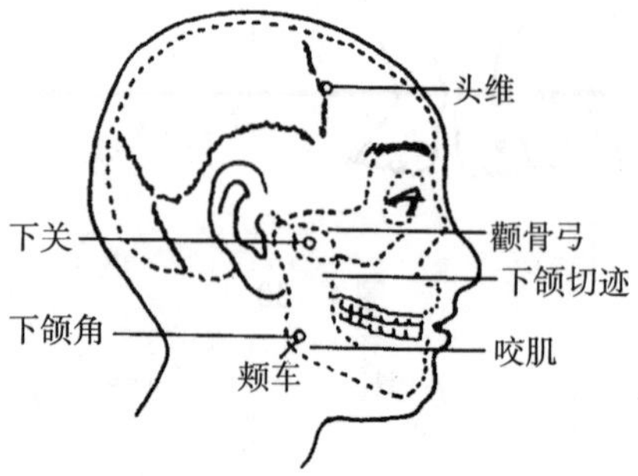

图4－33

层次解剖：皮肤→皮下组织→咬肌。布有耳大神经的分支、面神经下颌缘支的分支。

主治举例：面瘫、三叉神经痛、面肌抽搐、牙痛、腮腺炎等。

操作：直刺0.5～1.5寸或向地仓、颧髎透刺。

5. 下关（ST7）。

定位：耳屏前，颧弓与下颌切迹所形成的凹陷中（图4－33）。

层次解剖：皮肤→皮下组织→腮腺→咬肌与颞骨颧突之间→翼外肌。浅层有耳颞神经的分支、面神经颧支，面横动、静脉等结构。深层有上颌动、静脉，舌神经，下牙槽神经，脑膜中动脉和翼丛等。

主治举例：牙痛、颞下颌关节炎、三叉神经痛、耳聋、中耳炎等。

操作：直刺0.8～1.2寸或向听宫斜刺。

6. 头维（ST8）。

定位：在头侧部，额角发际上0.5寸，头正中线旁4.5寸（图4-33）。

层次解剖：皮肤→皮下组织→颞肌上缘的帽状腱膜→腱膜疏松结缔组织→颅骨外膜。布有耳颞神经的分支，面神经的颞支，颞浅动、静脉的额支等结构。

主治举例：头痛、眩晕、面瘫等。

操作：向后平刺0.5~1寸。

7. 天枢（ST25）。

定位：肚脐旁开2寸（图4-30）。

层次解剖：皮肤→皮下组织→腹直肌鞘前壁→腹直肌。浅层布有第九、十、十一胸神经前支的外侧皮支和前皮支及脐周静脉网。深层有腹壁上下动、静脉的吻合支和第九、十、十一胸神经前支的肌支。

主治举例：急慢性肠炎、急慢性胃炎、菌痢、肠麻痹、阑尾炎、婴幼儿腹泻、习惯性便秘、消化不良、腹肌瘫痪等。

操作：直刺0.6~1.2寸。

8. 髀关（ST31）。

定位：髂前上棘与髌骨外侧端的连线上，平臀横纹处（图4-30）。

层次解剖：皮肤→皮下组织→阔筋膜张肌与缝匠肌之间→股直肌→股外侧肌。浅层布有股外侧皮神经。深层有旋股外侧动、静脉的升支，股神经的肌支等。

主治举例：高位腰椎间盘突出症、髂胫束痉挛及髋关节疾患、下肢瘫痪等。

操作：直刺0.5~1寸。

9. 伏兔（ST32）。

定位：髌骨上6寸，髂前上棘与髌骨外侧端的连线上（图4-30）。

层次解剖：皮肤→皮下组织→股直肌→股中间肌。浅层布有股外侧静脉、股神经前皮支及股外侧皮神经。深层有旋股外侧动、静脉的降支，股神经的肌支痪等。

主治举例：高位腰椎间盘突出症、髂胫束痉挛、股外侧皮神经炎、疝气、腹股沟淋巴结炎、下肢瘫痪等。

操作：直刺0.5~1寸。

10. 梁丘（ST34）。

定位：髌骨外上缘上2寸凹陷处（图4-30）。

层次解剖：皮肤→皮下组织→股直肌腱与股外侧肌之间→股中间肌腱的外侧。浅层布有股神经的前皮支和股外侧皮神经。深层有旋股外侧动、静脉的降支和股神经的肌支。

主治举例：急性胃炎、胃痉挛、腹泻、乳腺炎、膝关节及周围软组织疾患等。

操作：直刺0.5~1.2寸。

11. 足三里（ST36）。

定位：犊鼻（髌韧带外侧凹陷）下3寸，胫骨前缘外侧一横指（图4-30）。

层次解剖：皮肤→皮下组织→胫骨前肌→小腿骨间膜→胫骨后肌。浅层布有腓肠外侧皮神经等结构。深层有胫前动、静脉的分支或属支等。

主治举例：急慢性胃炎、急慢性肠炎、胃痉挛、急慢性胰腺炎、胃或十二指肠溃疡、肝炎、消化不良、细菌性痢疾、阑尾炎、便秘、休克、神经性头痛、神经衰弱、动脉硬化、白细胞减少症、高血压、乳腺炎、坐骨神经痛、下肢瘫痪、支气管哮喘等。

操作：直刺0.5~1.5寸。

12. 上巨虚（ST37）。

定位：犊鼻（髌韧带外侧凹陷）下6寸，胫骨前缘一横指（图4-30）。

层次解剖：皮肤→皮下组织→胫骨前肌→小腿骨间膜→胫骨后肌。浅层布有腓肠外侧皮神经。深层有胫前动、静脉和腓深神经。如深刺可能刺中胫后动、静脉和胫神经。

主治举例：阑尾炎、痢疾、急慢性肠炎、下肢疼痛、瘫痪等。

操作：直刺0.5~1.2寸。

13. 条口（ST38）。

定位：犊鼻（髌韧带外侧凹陷）下8寸，胫骨前缘一横指（图4-30）。

层次解剖：皮肤→皮下组织→胫骨前肌→小腿骨间膜→胫骨后肌。浅层布有腓肠外侧皮神经。深层有胫前动、静脉和腓深神经。如深刺可能刺中腓动、静脉。

主治举例：肩周炎、腰椎间盘突出症、膝关节炎、多发性神经炎、胃痛等。

操作：直刺0.5~1.2寸。

14. 丰隆（ST40）。

定位：犊鼻（髌韧带外侧凹陷）下8寸，胫骨前缘外侧二横指（图4-30）。

层次解剖：皮肤→皮下组织→趾长伸肌→长伸肌→小腿骨间膜→胫骨后肌。浅层布有腓肠外侧皮神经。深层有胫前动、静脉的分支或属支和腓深神经的分支。

主治举例：支气管炎、哮喘、眩晕、精神病、癫痫、腓肠肌痉挛，下肢疼痛、麻木、瘫痪、消化不良、便秘等。

操作：直刺0.5~1.2寸。

参考：《肘后歌》，哮喘发来寝不得，丰隆刺人三分深。

15. 解溪（ST41）。

定位：足背、踝关节横纹中点，跗长伸肌腱和趾长伸肌腱之间（图4-30）。

层次解剖：皮肤→皮下组织→跗长伸肌腱与趾长伸肌腱之间→距骨。浅层布有足背内侧皮神经及足背皮下静脉。深层有腓深神经和胫前动、静脉。

主治举例：头痛、下肢瘫痪、踝关节及周围软组织疾患等。

操作：直刺0.4~0.8寸。

16. 内庭（ST44）。

定位：在足背，第二、三趾间，趾蹼后方赤白肉际处（图4-30）。

层次解剖：皮肤→皮下组织→在第二与第三趾的趾长、短伸肌腱之间→第二、第三趾骨头之间。浅层布有足背内侧皮神经的趾背神经和足背静脉网。深层有趾背动、静脉网。

主治举例：牙痛、喉炎、鼻出血、角膜炎、发热、急慢性肠炎、足背痛、面瘫等。

操作：直刺0.5~1.2寸。

4.3.10.4　次常用穴位

巨髎（ST3）：瞳孔直下，平鼻翼下缘处，当鼻唇沟外侧。

大迎（ST5）：下颌角前方，咬肌附着部的前缘，面动脉搏动处。

人迎（ST9）：喉结旁，胸锁乳突肌的前缘，颈总动脉搏动处。

缺盆（ST12）：在锁骨上窝中央，距前正中线4寸。

梁门（ST21）：脐上4寸，距前正中线2寸。

大巨（ST27）：脐下2寸，距前正中线2寸。

水道（ST28）：脐下3寸，距前正中线2寸。

归来（ST29）：脐下4寸，距前正中线2寸。

阴市（ST33）：髌骨外上缘上3寸，髂前上棘与髌骨外侧端的连线上。

犊鼻（ST35）：髌韧带外侧凹陷中。

下巨虚（ST39）：犊鼻下9寸，距胫骨前缘一横指（中指）。

冲阳（ST42）：在足背最高处，当𧿹长伸肌腱与趾长伸肌腱之间，足背动脉搏动处。

陷谷（ST43）：第二、三跖骨结合部前方凹陷处。

4.3.11　足少阳胆经

4.3.11.1　概况

本经从头至足，首穴瞳子髎，末穴足窍阴，单侧共44穴。主要治疗头、身侧面的病症及肝胆疾病。如偏头痛、耳鸣、耳聋、眼病、胁肋和下肢外侧的疾患，以及肝炎、胆囊炎等。

4.3.11.2　主要循行线

起于眼角，到达颞部，经耳后循颈部和少阳经前方，抵肩部，交叉到手少阳经之后，进入锁骨窝。直行的经脉从锁骨窝下行。经胁部到达髋关节部；其内行线联络肝，属于胆，经过前阴部，至髋关节部与体表循行的经脉会合。再沿下肢外侧，止于足第四趾端。支脉与足厥阴肝经相连（图4－34）。

4.3.11.3　常用穴位

1. 听会（GB2）。

定位：耳屏间切迹前方，下颌髁状突的后缘，张口有凹陷处取穴（图4－34）。

层次解剖：皮肤→皮下组织→腮腺囊→腮腺。浅层布有耳颞神经和耳大神经。深层有颞浅动、静脉和面神经丛等结构。

主治举例：耳聋、耳鸣、中耳炎、头痛、咀嚼肌痉挛、下颌关节炎、面瘫等。

操作：直刺0.5～0.8寸。

2. 率谷（GB8）。

定位：耳尖直上入发际1.5寸（图4－34）。

层次解剖：皮肤→皮下组织→耳上肌→颞筋膜→颞肌。布有耳颞神经和枕大神经会合支及颞浅动、静脉顶支。

主治举例：偏头痛、眩晕、结膜炎、角膜炎、面神经麻痹、小儿惊厥等。

操作：沿皮刺0.5～1寸。

3. 阳白（GB14）。

定位：眉毛正中上1寸，眼平视直对瞳孔（图4－35）。

层次解剖：皮肤→皮下组织→枕额肌额腹。布有眶上神经外侧支和眶上动、静脉外侧支。

主治举例：面瘫、头痛、眩晕、三叉神经痛、眼睑下垂、夜盲、近视等。

操作：沿皮刺0.4～0.8寸。

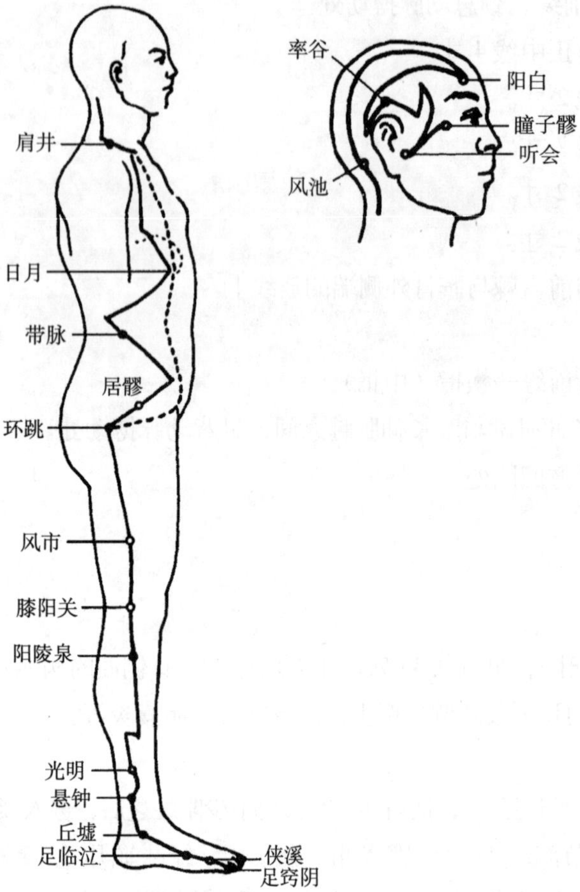

图 4－34

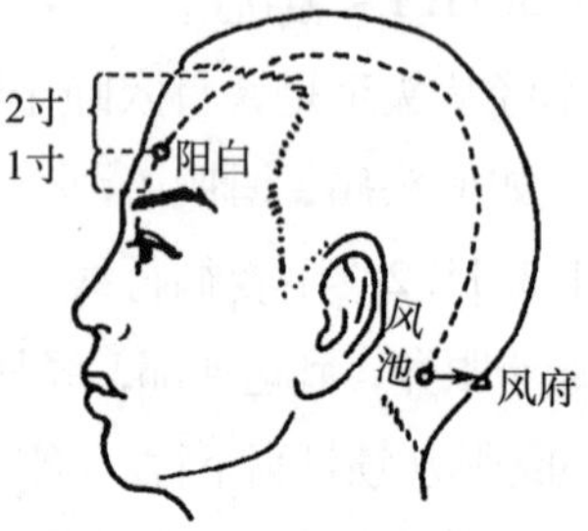

图 4－35

4. 风池（GB20）。

定位：枕骨粗隆直下凹陷处与乳突之间，斜方肌与胸锁乳突肌上端之间的凹陷中取穴（图 4－35）。

层次解剖：皮肤→皮下组织→斜方肌和胸锁乳突肌之间→头夹肌→头半棘肌→头后直肌与头上斜肌之间。浅层布有枕小神经和枕动、静脉分支或属支。深层有枕下神经等结构。

主治举例：感冒、眩晕、头痛、鼻炎、外眼炎症、视神经萎缩、失眠、高血压等。

操作：向对侧眼睛方向斜刺 0.5～0.8 寸。本穴深部中间为延髓，必须严格掌握针刺的角度和深度（图 4－36）。

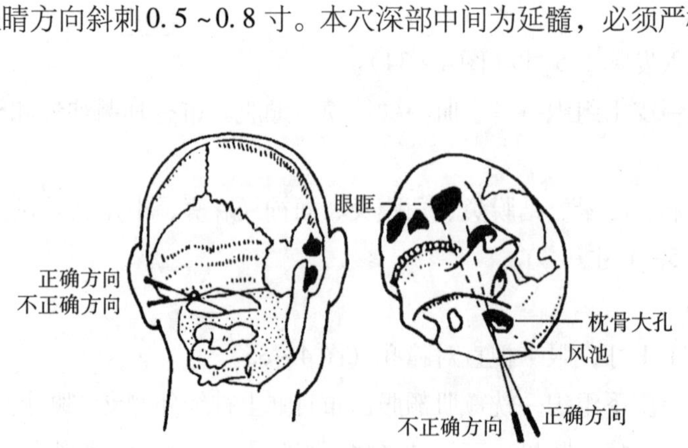

图 4－36

5. 肩井（GB21）。

定位：大椎与肩峰连线的中点处（图4－37）。

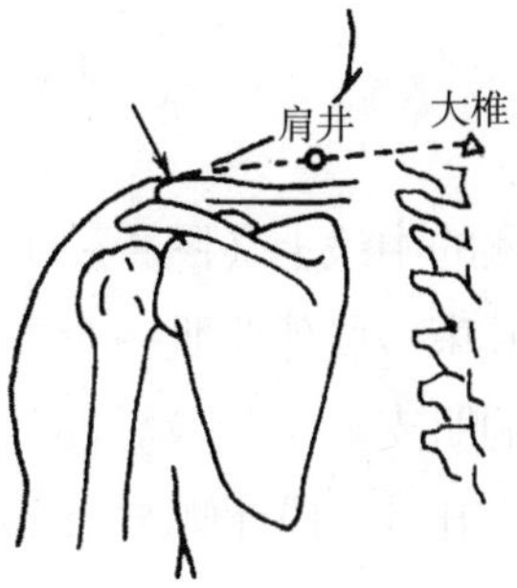

图4－37

层次解剖：皮肤→皮下组织→斜方肌→肩胛提肌。浅层布有锁骨上神经及颈浅动、静脉的分支或属支。深层有颈横动、静脉分支或属支和肩胛背神经的分支。

主治举例：肩背疼痛、乳腺炎等。

操作：直刺0.6～0.8寸。本穴内为肺尖，不可深刺。

参考：《类经图翼》，孕妇禁针；配天宗、少泽治乳腺炎，配灸中极治胞衣不下。

6. 日月（GB24）。

定位：乳头直下，第七肋间隙，前正中线旁开4寸（图4－34）。

层次解剖：皮肤→皮下组织→腹外斜肌→肋间外肌。浅层布有第六、七、八肋间神经外侧皮支和伴行的动、静脉。深层有第七肋间神经和第七肋间后动、静脉。

主治举例：急慢性肝炎、胆囊炎、胃溃疡、膈肌痉挛、呕吐等。

操作：斜刺0.5～0.8寸。

7. 居髎（GB29）。

定位：髂前上棘与股骨大转子最凸点连线的中点处（图4－34）。

层次解剖：皮肤→皮下组织→阔筋膜→臀中肌→臀小肌。浅层布有臀上皮神经和髂腹下神经外侧支皮支。深层有臀上动、静脉的分支或属支和臀上神经。

主治举例：髋关节炎、股外侧皮神经炎、膀胱炎、睾丸炎、中风后遗症等。

操作：直刺1.2～1.5寸。

8. 环跳（GB30）。

定位：股骨大转子最高点与骶骨裂孔连线上，外1/3与中1/3交点处（图4－38）。

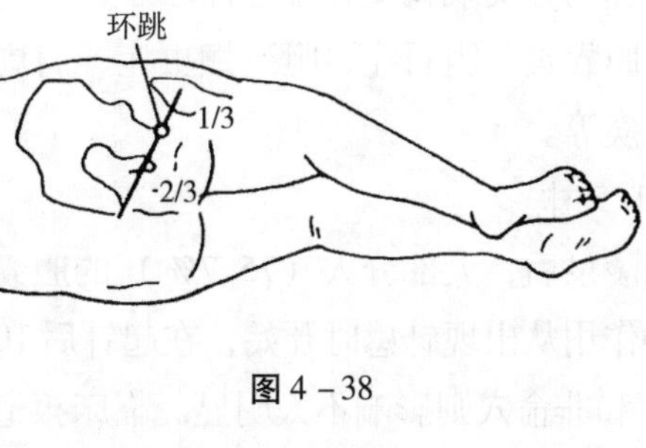

图4－38

层次解剖：皮肤→皮下组织→臀大肌→坐骨神经→股方肌。浅层布有臀上皮神经。深层有坐骨神经，臀下神经，股后皮神经和臀下动、静脉。

主治举例：坐骨神经痛、腰椎间盘突出症、梨状肌综合征、骶髂关节损伤、髋关节炎、中风后遗症等。

操作：直刺1.5～3寸。

9. 风市（GB31）。

定位：腘横纹上7寸，在大腿外侧的中线上（图4－34）。

层次解剖：皮肤→皮下组织→髂胫束→股外侧肌→股中间肌。浅层布有股外侧皮神经，深层有旋股外侧动脉降支的肌支和股神经的肌支。

主治举例：坐骨神经痛、腰椎间盘突出症、股外侧皮神经炎、膝关节炎、中风后遗症、荨麻疹等。

操作：直刺0.8～1.5寸。

10. 膝阳关（GB33）。

定位：阳陵泉上3寸，股骨外上髁上方的凹陷处（图4－34）。

层次解剖：皮肤→皮下组织→髂胫束后缘→腓肠肌外侧头前方。浅层布有股外侧皮神经。深层有膝上外侧动、静脉。

主治举例：膝关节炎、坐骨神经痛等。

操作：直刺0.8～1.5寸。

11. 阳陵泉（GB34）。

定位：腓骨小头前下方凹陷处（图4－39）。

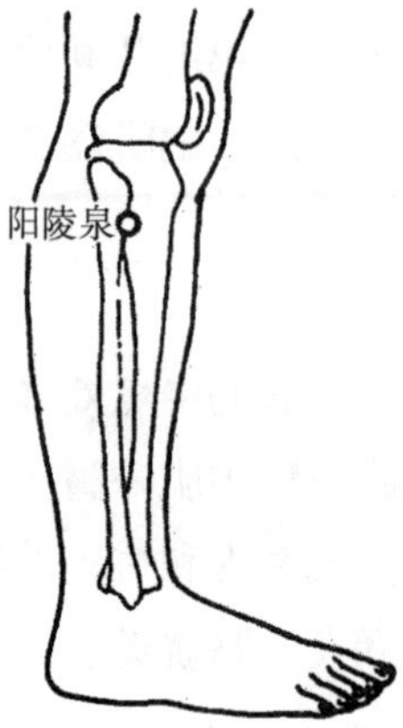

图4－39

层次解剖：皮肤→皮下组织→腓骨长肌→趾长伸肌。浅层布有腓肠外侧皮神经。深层有胫前返动、静脉，膝下外侧动、静脉的分支或属支和腓总神经分支。

主治举例：病毒性肝炎、胆囊炎、胆石症、胆道蛔虫症、肩周炎、膝关节炎、腰椎间盘突出症、下肢外侧疼痛、麻木或瘫痪等。

操作：直或斜向下刺1～1.5寸。

参考：实验报道，针刺阳陵泉后，大部分人（75.7%）的胆囊影像明显缩小，表明针刺能增强胆囊运动和排空能力。这种作用从出现针感时开始，在起针后10分钟更为明显。而针刺非胆经俞穴（如侠白、尺泽、太渊）和非俞穴则影响不太明显。临床报道，深刺阳陵泉对肝、脾脏的疼痛及绞痛有明显的镇痛效果（要求透刺阴陵泉，针感达足背部，留针20分钟）。若在本穴施行埋线疗法效果更佳。在本穴注射复方冬眠灵，对胆绞痛有较好的效果。

12. 光明（GB37）。

定位：外踝尖上5寸，腓骨前缘（图4－34）。

层次解剖：皮肤→皮下组织→腓骨短肌→前肌间隔→趾长伸肌→䠯长伸肌→小腿骨间膜→胫骨后肌。浅层布有腓浅神经和腓肠外侧皮神经。深层有腓深神经和胫前动、静脉。

主治举例：视神经萎缩、白内障、坐骨神经痛、腓总神经损伤、乳腺炎等。

操作：直刺0.5～0.8寸。

13. 悬钟（绝骨）（GB39）。

定位：外踝高点上3寸，腓骨前缘（也有许多文献定位于腓骨后缘）（图4－34）。

层次解剖：皮肤→皮下组织→趾长伸肌→小腿骨间膜。浅层布有腓肠外侧皮神经。深层有腓深神经的分支。如穿透小腿骨间膜可刺中腓动、静脉。

主治举例：落枕、颈椎病、胸胁痛、下肢疼痛、麻木或瘫痪、淋巴结肿大、小儿舞蹈病、动脉硬化症等。

操作：直刺0.5～1寸。

14. 丘墟（GB40）。

定位：足外踝前下方凹陷处（图4－34）。

层次解剖：皮肤→皮下组织→趾短伸肌→距跟外侧韧带→跗骨窦。布有足背浅静脉，足背外侧皮神经，足背中间皮神经，外踝前动、静脉。

主治举例：踝关节扭伤、足下垂、胆囊炎、颈椎病等。

操作：直刺0.5～1寸。

4.3.11.4 次常用穴位

瞳子髎（GB1）：目外眦旁，眶外侧缘处。

上关（GB3）：在耳前，下关直上，颧弓的上缘凹陷处。

颔厌（GB4）：头部鬓发上，头维与曲鬓弧形连线的1/4与下3/4交点处。

悬颅（GB5）：头部鬓发上，头维与曲鬓弧形连线的中点处。

悬厘（GB6）：头部鬓发上，头维与曲鬓弧形连线的3/4与下1/4交点处。

曲鬓（GB7）：耳前鬓角发际后缘的垂线与耳尖水平线交点处。

头窍阴（GB11）：耳后乳突的后上方，天冲与完骨的中1/3与下1/3交点处。

完骨（GB12）：耳后乳突的后下方凹陷处。

本神（GB13）：前额外侧，前发际上0.5寸，神庭旁开3寸。

头临泣（GB15）：瞳孔直上入前发际0.5寸，神庭与头维连线的中点处。

脑空（GB19）：枕外隆凸的上缘外侧，头正中线旁开2.25寸，平脑户。

京门（GB25）：章门后1.8寸，十二肋骨游离端的下方。

带脉（GB26）：第十一肋骨上游离端下方垂线与脐水平线的交点上。

外丘（GB36）：外踝尖上7寸，腓骨前缘。

阳辅（GB38）：外踝尖上4寸，腓骨前缘稍前方。

足临泣（GB41）：足第四跖趾关节的后方，小趾伸肌腱的外侧凹陷处。

侠溪（GB43）：第四、五趾间，趾蹼缘后方赤白肉际处。

足窍阴（GB44）：在足第四趾末节外侧，距趾甲角0.1寸。

4.3.12 足太阳膀胱经

4.3.12.1 概况

本经从头面走向下肢，首穴睛明，末穴至阴。单侧共67穴。主治眼、头、项、背、腰骶部、下肢疾病，痔疮、脱肛及精神病、癫痫等。"背俞穴"主治与有关内脏及与脏腑功能有关的组织器官病症。

4.3.12.2 主要循行线

起于目内眦，上头顶，向下到项后分开，一支脉沿脊柱两侧到腰部，从脊旁进入内脏，联络肾，属于膀胱，再向下通过臀部进入腘窝中央，另一支脉从肩胛骨的内侧缘下行，经过臀部，沿大腿外侧向下与腰部下行的支脉会合于腘窝中央，再沿小腿后面和足背外侧，止于足小趾外侧端（图4-40）。

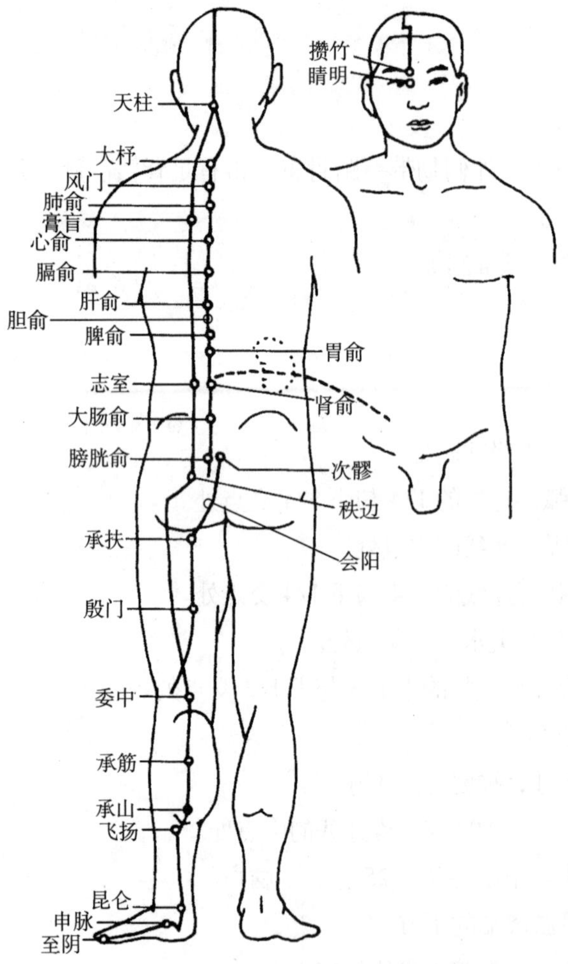

图4-40

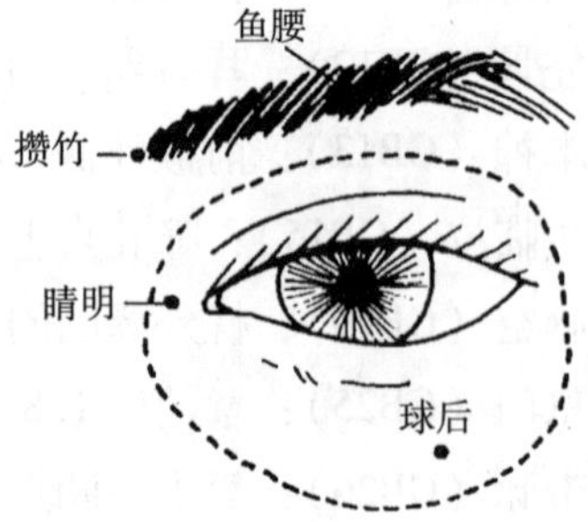

图4-41

4.3.12.3　常用穴位

1. 睛明（BL1）。

定位：目内眦的上方0.1寸，靠近眼眶骨内缘处（图4－41）。

层次解剖：皮肤→皮下组织→眼轮匝肌→上泪小管上方→内直肌与筛骨眶板之间。浅层布有三叉神经眼支的滑车上神经，有内眦动、静脉的分支或属支。深层有眼动、静脉的分支或属支，眼神经分支和动眼神经的分支。

主治举例：急性结膜炎、近视、斜视、青光眼、视神经炎、视神经萎缩、视网膜炎、脑炎后遗症失明等。

操作：沿眼眶边缘缓缓刺入0.3～0.5寸，不宜做大幅度提插；出针后按压局部1～2分钟，以防出血。禁灸。

参考：《席弘赋》，睛明治眼未效时，合谷光明安可缺。配伍：配太阳、球后、翳明、少泽、合谷治白内障、角膜白斑；配球后、风池、太冲治青光眼。

2. 攒竹（BL2）。

定位：当目内眦直上眉毛内侧端（图4－41）。

层次解剖：皮肤→皮下组织→眼轮匝肌。浅层布有额神经的滑车上神经，眶上动、静脉的分支或属支。深层有面神经的颞支和颧支。

主治举例：头痛、三叉神经痛、面瘫、面肌抽搐、结膜炎、视神经萎缩、夜盲、近视等。

操作：治疗眼病，可向下斜刺0.3～0.5寸；治疗头痛、面瘫，可平刺透鱼腰。禁灸。

3. 天柱（BL10）。

定位：斜方肌外缘之后发际凹陷中，约后发际正中旁开1.3寸（图4－40）。

层次解剖：皮肤→皮下组织→斜方肌→头夹肌的内侧→头半棘肌。浅层布有第三颈神经后支的内侧支和皮下静脉等结构。深层有枕大神经。

主治举例：头痛、眩晕、咽喉炎、颈椎病、枕大神经痛、肩背痛等。

操作：直刺0.5～1.2寸。

4. 大杼（BL11）。

定位：第一胸椎棘突下，旁开1.5寸（图4－40）。

层次解剖：皮肤→皮下组织→斜方肌→菱形肌→上后锯肌→颈夹肌→竖脊肌。浅层布有第一、二胸神经后支的内侧皮支和伴行的肋间后动、静脉背侧支的内侧皮支。深层有第一、二胸神经后支的肌支和相应的肋间后动、静脉背侧支的分支等结构。

主治举例：肩背痛、颈椎病、头痛、哮喘、咽喉炎、癫痫等。

操作：直刺0.5～1.2寸。

5. 风门（BL12）。

定位：第二胸椎棘突下，旁开1.5寸（图4－40）。

层次解剖：皮肤→皮下组织→斜方肌→菱形肌→上后锯肌→颈夹肌→竖脊肌。浅层布有第二、三胸神经后支的内侧皮支和伴行的肋间后动、静脉背侧支的内侧皮支。深层有第二、第三胸神经后支的肌支和相应的肋间后动、静脉背侧支的分支等结构。

主治举例：支气管炎、肺炎、百日咳、感冒、发热、荨麻疹、颈椎病、胸背痛等。

操作：直刺0.5～1.2寸。

6. 肺俞（BL13）。

定位：第三胸椎棘突下旁开 1.5 寸（图 4－42）。

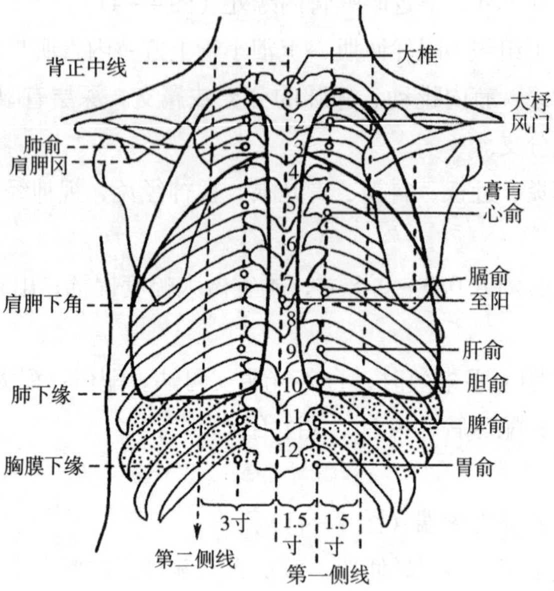

图 4－42

层次解剖：皮肤→皮下组织→斜方肌→菱形肌→上后锯肌→竖脊肌。浅层布有第三、四胸神经后支的内侧皮支和伴行的肋间后动、静脉背侧支的内侧皮支。深层有第三、四胸神经后支的肌支和相应的肋间后动、静脉背侧支的分支或属支。

主治举例：呼吸系统疾病、荨麻疹、背部软组织劳损等。

操作：向脊柱侧斜刺 0.5～0.8 寸。

注意：肺俞、心俞、肝俞等穴，位于第十胸椎以上，在肺区范围内，不宜针刺过深。

7. 心俞（BL15）。

定位：第五胸椎棘突下旁开 1.5 寸（图 4－42）。

层次解剖：皮肤→皮下组织→斜方肌→菱形肌下缘→竖脊肌。浅层布有第五、六胸神经后支的内侧皮支及伴行的动、静脉。深层有第五、六胸神经后支的肌支和相应肋间后动、静脉背侧支的分支或属支。

主治举例：心血管疾病、肋间神经痛、癔症、精神病、神经衰弱等。

操作：向脊柱侧斜刺 0.5～0.8 寸。

8. 膈俞（BL17）。

定位：第七胸椎棘突下，旁开 1.5 寸（图 4－42）。

层次解剖：皮肤→皮下组织→斜方肌→背阔肌→竖脊肌。浅层布有第七、八胸神经后支的内侧皮支和伴行的动、静脉。深层有第七、八胸神经后支的肌支和相应的肋间后动、静脉背侧支的分支等结构。

主治举例：胃炎、肠炎、膈肌痉挛、黄疸型肝炎、胆囊炎、荨麻疹、背痛等。

操作：向脊柱侧斜刺 0.5～0.8 寸。

9. 肝俞（BL18）。

定位：第九胸椎棘突下旁开1.5寸（图4－42）。

层次解剖：皮肤→皮下组织→斜方肌→背阔肌→下后锯肌→竖脊肌。浅层布有第九、十胸神经后支的皮支及伴行的动、静脉。深层有第九、十胸神经后支的肌支和相应的肋间后动、静脉的分支或属支。

主治举例：肝胆疾病、胃炎、眼科疾病、神经衰弱、精神病、月经不调等。

操作：向脊柱侧斜刺0.5～0.8寸。

10. 胆俞（BL19）。

定位：第十胸椎棘突下，旁开1.5寸（图4－42）。

层次解剖：皮肤→皮下组织→斜方肌→背阔肌→下后锯肌→竖脊肌。浅层布有第十、十一胸神经后支的皮支和伴行的动、静脉。深层有第十、十一胸神经后支的肌支和相应的肋间后动、静脉的分支和属支。

主治举例：黄疸型肝炎、胆囊炎、胆道蛔虫症、肋间神经痛、背痛等。

操作：向脊柱侧斜刺0.5～0.8寸。

11. 脾俞（BL20）。

定位：第十一胸椎棘突下，旁开1.5寸（图4－42）。

层次解剖皮肤→皮下组织→背阔肌→下后锯肌→竖脊肌。浅层布有第十一、十二胸神经后支的内侧皮支和伴行的动、静脉。深层有第十一、十二胸神经后支的肌支和相应的肋间、肋下动、静脉的分支和属支。

主治举例：胃肠疾患、肝炎、水肿、背腰痛、贫血、糖尿病等。

操作：向脊柱侧斜刺0.5～0.8寸。

12. 胃俞（BL21）。

定位：第十二胸椎棘突下，旁开1.5寸（图4－42）。

层次解剖：皮肤→皮下组织→胸腰筋膜浅层和背阔肌腱膜→竖脊肌。浅层布有第十二胸神经和第一腰神经后支的皮支和伴行的动、静脉。深层有第十二胸神经和第一腰神经后支的肌支和相应的动、静脉背侧支的分支或属支。

主治举例：胃溃疡、胃下垂、胃痉挛、胰腺炎、糖尿病等。

操作：直刺0.5～0.8寸。

13. 肾俞（BL23）。

定位：第二腰椎棘突下，旁开1.5寸（图4－43）。

层次解剖：皮肤→皮下组织→背阔肌腱膜和胸腰筋膜浅层→竖脊肌。浅层布有第二、三腰神经后支的皮支和伴行的动、静脉。深层有第二、三腰神经后支的肌支和相应的腰动、静脉背侧支的分支或属支。

主治举例：泌尿生殖系统疾病、腰背痛等。

操作：直刺0.5～1寸。

14. 大肠俞（BL25）。

定位：第四腰椎棘突下，旁开1.5寸（图4－43）。

层次解剖：皮肤→皮下组织→背阔肌腱膜和胸腰静脉浅层→竖脊肌。浅层布有第四、五腰神经后支的皮支和伴行的动、静脉。深层有第四、五腰神经后支的肌支和有关的动、静脉背侧支的分支或属支。

主治举例：肠道疾病、腰背痛等。

操作：直刺0.5~1.5寸。

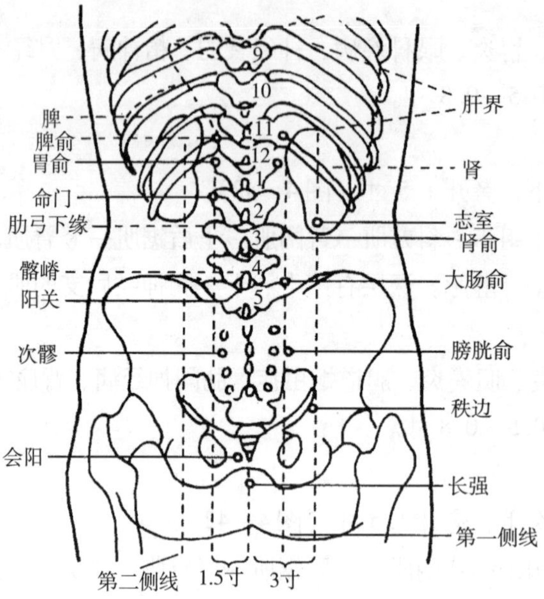

图4-43

15. 次髎（BL32）。

定位：第二骶后孔凹陷中（图4-43）。

层次解剖：皮肤→皮下组织→竖脊肌→第二骶后孔。浅层布有臀中皮神经。深层有第二骶神经和骶外侧动、静脉后支。

主治举例：盆腔疾病、腰腿痛等。

操作：直刺0.8~1.5寸。

16. 会阳（BL35）。

定位：尾骨端旁开0.5寸（图4-43）。

层次解剖：皮肤→皮下组织→臀大肌→提肛肌腱。浅层布有臀中皮神经。深层有臀下动、静脉的分支或属支和臀下神经。

主治举例：阳痿、遗精、前列腺炎、附件炎、月经不调、痔疮等。

操作：直刺1~1.5寸。

17. 承扶（BL36）。

定位：在大腿后面，臀下横纹的中点（图4-40）。

层次解剖：皮肤→皮下组织→臀大肌→股二头肌长头及半腱肌。浅层布有股后皮神经及臀下皮神经的分支。深层有股后皮神经干、坐骨神经及其伴行动、静脉。

主治举例：腰椎间盘突出、梨状肌综合征、痔疮等。

操作：直刺1~1.5寸。

18. 委中（BL40）。

定位：腘窝横纹中央（图4－40）。

层次解剖：皮肤→皮下组织→腓肠肌内、外侧头之间。浅层布有股后皮神经和小隐静脉。深层有胫神经，腘动、静脉和腓肠动脉等。

主治举例：急慢性腰痛、坐骨神经痛、下肢瘫痪等。

操作：直刺1～1.5寸或刺出血。

参考：配龈交、阿是穴治急性腰扭伤；配太溪治项后发际疮；配曲泽均用刺络放血，治急性胃肠炎、吐泻。

19. 秩边（BL54）。

定位：平第四骶后孔，骶正中嵴旁开3寸（图4－40）。

层次解剖：皮肤→皮下组织→臀大肌→臀中肌→臀小肌。浅层布有臀中皮神经和臀下皮神经。深层有臀上、下动、静脉和臀上、下神经。

主治举例：腰椎间盘突出症、梨状肌综合征、骶髂关节损伤等。

操作：直刺1～1.5寸。

20. 承山（BL57）。

定位：委中与昆仑之间，伸直小腿或足跟上提时腓肠肌肌腹下出现尖角凹陷处（图4－40）。

层次解剖：皮肤→皮下组织→腓肠肌→比目鱼肌。浅层布有小隐静脉和腓肠内侧皮神经。深层有胫神经和胫后动、静脉。

主治举例：腰腿痛、腓肠肌痉挛、下肢瘫痪、痔疮、脱肛等。

操作：直刺0.5～1.2寸。

21. 昆仑（BL60）。

定位：跟腱与外踝之间凹陷处，平外踝中点取穴（图4－40）。

层次解剖：皮肤→皮下组织→跟腱前方的疏松结缔组织中。浅层布有腓肠神经和小隐静脉。深层有腓动、静脉的分支或属支。

主治举例：头痛、落枕、腰背痛、鼻出血、下肢后面及踝关节病症等。

操作：直刺0.5～1寸。

22. 至阴（BL67）。

定位：足小趾外侧，距趾甲角0.1寸（图4－40）。

层次解剖：皮肤→皮下组织→甲根。布有足背外侧皮神经的趾背神经和趾背动、静脉网。

主治举例：胎位不正（灸）、难产、头痛、鼻炎等。

操作：毫针浅刺。

4.3.12.4　次常用穴位

眉冲（BL3）：攒竹直上入发际0.5寸。

通天（BL7）：前发际正中直上4寸，旁开1.5寸。

玉枕（BL9）：后发际正中直上2.5寸，旁开1.3寸，平枕外隆凸上缘的凹陷处。

厥阴俞（BL14）：第四胸椎棘突下，旁开1.5寸。

督俞（BL16）：第六胸椎棘突下，旁开1.5寸。

三焦俞（BL22）：第一腰椎棘突下，旁开1.5寸。

气海俞（BL24）：第三腰椎棘突下，旁开1.5寸。

关元俞（BL26）：第五腰椎棘突下，旁开1.5寸。

小肠俞（BL27）：骶正中嵴旁1.5寸，平第一骶后孔。

膀胱俞（BL28）：骶正中嵴旁1.5寸，平第二骶后孔。

上髎（BL31）：髂后上棘与后正中线之间，适对第一骶后孔处。

中髎（BL33）：次髎下内方，适对第三骶后孔处。

下髎（BL34）：中髎下内方，适对第四骶后孔处。

殷门（BL37）：承扶下6寸，承扶与委中的连线上。

委阳（BL39）：在腘横纹外侧端，股二头肌腱的内侧。

膏肓（BL43）：第四胸椎棘突下，旁开3寸。

神堂（BL44）：第五胸椎棘突下，旁开3寸。

膈关（BL46）：第七胸椎棘突下，旁开3寸。

志室（BL52）：第二腰椎棘突下，旁开3寸。

飞扬（BL58）：昆仑穴直上7寸，承山外下方1寸处。

跗阳（BL59）：外踝后，昆仑穴直上3寸。

仆参（BL61）：外踝后下方，昆仑直下，跟骨外侧赤白肉际处。

申脉（BL62）：外踝直下凹陷中。

金门（BL63）：外踝前缘直下，骰骨下缘处。

京骨（BL64）：第五跖骨粗隆下方，赤白肉际处。

束骨（BL65）：足第五跖趾关节的后方，赤白肉际处。

足通谷（BL66）：足第五跖趾关节的前方，赤白肉际处。

4.3.13 任　脉

4.3.13.1 概况

本经首穴会阴，末穴承浆，共24穴。主治胸腹部及其相应的内脏器官病症。

4.3.13.2 主要循行线

起于小腹内，出会阴部，上入毛际，经过腹部、胸部的正中线上行到达咽喉，再向上经过颈部、面部进入眼眶内（图4-44）。

4.3.13.3 常用穴位

1. 关元（RN4）。

定位：前正中线上，肚脐下3寸（图4-44）。

层次解剖：皮肤→皮下组织→腹白线→腹横筋膜→腹膜外脂肪→壁腹膜。浅层主要有第十二胸神经前支的前皮支和腹壁浅动、静脉的分支或属支。深层主要有第十二胸神经前支的分支。

主治举例：遗精、阳痿、月经不调、盆腔炎、子宫脱垂、尿潴留、遗尿、全身衰弱等。

操作：直刺0.5~1.2寸，需要排尿后进行针刺。

参考：《扁鹊心书》，每夏秋之交，即灼（灸）关元千壮，久久不畏寒暑。《太平圣惠方》，若怀胎，必不针。研究表明，针刺中极、关元、曲骨等穴对尿潴留患者膀胱功能有影响，发现膀胱神经支配完整的患者，每次捻针时膀胱逼尿肌即收缩，内压上升；不捻针时，逼尿肌又复松弛，膀胱内压下降。但在骶神经损伤仍然处于脊髓休克期的病人，针刺对膀胱的影响则完全消失。本穴和气海穴均有强壮的作用，为保健要穴。

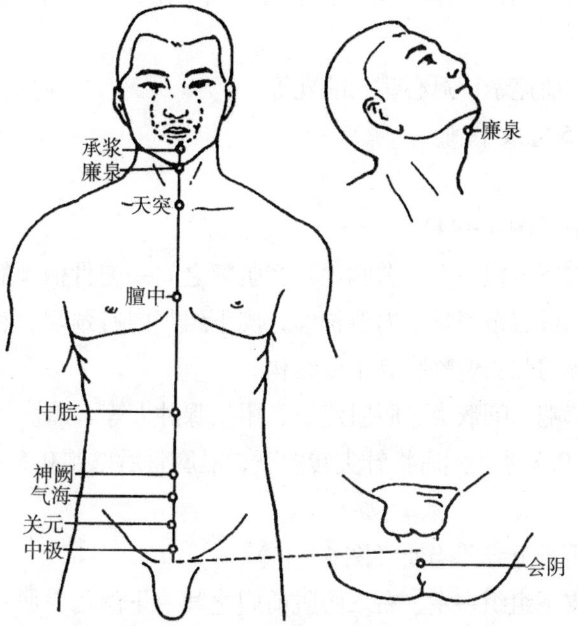

图4－44

2. 气海（RN6）。

定位：前正中线上，肚脐下1.5寸（图4－44）。

层次解剖：皮肤→皮下组织→腹白线→腹横筋膜→腹膜外脂肪→壁腹膜。浅层主要有第十一胸神经前支的前皮支和脐周静脉网。深层主要有第十一胸神经前支的分支。

主治举例：急慢性肠炎、痢疾、急性肠麻痹、尿路感染、尿潴留、遗尿、阳痿、早泄、月经不调、子宫脱垂、胃下垂、脱肛以及全身衰弱等。

操作：直刺0.5～1.2寸。孕妇慎用。

3. 神阙（RN8）。

定位：肚脐正中（图4－44）。

层次解剖：皮肤→结缔组织→壁腹膜。浅层主要有第十胸神经前支的前皮支和腹壁脐周静脉网。深层主要有第十胸神经前支的分支。

主治举例：胃肠炎及虚脱证候等。

操作：古时本穴因不易消毒而禁针，多用隔盐灸。

4. 中脘（RN12）。

定位：前正中线上，肚脐上4寸（图4－44）。

层次解剖：皮肤→皮下组织→腹白线→腹横筋膜→腹膜外脂肪→壁腹膜。浅层主要有第八胸神经前支的前皮支和腹壁浅静脉的属支。深层主要有第八胸神经前支的分支。

主治举例：溃疡病、胃痉挛、胃下垂、胃炎、膈肌痉挛、食欲不振、肠炎等胃肠疾病等。

操作：直刺0.5～1.2寸。

5. 膻中（RN17）。

定位：胸骨中线上，平第四肋间隙，两乳头之间（图4－44）。

层次解剖：皮肤→皮下组织→胸骨体。主要布有第四肋间神经前皮支和胸廓内动、静脉的穿支。

主治举例：哮喘、膈肌痉挛、冠心病、缺乳等。

操作：直刺0.3～0.5寸或平刺。

6. 天突（RN22）。

定位：胸骨上窝正中（图4－44）。

层次解剖：皮肤→皮下组织→左、右胸锁乳突肌腱之间→胸骨柄颈静脉切迹上方→左、右胸骨甲状肌→气管前间隙。浅层布锁骨上内侧神经，皮下组织内有颈阔肌和颈静脉弓。深层有头臂干、左颈总动脉、主动脉弓和头臂静脉等重要结构。

主治举例：咳嗽、哮喘、咽喉炎、膈肌痉挛、甲状腺肿大等。

操作：先直刺0.2～0.3寸，然后将针尖转向下，沿胸骨后壁刺0.5～1寸。

7. 廉泉（RN23）。

定位：喉结上方，舌骨上缘凹陷处（图4－44）。

层次解剖：皮肤→皮下组织→左、右二腹肌前腹之间→下颌舌骨肌→颏舌骨肌→颏舌肌。浅层布有面神经颈支和颈横神经上支的分支。深层有舌动、静脉的分支或属支，舌下神经的分支和下颌舌骨肌神经等。

主治举例：失音、运动性失语、慢性咽喉炎及吞咽困难等病症。

操作直刺0.5～1寸。

8. 承浆（RN24）。

定位：颏唇沟的正中凹陷处（图4－44）。

层次解剖：皮肤→皮下组织→口轮匝肌→降下唇肌→颏肌。布有下牙槽神经的终支颏神经和颏动、静脉。

主治举例：面瘫、口疮、齿神经痛、癔症性失语、糖尿病等。

操作：斜刺0.3～0.5寸。

4.3.13.4　次常用穴位

中极（RN3）：前正中线上，肚脐下4寸。

石门（RN5）：前正中线上，肚脐下2寸。

阴交（RN7）：前正中线上，肚脐下1寸。

水分（RN9）：前正中线上，肚脐上1寸。

下脘（RN10）：前正中线上，肚脐上2寸。

建里（RN11）：前正中线上，肚脐上3寸。

上脘（RN13）：前正中线上，肚脐上5寸。

巨阙（RN14）：前正中线上，肚脐上6寸。

鸠尾（RN15）：前正中线上，胸剑结合部下1寸。

璇玑（RN21）：前正中线上，天突下1寸。

4.3.14 督 脉

4.3.14.1 概况

首穴长强，末穴龈交，共28穴。主治发热、昏迷、精神病及与五脏有关的疾病。

4.3.14.2 主要循行线

起于小腹，出会阴部，向后沿脊柱之内上行到达风府穴处，进入脑内，再上行头顶，沿前额下行鼻柱，到唇系带处（图4－45）。

4.3.14.3 常用穴位

1. 腰阳关（DU3）。

定位：第四腰椎棘突下凹陷中（图4－45）。

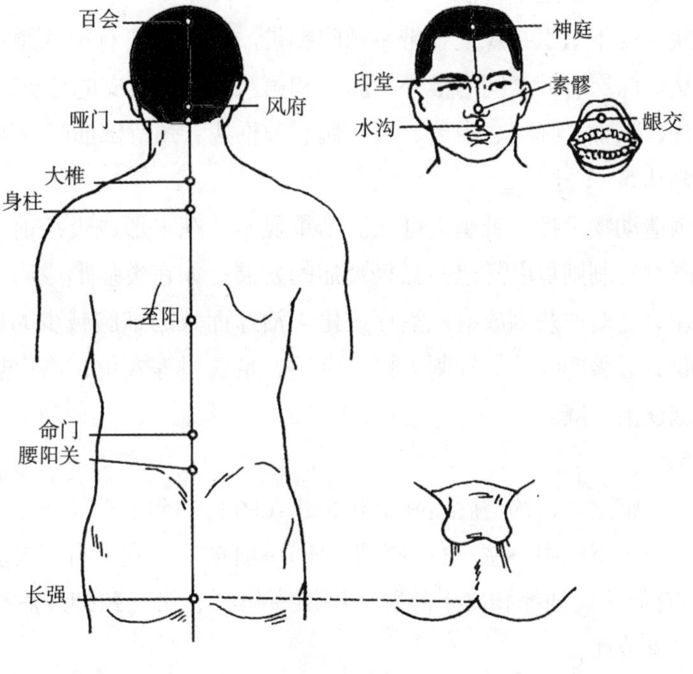

图4－45

层次解剖：皮肤→皮下组织→棘上韧带→棘间韧带→弓间韧带。浅层主要有第四腰神经后支的内侧支和伴行的动、静脉。深层有棘突间的椎外静脉丛，第四腰神经后支的分支和第四腰动、静脉背侧支的分支或属支。

主治举例：遗精、阳痿、月经不调、盆腔炎、慢性腰痛、强直性脊柱炎、类风湿病、小儿麻痹症、截瘫等。

操作：直刺0.5～1寸。

2. 命门（DU4）。

定位：第二腰椎棘突下凹陷中（图4－45）。

层次解剖：皮肤→皮下组织→棘上韧带→棘间韧带→弓间韧带。浅层主要有第二腰神经后支的内侧支和伴行的动、静脉。深层有棘突间的椎外静脉丛，第一腰神经后支的分支和第一腰动、静脉背侧支的分支或属支。

主治举例：遗精、阳痿、前列腺炎、月经不调、盆腔炎、慢性肠炎、慢性腰痛、慢性消耗性疾病等。

操作：直刺0.5～1寸。

3. 身柱（DU12）。

定位：第三胸椎棘突下凹陷中（图4－45）。

层次解剖：皮肤→皮下组织→棘上韧带→棘间韧带。浅层主要有第三胸神经后支的内侧皮支和伴行的动、静脉。深层有棘突间的椎外静脉丛，第三胸神经后支的分支和第三肋间后动、静脉背侧支的分支或属支。

主治举例：咳嗽、支气管哮喘、神经衰弱、癫痫、癔症、颈背肌筋膜炎等。

操作：直刺0.5～1寸。

4. 大椎（DU14）。

定位：第7颈椎棘突下凹陷中（图4－45）。

层次解剖：皮肤→皮下组织→棘上韧带→棘间韧带。浅层主要有第八颈神经后支的内侧皮支和棘突间皮下静脉丛。深层有棘突间的椎外静脉丛和第八颈神经后支的分支。

主治举例：发热、咳嗽、哮喘、中暑、精神病、颈椎病、颈背部筋膜炎等。

操作：向上斜刺0.5～1寸。

参考：用人工创造动物炎症，针刺大椎穴。结果显示，在未形成炎症前，可以预防炎症的发生；在形成炎症的同时针刺则可以延迟并减轻炎症的发展；如在炎症形成后针刺，则可以加速消炎过程，提前修复痊愈。对一些因放射线治疗或化学治疗而致的细胞减少的病人，针刺大椎、合谷、足三里等，可收到显著的疗效。针刺大椎、合谷、足三里等穴位，治疗热带嗜酸性细胞增生症。针后嗜酸性细胞逐渐下降。

5. 哑门（DU15）。

定位：第一、二颈椎之间，约当后发际上0.5寸（图4－45）。

层次解剖：皮肤→皮下组织→左、右斜方肌之间→项韧带（左、右头夹肌之间→左、右头半棘肌之间）。浅层布有第三枕神经和皮下静脉。深层有第二、第三颈神经后支的分支，椎外静脉丛和枕动、静脉的分支或属支。

主治举例：中风后遗症失语、舌骨肌麻痹、聋哑、精神病、癫痫等。

操作：微低头进针，针尖向下颌骨方向刺入0.5～1寸；本穴深部接近延髓，必须严格掌握角度和深度，以不刺进硬脊膜为度。行针时不宜大幅度提插。不宜灸（图4－46）。

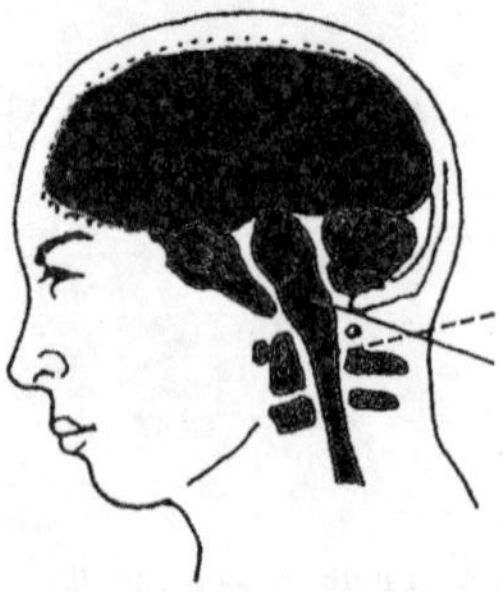

图4－46

6. 风府（DU16）。

定位：后发际正中直上1寸凹陷中（图4－45）。

层次解剖：皮肤→皮下组织→左、右斜方肌之间→项韧带（左、右头半棘肌之间）→左、右头后大、小直肌之间。浅层布有枕大神经和第三颈神经的分支及枕动、静脉分支或属支。深层有枕下神经的分支。

主治举例：感冒、头痛、眩晕、运动性失语、舌骨肌麻痹、颈椎病、精神病、癫痫等。

操作：微低头进针，针尖向下颌骨方向刺入0.5～1寸；针尖不可向上，以免刺入枕骨大孔，误伤延髓。不宜灸。

7. 百会（DU20）。

定位：后发际上7寸或于头部中线与两耳尖连线的交点处取穴（图4－45）。

层次解剖：皮肤→皮下组织→帽状腱膜→腱膜下疏松结缔组织。布有枕大神经及额神经分支和左、右颞浅动、静脉及枕动、静脉吻合网。

主治举例：头痛、眩晕、高血压、中风后遗症、失眠、神经衰弱、老年性痴呆、精神病、癔症、内脏下垂（灸）、免疫功能低下（灸）、休克等。

操作：向前或向后横刺0.5～1寸。

8. 神庭（DU24）。

定位：前发际正中上0.5寸（图4－45）。

层次解剖：皮肤→皮下组织→左右枕额肌额腹之间→腱膜下疏松结缔组织。布有额神经的滑车上神经分支和额动、静脉的分支或属支。

主治举例：头痛、眩晕、失眠、神经官能症、精神病、癫痫、鼻炎、结膜炎等。

操作：平刺0.5～1寸。

9. 素髎（DU25）。

定位：鼻尖的正中央（图4－45）。

层次解剖：皮肤→皮下组织→鼻中隔软骨和鼻外侧软骨。布有筛前神经鼻外支和面动、静脉的鼻背支。

主治举例：鼻炎、鼻息肉、休克、低血压、新生儿窒息等。

操作：向上斜刺0.3～0.5寸。

10. 水沟（人中）（DU26）。

定位：人中沟上1/3与下2/3交点处（图4－45）。

层次解剖：皮肤→皮下组织→口轮匝肌。布有眶下神经支和唇上动、静脉。

主治举例：昏迷、呼吸衰竭、面瘫、精神病、癔症、急性腰扭伤等。

操作：向上斜刺0.3～0.5寸，或用指甲按掐。

4.3.14.4　次常用穴位

长强（DU1）：在尾骨端下，尾骨端与肛门连线的中点处。

腰俞（DU2）：后正中线上，正对骶管裂孔。

悬枢（DU5）：后正中线上，第一腰椎棘突下凹陷中。

脊中（DU6）：后正中线上，第十一胸椎棘突下凹陷中。

中枢（DU7）：后正中线上，第十胸椎棘突下凹陷中。

筋缩（DU8）：后正中线上，第九胸椎棘突下凹陷中。

至阳（DU9）：后正中线上，第七胸椎棘突下凹陷中。

灵台（DU10）：后正中线上，第六胸椎棘突下凹陷中。

神道（DU11）：后正中线上，第五胸椎棘突下凹陷中。

陶道（DU13）：后正中线上，第一胸椎棘突下凹陷中。

脑户（DU17）：后发际正中直上2.5寸（风府上1.5寸），枕外隆凸的上缘凹陷处。

强间（DU18）：后发际正中直上4寸（脑户上1.5寸）。

前顶（DU21）：前发际正中直上3.5寸（百会前1.5寸）。

上星（DU23）：前发际正中上1寸。

龈交（DU28）：在上唇内，唇系带与上齿龈的相接处。

4.4 经外奇穴

经外奇穴是指十四经穴之外的经验效穴，历代记载颇多，仅唐朝《备急千金要方》就载187穴之众，本书介绍较常用的19个。此类穴位，有些位置偏离十四经，有些位置特殊、一名多穴而无法划归于某一经；还有许多则完全分布于十四经的循行线上，与十四经穴的界限很难区别。经外奇穴的这些特点，从另一侧面提示了现有的经络理论存在可修正、补充之处，为现代经络理论的创新提供有益的启示。

4.4.1 头颈部

4.4.1.1 四神聪（EX－HN1）

定位：头顶部，百会前后左右各1寸，共四穴（图4－47）。

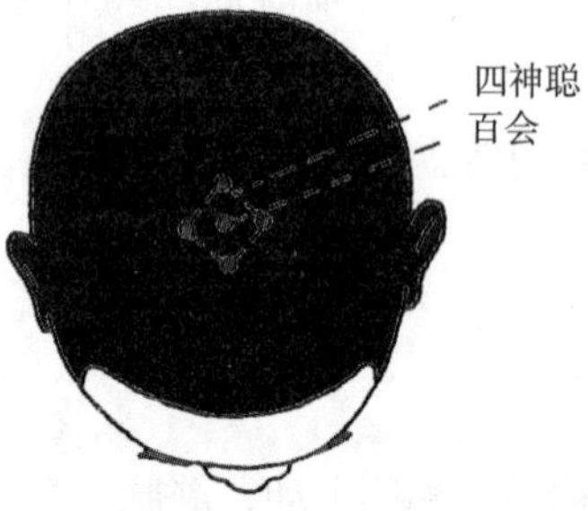

图4－47

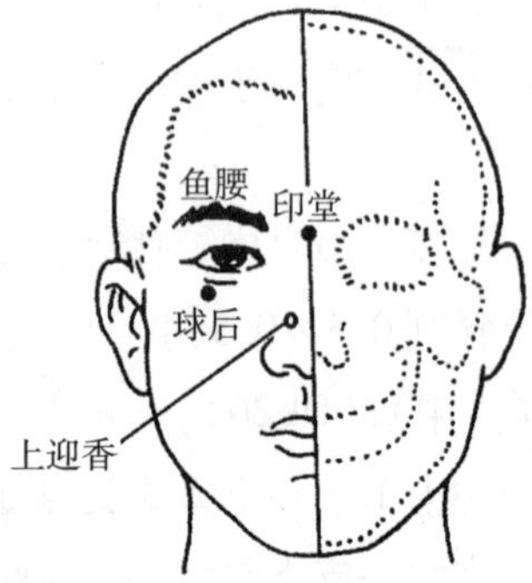

图4－48

层次解剖：皮肤→皮下组织→帽状腱膜→腱膜下疏松结缔组织。该处布有枕动、静脉，颞浅动、静脉顶支和眶上动、静脉的吻合网，有枕大神经、耳颞神经及眶上神经的额分支。

主治举例：神经衰弱、神经性头痛、眩晕、失眠、脑瘫、大脑发育不全、偏瘫、癫痫等。

操作：平刺0.5～1寸。

4.4.1.2 印堂（EX－HN3）

定位：两眉头的中间（图4－48）。

层次解剖：皮肤→皮下组织→降眉间肌。布有额神经的分支滑车上神经、眼动脉的分支、额动脉及伴行的静脉。

主治举例：神经性头痛、神经衰弱、眩晕、急性结膜炎、鼻炎、面神经麻痹、高血压、痤疮等。

操作：向下平刺0.3~0.5寸。

4.4.1.3　鱼腰（EX-HN4）

定位：眼平视，当瞳孔直上眉毛中点处（图4-48）。

层次解剖：皮肤→皮下组织→眼轮匝肌→枕额肌额腹。布有眶上神经外侧支，面神经的分支和眶上动、静脉的外侧支。

主治举例：三叉神经痛、面神经麻痹、面肌抽搐、眼睑下垂、急性结膜炎、视网膜出血等。

操作：向内侧或外侧横刺0.4~0.6寸。

4.4.1.4　太阳（EX-HN5）

定位：眉梢与目外眦的中点，向后约1寸凹陷处（图4-49）。

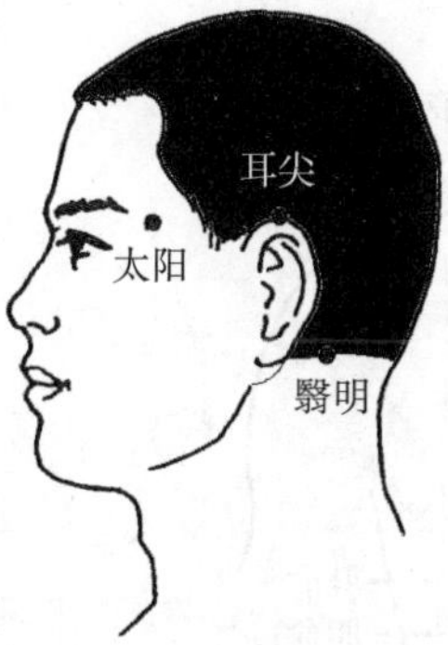

图4-49

层次解剖：皮肤→皮下组织→眼轮匝肌→颞筋膜→颞肌。该处布有颧神经的分支颧面神经，面神经的颞支和颧支，下颌神经的颞神经和颞浅动、静脉的分支或属支。

主治举例：神经血管性头痛、面神经麻痹、三叉神经痛、高血压、眩晕、急性结膜炎、眼睑炎、视神经萎缩、视网膜出血、睑腺炎、牙痛等。

操作：向下斜刺0.5~0.8寸。

4.4.1.5　耳尖（EX-HN6）

定位：在耳郭的上方，当折耳向前，耳郭上方的尖端处（图4-49）。

层次解剖：皮肤→皮下组织→耳郭软骨。布有颞浅动、静脉的耳前支，耳后动、静脉的耳后支。耳颞神经耳前支，枕小神经后支和面神经耳支等。

主治举例：沙眼、急性结膜炎、角膜炎、睑腺炎、偏头痛、痤疮等。

操作：直刺0.1~0.2寸或用三棱针点刺出血。

4.4.1.6　球后（EX-HN7）

定位：眼眶下缘外1/4与内3/4交界处（图4-48）。

层次解剖：皮肤→皮下组织→眼轮匝肌→眶脂体→下斜肌与眶下壁之间。浅层布有眶下神经，面神经的分支和眶下动、静脉的分支或属支。深层有动眼神经下支，眼动、静脉的分支或属支和眶下动、静脉等结构。

主治举例：急性结膜炎、近视、青光眼、视网膜炎、视神经萎缩、视神经炎、视网膜色素变性、早期白内障等。

操作：以左手食指将眼球推向内侧固定，沿眼眶下缘缓缓刺入0.5~1.5寸，出针时压迫局部

1~3分钟，以防出血。

4.4.1.7 上迎香（鼻通）（EX-HN8）

定位：在面部，鼻翼软骨与鼻甲的交界处，近鼻唇沟上端处（图4-48）。

层次解剖：皮肤→皮下组织→提上唇鼻翼肌。该处布有眶下神经，滑车下神经的分支，面神经的颊支和内眦动、静脉。

主治举例：急慢性鼻炎、鼻窦炎、鼻息肉、结膜炎、泪囊炎、痤疮等。

操作：向内上方斜刺0.3~0.5寸。

4.4.1.8 颈百劳（EX-HN15）

定位：大椎直上2寸，后正中线旁开1寸（图4-50）。

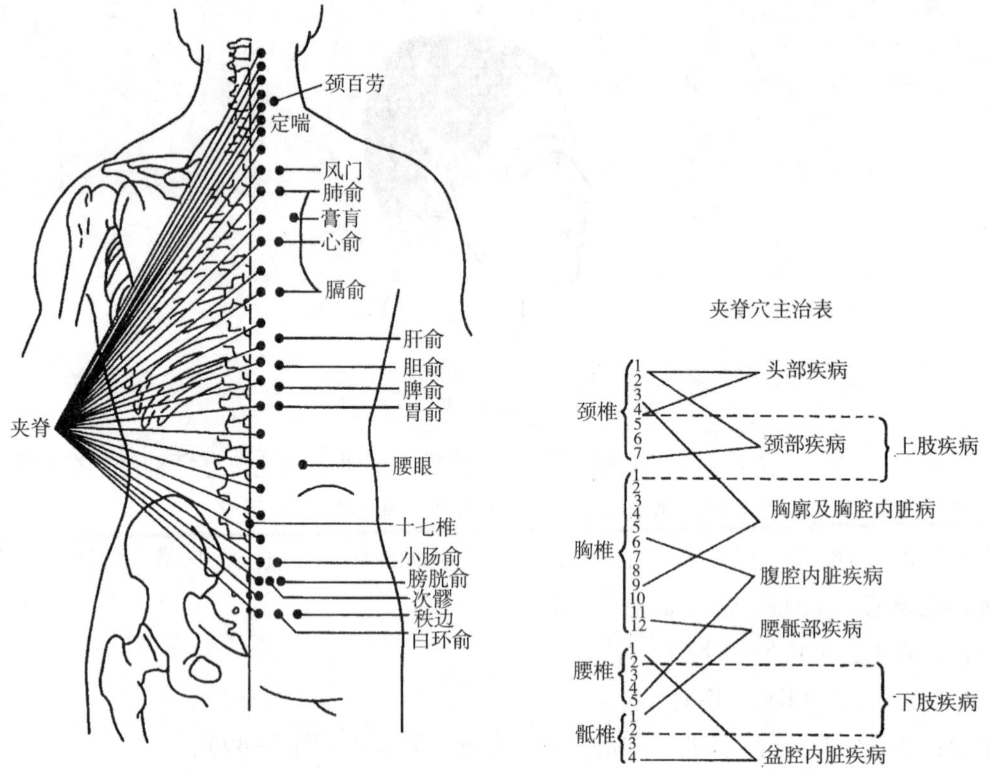

图4-50

层次解剖：皮肤→皮下组织→斜方肌→上后锯肌→头颈夹肌→头半棘肌→多裂肌。浅层布有第四、五颈神经后支的皮支。深层有第四、五颈神经后支的分支。

主治举例：支气管哮喘、百日咳、落枕、颈背肌筋膜炎、颈椎病、颈淋巴结肿大、神经衰弱等。

操作：直刺0.5~1寸。

4.4.2 胸背部

4.4.2.1 定喘（EX-B1）

定位：大椎旁0.5寸（图4-50）。

层次解剖：皮肤→皮下组织→斜方肌→菱形肌→上后锯肌→颈夹肌→竖脊肌。浅层主要布有第八颈神经后支的内侧皮支。深层有颈横动、静脉的分支或属支及第八颈神经，第一胸神经后支的肌支。

主治举例：慢性支气管炎、支气管哮喘、落枕、颈背肌筋膜炎、颈椎病、荨麻疹等。

操作：直刺0.6～1.2寸。

4.4.2.2　夹脊（华佗夹脊）（EX－B2）

定位：第一胸椎至第五腰椎，各椎棘突下旁开0.5寸（图4－50）。

层次解剖：因各穴位置不同，所涉及肌肉、血管、神经也不尽相同。一般的层次结构是：皮肤→皮下组织→浅层肌肉（斜方肌、背阔肌、菱形肌、上后锯肌、下后锯肌）→深层肌肉（竖脊肌、横突棘肌）。浅层内分别布有第一胸神经至第五腰神经后支的内侧皮支和伴行的动、静脉。深层布有第一胸神经至第五腰神经后支的肌支，肋间后动、静脉或腰动、静脉背侧支的分支或属支。

主治举例：上胸部的穴位治疗心肺、上肢疾病，下胸部的穴位治疗胃肠疾病，腰部的穴位治疗腰、腹及下肢疾病等。各穴均能治疗相应节段的脊柱病。

操作：向脊柱侧斜刺0.5～1.0寸。

4.4.2.3　腰眼（EX－B6）

定位：第四腰椎棘突下旁开3～4寸凹陷处（图4－50）。

层次解剖：皮肤→皮下组织→胸腰筋膜浅层和背阔肌腱膜→髂肋肌→胸腰筋膜深层→腰方肌。浅层布有臀上皮神经和第四腰神经后支的皮支。深层主要有第四腰神经后支的肌支和第四腰动、静脉的分支或属支。

主治举例：急慢性腰扭伤、髂腰韧带损伤、月经不调、前列腺炎、肾炎、糖尿病等。

操作：直刺0.5～1寸。

4.4.2.4　十七椎（EX－B7）

定位：第五腰椎棘突下凹陷中（图4－50）。

层次解剖：皮肤→皮下组织→棘上韧带→棘间韧带。浅层主要布有第五腰神经后支肠皮支和伴行的动、静脉。深层主要有第五腰神经后支和棘突间的椎外（后）静脉。

主治举例：腰骶痛、痛经、前列腺炎、遗尿等。

操作：直刺0.5～0.8寸。

4.4.3　上肢部

4.4.3.1　外劳宫（EX－UE8）

定位：手背第二、三掌骨间，指掌关节后约0.5寸，又称落枕穴（图4－51）。

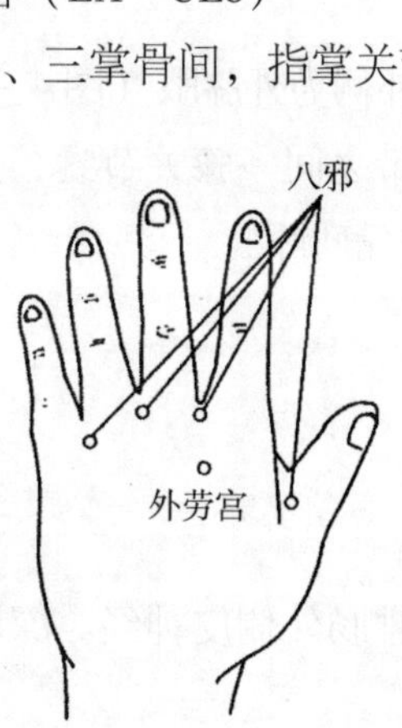

图4－51

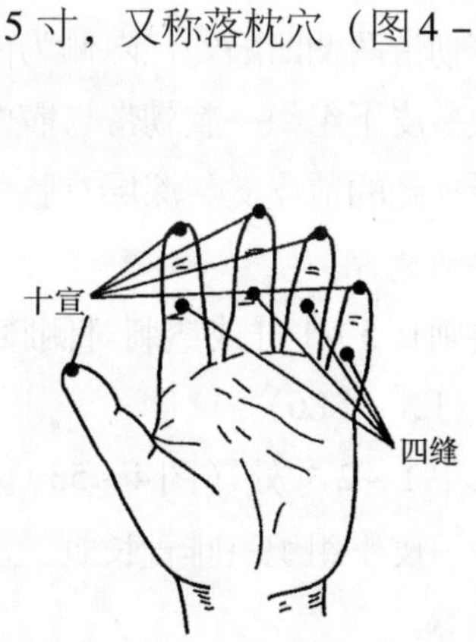

图4－52

层次解剖：皮肤→皮下组织→第二骨间背侧肌→第一骨间掌侧肌。布有桡神经浅支的指背神经、手背静脉网和掌背动脉。

主治举例：落枕、手指麻木、五指不能伸屈等。

操作：直刺0.5～0.8寸。

4.4.3.2　八邪（EX－UE9）

定位：手背各指间，指蹼缘后方赤白肉际处。左右共8穴（图4－51）。

层次解剖：皮肤→皮下组织→骨间背侧肌→骨间掌侧肌→蚓状肌。浅层布有掌背动、静脉或指背动、静脉和指背神经。深层有指掌总动、静脉或指掌固有动、静脉和指掌侧固有神经。

主治举例：指关节疾患，手背红肿、麻木，蛇咬伤（刺出血），颈椎病，肩背肌筋膜炎，咽炎，牙痛等。

操作：向掌骨间斜刺0.3～0.5寸或点刺出血。

4.4.3.3　四缝（EX－UE10）

定位：第二、三、四、五指掌面，近端指间关节横纹中点。一侧共4穴（图4－52）。

层次解剖：皮肤→皮下组织→指深屈肌腱。各穴的血管：指掌侧固有动、静脉的分支或属支和指皮下静脉。各穴的神经：食指和中指的四缝穴有正中神经的指掌侧固有神经分布，环指的四缝穴，桡侧的一支来自正中神经的指掌侧固有神经，尺侧的一支来自尺神经的指掌侧固有神经，小指的四缝穴有来自尺神经的指掌侧固有神经分布。

主治举例：小儿消化不良、营养不良、百日咳等。

操作：浅刺，从针孔中挤出少许黄白色透明液体。

4.4.3.4　十宣（EX－UE11）

定位：两手十指尖端，距指甲约0.1寸。左右共10穴（图4－52）。

层次解剖：皮肤→皮下组织。各穴的神经支配：拇指到中指的十宣穴有正中神经分布；环指的十宣穴有桡侧的正中神经和尺侧的尺神经双重分布；小指的十宣穴有尺神经分布。

主治举例：昏迷、发热、中暑、急性咽喉炎、指端麻木等。

操作：三棱针点刺出血。

4.4.4　下肢部

4.4.4.1　膝眼（EX－LE5）

定位：屈膝，髌韧带两侧凹陷处，内侧为内膝眼，外侧为外膝眼（图4－53）。

层次解剖：皮肤→皮下组织→髌韧带与髌内侧支持带之间→膝关节囊、翼状皱襞。浅层布有隐神经的髌下支和股神经的前皮支。深层有膝关节的动、静脉网。

主治举例：膝关节炎等。

操作：向膝中斜刺0.5～1寸或透刺对侧膝眼。

4.4.4.2　胆囊（EX－LE6）

定位：阳陵泉穴下1～2寸处（图4－53）。

层次解剖：皮肤→皮下组织→腓骨长肌。浅层布有腓肠外侧皮神经。深层布有腓浅神经，腓深神经和胫前动、静脉。

主治举例：急慢性胆囊炎、胆石症、胆道蛔虫症、胫神经卡压综合征等。

操作：直刺1～2寸。

4.4.4.3　阑尾（EX－LE7）

定位：足三里穴下约2寸，压痛点处（图4－53）。

层次解剖：皮肤→皮下组织→胫骨前肌→小腿骨间膜→胫骨后肌。浅层布有腓肠外侧皮神经和浅静脉。深层布有腓深神经和胫前动、静脉。

主治举例：单纯性阑尾炎、胃炎等。

操作：直刺1～1.5寸。

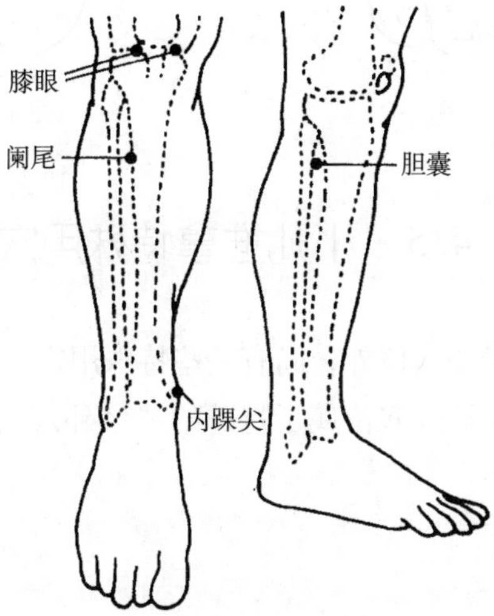

图4－53

4.4.4.4　内踝尖（EX－LE8）

定位：内踝的凸起处（图4－53）。

层次解剖：皮肤→皮下组织→内踝。布有隐神经的小腿内侧皮支的分支，胫前动脉的内踝网、内踝前动脉的分支和胫后动脉的内踝支。

主治举例：牙痛。

操作：禁刺，可灸。

4.4.4.5　八风（EX－LE10）

定位：足背的趾缝间，趾蹼缘后方赤白肉际处。左右共8穴（图4－54）。

主治举例：头痛、足背肿痛、趾端麻木、蛇咬伤（刺出血）、牙痛等。

操作：向上斜刺0.5～1寸。

4.4.4.6　独阴（EX－LE11）

定位：足第二趾的跖侧远侧趾间关节的中点（图4－55）。

层次解剖：皮肤→皮下组织→趾短、长屈肌腱。布有趾足底固有神经，趾底固有动、静脉的分支或属支。

主治举例：胸胁痛、呕吐、月经不调、睾丸炎、心绞痛、昏迷等。

操作：直刺0.1～0.2寸。

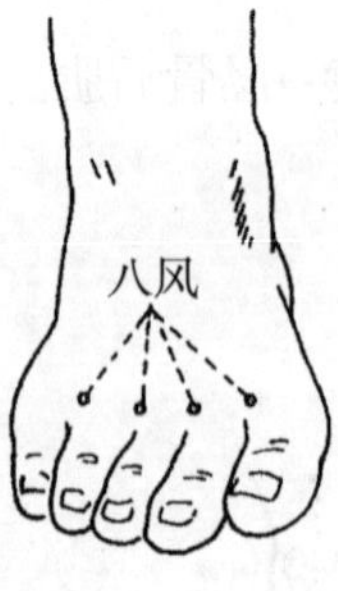

图4－54

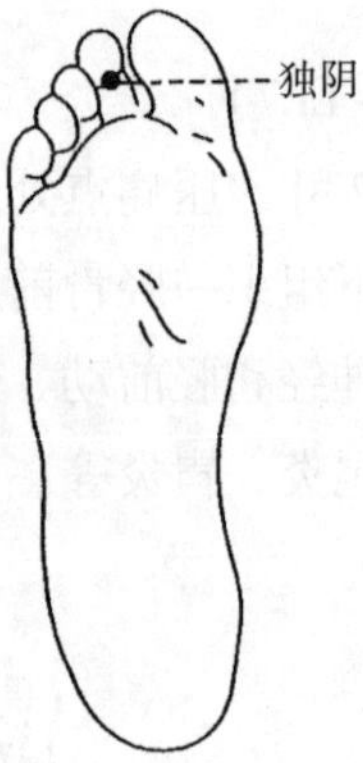

图4－55

4.5　小儿推拿特殊用穴

临床上除用于小儿推拿的通用穴位外，尚有一些特殊用穴。这些穴位不仅有“点”状，还有“线状”“面状”。从本质上看，这些穴位属于特殊的“经外穴”，常与特殊的小儿推拿手法配用，对于小儿疾病有特效。

4.5.1　头面部

4.5.1.1　天门（MA－HF1）

定位：两眉中央至前发际成一直线（图4－56）。

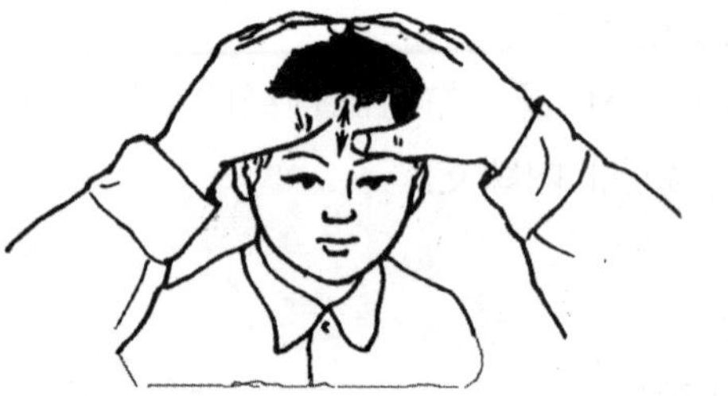

图4－56

主治举例：发热、感冒、头痛、精神萎靡、易惊等。

操作：常用两拇指，自下而上交替直推，称开天门，又称推攒竹。一般推30～50次。

注意：本穴又名攒竹，与足太阳膀胱经上的“攒竹”同名，但位置不同。

4.5.1.2　坎宫（MA－HF2）

定位：从两眉中央起，向两侧眉梢成一横线（图4－57）。

4.5.1.3　天柱骨（MA－HF3）

定位：颈后发际正中至大椎穴成一直线（图4－58）。

主治举例：恶心、呕吐、发热、咽炎、惊厥、落枕等。

操作：用拇指或食中指，自上向下直推。一般推50～100次。

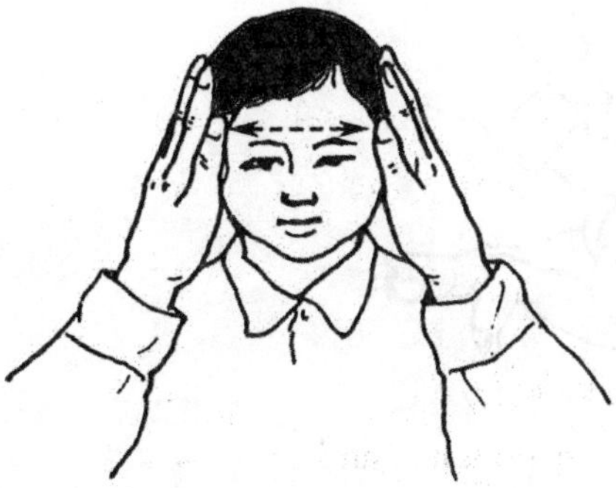

图4－57

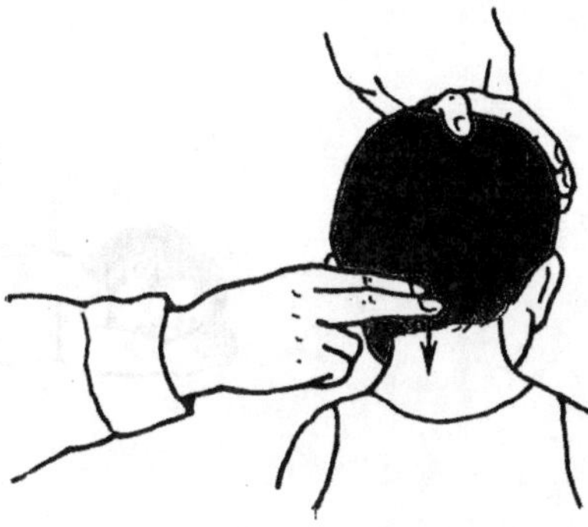

图4－58

4.5.2　躯干部

4.5.2.1　丹田（MA－T1）

定位：小腹部（脐下2寸与3寸之间）（图4－59）。

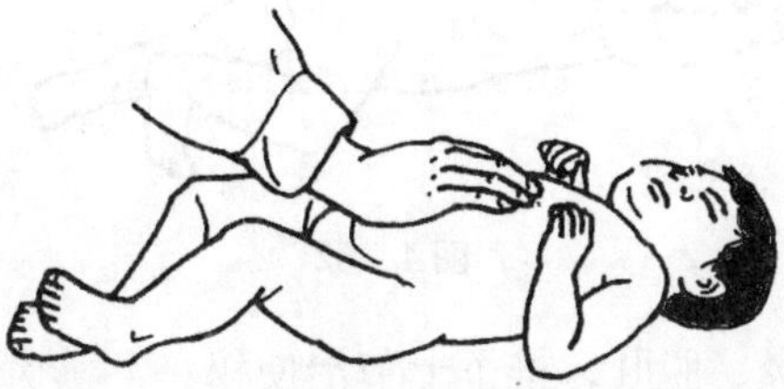

图4－59

主治举例：急慢性肠炎、遗尿、尿潴留、脱肛、疝气等。

操作：揉50～100次或按摩5分钟。

4.5.2.2　脊柱（MA－T2）

定位：大椎至长强，成一直线（图4－60）。

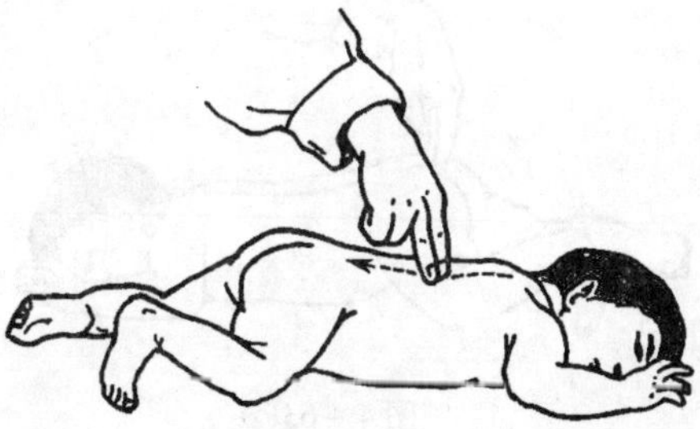

图4－60

主治举例：推脊治发热、小儿惊厥；捏脊治呕吐、肠炎、便秘等。也可用于小儿保健。

操作：用食、中二指面，自上而下做直推，称推脊，推50～100次；用捏法自下而上，称捏脊，捏3～5次（图4－61）。

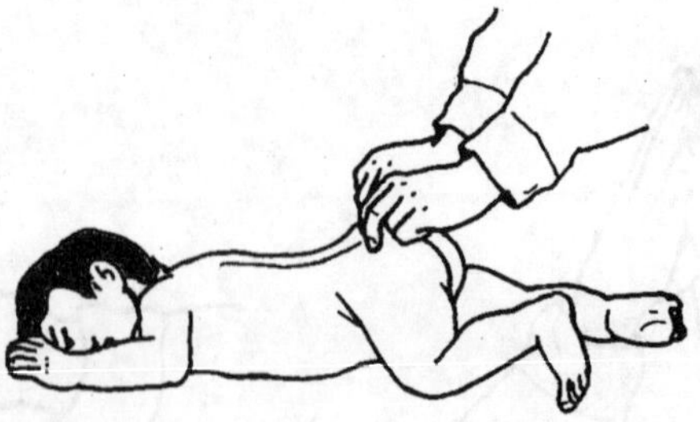

图4-61

4.5.2.3　七节骨（MA-T3）

定位：第四腰椎至尾骨端，成一直线（图4-62）。

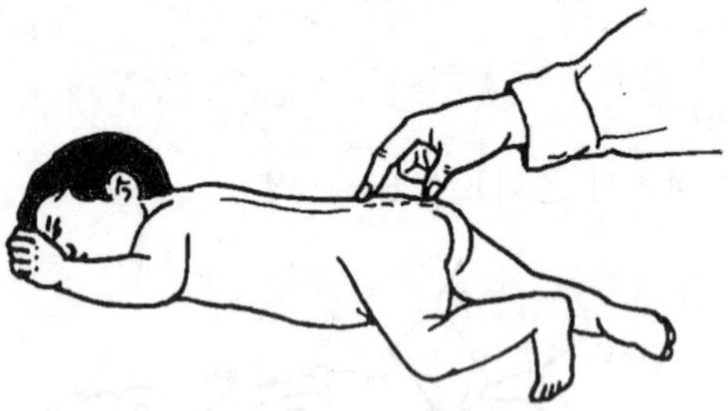

图4-62

主治举例：推上七节治肠炎、脱肛，推下七节治便秘。

操作：用食、中二指面，自下而上做直推，称推上七节；自上而下直推，称推下七节。推100～300次。

4.5.2.4　龟尾（MA-T4）

定位：尾骨端（图4-63）。

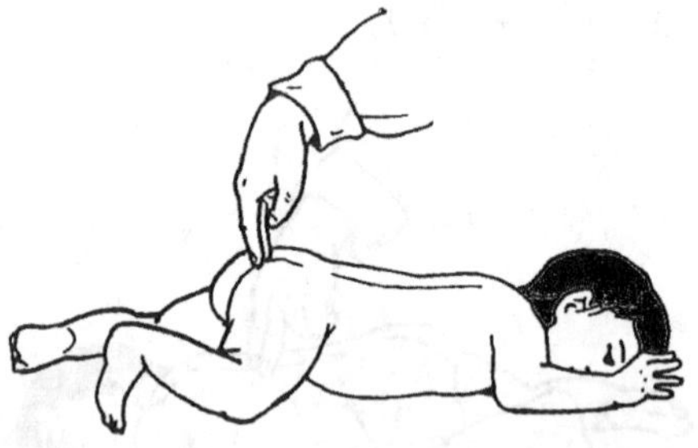

图4-63

主治举例：肠炎、便秘、脱肛、遗尿等。

操作：揉100～300次。

4.5.3　上肢部

4.5.3.1　脾经（MA-UE1）

定位：拇指末节螺纹面（图4-64）。

主治举例：肠炎、便秘、厌食等。

操作：旋推为补，称补脾经；由指端向指根方向直推为清，称清脾经。第二种补脾经法：将患儿拇指屈曲，循拇指桡侧边缘向掌根方向直推。以上操作，次数均为 100～500 次。

4.5.3.2　肝经（MA－UE2）

定位：食指末节螺纹面（图 4－64）。

主治举例：惊厥、目赤、口苦、咽干等肝经热证。

操作：旋推为补；向指根方向直推为清。肝经宜清不宜补。次数为 100～500 次。

4.5.3.3　心经（MA－UE3）

定位：中指末节螺纹面（图 4－64）。

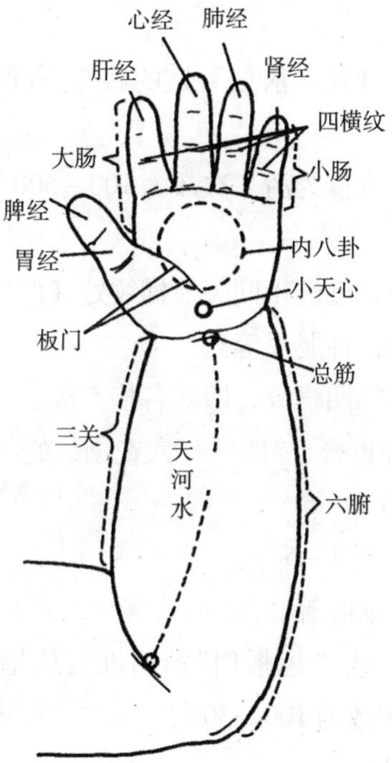

图 4－64

主治举例：高热（神昏）、口疮等。

操作：旋推为补，向指根方向直推为清。次数为 100～500 次。

4.5.3.4　肺经（MA－UE4）

定位：无名指末节螺纹面（图 4－64）。

主治举例：感冒、发热、咳嗽、哮喘等。

操作：旋推为补，向指根方向直推为清。次数为 100～500 次。

4.5.3.5　肾经（MA－UE5）

定位：小指末节螺纹面（图 4－64）。

主治举例：补肾经可主治先天不足、久病体虚、（肾虚）久泻、遗尿、虚喘等。清肾经可主治膀胱蕴热、小便刺痛等。

操作：由指根向指尖方向直推为补，向指根方向直推为清。次数为 100～500 次。

4.5.3.6　大肠（MA－UE6）

定位：食指桡侧缘，从食指到虎口成一直线（图4－64）。

主治举例：肠炎、痢疾、便秘等。

操作：从食指尖推到虎口为补；反之为清。次数为100～300次。

4.5.3.7　小肠（MA－UE7）

定位：小指尺侧缘，从指尖到指根成一直线（图4－64）。

主治举例：肠炎、遗尿等。

操作：从指尖推到指根为补；反之为清。次数为100～300次。

4.5.3.8　胃经（MA－UE8）

定位：拇指掌面近掌端第一节（在“脾经”穴的后方）（图4－64）。

主治举例：呕吐、厌食等。

操作：旋推为补；向指根方向直推为清。次数为100－500次。

4.5.3.9　四横纹（MA－UE9）

定位：二、三、四、五指掌面，近端指间关节横纹处（两手各有4穴）（图4－64）。

主治举例：小儿消化不良、急慢性肠炎等。

操作：常用拇指指甲掐揉，称掐四横纹，四穴各掐5次。

注意：本穴与“四缝”穴部分重叠，“四缝”穴在横纹的中点处。

4.5.3.10　板门（MA－UE10）

定位：手掌部的大鱼际平面（图4－64）。

主治举例：厌食、消化不良、呕吐等。

操作：指端揉，称“揉板门”或“运板门”；用推法从指根推向腕横纹，称“板门推向横纹”，反之称“横纹推向板门”。次数为100～300次。

4.5.3.11　内八卦（MA－UE11）

定位：手掌面，以掌心为圆心，从圆心到中指根横纹约2/3处为半径所作的圆周（图4－64）。

主治举例：咳嗽、哮喘、厌食、呕吐、腹胀等。

操作：顺时针方向摩动，称运八卦。次数为100～300次。

4.5.3.12　小天心（MA－UE12）

定位：大鱼际、小鱼际的交接处（图4－64）。

主治举例：小儿惊厥、夜啼、尿痛等。

操作：揉或掐100～300次。

4.5.3.13　总筋（MA－UE13）。

定位：手腕掌侧横纹中点（图4－64）。

主治举例：小儿惊厥、夜啼、口舌疮、牙痛等。

操作：揉100～300次，掐3～5次。

4.5.3.14　三关（MA－UE14）

定位：前臂桡侧，从腕背横纹正中，至曲池成一直线（图4－64）。

主治举例：病后体弱、腹痛、感冒等。

操作：用拇指桡侧面或食、中指面从腕推向肘，称“推三关”，做100~300次。

4.5.3.15 天河水（MA－UE15）

定位：前臂正中，总筋至曲泽成一直线（图4－64）。

主治举例：感冒发热、惊厥等一切热证。

操作：用食、中指指面从腕推向肘，称“清天河水”，做100~300次。

4.5.3.16 六腑（MA－UE16）

定位：前臂尺侧，神门至肘成一直线（图4－64）。

主治举例：高热、惊厥、扁桃体炎、腮腺炎、大便秘结等一切实热病症。

操作：用拇指面或食、中指指面从肘推向腕，称“退六腑”，做100~300次。

4.6 特定穴的应用

特定穴是指十四经中有特殊意义和作用的穴位，包括背俞穴、募穴、原穴、络穴、郄穴、下合穴、八脉交会穴、八会穴、五俞穴等12类。

4.6.1 背俞穴和募穴

背俞穴分布在背部脊柱两侧，属足太阳膀胱经，是与内脏病变关系密切的背部穴；募穴是与内脏病变关系密切且分布在胸腹部的穴位。当内脏病变时，会在相应的俞、募穴产生压痛等反应，临床取与病变内脏相应的俞穴和募穴相配，进行针刺或艾灸，称为俞募配穴法。与脏腑的关系见表4－3。

表4－3 俞、募配穴表

经脉	俞穴	募穴	经脉	俞穴	募穴
肺经	肺俞	中府	脾经	脾俞	章门
心包经	厥阴俞	膻中	肝经	肝俞	期门
心经	心俞	巨阙	肾经	肾俞	京门
大肠经	大肠俞	天枢	胃经	胃俞	中脘
三焦经	三焦俞	石门	胆经	胆俞	日月
小肠经	小肠俞	关元	膀胱经	膀胱俞	中极

穴位神经解剖学研究发现，募穴与其相关主治的脏器在神经节段分布上相当一致，见表4－4。

表4－4 俞穴和募穴与脏器在神经节段上的分布表

<table>
<tr><th colspan="2">相关脏器及所属节段</th><th colspan="2">俞穴及所属节段</th><th colspan="2">募穴及所属节段</th></tr>
<tr><td rowspan="2">肺</td><td rowspan="2">颈3~胸4</td><td>肺俞</td><td>胸1~3</td><td>中府</td><td>胸1</td></tr>
<tr><td>厥阴俞</td><td>胸2~4</td><td>膻中</td><td>胸4</td></tr>
</table>

续 表

相关脏器及所属节段		俞穴及所属节段		募穴及所属节段	
心	胸3~4	心俞	胸3~5	巨阙	
肝	胸7~10	肝俞	胸7~9	期门	胸8
肾	胸12~腰1	肾俞	胸11~ 腰1	京门	胸11
		脾俞	胸9~11	章门	胸10
胃	胸6~9	胃俞	胸10~12	中脘	胸9
大肠	胸11~12、腰1~3	大肠俞	腰3	天枢	胸10
胆	胸7~10	胆俞	胸8~10	日月	胸9
膀胱	胸11~腰2	膀胱俞	骶1~2	中极	胸12~腰1

4.6.2　原穴和络穴

原穴和络穴是十二经脉在肘膝关节以下的主要经穴。原穴是与内脏病变相关且分布于四肢末端的穴位；络穴是相表里的两经的交互联络点。当某一经发生病变时，可取本经的原穴，配合其对应的表里经的络穴，称为原络配穴法，可以起到加强治疗效果的作用（表4-5）。

表4-5　原穴络穴表

经 脉	原 穴	络 穴	经 脉	原 穴	络 穴
肺经	太渊	列缺	脾经	太白	公孙
心包经	大陵	内关	肝经	太冲	蠡沟
心经	神门	通里	肾经	太溪	大钟
大肠经	合谷	偏历	胃经	冲阳	丰隆
三焦经	阳池	外关	胆经	丘墟	光明
小肠经	腕骨	支正	膀胱经	京骨	飞扬

4.6.3　下合穴

下合穴是与六腑病变关系较为密切且分布在下肢部的穴位。如上巨虚治大肠病，阳陵泉治胆病等（表4-6）。

表4-6　下合穴表

经 脉	下合穴	经 脉	下合穴
手阳明大肠经	上巨虚	足阳明胃经	足三里
手少阳三焦经	委阳	足少阳胆经	阳陵泉
手太阳小肠经	下巨虚	足太阳膀胱经	委中

4.6.4 郄 穴

古人认为郄穴是经脉气血汇集的孔隙，十二经各有一个郄穴，奇经中的阴维、阳维、阴跷、阳跷也各有一个郄穴，共计十六郄穴。临床上郄穴常用于治疗急性病和剧烈的疼痛（表4－7）。

表4－7 十六郄穴表

经 脉	郄 穴	经 脉	郄 穴
肺经	孔最	肾经	水泉
心包经	郄门	胃经	梁丘
心经	阴郄	胆经	外丘
大肠经	温溜	膀胱经	金门
三焦经	会宗	阴维	筑宾
小肠经	养老	阳维	阳交
脾经	地机	阴跷	交信
肝经	中都	阳跷	跗阳

4.7 耳 针

耳针疗法是用针刺或其他方法刺激耳穴，以防治疾病的一种方法。该方法具有操作简便、适应证广、对许多病症疗效较好等优点。

4.7.1 耳郭解剖标志

耳郭表面的解剖标志（图4－65）。

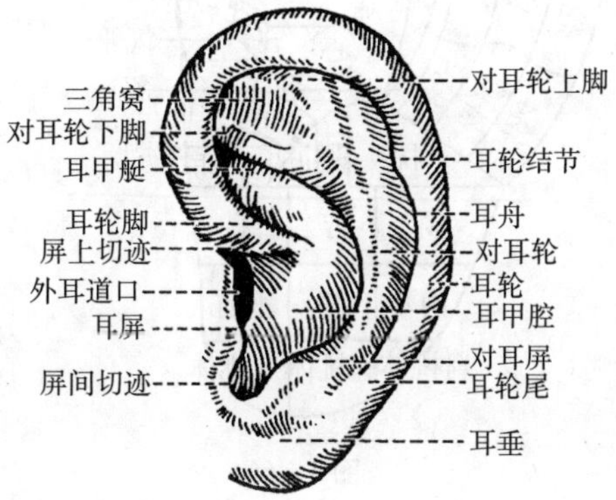

图4－65

4.7.1.1 耳轮和对耳轮

耳郭最外缘的卷曲部分叫耳轮，其深入耳腔的横行突起部叫耳轮脚。在耳轮的内侧，与耳轮相对的隆起部为对耳轮；对耳轮上部有两分叉，分别叫对耳轮上脚和对耳轮下脚。

4.7.1.2 耳垂、耳屏、对耳屏

耳郭下部柔软的皮垂叫耳垂；耳郭前面瓣状突起部为耳屏；耳垂上方与耳屏相对的隆起为对

耳屏。

4.7.1.3　三角窝、耳甲艇、耳甲腔

三角窝为对耳轮上脚和下脚之间的三角形凹窝；耳甲艇为耳轮脚与对耳轮下脚之间的橄榄形凹陷区；耳甲腔为耳轮脚以下的凹陷区。

4.7.1.4　耳舟、耳轮结节

耳舟为耳轮与对耳轮之间的凹沟；耳轮结节在耳轮后上方稍突出处。

4.7.1.5　屏上切迹、屏间切迹、轮屏切迹

屏上切迹为屏上缘与耳轮脚之间的凹陷；屏间切迹为耳屏与对耳屏之间的凹陷；轮屏切迹在对耳轮与对耳屏之间稍凹陷处。

4.7.2　常用耳穴

耳穴分布图很像胎儿在母腹中的倒立图（图4－66）。由下向上顺序为：耳垂代表头部，对耳屏为颅腔，耳甲腔为胸腔，耳轮脚为胸膈，耳甲艇为腹腔，三角窝为盆腔，对耳轮中下部代表躯干及颈、胸、腰、骶、尾椎，对耳轮上、下脚代表下肢，耳舟代表上肢。常用穴位的定位和主治见图4－66和表4－8。

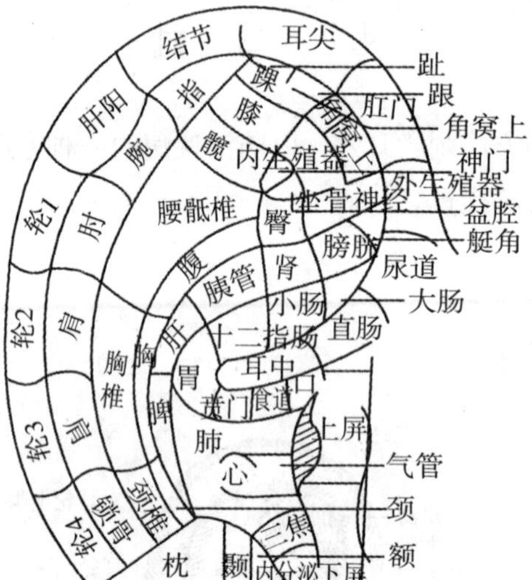

图4－66

表4-8 常用穴位的定位和主治

解剖	穴名	定位	主治
耳轮11穴	耳中（HX1）	耳轮脚	呃逆，荨麻疹，神经性皮炎，小儿遗尿，咯血
	直肠（HX2）	耳轮脚棘前上方的耳轮	便秘，腹泻，脱肛，痔疮
	尿道（HX3）	“直肠”上方耳轮	尿路感染，尿潴留
	外生殖器（HX4）	对耳轮下脚前方的耳轮	睾丸炎，附睾炎，外阴瘙痒症
	肛门（HX5）	三角窝前方的耳轮	痔疮，肛裂
	耳尖（HX6）	耳郭向前对折的上部尖端	发热，高血压，急性结膜炎，睑腺炎
	结节（HX7）	耳轮结节	头晕，头痛
	轮1~4（HX9-12）	耳轮结节下方的耳轮顺次向下	上呼吸道感染
耳舟6穴	指（SF1）	耳舟上方	甲沟炎，手指疼痛麻木
	腕（SF2）	“指”区下方	腕部疼痛
	风溪（SF1，2i）	耳轮结节前方，“指”“腕”之间	荨麻疹，神经性皮炎，过敏性鼻炎
	肘（SF3）	“腕”区下方	肘部疼痛
	肩（SF4，5）	“肘”区下方	肩关节周围炎
	锁骨（SF6）	“肩”区下方	肩关节周围炎
对耳轮14穴	跟（AH1）	对耳轮上脚前上部	足扭伤，足跟痛
	趾（AH2）	耳尖下方对耳轮上脚后上部	甲沟炎，趾部疼痛
	踝（AH3）	“趾”“跟”区下方	踝关节扭伤
	膝（AH4）	对耳轮上脚中1/3	膝关节痛
	髋（AH5）	对耳轮上脚下1/3	髋关节痛，坐骨神经痛
	坐骨神经（AH6）	对耳轮下脚前2/3	坐骨神经痛
	交感（AH6a）	对耳轮下脚末端与耳轮内缘相交	胃肠痉挛，心胆绞痛，尿路结石，自主神经功能紊乱
	臀（AH7）	对耳轮下脚后1/3	坐骨神经痛，臀筋膜炎
	腹（AH8）	对耳轮体前部上2/5	腹痛，急性腰扭伤，痛经，产后宫缩痛
	腰骶椎（AH9）	“腹”区后方	腰骶部疼痛
	胸（AH10）	对耳轮体前部中2/5	胸胁疼痛，胸闷，乳腺炎
	胸椎（AH11）	“胸”区后方	胸胁疼痛，乳腺炎，经前乳房胀痛，产后泌乳不足
	颈（AH12）	对耳轮体前部下1/5	落枕，颈椎病
	颈椎（AH13）	“颈”区后方	落枕，颈椎病

续 表

解剖	穴名	定位	主治
三角窝5穴	角窝上（TF1）	三角窝前1/3的上部	高血压
	内生殖器（TF2）	三角窝前1/3的下部	痛经，月经不调，功血，带下，遗精，早泄
	角窝中（TF3）	三角窝中1/3	哮喘
	神门（TF4）	三角窝后1/3的上部	失眠，多梦，痛经，戒断综合征
	盆腔（TF5）	三角窝后1/3的下部	盆腔炎
耳屏9穴	上屏（TG1）	耳屏外侧面上1/2处	咽炎，鼻炎
	下屏（TG2）	耳屏外侧面下1/2处	鼻炎
	外耳（TG10）	屏上切迹前方近耳轮处	外耳道炎，中耳炎，耳鸣
	屏尖（TG1P）	耳屏游离缘上部尖端	发热，牙痛
	外鼻（TG1，2i）	耳屏外侧面中部，上下屏之间	鼻炎，鼻窦炎
	肾上腺（TG2P）	耳屏游离缘下部尖端	低血压，风湿性关节炎，腮腺炎，链霉素中毒
	咽喉（TG3）	耳屏内侧面上1/2处	咽喉炎，扁桃体炎，声音嘶哑
	内鼻TG4	耳屏内侧面下1/2处	鼻炎，副鼻窦炎
	屏间前（TG21）	屏间切迹前方耳屏最下部	口腔炎，咽炎
对耳屏8穴	额（AT1）	对耳屏外侧面前部	头痛，头晕，失眠，多梦
	屏间后（AT11）	屏间切迹后方，对耳屏前下部	额窦炎
	颞（AT2）	对耳屏外侧面中部	偏头痛
	枕（AT3）	对耳屏外侧面后部	头痛，眩晕，哮喘，癫痫，神经衰弱
	皮质下（AT4）	对耳屏内侧面	痛症，间日疟，神经衰弱，假性近视，失眠
	对屏尖（AT1，2，4i）	对耳屏游离缘的尖端	哮喘，腮腺炎，神经性皮炎，睾丸炎，附睾炎
	缘中（AT2，3，4i）	对耳屏游离缘上，对屏尖与屏轮切迹中点	遗尿，内耳眩晕症
	脑干（AT 3，4i）	屏轮切迹处	后头痛，眩晕，假性近视
对耳轮穴11穴	口（CO1）	耳轮脚下方前1/3处	面瘫，口腔炎，胆石症，胆囊炎，戒断综合征
	食道（CO2）	耳轮脚下方中1/3处	食道炎，食道痉挛
	贲门（CO3）	耳轮脚下方后1/3处	贲门痉挛，神经性呕吐
	胃（CO4）	耳轮脚消失处	胃痉挛，胃炎，胃溃疡，消化不良，失眠，牙痛
	十二指肠（CO5）	耳轮脚上方后部	十二指肠溃疡，胆石症，胆囊炎，幽门痉挛

续　表

解剖	穴名	定位	主治
对耳轮穴11穴	小肠（CO6）	耳轮脚上方中部	消化不良，腹痛，心动过速，心律不齐
	大肠（CO7）	耳轮脚上方前部	腹泻，便秘
	阑尾（CO6，7i）	“大肠”和“小肠”区之间	腹泻，单纯性阑尾炎
	艇角（CO8）	对耳轮下脚下方前部	前列腺炎，尿道炎
	膀胱（CO9）	对耳轮下脚下方中部	膀胱炎，遗尿，尿潴留，后头痛，腰痛，坐骨神经痛
	肾（CO10）	对耳轮下脚下方后部	耳鸣，肾盂肾炎，遗尿，遗精早泄，月经不调，哮喘
耳甲10穴	输尿管（CO9，10i）	“肾”和“膀胱”区之间	输尿管结石
	胰胆（CO11）	耳甲艇的后上部	胆石症，胆囊炎，胆道蛔虫，偏头痛，胰腺炎，耳病
	肝（CO12）	耳甲艇的后下部	胁痛，高血压，假性近视，月经不调，更年期综合征
	艇中（CO6，10i）	“小肠”和“肾”区之间	腹痛，腹胀，胆道蛔虫症
	脾（CO13）	耳甲腔的后上部	腹胀，腹痛，便秘，食欲不振，功血，白带过多，内耳眩晕症
	心（CO15）	耳甲腔正中凹陷处	心动过速，心律不齐，心绞痛，神经衰弱，舌疮
	气管（CO16）	“心”区和外耳门之间	哮喘，支气管炎
	肺（CO14）	“心”“气管”区周围处	咳嗽，声音嘶哑，痤疮，便秘，荨麻疹，戒断综合征
	三焦（CO17）	外耳门后下，“肺”和“内分泌”间	便秘，腹胀，腹痛
	内分泌（CO18）	屏间切迹内，耳甲腔的前下部	痛经，月经不调，更年期综合征，痤疮，间日疟
耳垂8穴	牙（LO1）	耳垂正面前上部	牙痛，牙周炎，低血压
	舌（LO2）	耳垂正面中上部	舌炎，口腔炎
	颌（LO3）	耳垂正面后上部	牙痛，颞颌关节功能紊乱
	垂前（LO4）	耳垂正面前中部	神经衰弱，牙痛
	眼（LO5）	耳垂正面中央部	急性结膜炎，麦粒肿，假性近视，电光性眼炎
	内耳（LO6）	耳垂正面后中部	内耳眩晕症，耳鸣，听力减退
	面颊（LO5，6i）	耳垂正面，“眼”与“内耳”区间	面肌抽搐，三叉神经痛，扁平疣，痤疮
	扁桃体（LO7，8，9）	耳垂正面下部	扁桃体炎，咽炎

续 表

解 剖	穴 名	定 位	主 治
耳背6穴	耳背心（P1）	耳背上部	冠心病，失眠，多梦
	耳背肺（P2）	耳背中内部	哮喘，神经性皮炎
	耳背脾（P3）	耳背中央部	胃痛，消化不良，食欲不振
	耳背肝（P4）	耳背中外部	胆石症，胆囊炎，胁痛
	耳背肾（P5）	耳背下部	头痛，头晕，神经衰弱
	耳背沟（PS）	对耳轮沟与对耳轮上下脚沟处	高血压，神经性皮炎
耳根穴3穴	上耳根（R1）	耳根最上处	鼻衄
	耳迷根（R2）	耳轮脚后沟的耳根处	胆石症，胆囊炎，鼻塞，心动过速，腹泻，腹痛
	下耳根（R3）	耳根最下处	低血压

4.7.3 耳穴的应用

4.7.3.1 选穴处方原则

1. 主穴：病变的对应耳区。

2. 配穴：发生了病理反应的病变的非对应耳区或与疾病有关的其他耳区。

4.7.3.2 操作

1. 寻找反应点：根据疾病需要确定处方后，在选用的耳区内寻找反应点，如压痛点、低电阻点等。

2. 治疗：常规消毒后，用0.5寸毫针进行针刺或选用磁珠、王不留行子进行压籽，或皮内针埋针、穴位注射等刺激方法。针刺进深度以穿破软骨但不透过对侧皮肤为度，刺激强度以病人耐受为宜，一般留针30分钟，可带电针。压籽、皮内针一般每次贴压一侧耳穴，两耳轮流，3天1换；留置期间，每日按压2～4次，每穴每次1～2分钟。夏季留置时间可适当缩短。

4.7.3.3 注意事项

1. 严格消毒，预防感染。有皮肤损害的部位禁止用针刺、压籽等刺激。

2. 有习惯性流产史的孕妇禁针；高血压、动脉硬化的老年患者，针刺前后要适当休息。

3. 也可能发生晕针，防治措施同体针疗法。

Chapter 4 Acupuncture and Moxibustion

The purpose of acupuncture and moxibustion is to relief tiredness, prevent and treat disease by stimulating meridians and acupoints. Needles and Artemisia vulgaris are used in acupuncture and moxibustion respectively for stimulation.

4.1 The Meridian System

The Meridian theory is the basic theory of the science of acupuncture, moxibustion and Chinese massage. Meridian System consists of the pathways that connect organs with other parts of the body, and transport Qi and blood. The Meridian System consists of both meridians and collaterals. The meridians, meaning paths, are the main trunks that run longitudinally and interiorly-exteriorly, while the collaterals, meaning net works, are thinner and smaller than meridians. The Meridian System connects to the Zang-fu organs interiorly, and extends to the extremities exteriorly. The Meridian System integrates the Zang-fu, tissues, and organs into an organic whole, and keeps the functions and activities of all parts of the body in harmony and relative balance. The theory of Meridian System has directed the clinical practice of Chinese Traditional Medicine for thousands of years and provides the theoretical base for acupuncture, moxibustion, Tuina and Qigong.

Acupoints are specific anatomical points along the meridians. They are not isolated points on the skin, but rather, are connected with organs inside the body. Stimulation of acupoints can treat diseases by regulating organ function, passing Qi and blood through the Meridian System, and improving the ability of the body to resist disease.

4.1.1 The composition of the Meridian System

The famous ancient work, *Huangdi's Internal Classic*, describes a very complicated Meridian System, meridians and collaterals. The meridians include the Twelve Regular Meridians, the Eight Extra Meridians, the twelve divergent meridians, the twelve muscle regions, and the twelve cutaneous regions, etc. the collaterals, include the fifteen collaterals, the superficial collaterals, and the minute collaterals, etc. The most important parts of the system are the twelve regular meridians and the eight extra meridians, which will be mentioned below.

4.1.2 The Twelve Regular Meridians and Eight Extra Meridians

4.1.2.1 The Twelve Regular Meridians

There are twelve symmetrical meridians on each side of the body. They include the following: the

Lung Meridian of Hand-Taiyin, the Pericardium Meridian of Hand-Jueyin, the Heart Meridian of Hand-Shaoyin, the Large Intestine Meridian of Hand-Yangming, the Sanjiao Meridian of Hand-Shaoyang, the Small Intestine Meridian of Hand-Taiyang, the Spleen Meridian of Foot-Taiying, the Liver Meridian of Foot-Jueyin, the Kidney Meridian of Foot-Shaoyin, the Stomach Meridian of Foot-Yangming, the Gallbladder Meridian of Foot-Shaoyang and the Bladder Meridian of Foot-Taiyang.

The body-surface distribution of the Twelve Meridians is an important content here. Yin meridians are distributed on the medial aspects of the four limbs, and on the thoracic and abdominal regions. Yang meridians are distributed on the lateral aspects of the four limbs, the head and face, and the back and lumbar region. The three Yin meridians of hand and foot are arranged in a sequence, in which Taiyin meridian is the anterior one, Jueyin meridian the middle one, and Shaoyin meridian the posterior one. With respect to the three Yang meridians of hand and foot, Yangming meridian is the anterior one, Shaoyang meridian, the middle one, and Taiyang meridian, the posterior one (Table 4 – 1, Fig. 4 – 1).

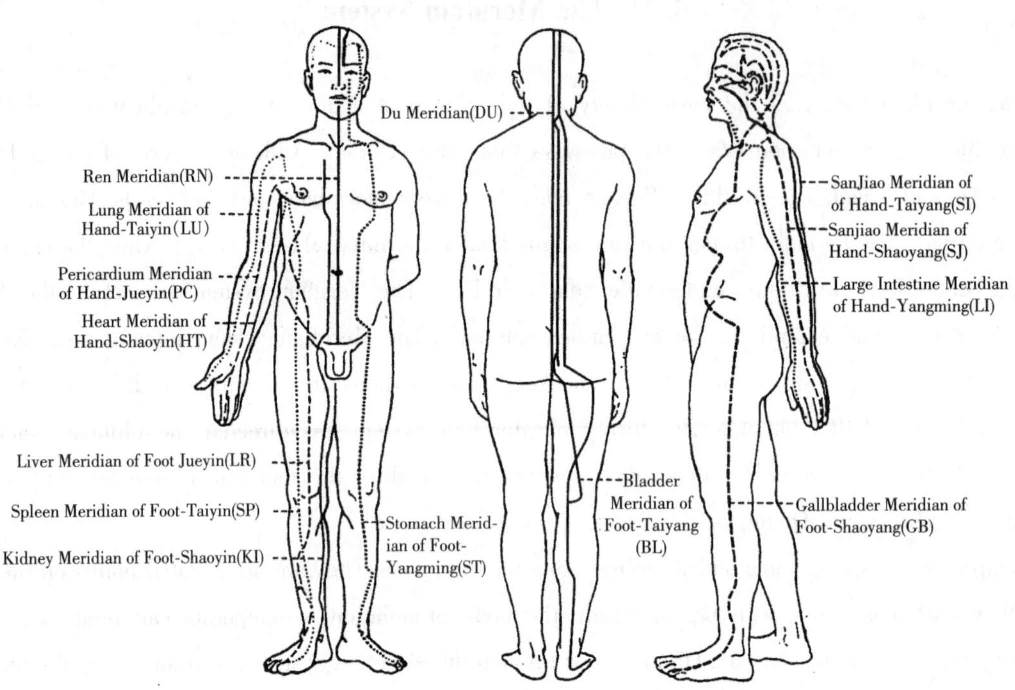

Fig. 4 – 1

Table 4 – 1 **Distribution of the Twelve Meridians Yin meridians Pathway and Yang (meridians) Pathway**

Yin meridians	Pathway	Yang meridians	Pathway
Lung	Chest, anterior edge of interior aspects of upper limbs	Large intestine	Head and face, anterior lateral aspects of upper limbs
Pericardium	Chest, medial area of interior aspects of upper limbs	Sanjiao	Neck and ear, middle lateral aspects of upper limbs
Heart	Chest, posterior edge of interior aspects of upper limbs	Small intestine	Shoulder, posterior lateral aspects of upper limbs

Yin meridians	Pathway	Yang meridians	Pathway
Spleen	Abdomen, anterior edge of interior aspects of legs *	Stomach	Chest, abdomen, head and face, anterior lateral aspects of legs
Liver	Abdomen, middle area of interior aspects of legs *	Gallbladder	Hypochondrium, middle lateral aspects of legs
Kidney	Chest and abdomen, posterior medial aspects of legs	Bladder	Back, posterior lateral aspects of legs

* Under the level of 8 *cun* above the medial malleolus, Liver Meridian is anterior and the Spleen Meridian is in the middle.

Above the level of 8 *cun* above the medial malleolus, Liver Meridian is in the middle and the Spleen Meridian is in the anterior.

The Lung Meridian of Hand-Taiyin (Lung Meridian) and the Large Intestine Meridian of Hand Yangming (Large Intestine Meridian) pass anteriorally along the medial and lateral sides of the upper limbs respectively. This relationship is an example of an "inside and outside" relationship. Other meridian pairs in the above table are also inside and outside meridians. These meridian pairs have a close relationship in the treatment of disease. When one of the Twelve Meridians has a problem, there will be some symptoms related to the meridian, such as cough, asthma, or chest pain for the Lung Meridian, and pain along the Lung Meridian. We can choose appropriate acupoints along the Lung and Large Intestine Meridians to treat it. When there is a problem with the Pericardium Meridian of Hand-Jueyin, the patient may have symptoms such as cardiac pain, palpitation, insomnia, endless laughter and other cardiac and mental symptoms.

4. 1. 2. 2 The Eight Extra Meridians

The Eight Extra Meridians are the Ren, Du, Chong, Dai, Yinwei, Yangwei, Yinqiao, and Yangqiao meridians. They are complementary to the Twelve Regular Meridians, but unlike the Twelve Regular Meridians, none of them pertain to the Zang-fu organs, and they are not exteriorly – interiorly related.

The Ren and Du meridians have their own related acupoints, and together with the Twelve Regular Meridians, they make up the "Fourteen Meridians" (Fig. 4 – 1). The Fourteen Meridians have their own pathways, acupoints and indications for disease. They comprise the most important part of the Meridian System, and are the basis for the clinical practice of acupuncture, moxibustion and Chinese massage.

4. 1. 3 Basic concepts on the theory of the meridian system

4. 1. 3. 1 Yin and yang

Yin and yang is a very important concept in Chinese Traditional Medicine. It is a kind of abstract classification of human body and disease in traditional Chinese culture. They have different meanings in different classifications. In Meridian System, the main interpretation of yin and yang is symmetry.

1. Inside and outside meridians: The six yin meridians are located in the medial part of the

extremities while the six yang meridians are in the lateral part. They are called "inside and outside" meridians. They can be chosen together to treat diseases related to the particular meridian pair. It is recorded in the book *Miraculous Pivot* (*Fainting Diseases*), a classic of Acupuncture and Moxibustion that "in the case of abdominal distension and severe cardiac pain, it is called stomach-heart pain. The acupoints of Dadu and Taibai can be chosen for treatment". This is one example of choosing corresponding inside-outside meridians.

2. Same name meridians: The Lung Meridian of Hand-Taiyin passes through the anterior part of the medial aspect of the upper limbs, while the Spleen Meridian of Foot-Taiyin passes through the anterior part of the medial aspect of the leg. They have up and down symmetry, and are called "same name" meridians. The three yin meridians and the three yang meridians in the upper limbs and legs are all called same name meridians. They have up and down symmetry. For disease occurance along one meridian, the acupoints along its same-name meridian are often chosen for treatment. It is said in *Miraculous Pivot* (*Miscellaneous Diseases*) that: "In the case of pharyngitis, if the patient cannot speak, Foot-Yangming Meridian is adopted. If the patient can speak, Hand-Yangming Meridian is adopted. When nose bleeding occurs, if the blood is not coagulated, adopt Foot-Taiyang Meridian; if the blood is coagulated, adopt Hand-Taiyang Meridian. These are some examples of applying the rule."

3. Left and right symmetry: The Twelve Regular Meridians have right and left symmetry. Wang Bing made comments on "Plain Questions" and said: "When you perform acupuncture on meridians to treat pain if pain is on the left side, you should needle the right meridian. If the pain is on the right side, you should needle the left meridian." Symmetry is a common occurrence in human body. It is obvious that gross anatomical symmetry exists, such as in the face, extremities, and trunk; but symmetry extends to the microlevel as well. E. g. the DNA molecule has a symmetrical double spiral structure.

4.1.3.2 Zang-fu organs

Another name is five Zang-organs and six Fu-organs. Five Zang-organs include lung, heart (pericardium), liver, spleen and kidney. Six Fu-organs are large intestine, small intestine, Sanjiao, gallbladder, stomach and bladder. Most of them have corresponding anotomic organs and functions. However, pericardium and Sanjiao are unique concepts in TCM. Especially, Sanjiao does not have corresponding organ. In the integrated studies of TCM and western medicine, it should be noticed that Zang-fu organs are not equivalent anotomic objects. For example, "heart" in TCM is not completely equal to the concept of "heart" in western medicine. In TCM, besides cardiovascular system, heart also include mental and neuro scope, which has the functions of brain and spinal marrow. "Spleen" in TCM is corresponding to stomach, rather than the familiar immue organ in western medicine. It has close relationship with digestive functions and some diseases of urinary system. Therefore, Zang-fu organs are more bridges between meridians and diseases rather than anotomic organs. The essence of Zang-fu theory is that it reveals that "internal organs are related to surface of the body" and such relationship has been proved by the experiments of neuro anotomy and physiology. The focus of future researches is to find clues of clinical experiences of ancient people in thousands of years, and then describe its mechanisms by using modern languages.

4.1.3.3 Qi and blood

Qi and blood are very important concepts in Traditional Chinese Medicine. They have different meanings in different fields. In meridians theory, the meaning of Qi originates from the needle-induced sensation passing through the meridians in acupuncture. Traditionally, this feeling is called the "Arrival of Qi". In meridian theory, "Passage of Qi and Blood" means "transmitting stimulating message, accelerating blood circulation".

4.2 Acupoints

4.2.1 Classification

Acupoints are also called acupuncture points, which can be classified into three kinds.

1. Acupoints of the Fourteen Meridians: These are also known as "regular points". The acupoints are distributed along the Twelve Regular Meridians and the Ren and Du Meridians. There are 361 acupoints comprising 309 pairs of double acupoints and 52 single acupoints.

2. Extraordinary Acupoints: "These are points with regular names and regular locations, but are not in the Fourteen Meridians."

3. Ashi Acupoints: They are the tender spots and other sensitive points, which exist on the patient's body. These acupoints do not have specific names or definite locations.

4.2.2 Therapeutic Properties

1. Local and adjacent therapeutic properties. Each acupoint located on a particular site is able to treat disorders of the area or nearby tissues and organs. All the acupoints in the body share this common therapeutic property like Jingming (BL1), Sibai (ST2) for eye diseases, and Zhongwan (RN12), Xiawan (RN10) for gastritis.

2. Remote therapeutic properties. Some acupoints are able to treat disorders at remote areas. For example, acupoints located below the elbow and knee joints can treat disorders in the face, head, chest and abdomen. Examples include the Hegu (LI4) to treat disorders in the face and head, and the Zusanli (ST36) to treat diseases of the digestive system.

3. Special therapeutic properties. Some acupoints have a biphasic beneficial effect. For instance, puncturing the Tianshu (ST25) relieves both diarrhea and constipation; puncturing Neiguan (PC6) relieves both bradycardia and tachycardia. In addition, the therapeutic properties of some acupoints show relative specialty. For example, Dazhui (DU14), has an antipyretic effect, and Zhiyin (BL67) helps to correct the malposition of a fetus.

4.2.3 Methods of Locating

4.2.3.1 Anatomical marks

This method is divided into two types, fixed marks and movable marks.

1. Fixed marks: Fixed marks are the anatomic body surface marks which do not change with body movement, such as the five sense organs, eyebrows and hair on the face, vertebral spines, spealbone,

rib and ilium on the back; nipple, sternum, umbilical opening and pubis symphysis on the chest and abdomen, joints and apophysis on the limbs. Some commonly used fixed marks are T3, T7 and L4 (Fig. 4 -2).

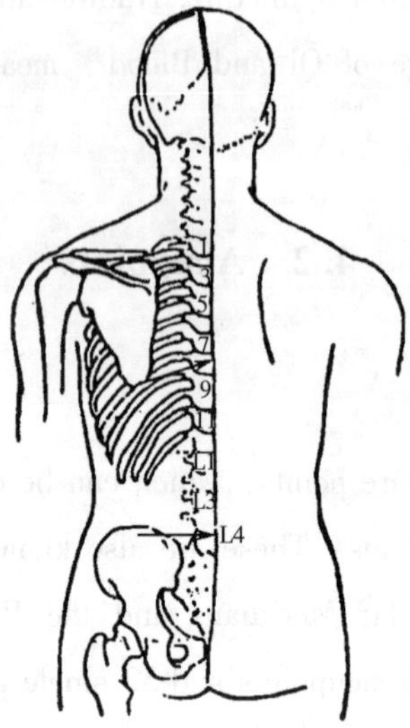

Fig. 4 -2

2. Movable marks: Movable marks will appear while the body is in a special posture. For instance, when we stand up and drop our hands, the points on the thighs where the middle fingers touch are Fengshi (GB31). When we hold the two palms together by touching the two webs near the thumb together, the dent, which the index finger can feel, is Lieque (LU7, Fig. 4 -9).

4. 2. 3. 2 Fingers Measurement

The length and width of the patient's finger (s) are taken as a standard for acupoint location. If the doctor's and patient's fingers are similar, the doctor's fingers can be used as a standard for point location. The following three methods are commonly used in clinical practice:

1. Middle finger measurement: When the patient's middle finger is bended, the distance between the two medial ends of the creases of the interphalangeal joint is taken as 1 *cun*. This method is employed for measuring vertical distances to locate limb acupoints, or for measuring horizontal distances to locate acupoints on the back (Fig. 4 -3).

2. Thumb measurement: The width of the interphalangeal joint of the patient's thumb is taken as 1 *cun*. This method is also employed for measuring vertical distances to locate acupoints on the limbs (Fig. 4 -4).

3. Four-finger measurement: To bring the index, middle, ring and little fingers close together side by side, the width of the four fingers at the level of the dorsal skin crease of the proximal interphalangel joint of the middle finger is taken as 3 *cun* (Fig. 4 -5).

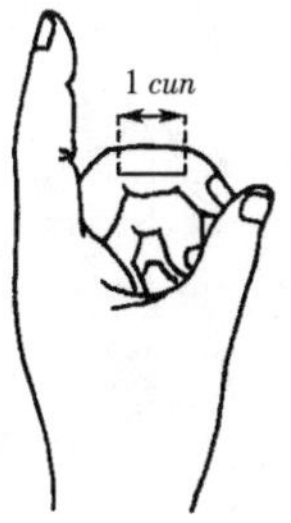

Fig. 4 – 3

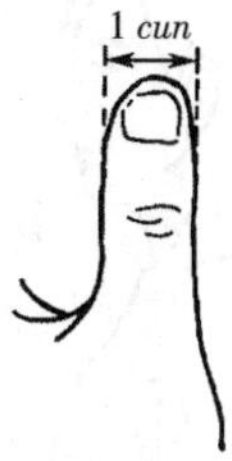

Fig. 4 – 4

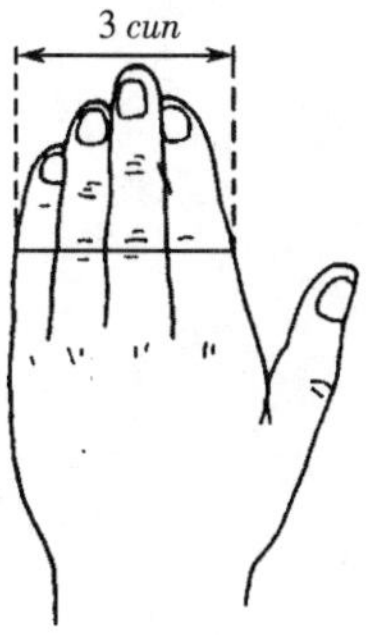

Fig. 4 – 5

4. 2. 3. 3 Proportional Measurement

Proportional measurements define the width or length of each part of human body. Equal proportions are made to define one personal *cun*. Examples are shown in the following Table 4 – 2 and in Fig. 4 – 6.

Table 4 – 2 Standards for Proportional Measurements

Body	Distance	Proportional Unit
Head	From the anterior hairline to the posterior hairline	12 *cun*
Chest and abdomen	From the suprasternal fossa to the sternocostal angle From the sternocostal angle to the center of the umbilicus Between the center of the umbilicus and the upper rim of symphysis pubis Between the two nipples	9 *cun* 8 *cun* 5 *cun* 8 *cun*
Back	From process of C7 to the coccyx Between the medial rims of scapulas	21 vertebra 6 *cun*
Upper limbs	Between the end of the axillary fold and the transverse cubital crease Between the transverse cubital crease and the transverse wrist crease	9 *cun* 12 *cun*
Lower limbs	From the level of the border of symphysis pubis to the medial epicondyle of femur From the lower border of the medial condyle of tibia to the tip of medial malleolus From the prominence of the great trochanter to the middle of patella From the center of patella to the tip of lateral malleolus	18 *cun* 13 *cun* 19 *cun* 16 *cun*

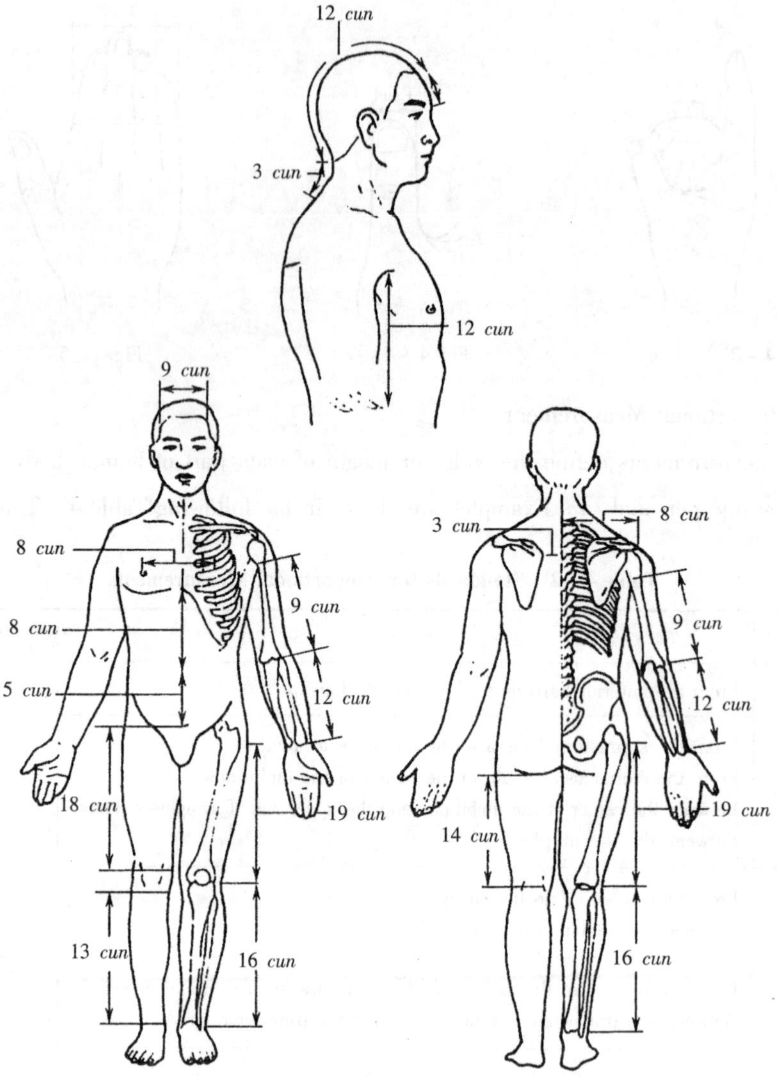

Fig. 4 – 6

4.3 The Fourteen Meridians and Their Acupoints

This section will introduce the Fourteen Meridians according to their distribution law. The introduction sequence is from three-Yin to three-Yang meridians in the hands, then from three – Yin to three-Yang meridians in the legs, and finally the Ren and Du meridians. The number of acupoints was 349 in *A – B Classic of Acupuncture and Moxibustion* and it increased gradually in different dynasties. By Qing Dynasty, Li Xuechuan listed 361 in his book *Acupuncture and Moxibustion on the Source*, which has been used till now. We will introduce some of the commonly used and some of the less commonly used acupoints in this book. The location and English code of the acupoints follow the national standards that was introduced in 1991. The references to the manipulation of the needle in an acupoint means manipulation at the regular depth and angle. The Chinese massage on acupoints presented in this section adopt Digital-pressing, Pressing-kneading, One-finger Zen Pushing manipulations etc. Only some special manipulations will be introduced in this section.

4. 3. 1 Lung Meridian of Hand-Taiyin (LU)

4. 3. 1. 1 General information

This meridian goes from chest to hand. The first acupoint is Zhongfu, and the last acupoint is Shaoshang. There are a total of 11 acupoints. Locations of most acupoints are the same as those described in the book "Compendium of Acupuncture and Moxibustion"; only a few are different. The main indications include respiratory system diseases, such as cough, asthma, emptysis, sore throat, chest pain, and pain which locates in the medial anterior side of the hand.

4. 3. 1. 2 Main course of the meridian

This meridian originates in the stomach and runs downwards to connect with the large intestine. It then winds back, enters the lung, its pertaining organ, and passes along the trachea. From here it goes to the lateral aspect of the forearm, descends along the radial border of the medial aspect of the upper arm and ends at the radial side of the thumb. The branch connects with Large Intestine Meridian of Hand-Yangming (Fig. 4 – 7).

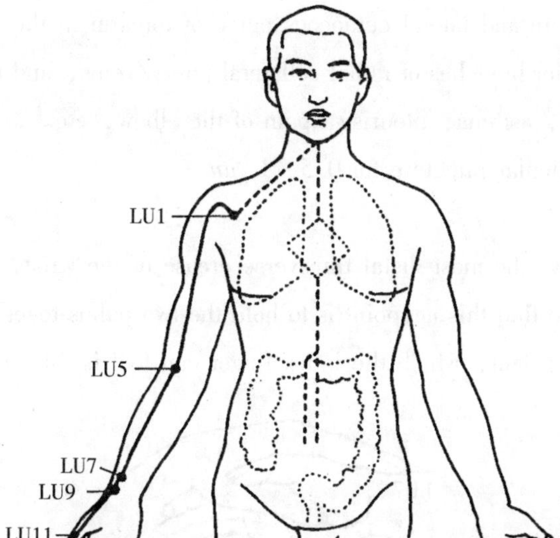

Fig. 4 – 7

4. 3. 1. 3 Commonly used acupoints

1. Zhongfu (LU1).

Location: 6 *cun* laterals to the midline of the chest, in the first intercostals space, near the coracoid process (Fig. 4 – 8).

Layers of dissection: Skin→Subcutaneous tissue→Great pectoral muscle→Lesser pectoral muscle – Thoracic cavity. In the superficial layer are intermediate supraclavicular nerve, lateral cutaneous branch of the first intercostals nerve, and cephalic vein. In the deep layer are thoracoacromial artery/vein, Medial/Lateral pectoral nerve.

Indications: Bronchitis, asthma, pneumonia, chest pain, shoulder pain, and backache, etc.

Manipulation: Oblique or horizontal puncture for 0.5 ~ 0.8 *cun* towards the lateral side. Puncturing deep and towards the medial side may penetrate the lung.

2. Chize (LU5).

Location: At the elbow crease, on the radial side of the tendon of the biceps brachial muscle (Fig. 4 – 8).

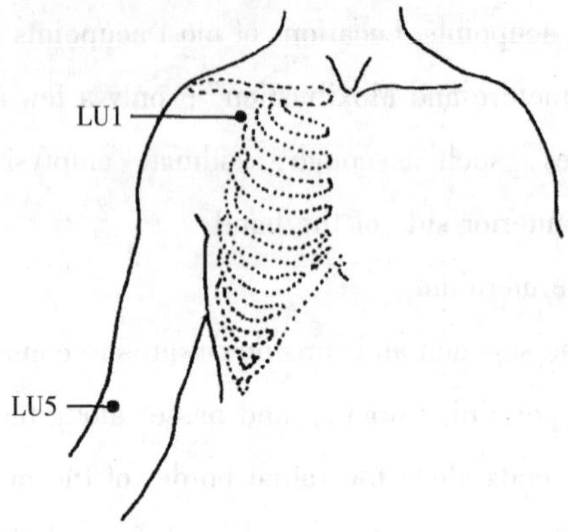

Fig. 4 – 8

Layers of dissection: Skin → Subcutaneous tissue → Brachioradial muscle → Radial nerve → Brachial muscle. There are cephalic vein and lateral cutaneous nerve of forearm in the superficial layer. In the deep layer are radial nerve, anterior branches of radial collateral artery/veins, and radial recurrent artery/veins.

Indications: Bronchitis, asthma, pleurisy, pain of the elbow, etc.

Manipulation: Perpendicular puncture for 0.5 ~ 1 *cun*.

3. Lieque (LU7).

Location: 1.5 *cun* above the most distal transverse crease of the wrist, above the styloid process of the radius. The simple way to find this acupoint is to hold the two palms together by touching the two webs near the thumb together; the dent, which the index finger can feel is this acupoint (Fig. 4 – 9).

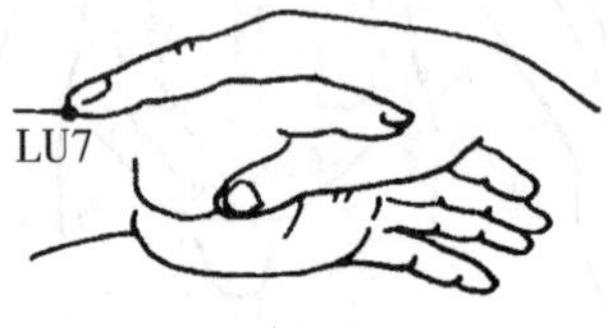

Fig. 4 – 9

Layers of dissection: Skin → Subcutaneous tissue → the tendon of long abductor muscle of thumb → the tendon of brachioradial muscle → Quadrate pronator muscle. There are cephalic vein, lateral cutaneous nerve of forearm, and superficial branch of radial nerve in the superficial layer. In the deep layer are branches of radial artery veins.

Indications: Common cold, bronchitis, asthma, headache, facial paralysis, stiff neck, urticaria, and weakness of the wrist, etc.

Manipulation: Oblique puncture towards elbow for 0.5 ~ 1 *cun*.

4. Taiyuan (LU9).

Location: On the most distal transverse crease of the wrist, on the lateral border of the radial artery (Fig. 4 – 7).

Layers of dissection: Skin→Subcutaneous tissue→between the tendon of radial flexor muscle of wrist and the tendon of long abductor muscle of thumb. There are lateral cutaneous nerve of forearm, superficial branch of radial nerve in the superficial layer. In the deep layer are radial artery/veins.

Indications: Common cold, bronchitis, asthma, chest pain, intercostal neuralgia, acrotism, pain in the wrist, etc.

Manipulation: Perpendicular puncturing for 0.5 *cun*, avoid artery.

5. Shaoshang (LU11).

Location: On the radial side of the thumb, about 0.1 *cun* behind the corner of the nail (Fig. 4 – 7).

Layers of dissection: Skin→Subcutaneous tissue→Root of fingernail. In this area there are the dorsal digital branches of proper palmar digital nerves (branches of median nerve), the rete, which is composed of the branches of the principal artery and vein of the thumb, and the first dorsal metacarpal artery and vein.

Indications: Fever, pneumonia, mumps, acute faucitis, acute tonsillitis, coma, and manic-depressive disorders, etc.

Manipulation: Oblique puncture upwards for 0.1 *cun*. Induce bleeding if the case is acute and serious.

4.3.1.4 Less commonly used acupoints

Kongzui (LU6): 7 *cun* above the transverse crease of the wrist, along the line of LU5 to LU9.

Jingqu (LU8): 1 *cun* above the transverse crease of the wrist, on the lateral border of the radial artery.

Yuji (LU10): At the middle of the first metecarpal bone, at the conjunction of the red and white skin.

4.3.2 Pericardium Meridian of Hand-Jueyin (PC)

4.3.2.1 General information

This meridian goes from chest to hand. The first acupoint is Tianchi and the last one is Zhongchong. There are 9 acupoints on each side. The main indications include cardiovascular and mental diseases, such as angina pectoris, arrhythmia, coma, acrotism, stomach problem, vomiting, and diaphragm spasm, etc.

4.3.2.2 Main course of the meridian

This meridian originates in the chest. It belongs to pericardium and descends to connect with Sanjiao Meridian. One branch arising from the chest, ascends to the axilla, and then passes in the middle of the medial aspect of the upper arm. Entering the palm, it ends at the end of the middle finger. Another branch links with the Sanjiao Meridian of Hand-Shaoyang (Fig. 4 – 10).

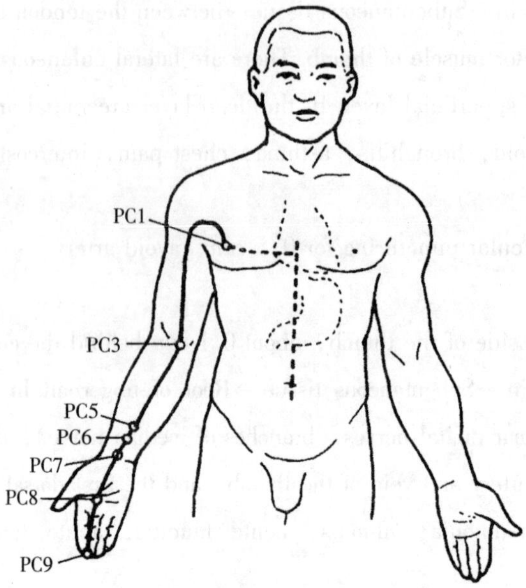

Fig. 4 – 10

4.3.2.3 Commonly used acupoints

1. Quze (PC3).

Location: Along the elbow crease at the ulnar side of the tendon of the biceps brachia muscle (Fig. 4 – 11):

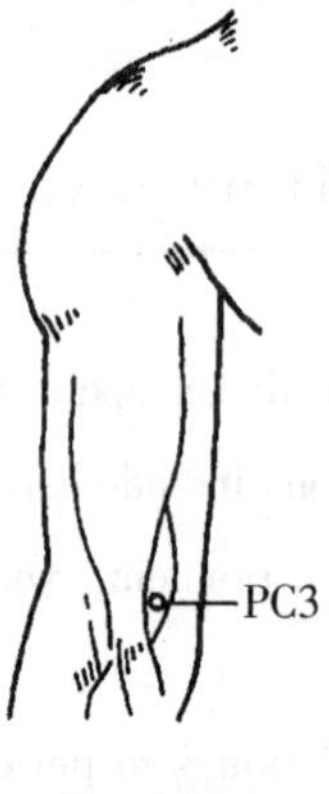

Fig. 4 – 11

Layers of dissection: Skin→Subcutaneous tissue→Median nerve→Brachial muscle. There are median cubital vein and medial cutaneous nerve of forearm in the superficial layer. In the deep layer are brachial artery/veins, rete composed of anterior branches of ulnar recurrent artery/veins and anterior branches of inferior ulnar collateral artery/veins, trunk of median nerve.

Indications: Acute gastroenteritis, bronchitis, sunstroke, high fever, angina pectoris, rheumatic heart diseases, pediatric chorea, and pain located in the medial side of elbow, etc.

Manipulation: Perpendicular puncture for 0.5 ~ 1 *cun*. You can cause the acupoint bleeding to treat acute vomiting and diarrhea.

2. Neiguan (PC6).

Location: 2 *cun* above the most distal transverse crease of the wrist, between the two tendons of the palmaris longus muscle and flexor carpi radialis muscle (Fig. 4-10).

Layers of dissection: Skin→Subcutaneous tissue→between the tendon of radial flexor muscle of wrist and the tendon of long palmar muscle→Superficial flexor muscle of fingers→Deep flexor muscle of fingers →Quadrate pronator muscle. There are medial cutaneous nerve of forearm, lateral cutaneous nerve of forearm and median antebrachial vein in the superficial layer. In the deep layer are median nerve and following artery/veins lain among superficial flexor muscle of fingers, long flexor muscle of thumb and deep flexor muscle of fingers. There are anterior interosseous artery/veins and anterior interosseous nerve in front of interosseous membrane of forearm.

Indications: Tachycardia or bradycardia, angina pectoris, myocarditis, neurosis, gastritis, vomiting, hiccup, acute cholecystitis, hyperthyroidism, angitis, and migraine, etc.

Manipulation: Perpendicular puncture or oblique puncture upwards for 0.5 ~ 1.2 *cun*.

3. Daling (PC7).

Location: In the middle of the most distal transverse crease of the wrist, between the two tendons of palmaris longus muscle and flexor carpi radialis muscle (Fig. 4-10).

Layers of dissection: Skin→Subcutaneous tissue→between the tendon of long palmar muscle and the tendon of radial flexor muscle of wrist→among the tendon of long flexor muscle of thumb, the tendon of superficial flexor muscle of fingers and deep flexor muscle of fingers→in front of radiocarpal joint. There are medial/lateral cutaneous nerve of forearm, palmar branch of median nerve and palmar carpometacarpal venous rete in the superficial layer. In the deep layer is median nerve lain in the deep layer of long palmar muscle and radial flexor muscle of wrist, etc.

Indication: Tachycardia, angina pectoris, arrhythmia, gastritis, tonsillitis, pain of wrist, and mental disorder.

Manipulation: Perpendicular puncturing for 0.3 ~ 0.5 *cun*.

4.3.3 Heart Meridian of Hand-Shaoyin (HT)

4.3.3.1 General information

This meridian goes from the chest to the hand. The first acupoint is Jiquan, and the last acupoint is Shaochong. There are 9 acupoints on each side. The main indications include cardiovascular and nervous system diseases, mental disorder, and also for local diseases, such as tachycardia, bradycardia, angina pectoris, insomnia, mental problem, epilepsy, hysteria, and pain which is located on the medial side of the hand, etc.

4.3.3.2 Main course of the meridian

It originates in the heart and then passes downwards to connect with the small intestine. The straight portion of the meridian goes upwards to the lung. Then it runs downwards and emerges from the axilla. From there it goes along the ulnar side of the medial aspect of the upper arm and passes between the 4th and 5th metacarpal, and then ends at the radial side of the little finger (Fig. 4-12).

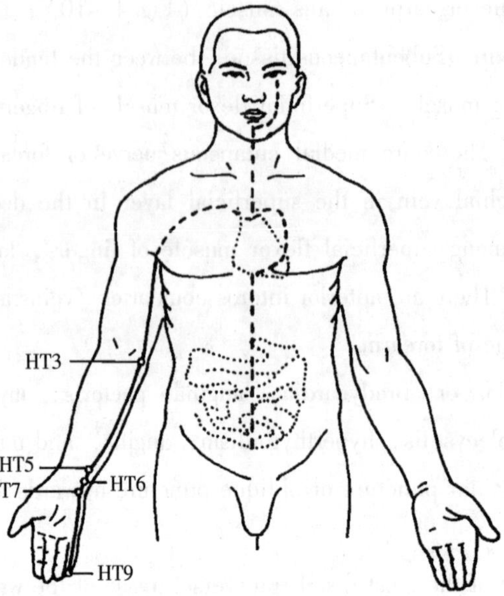

Fig. 4 – 12

4. 3. 3. 3 Commonly used acupoints

1. Jiquan (HT1).

Location: In the center of the axilla and on the medial aspect of the axillary artery (Fig. 4 – 13).

Layers of dissection: Skin→Subcutaneous tissue→brachial plexus, axillary artery/vein→the tendon of broadest muscle of back→Greater round muscle. There is intercostobrachial nerve in the superficial layer. In the deep layer are median nerve, radial nerve, ulnar nerve, medial cutaneous nerve of forearm, medial cutaneous nerve of arm, and axillary artery/vein.

Indications: Intercostal neuralgia, hand paralysis, and scrofula of neck, etc.

Manipulation: Perpendicular puncture for 0. 5 ~0. 8 *cun*.

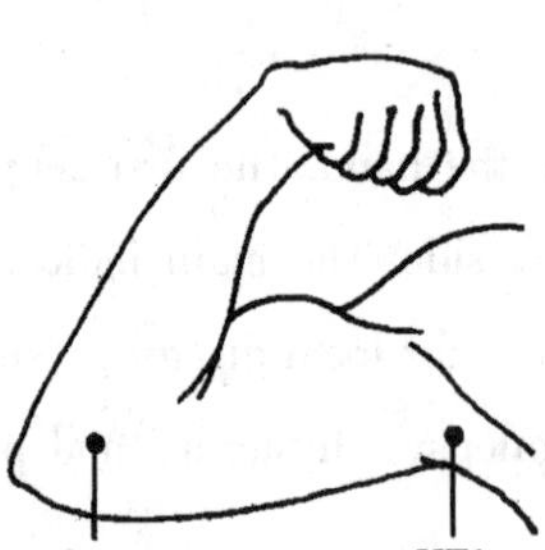

Fig. 4 – 13

2. Shaohai (HT3).

Location: When the elbow is flexed, the acupoint is at the dent, which is located at the end of the transverse cubital crease on the ulnar side (Fig. 4 – 13).

Layers of dissection: Skin→Subcutaneous tissue→Round pronator muscle→Brachial muscle. There are medial cutaneous nerve of forearm and basilic vein in the superficial layer. In the deep layer are median nerve, anastomotic branches of ulnar recurrent artery/veins, and inferior ulnar collateral artery/veins.

Indications: Angina pectoris, epilepsy, mental disorder, ulnar nerve paralysis, intercostal neuralgia, scrofula of neck, hand tremor, hand numbness, and elbow pain, etc.

Manipulation: Perpendicular puncture for 0.5 ~ 1 *cun*.

3. Tongli (HT5).

Location: 1 *cun* above the most distal transverse crease of the wrist, on the radial side of the tendon of flexor carpi ulnaris muscle (Fig. 4 – 12).

Layers of dissection: Skin → Subcutaneous tissue → between ulnar flexor muscle of wrist and superficial flexor muscle of fingers→Deep flexor muscle of fingers→Quadrate pronator muscle. There are medial cutaneous nerve of forearm and branches of basilic vein in the superficial layer. In the deep layer are ulnar artery/veins and ulnar nerve.

Indications: Bradycardia, angina pectoris, neurosis, hysteria, tonsillitis, aphasia, and pain in the wrist, etc.

Manipulation: Perpendicular puncture for 0.3 ~ 0.5 *cun*.

4. Yinxi (HT6).

Location: 0.5 *cun* above the most distal transverse crease of the wrist, on the radial side of the tendon of flexor carpi ulnaris muscle (Fig. 4 – 12).

Layers of dissection: Skin→Subcutaneous tissue→radial margin of the tendon of ulnar flexor muscle of wrist→ulnar nerve. There are medial cutaneous nerve of forearm and branches of basilic vein in the superficial layer. In the deep layer are ulnar artery and veins.

Indications: Tachycardia, angina pectoris, arrhythmia, hematemesis, rhinorrhagia, neurosis, and hectic fever, etc.

Manipulation: Perpendicular puncture for 0.5 *cun*.

5. Shenmen (HT7).

Location: Along the most distal transverse crease of the wrist, on the radial side of the tendon of flexor carpi ulnaris muscle (Fig. 4 – 12).

Layers of dissection: Skin→Subcutaneous tissue→radial part of the tendon of ulnar flexor muscle of wrist. There are medial cutaneous nerve of forearm, branches of basilic vein and palmar branch of ulnar nerve in the superficial layer. In the deep layer are ulnar artery/veins and ulnar nerve.

Indications: Tachycardia, angina pectoris, arrhythmia, insomnia, neurosis, hysteria, and mental disorder.

Manipulation: Perpendicular puncture for 0.3 ~ 0.5 *cun*.

6. Shaochong (HT9).

Location: About 0.1 *cun* behind the corner of the nail on the radial side of the little finger (Fig. 4 – 12).

Layers of dissection: Skin→Subcutaneous tissue→Root of nail. There are dorsal digital branches of proper palmar digital nerves and rete composed of dorsal digital branches of proper palmar digital artery/veins in the area.

Indications: Angina pectoris, mental disorder, coma, and febrile diseases, etc.

Manipulation: Induce bleeding.

4. 3. 4 Large Intestine Meridian of Hand – Yangming (LI)

4. 3. 4. 1 General information

This meridian goes from hand to the head and face. The first acupoint is Shangyang and the last acupoint is Yingxiang. There are 20 acupoints on each side. The main indications include diseases of the head, face, five sense organs and large intestine and other diseases in the regions along the course of this meridian such as headache, trigeminal neuralgia, facial paralysis, eye diseases, toothache, stuffed nose, sore throat, goitre, gastrointestinal diseases, pain, numbness and paralysis of hand.

4. 3. 4. 2 Main course of the meridian

It starts from the radial side of the index finger and passes through the interspace of the 1st and 2nd metacarpal bones. Then it ascends along the lateral side of the wrist and elbow to the shoulder. It passes through supraclavicular fossa and connects with lung and large intestine. One branch ascends along the cheek and enters the lower gums. Then it turns back to the upper lip. From there, the left meridian goes to the right and the right meridian to the left. Both end at the contralateral sides of the nose (Fig. 4 – 14).

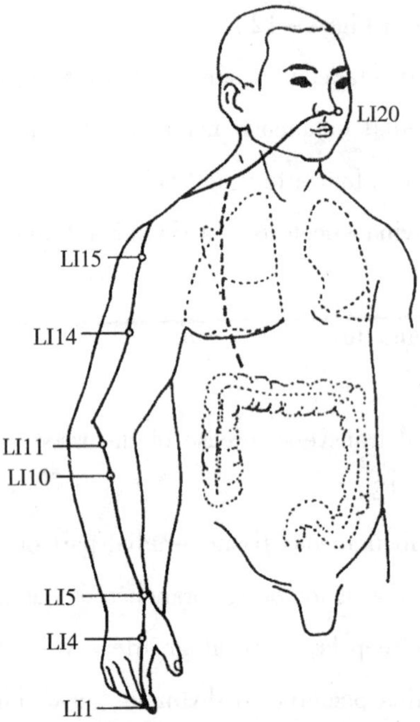

Fig. 4 – 14

4. 3. 4. 3 Commonly used acupoints

1. Shangyang (LI1).

Location: On the radial side of the index finger, about 0. 1 *cun* behind the corner of the nail (Fig. 4 – 14).

Layers of dissection: Skin → Subcutaneous tissue → the root of fingernail. There are dorsal digital branches of proper palmar digital nerves (branches of median nerve) and the rete composed of the branches of dorsal radial artery/vein of index finger and the first dorsal metacarpal artery/vein in this area.

Indications: Febrile diseases, coma, acute faucitis, tonsillitis, mumps, and stomatitis, etc.

Manipulation: shallow puncture or quick puncture by three-edged needle.

2. Hegu (LI4).

Location: Over the dorsum of the hand, between the first and second metacarpal bones, near the middle of the second metacarpal bone on the radial side (Fig. 4 – 15).

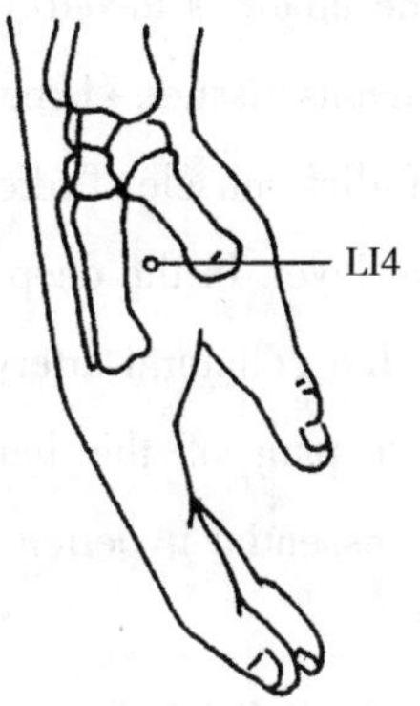

Fig. 4 – 15

Layers of dissection: Skin→Subcutaneous tissue→the first dorsal interosseal muscle→Adductor muscle of thumb. There are superficial branch of radial nerve, a radial part of dorsal venous rete of hand and branches of the first dorsal metacarpal artery/vein in the superficial layer. In the deep layer is the deep branch of ulnar nerve.

Indications: Common cold, tonsillitis, mumps, headache, facial paralysis, facial muscle spasm, trigeminal neuralgia, glossitis, gingivitis, myopia, hypertension, stroke sequela, polyneuritis, gastroenteritis, appendicitis, constipation, dysmenorrhea, dystocia, and nettle rash, etc.

Manipulation: Perpendicular puncture for 0.5 ~ 1 *cun*.

3. Shousanli (LI10).

Location: 2 *cun* below Quchi, between the line of Quchi (LI11) and Jianyu (LI15) (Fig. 4 – 16).

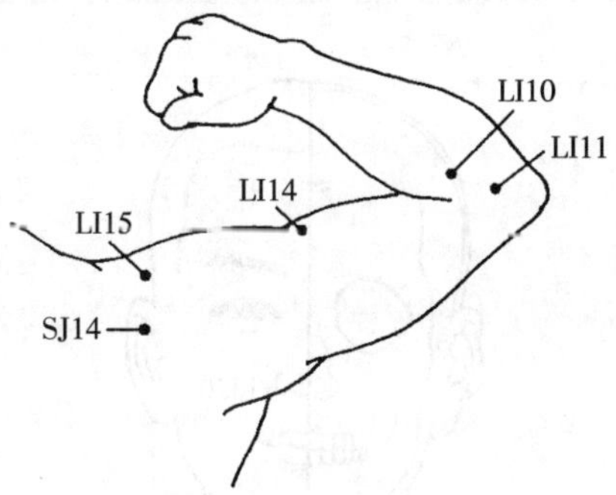

Fig. 4 – 16

Layers of dissection: Skin→Subcutaneous tissue→Long radial extensor muscle of wrist→Short radial extensor muscle of wrist→front of extensor muscle of fingers→Supinator muscle. There are lateral cutaneous nerve of forearm, posterior cutaneous nerve of forearm in the superficial layer. In the deep layer are branches of radial recurrent artery/vein and deep branch of radial nerve.

Indications: Bellyache, diarrhea, toothache, cervical spondylopathy, sequel of stroke, acute faucitis, pain of the elbow and arm.

Manipulation: Perpendicular puncture for 0.8 ~ 1.5 *cun.*

4. Quchi (LI11).

Location: At the midpoint of the line joining the external end of the elbow transverse crease and the lateral epicondyle of the humerus, when the elbow is flexed (Fig. 4 – 16).

Layers of dissection: Skin→Subcutaneous tissue→Long radial extensor muscle of wrist and Short radial extensor muscle of wrist→Brachioradial muscle. There are branches of cephalic vein, posterior cutaneous nerve of forearm in the superficial layer. In the deep layer is radial nerve, anastomotic branches between radial recurrent artery/vein and radial collateral artery/vein.

Indications: Paralysis, numbness and pain of the hand, nettle rash, eczema, gastroenteritis, common cold, tonsillitis, malaria, fever, essential hypertension, neurosis, epilepsy, mental disorder, sequela of polio, and goitre etc.

Manipulation: Perpendicular puncture for 0.8 ~ 1.5 *cun.*

5. Jianyu (LI15).

Location: At the antero-inferior part of the acromion, where two depressions are formed when the arm is raised horizontally. The anterior depression is this acupoint (Fig. 4 – 16).

Layers of dissection: Skin→Subcutaneous tissue→Deltoid muscle→Subdeltoid bursa→the tendon of Supraspinous muscle. There are lateral supraclavicular nerves, Superior lateral cutaneous nerve of arm in the superficial layer. In the deep layer are branches of posterior circumfler humeral artery/vein and Axillary nerve.

Indications: Paralysis of hand, and periarthritis of shoulder.

Manipulation: When the arm is raised horizontally, perpendicular puncture for 1 ~ 1.5 *cun.* If the arm cannot be raised, use oblique puncture downwards.

6. Yingxiang (LI20).

Location: Beside the midpoint of the outer side of the ala nasi, in the nasolabial groove (Fig. 4 – 17).

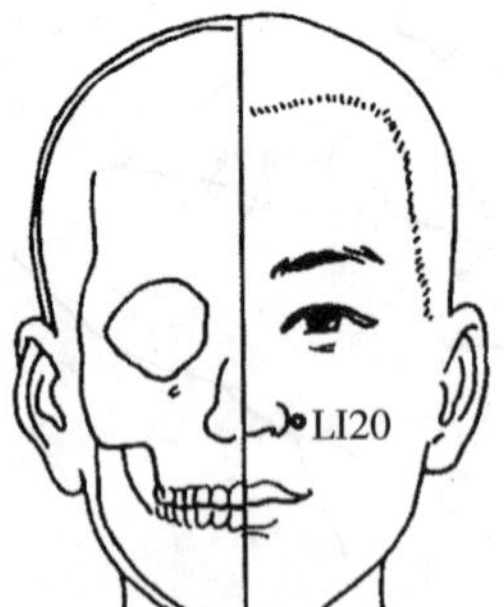

Fig. 4 – 17

Layers of dissection: Skin→Subcutaneous tissue→Levator muscle of upper lip. There are branches of infraorbital nerve (a branch of maxillary nerve) in the superficial layer. In the deep layer are buccal branches of facial nerve, branches of facial artery/vein.

Indications: Chronic rhinitis, facial paralysis, and trigeminal neuralgia.

Manipulation: Oblique puncture toward the nose root for 0. 5 ~ 1 *cun*.

4. 3. 4. 4 Less commonly used acupoints

Erjian (LI2): The fist being lightly closed, on the dorsum of the hand, at the radial side of the distal end of the index finger.

Sanjian (LI3): The fist being lightly closed, on the dorsum of the hand, at the radial side of the proximal part of the index finger.

Yangxi (LI5): Over the wrist joint, in the depression between the tendons of the extensor pollicis brevis muscle and extensor pollicis longus muscle.

Pianli (LI6): Along the line of LI5 to LI11, 3 *cun* above the transverse crease of the wrist.

Wenliu (LI7): Along the line of LI5 to LI11, 5 *cun* above the transverse crease of the wrist.

Xialian (LI8): Along the line of LI5 to LI11, 4 *cun* below the elbow crease.

Shanglian (LI9): Along the line of LI5 to LI11, 3 *cun* below the elbow crease.

Zhouliao (LI12): When the elbow is flexed, 1 *cun* above the external part of LI11, beside the humerus.

Shouwuli (LI13): Along the line of LI11 to LI15, 3 *cun* above LI11.

Jugu (LI16): At the depression between the acromial end of the clavicle and the upper part of the spine of the scapula.

Tianding (LI17): At the posterior margin of the sternocleidomastoid muscle and between the midpoint of LI18 and the supraclavicular fossa.

Futu (LI18): Laterally from the middle of the laryngeal prominence, just between the two head of the sternocleidomastoid muscle.

4. 3. 5 Sanjiao Meridian of Hand-Shaoyang (SJ)

4. 3. 5. 1 General information

This meridian goes from the hand to the head. The first acupoint is Guanchong and the last acupoint is Sizhukong. There are 23 acupoints on each side. The main indications include diseases on the ear, the lateral side of the head, and hypochondria as well as diseases of eye and throat, such as tinnitus, deafness, otitis media, conjunctivitis, myopia, sore throat, fever and pain which locates in the lateral side of the hand and shoulder.

4. 3. 5. 2 Main course of the meridian

This meridian starts from the tip of the ring finger, running upwards in the middle of the dorsal aspect of the upper extremity to the shoulder. Then it winds over to the supraclavicular fossa and connects with the pericardium. One branch originates from the chest. Running upwards, it ascends to the neck along the posterior boarder of the ear and reaches the upper corner of the ear. Then, it runs downwards to the cheek and terminates in the infraorbital region. Another branch connects with the Gallbladder Meridian of Foot-Shaoyang (Fig. 4 – 18).

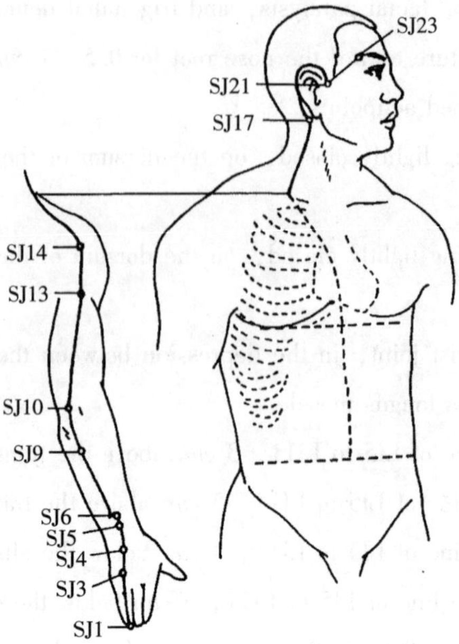

Fig. 4 – 18

4. 3. 5. 3 Commonly used acupoints

1. Guanchong (SJ1).

Location: About 0. 1 *cun* from the corner of the nail on the ulnar side of the ring finger (Fig. 4 – 18).

Layers of dissection: Skin→Subcutaneous tissue→Root of nail. There are dorsal digital branches of proper palmar digital nerve of ulnar nerve and rete of dorsal digital branches of proper palmar digital artery/veins in the subcutaneous tissue.

Indications: Common cold, fever, keratitis, acute faucitis, tonsillitis, mumps, deafness, coma and sunstroke.

Manipulation: Shallow puncture for 0. 1 *cun*, or induce bleeding by three-edged needle.

2. Zhongzhu (SJ3).

Location: Between the 4th and 5th metacarpal bones, in the dent behind the metacarpo – phalangeal joints (Fig. 4 – 18).

Layers of dissection: Skin→Subcutaneous tissue→Dorsal interosseal muscle IV. There are dorsal digital nerves of ulnar nerve and ulnar part of dorsal venous rete of hand in the superficial layer. In the deep layer is dorsal metacarpal artery IV.

Indications: Deafness, tinnitus, temporomandibular joint syndrome (Costen's Syndrome), stiff neck, intercostal neuralgia, and numbness of little finger.

Manipulation: Perpendicular or oblique puncture for 0. 3 ~ 0. 8 *cun*.

3. Waiguan (SJ5).

Location: 2 *cun* above the transverse crease on the back of the wrist, between the ulnar and radius (Fig. 4 – 18).

Layers of dissection: Skin→Subcutaneous tissue→extensor muscle of little finger and extensor muscle of fingers→long extensor muscle of thumb and extensor muscle of index finger. There are posterior cutaneous nerve of forearm, branches of cephalic vein and basilic vein in the superficial layer. In the deep layer are posterior interosseous artery/veins and posterior interosseous nerve.

Indications: Common cold, fever, deafness, tinnitus, migraine, intercostal neuralgia, hypertension, paralysis of hand, sequela of polio, and pain of finger and wrist.

Manipulation: Perpendicular puncture for 0.5 ~ 1 *cun*.

Reference: Puncturing SJ5 through Neiguan (PC6) combining with Yang/ao (SJ6) can treat pain of the wrist. To treat constipation, combine with Daling (PC7) and Zhigou (SJ6).

4. Zhigou (SJ6).

Location: 3 *cun* above the transverse crease on the back of the wrist, between the ulnar and radius (Fig. 4 - 18).

Layers of dissection: Skin→Subcutaneous tissue→extensor muscle of little finger→Long extensor muscle of thumb→Interosseous membrane of forearm. There are posterior cutaneous nerve of forearm, branches of cephalic vein and basilic vein in the superficial layer. In the deep layer are Posterior interosseous artery/veins and posterior interosseous nerve.

Indications: Deafness, tinnitus, constipation, fever, intercostal neuralgia, finger tremor and pain of elbow and hand.

Manipulation: Perpendicular puncture for 0.5 ~ 1 *cun*.

5. Sidu (SJ9).

Location: 5 *cun* below the tip of elbow on the back of the forearm, on the line connecting Yangchi (SJ4) and the tip of elbow, between the ulnar and radius (Fig. 4 - 18).

Layers of dissection: Skin→Subcutaneous tissue→extensor muscle of little finger and ulnar extensor muscle of wrist→long abductor muscle of thumb and long extensor muscle of thumb. There are posterior cutaneous nerve of forearm, branches of cephalic vein and basilica vein in the superficial layer. In the deep layer are posterior interosseous artery/veins and posterior interosseous nerve.

Indications: Cervical spondylopathy, deafness (especially sudden deafness), hoarseness, and paralysis of hand.

Manipulation: Perpendicular puncture for 0.5 ~ 1 *cun*.

6. Jianliao (SJ14).

Location: At the postero - inferior side of the acromion, posterior to Jianyu (LI15), where a depression is formed when the arm is raised (Fig. 4 - 18).

Layers of dissection: Skin→Subcutaneous tissue→Deltoid muscle→Lesser round muscle→Greater round muscle→tendon of broadest muscle of back. There is lateral supraclavicular nerve in the superficial layer. In the deep layer are axillary nerve and posterior circumflex humeral artery/veins.

Indications: Diseases of shoulder and lateral side of hand.

Manipulation: Perpendicular or oblique puncture for 0.6 ~ 1.2 *cun*.

7. Yifeng (SJ17).

Location: Behind the lobule of the auricle, in the depression between the mastoid process and the mandible (Fig. 4 - 18).

Layers of dissection: Skin→Subcutaneous tissue→Parotid gland. There are great auricular nerve and branches of external jugular vein in the superficial layer. In the deep layer is posterior auricular artery and facial nerve.

Indications: Deafness, tinnitus, otitis media, mumps, temporomandibular joint diseases, facial paralysis and migraine.

Manipulation: Perpendicular puncture for 0. 8 ~ 1. 2 *cun*.

8. Ermen (SJ21).

Location: In front of the superior notch of the auricula, where a depression is formed when the mouth is opened (Fig. 4 - 18).

Layers of dissection: Skin→Subcutaneous tissue→Parotid gland. There are auriculotemporal nerve, anterior auricular branches of superficial temporal artery/veins and temporal branches of facial nerve in this area.

Indications: Deafness, tinnitus, otitis media, temporomandibular joint syndrome, and toothache.

Manipulation: Open the mouth, then perpendicular puncture for 0. 5 ~ 1 *cun*.

9. Sizhukong (SJ23).

Location: At the lateral end of the eyebrow (Fig. 4 - 18).

Layers of dissection: Skin→Subcutaneous tissue→Obicular muscle of eye. There are supraobital nerve, zygomatic and temporal branches of facial nerve, frontal branch of superficial temporal artery/vein in this area.

Indications: Migraine, vertigo, keratitis, optic atrophy, chalazion, myopia, extraocular fatigability or spasm, toothache, mental disorder, etc.

Manipulation: Horizontal perpendicular puncture for 0. 5 ~ 1 *cun*.

4. 3. 5. 4 Less Commonly used acupoints

Yemen (SJ2): In the web at the junction of the red and white skin, between the ring finger and little finger.

Yangchi (SJ4): Middle of the skin crease on the back of the wrist, at the ulnar side of the tendon of extensor digitaorum communis muscle.

Huizong (SJ7): 3 *cun* above the transverse crease on the back of the wrist, on the ulnar side of SJ6, at the radial border of the ulnar bone.

Sanyangluo (SJ8): 4 *cun* above the transverse crease on the back of the wrist, at the radial border of the ulnar bone.

Tianjing (SJ10): In the depression 1 *cun* behind the upper part of the olecranon.

Naohui (SJ13): Between the line of the olecranon and Jianliao (SJ14), 3 *cun* below Jianliao (SJ14), just down the deltoid muscle.

4. 3. 6 Small Intestine Meridian of Hand-Taiyang (SI)

4. 3. 6. 1 General information

This meridian goes from the hand to head. The first acupoint is Shaoze, and the last acupoint is

Tinggong. There are 19 acupoints on each side. The main indications include pain of the head, neck, and back, and other diseases in the regions along the course of this meridian.

4.3.6.2 Main course of the meridian

The meridian starts from the ulnar side of the tip of the little finger. Following the ulnar side of the dorsum of the hand, it reaches the shoulder. Then circling around the scapular region, it meets Dazhui (Du14). Finally, turning downwards to the supra-clavicular fossa, it connects with the heart and enters the small intestine, its pertaining organ. One branch from the supraclavicular fossa ascends along the neck to the cheek. Via the outer canthus, it enters the ear. Another branch links with the Bladder Meridian of Foot-Taiyang (Fig. 4-19).

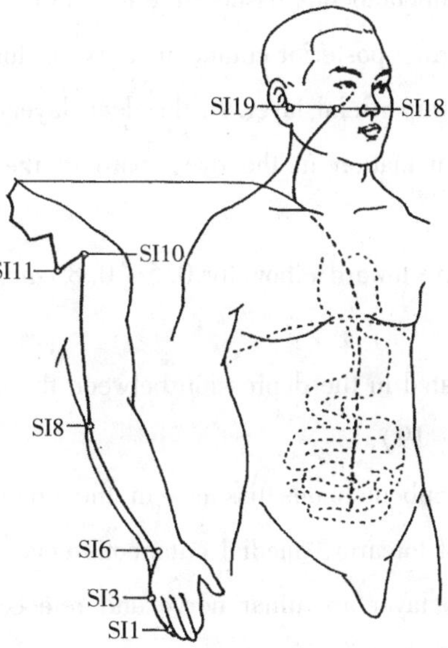

Fig. 4-19

4.3.6.3 Commonly used acupoints

1. Shaoze (SI1).

Location: About 0.1 *cun* proximal to the corner of the nail on the ulnar side of the little finger (Fig. 4-19).

Layers of dissection: Skin→Subcutaneous tissue→Root of nail. There are dorsal digital branches of proper palmar digital nerve (come from ulnar nerve) and rete composed of palmar ulnar artery/veins of finger V in the area.

Indications: Puerperal insufficient lactation, mastitis, coma, sun stroke, febrile diseases, numbness in the finger.

Manipulation: Shallow puncture or prick to induce bleeding.

2. Houxi (SI3).

Location: On the ulnar side proximal to the metacarpophalangeal joint of the little finger. The point is located at the end of the transverse crease of the palm, lying between the red and white skin, when the fist is slightly clenched (Fig. 4-19).

Layers of dissection: Skin→Subcutaneous tissue→Abductor muscle of little finger→Short flexor muscle of little finger. There are dorsal branch of ulnar nerve, palmar branch of ulnar nerve and cutaneous vein in the superficial layer. In the deep layer are proper palmar artery/veins of little finger and proper palmar digital nerves.

Indications: Headache, epilepsy, stiff neck, deafness, tinnitus, keratitis, tonsillitis, pain of the shoulder and back, acute lumbar muscle sprain.

Manipulation: Perpendicular puncture for 0.6 ~ 1.5 *cun*.

3. Yanglao (SI6).

Location: The point is located along the seam on the radial side of the distal head of the ulna, when the palm faces to the chest (Fig. 4 – 19).

Layers of dissection: Skin→Subcutaneous tissue→the tendon of ulnar extensor muscle of wrist. There are medial cutaneous nerve of forearm, posterior cutaneous nerve of forearm, dorsal branch of ulnar nerve and branches of basilic vein in the superficial layer. In the deep layer is dorsal venous rete of hand.

Indications: Poor vision, inflammation in the eye, pain in the shoulder and back, acute lumbar muscle sprain.

Manipulation: Oblique puncture toward elbow for 0.5 ~0.8 *cun*, when the palm faces to the chest.

4. Xiaohai (SI8).

Location: The acupoint is located in the depression between the olecranon of the ulna and the medial epicondyle of the humerus (Fig. 4 – 19).

Layers of dissection: Skin→Subcutaneous tissue→in the groove for ulnar nerve. There are ulnar branch of medial cutaneous nerve of forearm, medial cutaneous nerve of arm and branches of basilic vein in the superficial layer. In the deep layer are ulnar nerve and rete composed of superior ulnar collateral artery/veins and posterior branch of ulnar recurrent artery/veins.

Indications: Ulnar neuralgia, epilepsy, neurosis, mental disorder, tinnitus, deafness.

Manipulation: Perpendicular puncture for 0.5 ~ 1 *cun*.

5. Tianzong (SI11).

Location: In the center of the infraspinus fossa of the scapular (Fig. 4 – 19).

Layers of dissection: Skin→Subcutaneous tissue→Trapezius muscle→Infraspinous muscle. There are cutaneous branches of dorsal branches of thoracic nerve Ⅳ and following artery/veins in the superficial layer. In the deep layer are branches of suprascapular nerve and branches of circumflex artery/veins of scapula.

Indications: Periarthritis of shoulder, musculus supraspinatus tendinitis, fascitis of muscle in shoulder and back, cervical spondylopathy, asthma, mastitis.

Manipulation: Perpendicular or oblique puncture for 0.8 ~ 1.2 *cun*.

6. Tinggong (SI19).

Location: In between the middle of the tragus and the mandibular joint, where a depression is formed when the mouth is opened (Fig. 4 – 19).

Layers of dissection: Skin → Subcutaneous tissue → Cartilage of acoustic meatus. There are auriculotemporal nerve and branches of anterior auricular branches of superficial temporal artery in this area.

Indications: Deafness, tinnitus, tympanitis, temporomandibular joint disorder, deaf-mute, etc.

Manipulation: Perpendicular puncture for 0.5 ~ 1 *cun*.

4.3.6.4 Less commonly used acupoints

Qiangu (SI2): Clench the fist slightly. The acupoint is just in front of the 5th metacarpophalangeal joint, at the juncture of red and white skin.

Wangu (SI4): On the ulnar side of the palm, between the base of 5th metacarpal bone and the hamate bone, the point is located at the junction of red and white skin.

Yanggu (SI5): On the ulnar side of the ulnocarpal joint, between the styloid process of the ulnar and the triquetral bone.

Zhizheng (SI7): Along the line of SI5 to SI8, 5 *cun* above dorsum transverse crease of the wrist.

Jianzhen (SI9): 1 *cun* above the end of posterior axillary fold, at the infero – posterior part of the shoulder joint.

Naoshu (SI10): Above SI9, in the depression below spine of the scapular.

Bingfeng (SI12): Middle of the supraspinatous fossa, directly above SI11.

Jianwaishu (SI14): 3 *cun* lateral to the lower border of the spinous process of the first thoracic vertebra.

Jianzhongshu (SI15): 2 *cun* lateral to the lower border of the spinous process of the seventh thoracic vertebra.

Quanliao (SI18): Directly below the external canthus on the lower bonder of the zygomatic bone.

4.3.7 Spleen Meridian of Foot-Taiyin (SP)

4.3.7.1 General information

This meridian goes from the foot to the stomach. The first acupoint is Yinbai and the last acupoint is Dabao. There are totally 21 acupoints on each side. The main indications include digestive and urinary system diseases. Disease, which has relationship with bleeding problem, and diseases which locate near the meridian, such as dyspepsia, dysentery, enteritis, retention of urine, bed-wetting, metrorrhagia, bloody stools, knee pain, etc.

4.3.7.2 Main course of the meridian

This meridian starts from the medial side of the big toe. It runs along the medial aspect of the foot and ascends to the front of the medial malleolus and further up to the posterior aspect of the tibia. It passes through the front of the Liver Meridian of Foot – Jueyin at the point, which is 8 *cun* above the medial malleolus. Going on along the anterior medial aspect of the knee and then the thigh, it enters the abdomen, reaches the spleen, its pertaining organ, and connects with the stomach. One branch connects with Heart Meridian of Hand-Shaoyin (Fig. 4 – 20).

4.3.7.3 Commonly used acupoints

1. Yinbai (SP1).

Location: About 0.1 *cun* behind the corner of the nail at the medial side of the big toe (Fig. 4 – 21).

Layers of dissection: Skin→Subcutaneous tissue→Root of nail. There are branches of medial dorsal cutaneous nerve, dorsal digital nerves and dorsal digital arteries/veins in the area.

Indications: Dyspepsia, acute or chronic enteritis, upper gastrointestinal bleeding, metrorrhagia, irregular menstruation (moxibustion), neurosis, mental disorder, coma, pain of toes, etc.

Manipulation: Shallow puncture.

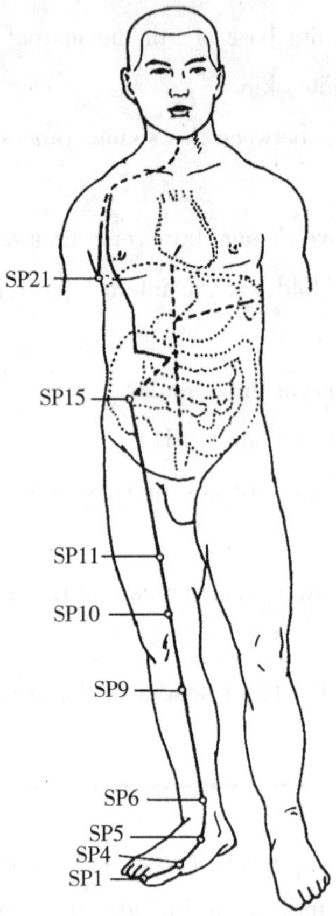

Fig. 4 – 20

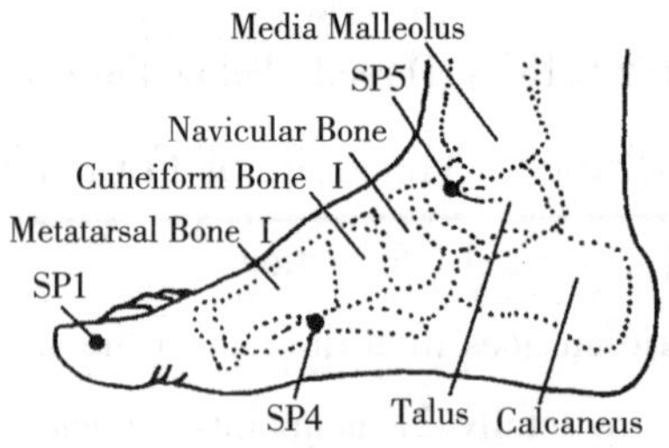

Fig. 4 – 21

2. Gongsun (SP4).

Location: In the medial of foot, depression distal and inferior to the base of the first metatarsal bone (Fig. 4 – 21).

Layers of dissection: Skin→Subcutaneous tissue→Abductor muscle of great toe→Short flexor muscle of great toe→the tendon of long flexor muscle of great toe. There are medial margin branches of foot (branches of saphenous nerve), branches of dorsal venous arch of foot in the superficial layer. In the deep layer are branches of medial plantar artery/veins, branches of medial plantar nerve.

Indications: Dyspepsia, vomitting, acute or chronic gastroenteritis, ascites, capsulitis of big toe, gout, etc.

Manipulation: Perpendicular puncture for 0. 5 ~ 1 *cun*.

3. Sanyinjiao (SP6).

Location: 3 *cun* above the apex of the medial malleolus, behind the tibia (Fig. 4 – 22).

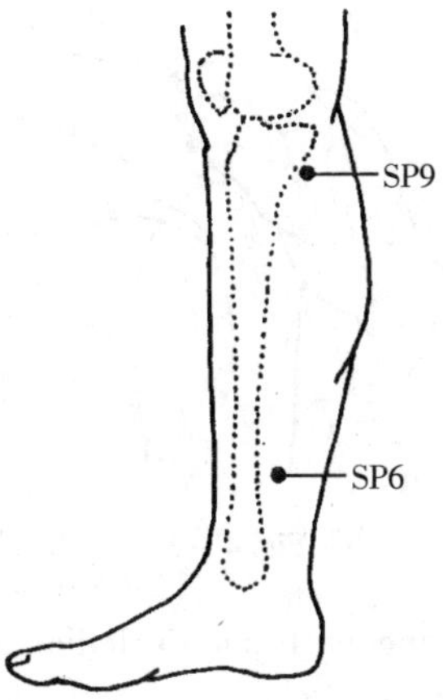

Fig. 4 – 22

Layers of dissection: Skin→Subcutaneous tissue→Long flexor muscle of toes→Posterior tibial muscle →long flexor muscle of great toes. There are medial crural cutaneous branches of saphenous nerve, branches of great saphenous vein in the superficial layer. In the deep layer are tibial nerve, posterior tibial artery/veins.

Indications: Abdominal pain, diarrhea, irregular menstruation, dysmenorrhea, amenorrhea, dystocia, enuresis, retention of urine, neurodermatitis, eczema, nettle rash, insomnia, paralysis of leg.

Manipulation: Perpendicular puncture for 0.5 ~ 1 *cun*.

Reference: ①According to ancient works, the acupoint is forbidden for acupuncture in pregnant women. ②It is commonly used for anaesthesia in operation to abdomen, such as caesarean delivery, complete hysterectomy, oophorectomy, ovariohysterectomy, cystolithotomy etc. ③ SP6 and Geshu (BL17) can treat mild hypertension, which is caused by microvascular spasm.

4. Yinlingquan (SP9).

Location: Under the medial condyle of the tibia, on the dent medial side below the knee (Fig. 4 – 22).

Layers of dissection: Skin→Subcutaneous tissue→the tendon of Semitendinous muscle→medial head of gastrocnemius muscle. There are medial crural cutaneous branches of saphenous nerve, great saphenous vein and branches of descending genicular artery in the superficial layer. In the deep layer are medial inferior genicular artery/veins.

Indications: Abdominal pain, diarrhea, edema, retention of urine, urethritis, enuresis, injury of knee joint and surrounding soft tissue.

Manipulation: Perpendicular puncture for 0.5 ~ 1 *cun*.

Reference: According to *Qianjin Yi Fang*, if the patient can not sleep due to edema, moxibustion on SP9 can relief edema.

5. Xuehai (SP10).

Location: 2 *cun* above the medial border of the patella over the protuberance of the medial thigh (Fig. 4 – 23).

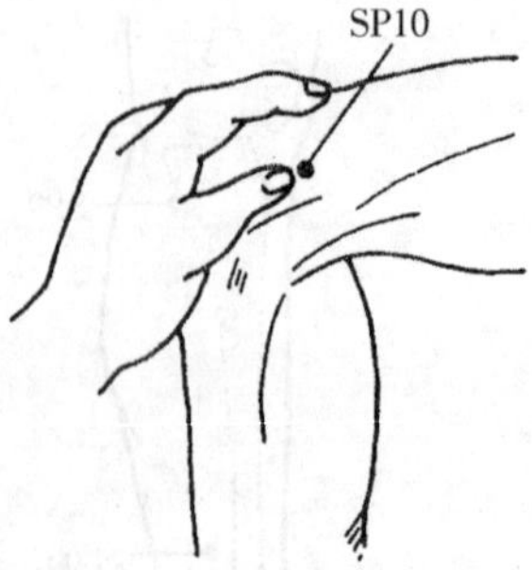

Fig. 4 – 23

Layers of dissection: Skin→Subcutaneous tissue→Medial great muscle of thigh. There are anterior cutaneous branches of femoral nerve, branches of great saphenous vein in the superficial layer. In the deep layer are muscular branches of femoral artery/veins, muscular branches of femoral nerve.

Indications: Menorrhagia, hematuria, nettle rash, eczema, knee pain.

Manipulation: Perpendicular puncture for 0.5 ~ 1 *cun*.

Reference: To treat nettle rash, combine with Quchi (LI11), Dingchuan (EX – B1) and Sanyinjiao (SP6).

4.3.7.4 Less commonly used acupoints

Dadu (SP2): On the medial side of the proximal end of the proximal phalange of the big toe, at the junction of the red and white skin.

Taibai (SP3): On the medial side of the distal end of the proximal phalange of the big toe, at the junction of the red and white skin.

Shangqiu (SP5): In the depression at the anterior part under the medial malleolus.

Lougu (SP7): 6 *cun* above the apex of the medial malleolus, behind the tibia.

Diji (SP8): 3 *cun* below SP9, behind the tibia.

Daheng (SP15): 4 *cun* lateral to the center of the umbilicus.

Dabao (SP21): In the 6th intercostals space, on the midaxillary line.

4.3.8 Liver Meridian of Foot-Jueyin (LR)

4.3.8.1 General information

This meridian goes from the foot to belly. The first acupoint is Dadun and the last acupoint is Qimen. There are totally 14 acupoints on each side. The main indications include diseases in the areas like the tip of head, lip, lower belly, external genitalia, eyes, liver, and gallbladder, such as dysmenorrhea, testitis, headache, facial paralysis, biliary tract infection, chronic hepatitis.

4.3.8.2 Main course of the meridian

This meridian starts from the big toe. Running upward along the dorsum of the foot, passing through the anterior side of the medial malleolus, it ascends to an area 8 *cun* above the medial malleolus, where it runs across and behind the Spleen Meridian. Then it runs in the middle of the medial side of the thigh, curves around the external genitalia and goes up to the lower abdomen. It then runs upward and curves around the stomach to enter the liver, its pertaining organ, connects with the gallbladder and branches out in the costal and hypochondriac region. Then it ascends along the posterior aspect of the throat and connects with the eye. Running further upward, it emerges from the forehead. One branch links with the Lung Meridian of Hand-Taiyin (Fig. 4 – 24).

4. 3. 8. 3 Commonly used acupoints

1. Dadun (LR1).

Location: On the lateral side of the dorsum of the big toe, 0. 1 *cun* posterior to the corner of the nail (Fig. 4 – 25).

Layers of dissection: Skin→Subcutaneous tissue→Root of nail. There are lateral dorsal nerve of deep peroneal nerve and dorsal digital artery/veins in this area.

Indications: Hernia, spermoneuralgia, penis pain, dysfunctional uterine bleeding, incontinence of urine, epilepsy, and coma, etc.

Manipulation: Shallow punctures or pricks to induce bleeding by using three-edged needle.

Reference: According to some reports, this acupoint has obvious effects to treat acute epididymitis and it is often chosen with the combination of Taichong, Qihai, Guilai and Ququan in clinical practice.

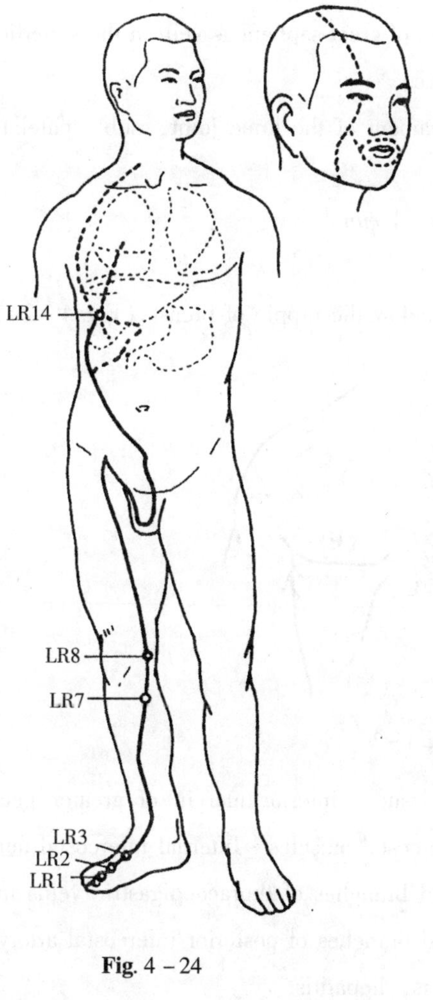

Fig. 4 – 24

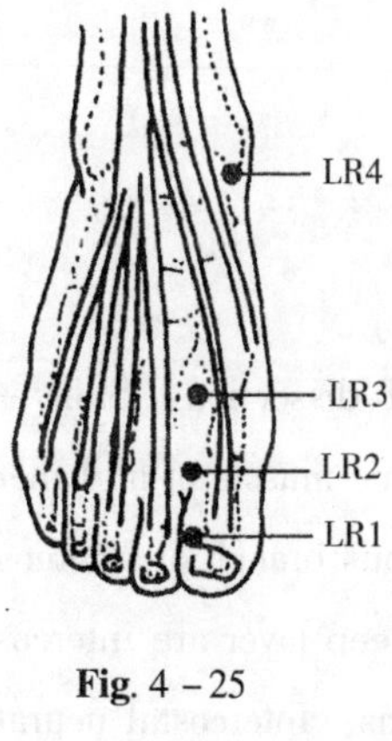

Fig. 4 – 25

2. Taichong (LR3).

Location: On the depression distal to junction of the first and second metatarsal bones (Fig. 4 – 25).

Layers of dissection: Skin→Subcutaneous tissue→between the tendon of long extensor muscle of toes and long extensor muscle of great toe → lateral part of short extensor muscle of great toe → Dorsal interosseous muscle. There are dorsal venous rete of foot and medial dorsal cutaneous nerve in the superficial layer. In the deep layer is deep fibular nerve and dorsal metatarsal artery/veins.

Indications: Headache, dizziness, hypertension, facial paralysis, facial spasm, capsulitis of big toe, gout, mental disorder, epilepsy, etc.

Manipulation: Perpendicular puncture for 0.5 ~ 1 *cun*.

Reference: ①In the patients who were undertaking operations like cholecystectomy, after injecting morphine, if LR3 is stimulated, the pressure in biliary tract would stop increasing but decreasing rapidly. ②Acupuncture on LR3 was more effective to relieve the spasm of Oddi's sphincter than Zusanli (ST36) and Yanglingquan (GL34). However, puncturing Weizhong and Qimen does not have similar effects.

3. Xiguan (LR7).

Location: 1 *cun* behind Yinlingquan (SP9), in the depression of the inferior and posterior side of the medial condyle of the tibia (Fig. 4 - 24).

Layers of dissection: Skin → Subcutaneous tissue → Gastrocnemius muscle. There are medial crural cutaneous branches of saphenous nerve and branches of great saphenous vein in the superficial layer. In the deep layer are popliteal artery/veins and tibial nerve.

Indications: Injury of the lateral collateral ligament of the knee joint, sub - patella bursitis, knee arthritis, acute or chronic faucitis.

Manipulation: Perpendicular puncture for 0.5 ~ 1 *cun*.

4. Qimen (LR14).

Location: In the 6th intercostal spaces, just below the nipple of breast (Fig. 4 - 26).

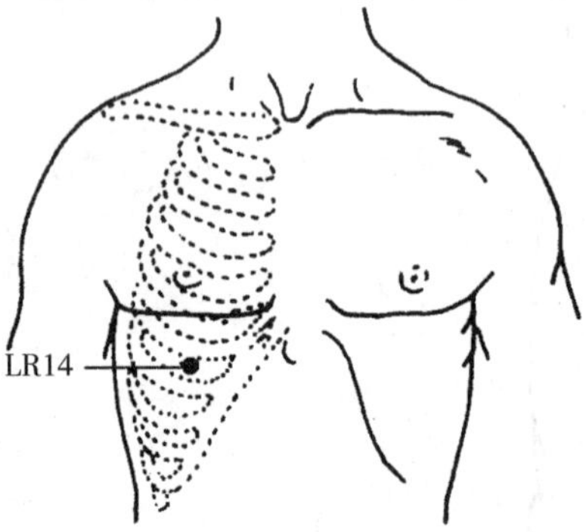

Fig. 4 - 26

Layers of dissection: Skin → Subcutaneous tissue → inferior margin of greater pectoral muscle → External oblique muscle of abdomen → External intercostal muscles → Internal intercostal muscles. There are lateral cutaneous branch of intercostal nerve VI and branches of thoracoepigastric veins in the superficial layer. In the deep layer are intercostal nerve VI and branches of posterior intercostal artery/veins VI.

Indications: Intercostal neuralgia, cholecystitis, hepatitis.

Manipulation: Oblique puncture for 0.3 ~ 0.5 *cun*.

4.3.8.4 Less commonly used acupoints

Xingjian (LR2): Behind the margin of the web of the big toe and second toe.

Zhongfeng (LR4): Anterior from the medial malleolus, in the depression of the tibialis anterior muscle, between SP5 and ST41.

Ligou (LR5): 5 *cun* above the medial malleolus on the medial border of the tibia.

Zhongdu (LR6): 7 *cun* above the medial malleolus beside the tibia.

Ququan (LR8): When the knee flexes, at the medial end of the knee crease, in front of the semimembranous muscle, behind medial condyle of the tibia.

Zhangmen (LR13): Below the end of the 11th rib.

4.3.9 Kidney Meridian of Foot-Shaoyin (KI)

4.3.9.1 General information

This meridian goes from the foot to the belly. The first acupoint is Yongquan and the last one is Shufu. There are 27 acupoints on each side. The main indications include the diseases of the urogenital system, the respiratory and neurology system, which are caused by deficiency of kidney function, such as seminal emission, impotence, premature ejaculation, edema, retention of urine, bed-wetting, asthma, cough, faucitis, insomnia, tinnitus, deafness, vertigo, backache.

4.3.9.2 Main course of the meridian

This meridian starts from the inferior aspect of the small toe and runs obliquely towards the sole. Running behind the medial malleolus, it enters the heel and goes further upward along the posteromedial aspect of the leg towards the vertebral column, where it enters the kidney, its pertaining organ, and connects with the bladder. The straight portion of the meridian ascends to the liver and enters the lung. Then, running along the throat, it terminates at the root of the tongue. One branch links with the Pericardium Meridian of Hand-Taiyin (Fig. 4-27).

4.3.9.3 Commonly used acupoints

1. Yongquan (KI1).

Location: At the junction between anterior one-third and posterior two-thirds of the sole (the length of the toe is not included), in the depression when the toes are flexed (Fig. 4-28).

Layers of dissection: Skin→Subcutaneous tissue→Plantar aponeurosis→Common plantar digital nerve of toe Ⅱ→Second lumbrical muscle. There are branches of medial plantar nerve in the superficial layer. In the deep layer are common plantar digital nerve of toe Ⅱ and common plantar artery/veins.

Indications: Coma, headache, dizziness, hypertension, neurosis, insomnia, dysuria, etc.

Manipulation: Perpendicular puncture for 0.5 ~ 1 *cun.*

Reference: With Guanyuan (RN4) and Fenglong (ST40), it can treat cough which is caused by weak syndrome. With Shuigou (DU26), Shixuan (EX - UE11) and Zusanli (ST36), it can treat coma, faint and convulsion.

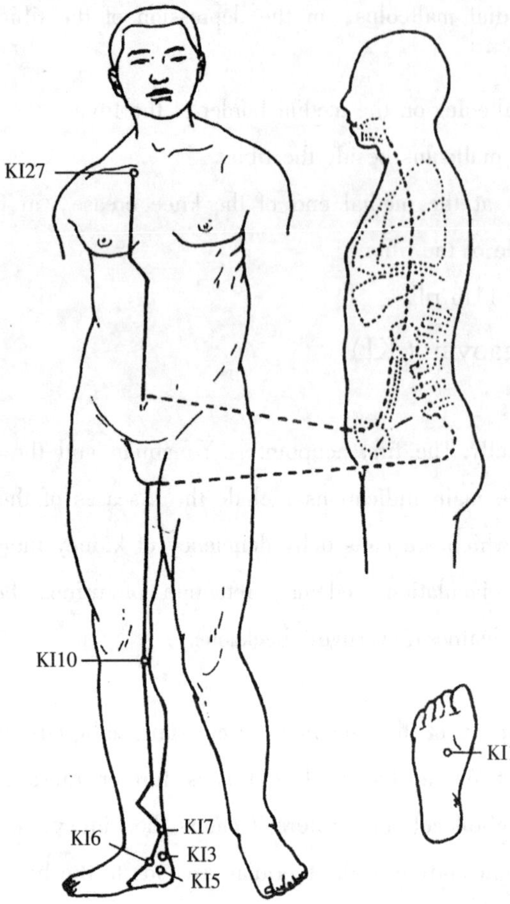

Fig. 4-27

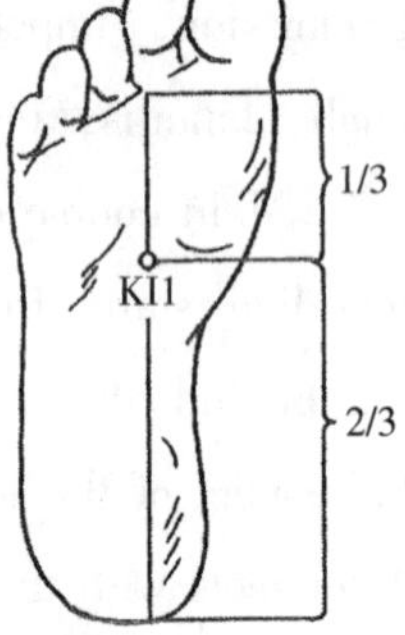

Fig. 4-28

2. Taixi (KI3).

Location: In the depression between the tip of medial malleolus and tendo calcaneus (Fig. 4-29).

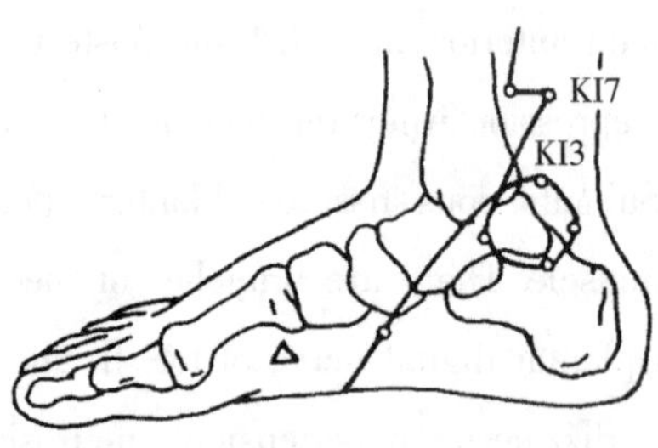

Fig. 4-29

Layers of dissection: Skin→Subcutaneous tissue→among the tendon of posterior tibial muscle, the tendon of long flexor muscle of toes, calcaneal tendon and the tendon of plantar muscle. There are medial crural cutaneous branches of saphenous nerve and branches of great saphenous vein in the superficial layer. In the deep layer are tibial nerve and posterior tibial artery/veins.

Indication: Headache, dizziness, tinnitus, poor vision, toothache, chronic faucitis, heel pain, seminal emission, impotence, chronic prostatitis, ankle strain.

Manipulation: Perpendicular puncture for 0.6 ~ 1 *cun*.

Reference: With Kunlun (BL60) and Shengmai (BL62), it can treat foot edema. With Shenmen

(HT7) and Sanyinjiao (SP6), it can treat insomnia or neurosis.

3. Fuliu (KI7).

Location: 2 *cun* directly above Taixi (KI3) in the medial side of leg (Fig. 4-29).

Layers of dissection: Skin→Subcutaneous tissue→in front of tendon of plantar muscle and calcaneal tendon→Long flexor muscle of great toe. There are medial crural cutaneous branches of saphenous nerve and branches of great saphenous vein in the superficial layer. In the deep layer is tibial nerve and posterior tibial artery/veins.

Indication: Chronic backache, nephritis, edema, peripheral neuritis.

Manipulation: Perpendicular puncture for 0.5 ~ 1 *cun*.

4.3.9.4 Less Commonly used acupoints

Rangu (KI2): In the depression on the inferior border of the tuberosity of the navicular bone, at the junction of the red and white skin.

Dazhong (KI4): In the postero-inferior part of the medial malleolus, in front of the tendo calcaneus, and above the calcaneus.

Shuiquan (KI5): 1 *cun* below KI3, on the medial border of the calcaneus.

Zhaohai (KI6): In the depression directly below the medial malleolus.

Jiaoxin (KI8): 2 *cun* above KI3, 0.5 *cun* in front of KI7, and just behind the medial border of the tibia.

Zhubin (KI9): 5 *cun* above KI3, in the line of KI3 to KI10, below the belly of the gastrocnemius muscle.

Yingu (KI10): At the medial side of the popliteal fossa, in between the semitendinous muscle and the semimembranous muscle, when the knee is flexed.

4.3.10 Stomach Meridian of Foot-Yangming (ST)

4.3.10.1 General information

This meridian goes from the head to the leg. The first acupoint is Chengqi and the last acupoint is Lidui. There are 45 acupoints on each side. The main indications include gastrointestinal diseases, diseases of the head, face, eye, nose and mouth, and other diseases in the regions along the course of this meridian, such as stomach diseases, enteritis, dyspepsia, headache, facial paralysis, toothache, faucitis, paralysis, numbness, pain of legs.

4.3.10.2 Main course of the meridian

This meridian starts from the lateral side of the nose. It ascends to the bridge of the nose, where it meets the Bladder Meridian. Turning downwards along the lateral side of the nose, it enters the upper gum. Reemerging, it curves round the lip and descends to the angle of the mandible. Then it ascends to the forehead. Its down-ward branch runs out from mandible and enters the supraclavicular fossa. Descending, it passes through the diaphragm, enters the stomach, its pertaining organ, and connects with the spleen. One branch from the orifice of the stomach descends inside the abdomen and reaches the groin. Then connecting with the meridian, which descends along the body surface, it continues downwards along the anterior aspect of the thigh, the lateral side of the tibia, passes through the dorsum of the foot and reaches the lateral side of the tip of the 2nd toe. One branch connects with the Spleen Meridian of Foot – Taiyin（Fig. 4 – 30）.

4. 3. 10. 3 Commonly used acupoints

1. Chengqi（ST1）.

Location：Directly below the pupil，between the infraorbital ridge and the eyeball，when the eyes look straight forward（Fig. 4 – 30）.

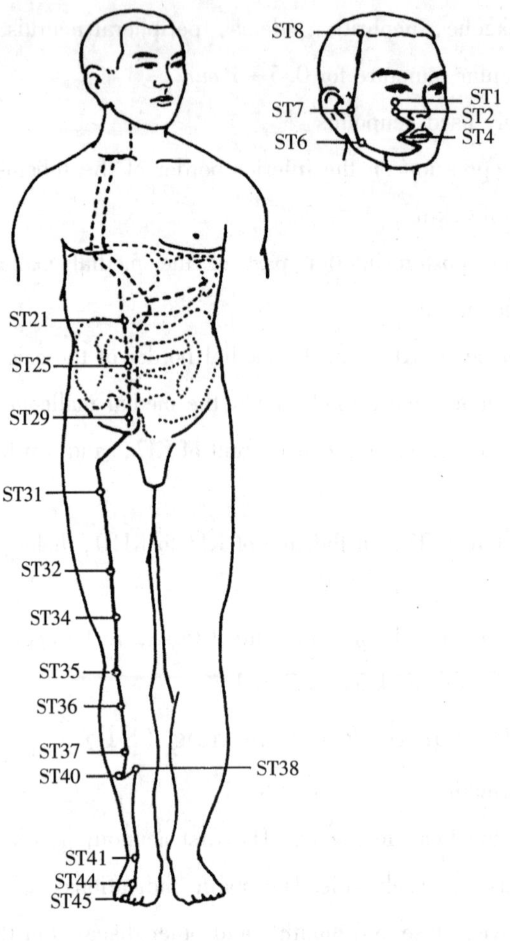

Fig. 4 – 30

Layers of dissection：Skin→Subcutaneous tissue→Orbicular muscle of eye→Adipose body of orbit→Inferior oblique muscle. There are branches of infraorbital nerve，zygomatic branches of facial nerve in the superficial layer. In the deep layer are branches of oculomotor nerve，ophthalmic artery/vein.

Indications：Keratitis，acute or chronic conjunctivitis，strabismus，cataract，glaucoma，night blindness，optic neuritis，optic atrophy，myopia，colour blindness，facial paralysis，twitching of eyelids，facial spasm，eyelid drop.

Manipulation：Puncture perpendicularly 0. 3 ~ 0. 5 *cun* along the infraorbital ridge. Don’ t twirl the needle in this acupoint（Fig. 4 – 31）.

2. Sibai（ST2）.

Location：Directly below the pupil，in the depression over the infraorbital foramen，when the eyes look straightforward (Fig. 4 -32).

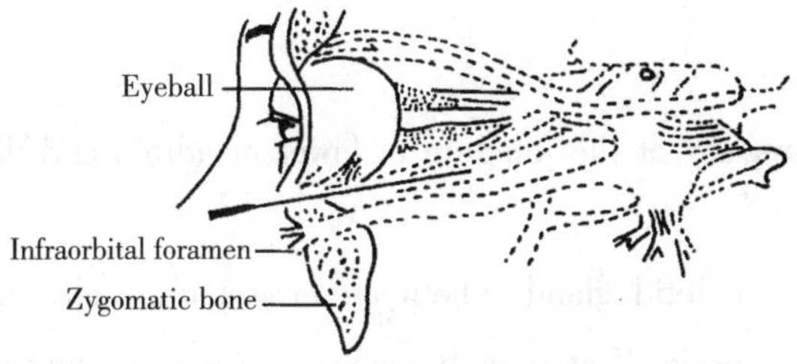

Fig. 4 -31

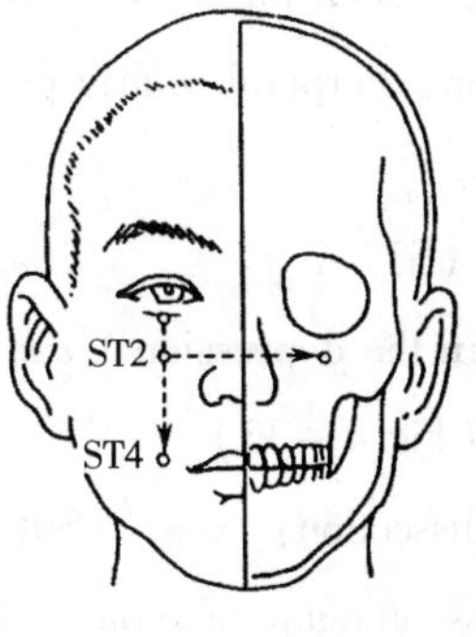

Fig. 4 -32

Layers of dissection: Skin→Subcutaneous tissue→Orbicular muscle of eye, Levator muscle of angle of mouth→Infraorbital foramen. There are branches of Infraorbital nerve, Zygomatic branches of Facial nerve in the superficial layer. In the profundity layer are Infraorbital artery/vein and Infraorbital nerve coming from Infraorbital foramen.

Indications: Facial paralysis, facial spasm, trigeminal neuralgia, myopia, keratitis, conjunctivitis, eyelid drop, glaucoma, rhinitis, biliary ascariasis, etc.

Manipulation: Perpendicularly puncture for 0. 4 ~0. 6 *cun*. Moxibustion is forbidden.

3. Dicang (ST4).

Location: Directly below the pupil, about 0. 4 *cun* from the angle of the mouth, when the eyes look straightforward (Fig. 4 -32).

Layers of dissection: Skin→Subcutaneous tissue→orbicular muscle of mouth→Depressor muscle of angle of mouth. There are branches of buccal nerve, Infraorbital nerve (coming from trigeminal nerve) and branches of facial artery/vein in the area.

Indications: Facial paralysis, trigeminal neuralgia, salivation.

Manipulation: Oblique or horizontal puncture for 0. 5 *cun*, or puncture toward Jiache (ST6) or Yingxiang (LI20).

4. Jiache (ST6).

Location: Over the masseter, 1 *cun* anterior and superior to the angle of the mandible (Fig. 4 -33).

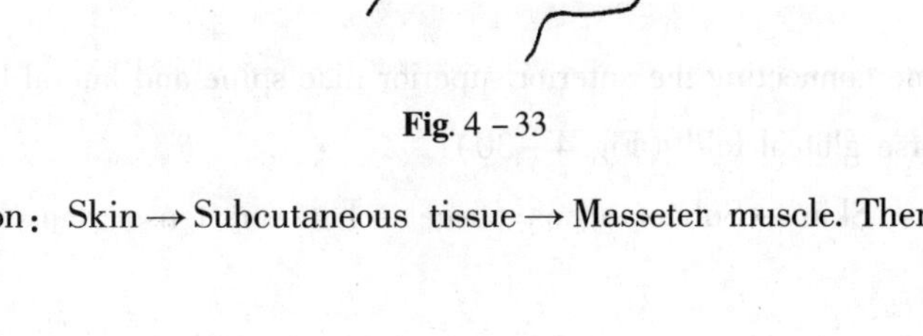

Fig. 4 -33

Layers of dissection: Skin → Subcutaneous tissue → Masseter muscle. There are branches of great auricular nerve and marginal mandibular branch of facial nerve in the area.

Indications: Facial paralysis, trigeminal neuralgia, toothache, facial spasm, mumps.

Manipulation: Perpendicularly puncture for 0.5 ~ 1.5 *cun*, or puncture toward Dicang (ST4) or Quanliao (SI18).

5. Xiaguan (ST7).

Location: In the depression 1 *cun* anterior to the tragus, at the juncture of lower mandible and the zygomatic arch (Fig. 4 – 33).

Layers of dissection: Skin → Subcutaneous tissue → Parotid gland → between masseter muscle and zygomatic process of temporal bone → Lateral pterygoid muscle. There are branches of Auriculotemporal nerve, zygomatic branches of facial nerve, and transverse artery/vein of face in the superficial layer. In the deep layer are maxillary artery/vein, lingual nerve, inferior alveolar nerve, middle meningeal artery, and pterygoid plexus.

Indications: Toothache, temporomandibular joint syndrome, trigeminal neuralgia, deafness, otitis media.

Manipulation: Perpendicularly puncture for 0.8 ~ 1.2 *cun*, or oblique puncture toward Tinggong (SI19).

6. Touwei (ST8).

Location: On the lateral side of the head, 0.5 *cun* directly above the hairline at the corner of the forehead, 4.5 *cun* lateral to the midline of the head (Fig. 4 – 33).

Layers of dissection: Skin → Subcutaneous tissue → epicranial aponeurosis on the superior margin of temporal muscle → loose connective tissue under aponeurosis → Pericranium. There are branches of auriculotemporal nerve, temporal branches of facial nerve and frontal branch of superficial temporal artery/veins in the area.

Indications: Headache, vertigo, facial paralysis, etc.

Manipulation: Puncture to the back for 0.5 ~ 1 *cun* subcutaneously.

7. Tianshu (ST25).

Location: 2 *cun* beside the umbilicus (Fig. 4 – 30).

Layers of dissection: Skin → Subcutaneous tissue → anterior layer of sheath of straight muscle of abdomen → Straight muscle of abdomen. There are lateral/anterior cutaneous branches of anterior branches of lumbar nerve Ⅸ, Ⅹ, Ⅺ and venous rete around navel in the superficial layer. In the deep layer are anastomotic branch of superior/inferior epigastric veins and muscular branches of anterior branches of lumbar nerve Ⅸ, Ⅹ, Ⅺ.

Indications: Acute or chronic enteritis or gastritis, bacillary dysentery, enteroparalysis, appendicitis, infant diarrhea, constipation, dyspepsia, abdominal muscle paralysis.

Manipulation: Perpendicular puncture for 0.6 ~ 1.2 *cun*.

8. Biguan (ST31).

Location: On the line connecting the anterior superior iliac spine and lateral border of the patella, at the same level as transverse gluteal fold (Fig. 4 – 30).

Layers of dissection: Skin → Subcutaneous tissue → between tensor muscle of broad fascia and sartorius muscle→straight muscle of thigh→Lateral great muscle of thigh. There is Lateral cutaneous nerve of thigh in the superficial layer. In the deep layer are ascending branch of lateral circumflex artery/vein, and muscular branches of femoral nerve.

Indication: Protrusion of the lumbar intervertebral disc, iliotibial muscle spasm, hip joint diseases, paralysis of legs.

Manipulation: Perpendicular puncture for 0.5 ~ 1 *cun*.

9. Futu (ST32).

Location: On the line connecting the anterior superior iliac spine and lateral border of the patella, 6 *cun* above the laterosuperior border of the patella (Fig. 4 – 30).

Layers of dissection: Skin → Subcutaneous tissue → Straight muscle of thigh → Intermediate great muscle of thigh. There are lateral veins of thigh, anterior cutaneous branches of femoral nerve and lateral cutaneous nerve of thigh in the superficial layer. In the deep layer are descending branches of lateral circumflex femoral artery/veins, and muscular branches of femoral nerve.

Indication: Protrusion of the lumbar intervertebral disc, iliotibial muscle spasm, inflammation of the nerves cutaneus femoris lateralis, hernia, inguinal lymphadenitis, paralysis of legs, etc.

Manipulation: Perpendicular puncture for 0.5 ~ 1 *cun*.

10. Liangqiu (ST34).

Location: Depression 2 *cun* above the patella, along the lateral margin (Fig. 4 – 30).

Layers of dissection: Skin→Subcutaneous tissue→between straight muscle of thigh and lateral great muscle of thigh → lateral part of the tendon of intermediate great muscle of thigh. There are anterior cutaneous branches of femoral nerve, Lateral cutaneous nerve of thigh in the superficial layer. In the deep layer are descending branch of lateral circumflex femoral artery/vein, muscular branches of femoral nerve.

Indications: Acute gastric pain, gastrospasm, diarrhea, mastitis, diseases of knee.

Manipulation: Perpendicular puncture for 0.5 ~ 1.2 *cun*.

11. Zusanli (ST36).

Location: 3 *cun* below the dent of lateral patella ligament, one fingerbreadth from the anterior crest of the tibia (Fig. 4 – 30).

Layers of dissection: Skin→Subcutaneous tissue→Anterior tibial muscle→Interosseous membrane of leg→Posterior tibial muscle. There is lateral cutaneous nerve of calf in the superficial layer. In the deep layer are branches of anterior tibial artery/vein, etc.

Indications: Acute or chronic gastritis or enteritis, gastral spasm, pancreatitis, gastral or duodenal ulcer, hepatitis, dyspepsia, bacillary dysentery, appendicitis, constipation, shock, headache, neurosis, arteriosclerosis, leukopenia, hypertension, mastitis, sciatica, paralysis of legs, Asthma.

Manipulation: Perpendicular puncture for 0.5 ~ 1.5 *cun*.

12. Shangjuxu (ST37).

Location: 6 *cun* below the dent of lateral patella ligament, one finger-breadth from the anterior crest of the tibia (Fig. 4 – 30).

Layers of dissection: Skin→Subcutaneous tissue→Anterior tibial muscle→Interosseous membrane of leg→Posterior tibial muscle. There is lateral cutaneous nerve of calf in the superficial layer. In the deep layer are anterior tibial artery/vein, deep peroneal nerve. If stab too deep, you might stab posterior tibial artery/vein and tibial nerve.

Indications: Appendicitis, dysentery, acute or chronic diarrhea, pain or paralysis of the lower extremities.

Manipulation: Perpendicular puncture for 0.5 ~ 1.2 *cun*.

13. Tiaokou (ST38).

Location: 8 *cun* below the dent of lateral patella ligament, one finger – breadth from the anterior crest of the tibia (Fig. 4 – 30).

Layers of dissection: Skin→Subcutaneous tissue→anterior tibial muscle →Interosseous membrane of leg→ Posterior tibial muscle. There is Lateral cutaneous nerve of calf in the superficial layer. In the profundity layer are anterior tibial artery/vein, and deep peroneal nerve. If you stab too deep, you might stab Fibular artery/vein.

Indications: Periarthritis of shoulder, protrusion of the lumbar intervertebral disc, knee arthritis, multiple neuritis, stomachache.

Manipulation: Perpendicular 0.5 ~ 1.2 *cun*.

14. Fenglong (ST40).

Location: 8 *cun* below the dent of lateral patella ligament, two finger-breadth from the anterior crest of the tibia (Fig. 4 – 30).

Layers of dissection: Skin→Subcutaneous tissue→Long extensor muscle of toes→Long extensor muscle of great toe→Interosseous membrane of leg→Posterior tibial muscle. There is lateral cutaneous nerve of calf in the superficial layer. In the deep layer are branches of anterior tibial artery/vein, and deep peroneal nerve.

Indications: Bronchitis, asthma, dizziness, mental disorder, epilepsy, systremma, numbness, pain or paralysis of the lower extremities, dyspepsia, constipation.

Manipulation: Perpendicular puncture for 0.5 ~ 1.2 *cun*.

Reference: *Standby Songs*: When a patient has asthma and can not fall asleep, give him puncture for 0.3 *cun* at Fenglong.

15. Jiexi (ST41).

Location: Over the dorsum of the foot, in the middle of the ankle transverse crease (Fig. 4 – 30).

Layers of dissection: Skin→Subcutaneous tissue→between the tendon of long extensor muscle of great toe and the tendon of long extensor muscle of toes→Talus. There are medial dorsal cutaneous nerve of foot, dorsal cutaneous venous of foot in the superficial layer. In the deep layer are deep peroneal nerve, and anterior fibial artery/vein.

Indications: Headache, paralysis of the lower extremities, diseases of ankle, etc.

Manipulation: Perpendicular puncture for 0.4 ~ 0.8 *cun*.

16. Neiting (ST44).

Location: Behind the vertical skin crease of the web between the 2nd and 3rd toes, on the junction of the red and white skin (Fig. 4 –30).

Layers of dissection: Skin→Subcutaneous tissue→between the tendon of long/short extensor muscle of toe Ⅱ and toe Ⅲ→between head of metatarsus of toe Ⅱ and toe Ⅲ. There are dorsal digital nerves of foot (branches of medial dorsal cutaneous nerve), dorsal venous rete of foot in the superficial layer. In the deep layer are dorsal digital arteries/veins.

Indication: Toothache, laryngitis, epistaxis, keratitis, fever, acute or chronic enteritis, pain of the dorsum of the foot, facial paralysis, etc.

Manipulation: Perpendicular puncture for 0.5 ~ 1.2 *cun*.

4.3.10.4 Less commonly used acupoints

Juliao (ST3): Directly below the middle of the eye, at a level with the inferior border of the ala of the nose.

Daying (ST5): In front of the angle of the mandible, on the anterior border of the masseter, near the beating facial artery.

Renying (ST9): By the side of the laryngeal prominence, just in the carotid artery.

Quepen (ST12): Middle of the superior border of the clavicle, 4 *cun* lateral to the anterior median line.

Liangmen (ST21): 4 *cun* above the umbilicus, 2 *cun* lateral to the anterior median line.

Daju (ST27): 2 *cun* below the umbilicus, and 2 *cun* lateral to the anterior median line.

Shuidao (ST28): 3 *cun* below the umbilicus, 2 *cun* lateral to the anterior median line.

Guilai (ST29): 4 *cun* below the umbilicus, 2 *cun* lateral to the anterior median line.

Yinshi (ST33): Along the line of the lateral margin of patella to the anterior prior iliac spine, 3 *cun* above the lateral margin of the patella.

Dubi (ST35): In the dent of lateral patella ligament.

Xiajuxu (ST39): 9 *cun* below ST35, one finger-breadth from the anterior crest of the tibia.

Chongyang (ST42): On the hump of the dorsum of the foot, by the side of the dorsalis pedis artery.

Xiangu (ST43): On the depression distal to junction of the second and third metatarsal bones.

4.3.11 Gallbladder Meridian of Foot-Shaoyang (GB)

4.3.11.1 General information

This meridian goes from the head to the foot. The first acupoint is Tongziliao and the last acupoint is Zuqiaoyin. There are 44 acupoints on each side. The main indications include diseases of the head, lateral side of the body, liver and gallbladder, such as migraine, tinnitus, deafness, eye diseases, diseases of lateral thorax and diseases of lateral lower limbs, hepatitis and cholecystitis, etc.

4.3.11.2 Main course of the meridian

This meridian starts from the outer canthus, ascends to the corner of the forehead, then curves downwards to the retroauricular region and runs along the side of the neck in front of the Sanjiao Meridian to the shoulder. Turning back, it traverses and passes behind the Sanjiao Meridian down to the supraclavicular fossa. The straight portion of the meridian runs downwards from the supraclavicular fossa, passes along the lateral aspect of the chest to the hip region. The inside part of the meridian connects with the liver and enters its pertaining organ, the gallbladder. It runs along the pubic area and goes transversely into the hip region, where it joins with the body surface part of the meridian. There, it descends along the lateral aspect of the leg to the tip of the 4th toe. One branch connects with the Liver Meridian of Foot-Tueyin (Fig. 4 -34).

4.3.11.3 Commonly used acupoints

1. Tinghui (GB2).

Location: In front of the intertragic notch, on the posterior margin of the condyloid process of the mandible, where a depression is formed when the mouth is wide open (Fig. 4 -34).

Layers of dissection: Skin → Subcutaneous tissue → Parotid capsule → Parotid gland. There are auriculotemporal nerve and great auricular nerve in the superficial layer. In the deep layer are superficial temporal artery/veins and plexus of facial nerve.

Indications: Deafness, tinnitus, otitis media, headache, masticatory muscle spasm, temporomandibular joint inflammation, facial paralysis.

Manipulation: Perpendicular puncture for 0.5 ~ 0.8 *cun*.

2. Shuaigu (GB8).

Location: directly above the apex auriculae, 1.5 *cun* above the hairline (Fig. 4 -34).

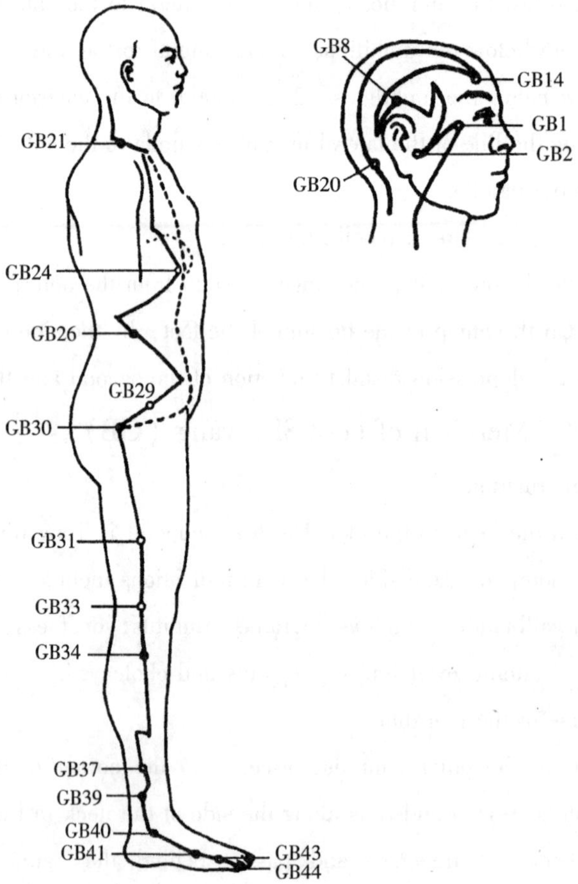

Fig. 4 -34

Layers of dissection: Skin → Subcutaneous tissue → Superior auricular muscle → Temporal fascia →

Temporal muscle. There are auriculotemporal nerve, greater occipital nerve and parietal branch of superficial temporal artery/veins in this area.

Indications: Migraine, vertigo, conjunctivitis, keratitis, facial paralysis, infantile convulsion.

Manipulation: Subcutaneous puncture for 0. 5 ~ 1 *cun*.

3. Yangbai (GB14).

Location: 1 *cun* above the middle of the eyebrow. When the eyes looking straight forward, directly above the pupil (Fig. 4 – 35).

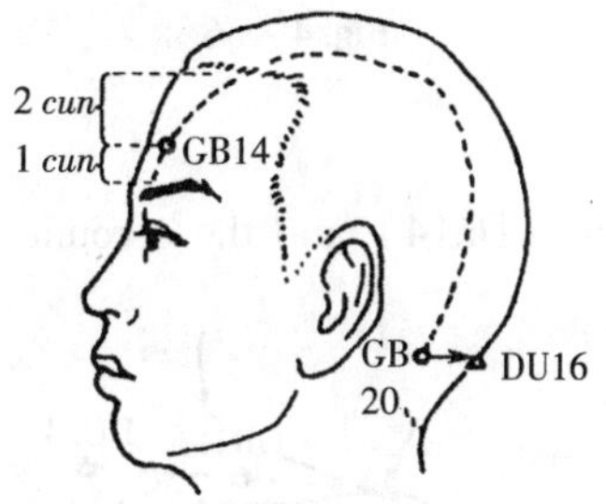

Fig. 4 – 35

Layers of dissection: Skin→Subcutaneous tissue→Frontal venter of occipitofrontal muscle. There are lateral branch of supraorbital nerve and lateral branch of supraorbital artery/vein in this area.

Indications: Facial paralysis, headache, vertigo, trigeminal neuralgia, eyelid drop, night blindness, myopia.

Manipulation: Subcutaneous puncture for 0. 4 ~0. 8 *cun*.

4. Fengchi (GB20).

Location: Below the occipital bone, in the depression between the upper part of the trapezius muscle and sternocleidomastoid muscle (Fig. 4 – 35).

Layers of dissection: Skin→Subcutaneous tissue→between trapezius muscle and sterno-cleidomastoid muscle→Splenius muscle of head→Semispinal muscle of head→between greater posterior straight muscle of head and superior oblique muscle of head. There are lesser occipital nerve and branches of occipital artery/veins in the superficial layer. In the deep layer is suboccipital nerve.

Indications: Common cold, dizziness, headache, rhinitis, inflammation in the eye, optic atrophy, insomnia, hypertension, etc.

Manipulation: Oblique puncture toward the eye which locates at the other side for 0. 5 ~ 0. 8 *cun*. Medulla oblongata is deep below this acupoint. Pay attention to the angle and depth of acupuncture on this acupoint to avoid hurting it (Fig. 4 – 36).

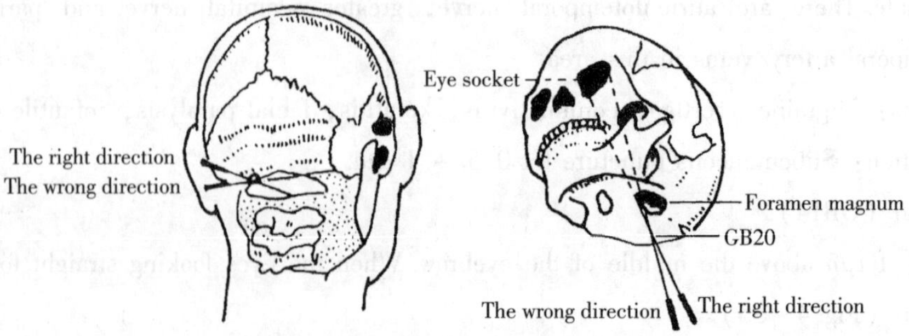

Fig. 4 – 36

5. Jianjing (GB21).

Location: Midway between Dazhui (Du14) and the acromion (Fig. 4 – 37).

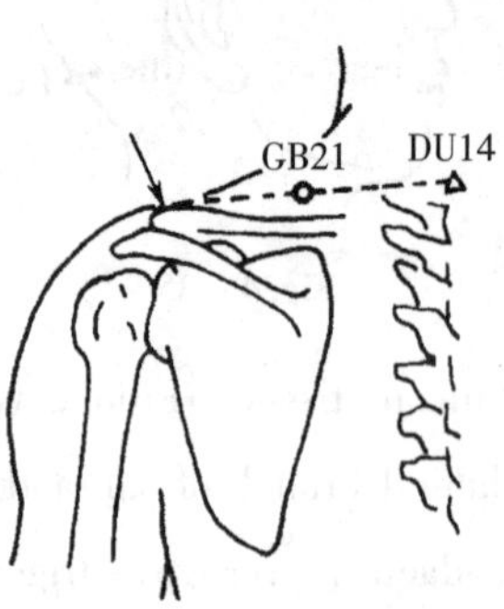

Fig. 4 – 37

Layers of dissection: Skin→Subcutaneous tissue→trapezius muscle→Levator muscle of scapula. There are supraclavicular nerves and branches of superficial cervical artery/vein in the superficial layer. In the deep layer are branches of transverse cervical artery/vein and branches of dorsal nerve of scapula.

Indications: Pain of back and shoulder, mastitis.

Manipulation: Perpendicular puncture for 0.6 ~ 0.8 *cun*. Don' t puncture too deep to hurt the apex of the lung, which is inside the acupoint.

Reference: *Figures of classified cannon* says: "The acupoint is forbidden for pregnant women". With Tianzong (SI11), Shaoze (SI1) for mastitis. With moxibustion on Zhongji (RN3) for helping placenta delivery.

6. Riyue (GB24).

Location: Below the nipple, in the 7th intercostals space, 4 *cun* lateral to the anterior median line (Fig. 4 – 34).

Layers of dissection: Skin→Subcutaneous tissue→External oblique muscle of abdomen→External intercostal muscles. There are lateral cutaneous branch of intercostals nerve Ⅵ, Ⅶ, Ⅷ and following artery/veins in the superficial layer. In the deep layer are intercostals nerve Ⅶ and posterior intercostals artery/veins Ⅶ.

Indications: Acute or chronic hepatitis, cholecystitis, gastric ulcer, phrenospasm, vomiting.

Manipulation: Oblique puncture for 0.5 ~ 0.8 *cun*.

7. Juliao (GB29).

Location: In the mid-point of the line between the anterosupeior iliac spine and the great trochanter of the femur (Fig. 4 – 34).

Layers of dissection: Skin → Subcutaneous tissue → Wide fascia → Middle gluteal muscle → Least gluteal muscle. There are superior cluneal nerves and lateral cutaneous branch of iliohypogastric nerve in the superficial layer. In the deep layer are branches of superior gluteal artery/veins and superior gluteal nerve.

Indications: Hip joint diseases, inflammation of nervus cutaneus femoris lateralis, cystitis, orchitis, sequela of stroke.

Manipulation: Perpendicular puncture for 1.2 ~ 1.5 *cun*.

8. Huantiao (GB30).

Location: At the junction of lateral one third and medial two thirds of the distance between the greater trochanter of the femur and the sacral hiatus (Fig. 4 – 38).

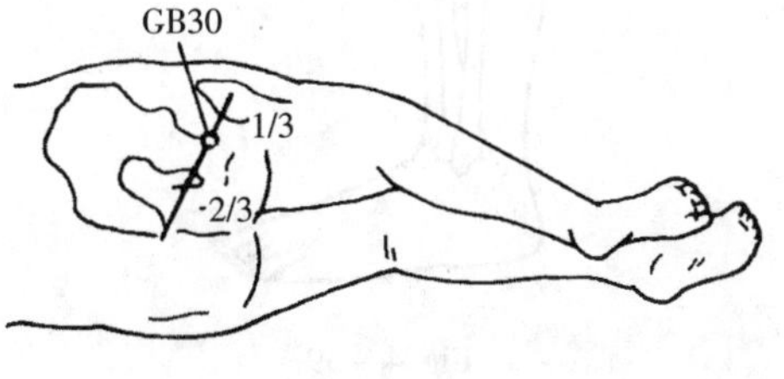

Fig. 4 – 38

Layers of dissection: Skin → Subcutaneous tissue → Greatest gluteal muscle → Ischiadic nerve → Quadrate muscle of thigh. There are superior cluneal nerves in the superficial layer. In the deep layer are ischiadic nerve, inferior gluteal nerve, posterior cutaneous nerve of thigh and inferior gluteal artery/veins.

Indications: Sciatica, protrusion of the lumbar intervertebral disc, piriform muscle syndrome, sacro – iliac joints injury, hip joint diseases, sequela of stroke.

Manipulation: Perpendicular puncture for 1.5 ~ 3.0 *cun*.

9. Fengshi (GB31).

Location: On the midline of the lateral aspect of the thigh, 7 *cun* above the transverse popliteal creasc (Fig. 4 34).

Layers of dissection: Skin→Subcutaneous tissue→Iliotibial tract→Lateral great muscle of thigh→ Intermediate great muscle of thigh. There is lateral cutaneous nerve of thigh in the superficial layer. In the deep layer are muscular branches of descending branch of lateral circumflex femoral artery and muscular branches of femoral nerve.

Indications: Sciatica, protrusion of the lumbar intervertebral disc, inflammation of nervus cutaneus femoris lateralis, knee arthritis, sequela of stroke, nettle rash.

Manipulation: Perpendicular puncture for 0.8 ~ 1.5 *cun*.

10. Xiyangguan (GB33).

Location: 3 *cun* above Yanglingquan (GB34), in the depression superior to the external epicondyle

(Fig. 4 – 34).

Layers of dissection: Skin→Subcutaneous tissue→Posterior margin of iliotial tract→in front of lateral head of gastrocnemius muscle. There is lateral cutaneous nerve of thigh in the superficial layer. In the deep layer are lateral superior genicular artery/veins.

Indications: Knee arthritis, sciatica.

Manipulation: Perpendicular puncture for 0. 8 ~ 1. 5 *cun*.

11. Yanglingquan (GB34).

Location: On the antero – infefior part of the capitulum of the fibula (Fig. 4 – 39).

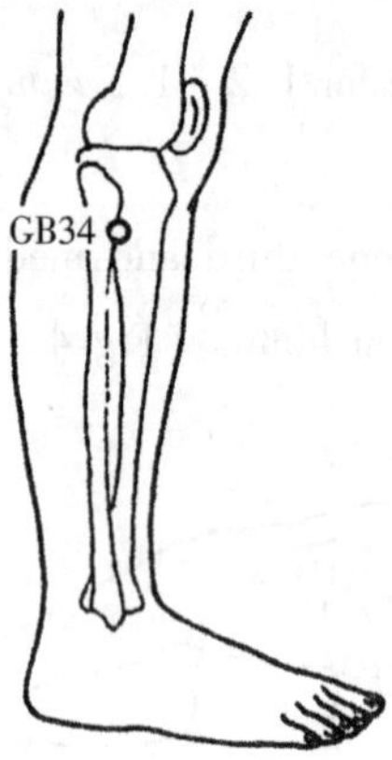

Fig. 4 – 39

Layers of dissection: Skin → Subcutaneous tissue → long fibular muscle → Long extensor muscle of toes. There is lateral cutaneous nerve of calf in the superficial layer. In the deep layer are anterior recurrent tibial artery/vein, branches of lateral inferior genicular artery/veins and branches of common fibular nerve.

Indications: Hepatitis, cholecystitis, cholelithiasis, biliary ascariasis, periarthritis of shoulder, knee arthritis, protrusion of the lumbar intervertebral disc, paralysis, numbness and pain of the lateral aspects of lower extremities.

Manipulation: Perpendicular or oblique downward puncture for 1 ~ 1. 5 *cun*.

Reference: It is reported that acupuncture on this acupoint can make gallbladder shrink obviously in 75. 7% people, which indicates that acupuncture on this acupoint can increase the cholecystic mobility and evacuation. This function appears when the needle sensation appears and becomes more obvious 10 minutes after the removal of the needle. Acupuncture on the acupoints (Xiabai, Chize, Taiyuan) which are not on the Gallbladder Meridian or on the points which are not acupoints has no similar function. Clinical experience has shown that deep acupuncture on GB34 has obvious analgesic function on the pain or colic of liver or spleen diseases (This demands the needle should puncture toward Yinlingquan; the needle sensation passes down to the dorsum of foot, and the needle should be retained in the body for 20 minutes). If we can practice suture imbedding in this acupoint, the effect will be better. Injection of chloromazine in this acupoint can relief biliary colic obviously.

12. Guangming (GB37).

Location: 5 *cun* above the tip of the external malleolus, on the anterior border of the fibula (Fig. 4 – 34).

Layers of dissection: Skin→Subcutaneous tissue→Short fibular muscle→Anterior intermuscular septum→Long extensor muscle of great toes→Interosseous membrane of leg→Posterior tibial muscle. There are superficial fibular nerve and lateral cutaneous nerve of calf in the superficial layer. In the deep layer are deep fibular nerve and anterior tibial artery/veins.

Indications: Optic atrophy, cataract, sciatica, injury of nervi fibularis communis, mastitis.

Manipulation: Perpendicular puncture for 0.5 ~ 0.8 *cun*.

13. Xuanzhong (GB39).

Location: 3 *cun* above the tip of the external malleolus, on the anterior border of the fibula (Many documents say that the acupoint is on the posterion border of the fibula) (Fig. 4 – 34).

Layers of dissection: Skin→Subcutaneous tissue→Long extensor muscle of toes→Interosseous membrane of leg. There is lateral cutaneous nerve of calf in the superficial layer. In the deep layer are branches of deep fibular nerve. If you pierce through interosseous membrane of leg, you may prick fibular artery/veins.

Indications: Stiff neck, cervical spondylopathy, pain of hypochondrium, paralysis, numbness and pain of lower extremities, lymphaden hypertrophy, chorea in children, arteriosclerosis.

Manipulation: Perpendicular puncture for 0.5 ~ 1 *cun*.

14. Qiuxu (GB40).

Location: In the depression which is antero-inferior to the external malleolus (Fig. 4 – 34).

Layers of dissection: Skin→Subcutaneous tissue→Short extensor muscle of toes→Lateral talocalcaneal ligament→Tarsal sinus. There are superficial dorsal veins of foot, lateral dorsal cutaneous nerve, intermediate dorsal cutaneous nerve and lateral anterior malleolar artery/veins in this area.

Indications: Ankle strain, foot drop, cholecystitis, cervical spondylopathy.

Manipulation: Perpendicular puncture for 0.5 ~ 1 *cun*.

4.3.11.4 Less commonly used acupoints

Tongziliao (GB1): Lateral to the external canthus.

Shangguan (GB3): On the anterior part of the ear and the upper margin of the zygomatic arch, right above ST7.

Hanyan (GB4): Within the temple, at the junction of upper 1/4 and lower 3/4 of the distance between ST8 and GB7.

Xuanlu (GB5): Within the temple, midway between ST8 and GB7.

Xuanli (GB6): Within the temple, at the junction of upper 3/4 and lower 1/4 of the distance between ST8 and GB7.

Qubing (GB7): In the temple on a level with the apex of the ear.

Touqiaoyin (GB11): On the posterior part of the mastoid process of the temporal bone.

Wangu (GB12): In the depression on the postero – inferior side of the mastoid behind the ear.

Benshen（GB13）：On the lateral part of the forehead，0. 5 *cun* within the natural line of the hair，3 *cun* lateral to DU24.

Toulinqi（GB15）：0. 5 *cun* within the natural line of the hair，midway between DU24 and ST8.

Naokong（GB19）：Laterally to the external occipital protuberance，2. 25 *cun* beside the posterior median line. Same level with DU17.

Jingmen（GB25）：Inferior to the extremity of the 12th rib. 1. 8 *cun* posterior to LR13.

Daimai（GB26）：Directly below the free end of the 11th rib，and same level with umbilicus.

Waiqiu（GB36）：7 *cun* above the lateral malleolus，in front of the fibula.

Yangfu（GB38）：4 *cun* above the lateral malleolus，in front of the fibula.

Zulinqi（GB41）：On the posterior lateral part of the head of the 4th metatarsal bone.

Xiaxi（GB43）：Behind the margin of the web between the 4th toe and the 5th toe，at the junction of the red and white skin.

Zuqiaoyin（GB44）：About 0. 1 *cun* beside the lateral corner of the vallum ungis of the 4th toe.

4. 3. 12　Bladder Meridian of Foot-Taiyang（BL）

4. 3. 12. 1　General information

This meridian goes from the head to the leg. The first acupoint is Jingming and the last acupoint is Zhiyin. There are 67 acupoints on each side. The main indications include diseases of the eye，head，nape，lumbar and sacral region，legs，hemorrhoid，prolapse of rectum，mental diseases and epilepsy，etc. The Beishu Acupoints are used to treat diseases of their relevant organs and tissues respectively.

4. 3. 12. 2　The maim course of the meridian

This meridian starts from the inner canthus. Ascending to the vertex of the head，it descends to the nape and breaks into two branches. One branch，which is parallel to the vertebral column，descends to the lumbar region，where it enters the body cavity to connect with the kidney and joins its pertaining organ，the urinary bladder. Through the hips，it descends to the center of popliteal fossa. The other branch runs straight downward along the medial border of the scapula. Passing through the gluteal region and going downward along the lateral aspect of the thigh，it meets the preceding branch descending from the lumbar region in the popliteal fossa. From there，it descends through the calf muscle to the lateral side of the dorsum of the foot and reaches the lateral side of the little toe（Fig. 4 –40）.

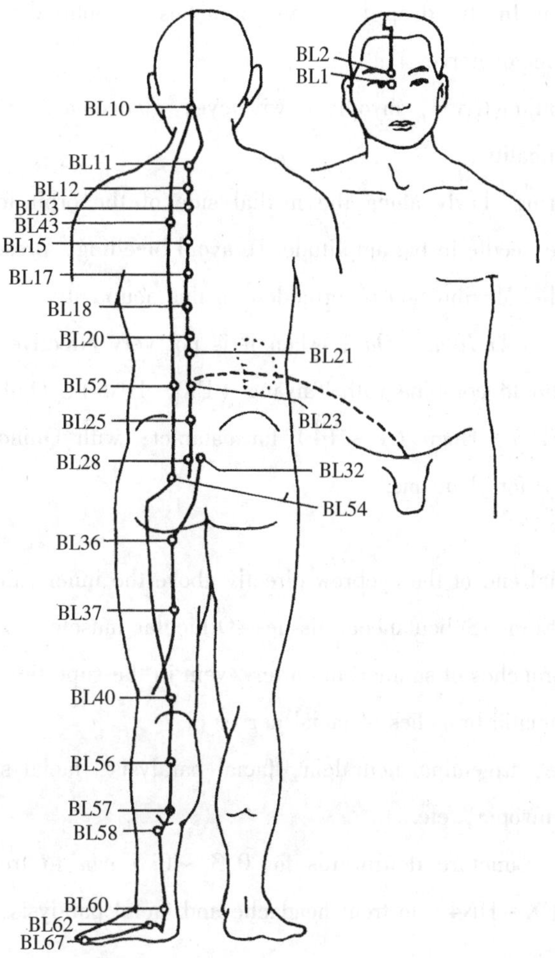

Fig. 4 – 40

4. 3. 12. 3 Commonly used acupoints

1. Jingming (BL1).

Location: About 0. 1 *cun* superior to the inner canthus, near the medial side of the orbitae (Fig. 4 – 41).

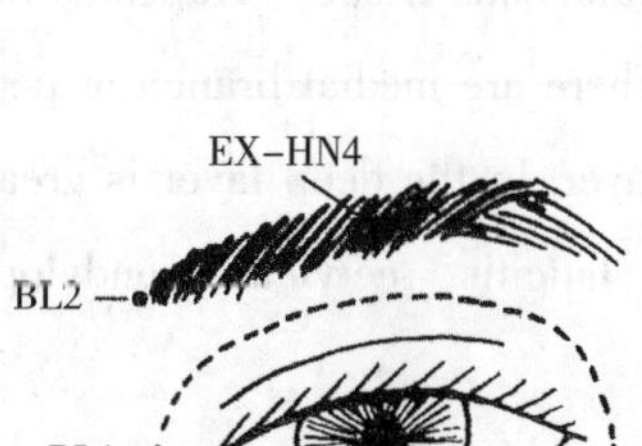

Fig. 4 – 41

Layers of dissection: Skin → Subcutaneous tissue → Orbicular muscle of eye → above the superior lacrimal canaliculus → between medial straight muscle and orbital plate of ethmoid bone. There are supratrochlear nerve of ophthalmic nerve (a branch of trigeminal nerve) and branches of angular artery/

vein in the superficial layer. In the deep layer are branches of ophthalmic artery/vein, branches of ophthalmic nerve and oculomotor nerve.

Indications: Acute conjunctivitis, myopia, swiveleye, glaucoma, optic atrophy, optic neuritis, retinitis, blindness of encephalitis.

Manipulation: Puncturing slowly along the medial side of the orbit for 0.3 ~ 0.5 *cun*. It is not advisable to lift or thrust the needle in big amplitude. To avoid bleeding, press this point for 1 ~ 2 minutes after withdrawal of the needle. Moxibustion is forbidden on this acupoint.

Reference: According to *Xi Hong's Ode*, when it is not very effective for puncturing BL1 to treat some optic diseases, we should combine with Taiyang (EX – HN5), Qiuhou (EX – HNT), Yiming (near GB20), Shaoze (SI1), Hegu (1 ~ 14) for cataract; with Qiuhou (EX – HN7), Fengchi (GB20), Taichong (LR3) for glaucoma.

2. Zanzhu (BL2).

Location: At the medial end of the eyebrow directly above the inner canthus (Fig. 4 – 41).

Layers of dissection: Skin→Subcutaneous tissue→Orbicular muscle of eye. There are supratrochlear nerve of frontal nerve and branches of supraorbital artery/vein in the superficial layer. In the deep layer are temporal branches and zygomatic branches of facial nerve.

Indications: Headache, trigeminal neuralgia, facial paralysis, facial spasm, conjunctivitis, optic atrophy, night blindness, myopia, etc.

Manipulation: Oblique puncture downwards for 0.3 ~ 0.5 *cun* to treat eye diseases, horizontal puncture towards Yuyao (EX – HN4) to treat headache and facial paralysis. Moxibustion is forbidden on this acupoint.

3. Tianzhu (BL10).

Location: Right on the natural line of the hair at the back of the head, on the lateral part of the margin of the trapezius muscle, 1.3 *cun* lateral to the midpoint of the natural line of the hair (Fig. 4 – 40).

Layers of dissection: Skin→Subcutaneous tissue→Trapezius muscle→medial part of splenius muscle of head→Semispinal muscle of head. There are medial branch of posterior branch of cervical nerve Ⅲ and subcutaneous veins in the superficial layer. In the deep layer is greater occipital nerve.

Indications: Headache, vertigo, faucitis, cervical spondylopathy, neuralgia of nervus occipitalis major, pain in the shoulder and back.

Manipulation: Perpendicular puncture for 0.5 ~ 1.2 *cun*.

4. Dashu (BL11).

Location: 1.5 *cun* beside the depression below the spinous process of the 1st thoracic vertebra (Fig. 4 – 40).

Layers of dissection: Skin→subcutaneous tissue→Trapezius muscle→Rhomboid muscles Superior posterior serratus muscle→Splenius muscle of neck→Erector spinal muscle. There are medial cutaneous branches of posterior branches of thoracic nerve Ⅰ, Ⅱ and following medial cutaneous branches of dorsal branches of posterior intercostal arteries/veins in the superficial layer. In the deep layer are muscular branches of posterior branches of thoracic nerve Ⅰ, Ⅱ and following dorsal branches of posterior intercostal arteries/veins.

Indications: Pain in the shoulder and back, cervical spondylopathy, headache, asthma, faucitis, epilepsy.

Manipulation: Perpendicular puncture for 0.5 ~ 1 *cun*.

5. Fengmen (BL12).

Location: 1.5 *cun* beside the depression below the spinous process of the 2nd thoracic vertebra (Fig. 4-40).

Layers of dissection: Skin→Subcutaneous tissue→Trapezius muscle→Rhomboid muscle→Superior posterior serratus muscle→Splenius muscle of neck→Erector spinal muscle. There are medial cutaneous branches of posterior branches of thoracic nerve Ⅱ, Ⅲ and following medical cutaneous branches of dorsal branches of posterior intercostal arteries/veins in the superficial layer. In the deep layer are muscular branches of posterior branches of thoracic nerve Ⅱ, Ⅲ and following dorsal branches of posterior intercostal arteries/veins.

Indication: Bronchitis, pneumonia, whooping cough, common cold, fever, nettle rash, cervical spondylopathy, pain in the chest and back.

Manipulation: Perpendicular puncture for 0.5 ~ 1.2 *cun*.

6. Feishu (BL13).

Location: 1.5 *cun* beside the depression below the spinous process of the 3rd thoracic vertebra (Fig. 4-42).

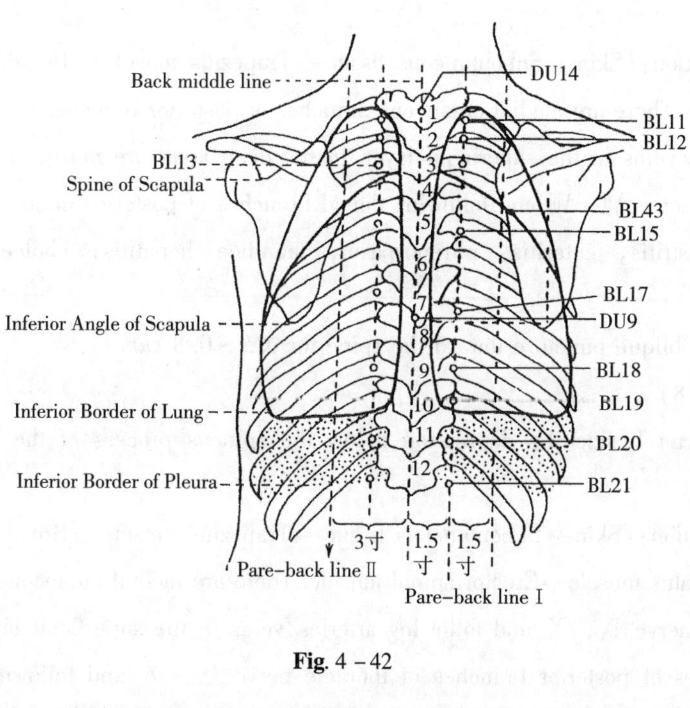

Fig. 4-42

Layers of dissection: Skin→Subcutaneous tissue→Trapezius muscle→Rhomboid muscle→Superior posterior serratus muscle → Erector spinal muscle. There are medial cutaneous branches of posterior branches of thoracic nerve Ⅲ, Ⅳ and following medical cutaneous branches of dorsal branches of posterior intercostal arteries/veins in the superficial layer. In the deep layer are muscular branches of posterior branches of thoracic nerve Ⅲ, Ⅳ and following dorsal branches of posterior intercostal arteries/veins.

Indications: Respiratory system diseases, nettle rash, backache.

Manipulation: Oblique puncture toward the spine for 0.5 ~ 0.8 *cun*.

Caution: BL11 ~ 19, are all locating above the 10th thoracic vertebra and in the area of lung. Don't puncture too deep.

7. Xinshu (BL15).

Location: 1.5 *cun* beside the depression below the spinous process of the 5th thoracic vertebra (Fig. 4 – 42).

Layers of dissection: Skin→Subcutaneous tissue→Trapezius muscle→inferior margin of rhomboid muscle→Erector spinal muscle. There are medial cutaneous branches of posterior branches of thoracic nerve Ⅴ, Ⅵ and following arteries/veins in the superficial layer. In the deep layer are muscular branches of posterior branches of thoracic nerve Ⅴ, Ⅵ and following dorsal branches of posterior intercostal arteries/veins.

Indications: Cardiovascular system diseases, intercostals neuralgia, hysteria, mental diseases, neurosis.

Manipulation: Oblique puncture toward the spine for 0.5 ~ 0.8 *cun*.

8. Geshu (BL17).

Location: 1.5 *cun* beside the depression below of the spinous process of the 7th thoracic vertebra (Fig. 4 – 42).

Layers of dissection: Skin→Subcutaneous tissue→Trapezius muscle→Broadest muscle of back→Erector spinal muscle. There are medial cutaneous branches of posterior branches of thoracic nerve Ⅶ, Ⅷ and following arteries/veins in the superficial layer. In the deep layer are muscular branches of posterior branches of thoracic nerve Ⅶ, Ⅷ and following dorsal branches of posterior intercostal arteries/veins.

Indications: Gastritis, enteritis, phrenospasm, jaundice hepatitis, cholecystitis, nettle rash, backache, etc.

Manipulation: Oblique puncture toward the spine for 0.5 ~ 0.8 *cun*.

9. Ganshu (BL18).

Location: 1.5 *cun* beside the depression below the spinous process of the 9th thoracic vertebra (Fig. 4 – 42).

Layers of dissection: Skin→Subcutaneous tissue→Trapezius muscle→Broadest muscle of back→Inferior posterior serratus muscle→Erector spinal muscle. There are medial cutaneous branches of posterior branches of thoracic nerve Ⅸ, Ⅹ and following arteries/veins in the superficial layer. In the deep layer are muscular branches of posterior branches of thoracic nerve Ⅸ, Ⅹ and following dorsal branches of posterior intercostal arteries/veins.

Indications: liver, gallbladder and eye diseases, gastritis, neurosis, mental disease, irregular menstruation.

Manipulation: Oblique puncture toward the spine for 0.5 ~ 0.8 *cun*.

10. Danshu (BL19).

Location: 1.5 *cun* beside the depression below the spinous process of the 10th thoracic vertebra (Fig. 4 - 42).

Layers of dissection: Skin→Subcutaneous tissue→Trapezius muscle→Broadest muscle of Back→Inferior posterior serrate muscle→Erector spinal muscle. There are medial cutaneous branches of posterior branches of thoracic nerve Ⅹ, Ⅺ and following arteries/veins in the superficial layer. In the deep layer are muscular branches of posterior branches of thoracic nerve Ⅹ, Ⅺ and following dorsal branches of posterior intercostal arteries/veins.

Indications: jaundice hepatitis, cholecystitis, biliary ascariasis, intercostals neuralgia, and backache, etc.

Manipulation: Oblique puncture toward the spine for 0.5 ~ 0.8 *cun*.

11. Pishu (BL20).

Location: 1.5 *cun* beside the depression below the spinous process of the 11th thoracic vertebra (Fig. 4 - 42).

Layers of dissection: Skin→Subcutaneous tissue→Broadest muscle of back→Inferior posterior serrate muscle→Erector spinal muscle. There are medial cutaneous branches of posterior branches of thoracic nerve Ⅺ, Ⅻ and following arteries/veins in the superficial layer. In the deep layer are muscular branches of posterior branches of thoracic nerve Ⅺ, Ⅻ and following dorsal branches of posterior intercostal arteries/veins.

Indications: Digestive system diseases, hepatitis, edema, pain of back, anemia, diabetes.

Manipulation: Oblique puncture toward the spine for 0.5 ~ 0.8 *cun*.

12. Weishu (BL21).

Location: 1.5 *cun* beside the depression below the spinous process of the 12th thoracic vertebra (Fig. 4 - 42).

Layers of dissection: Skin→Subcutaneous tissue→superficial layer of thoracolumbar fascia and aponeurosis of broadest muscle of back→Erector spinal muscle. There are cutaneous branches of posterior branches of thoracic nerve Ⅻ and lumbar nerve Ⅰ and following arteries/veins in the superficial layer. In the deep layer are muscular branches of posterior branches of thoracic nerve Ⅻ and lumbar nerve Ⅰ and following branches of arteries/veins.

Indications: Gastric ulcer, gastroptosis, gastrospasm, pancreatitis, diabetes, etc.

Manipulation: Perpendicular puncture for 0.5 ~ 0.8 *cun*.

13. Shenshu (BL23).

Location: 1.5 *cun* beside the depression below the spinous process of the 2nd lumbar vertebra (Fig. 4 - 43).

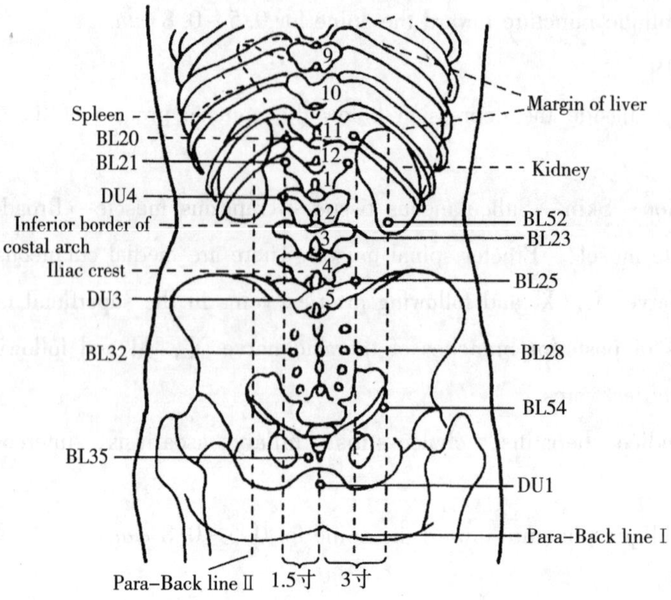

Fig. 4 – 43

Layers of dissection: Skin→Subcutaneous tissue→Aponeurosis of broadest muscle of back and superficial layer of thoracolumbar fascia→Erector spinal muscle. There are cutaneous branches of posterior branches of lumbar nerve Ⅱ, Ⅲ and following arteries/veins in the superficial layer. In the deep layer are muscular branches of posterior branches of lumbar nerve Ⅱ, Ⅲ and following dorsal branches of lumbar arteries/veins.

Indications: Urogenital system diseases, backache.

Manipulation: Perpendicular puncture for 0.5 ~ 1 *cun*.

14. Dachangshu (BL25).

Location: 1.5 *cun* beside the depression below the spinous process of the 4th lumbar vertebra (Fig. 4 – 43).

Layers of dissection: Skin→Subcutaneous tissue→Apneurosis of broadest muscle of back and superficial layer of thoracolumbar fascia→Erector spinal muscle. There are cutaneous branches of posterior branches of lumbar nerve Ⅳ, Ⅴ and following arteries/veins in the superficial layer. In the deep layer are muscular branches of posterior branches of lumbar nerve Ⅳ, Ⅴ and following branches of arteries/veins.

Indications: Intestinal diseases, backache.

Manipulation: Perpendicular puncture for 0.5 ~ 1.5 *cun*.

15. Ciliao (BL32).

Location: On the second posterior sacral foramen and inferior medial to the lower part of the posterior superior iliac spine (Fig. 4 – 43).

Layers of dissection: Skin→Subcutaneous tissue→Erector spinal muscle→Posterior sacral foramina Ⅱ. There are middle cluneal nerves in the superficial layer. In the deep layer are sacral nerve Ⅱ, posterior branches of lateral sacral arteries/veins.

Indications: pelvic disease, lower back and leg pain.

Manipulation: Perpendicular puncture for 0.8 ~ 1.5 *cun*.

16. Huiyang (BL35).

Location: 0.5 *cun* beside the coccyx (Fig. 4 -43).

Layers of dissection: Skin→Subcutaneous tissue→Greatest gluteal muscle→tendon of levator muscle of anus. There are middle cluneal nerves in the superficial layer. In the deep layer are branches of inferior gluteal artery/veins and inferior gluteal nerve.

Indications: Impotent, nocturnal emission, prostatitis, appendagitis, irregular menstruation, hemorrhoid.

Manipulation: Perpendicular puncture for 1 ~ 1.5 *cun*.

17. Chengfu (BL36).

Location: Right in the middle of the inferior cluneal transverse crease (Fig. 4 -40).

Layers of dissection: Skin→Subcutaneous tissue→Greatest gluteal muscle→long head of biceps muscle of thigh and semitendinous muscle. There are branches of posterior cutaneous nerve of thigh and inferior cluneal nerves in the superficial layer. In the deep layer are trunk of posterior cutaneous nerve of thigh, ischiadic nerve and following artery/veins.

Indications: Protrusion of lumbar intervertebral disc, piriform muscle syndrome, hemorrhoid.

Manipulation: Perpendicular puncture for 1 ~ 1.5 *cun*.

18. Weizhong (BL40).

Location: Right in the middle of the popliteal fossa (Fig. 4 -40).

Layers of dissection: Skin → Subcutaneous tissue → between medial head and lateral head of gastrocnemius muscle. There are branches of posterior cutaneous nerve of thigh and small saphenous vein in the superficial layer. In the deep layer are tibial nerve, popliteal artery/vein and sural arteries.

Indications: Acute or chronic backache, sciatica and lower extremities paralysis.

Manipulation: Perpendicular puncture for 1 ~ 1.5 *cun*, or induce bleeding.

Reference: With Yinjiao (RN7), Ashi acupoints for acute lumbar strain, with Taixi (KI3) for pyogenic infection on the nape hair line. Bleeding with Quze (PC3) for acute gastroenteritis, vomiting and diarrhea.

19. Zhibian (BL54).

Location: 3*cun* beside the lower end of the spinous process of the 4th sacral vertebra (Fig. 4 -40).

Layers of dissection: Skin→Subcutaneous tissue→Greatest gluteal muscle→Middle gluteal muscle→ Least gluteal muscle. There are middle cluneal nerves and inferior nerves in the superficial layer. In the deep layer is superior/inferior gluteal artery/vein and superior/inferior gluteal nerve.

Indications: Protrusion of lumbar intervertebral disc, piriform muscle syndrome and sacro-iliac joints injury.

Manipulation: Perpendicular puncture for 1 ~ 1.5 *cun*.

20. Chengshan (BL57).

Location: Below the belly of the gastrocnemius muscle, midway between Weizhong (BL40) and Kunlun (BL60) (Fig. 4 -40).

Layers of dissection: Skin→Subcutaneous tissue→Gastrocnemius→Soleus muscle. There are small saphenous vein and medial cutaneous nerve of calf in the superficial layer. In the deep layer are tibial nerve and posterior tibial artery/veins.

Indications: leg pain, calf muscle spasm, lower extremities paralysis, hemorrhoids and proctoptosis.

Manipulation: Perpendicular puncture for 0.5 ~ 1.2 *cun*.

21. Kunlun (BL60).

Location: In the depression between the tendo calcaneus and the lateral malleolus, at the same level as the apex of the lateral malleolus (Fig. 4 – 40).

Layers of dissection: Skin → Subcutaneous tissue → loose connective tissue in front of calcaneal tendon. There are sural nerve and small saphenous vein in the superficial layer. In the deep layer are branches of fibular artery/veins.

Indications: Headache, stiff neck, backache, epistaxis (nose bleeding), leg and ankle diseases.

Manipulation: Perpendicular puncture for 0.5 ~ 1*cun*.

22. Zhiyin (BL67).

Location: About 0.1*cun* behind the lateral corner of the nail of the little toe (Fig. 4 – 40).

Layers of dissection: Skin→Subcutaneous tissue→Root of nail. There are dorsal digital nerves of foot of lateral dorsal cutaneous nerve and rete of dorsal digital arteries/veins in this area.

Indications: Malposition of fetus (moxibustion), dystocia (difficult labor), headache, rhinitis.

Manipulation: Shallow puncture.

4.3.12.4 Less commonly used acupoints

Meichong (BL3): 0.5 *cun* within the natural line of the hair, right above BL2.

Tongtian (BL7): 4 *cun* above the natural line of the hair, and 1.5 *cun* beside the median line.

Yuzhen (BL9): On the lateral part of the upper margin of the external occipital protuberance, and 1.3 *cun* beside the median line.

Jueyinshu (BL14): 1.5 *cun* beside the lower end of the spinous process of the 5th thoracic vertebras.

Dushu (BL16): 1.5 *cun* beside the lower end of the spinous process of the 6th thoracic vertebra.

Sanjiaoshu (BL22): 1.5 *cun* beside the lower end of the spinous process of the 1st lumbar vertebra.

Qihaishu (BL24): 1.5 *cun* beside the lower end of the spinous process of the 3rd lumbar vertebra.

Guanyuanshu (BL26): 1.5 *cun* beside the lower end of the spinous process of the 5th lumbar vertebra.

Xiaochangshu (BL27): 1.5 *cun* beside the spinous process of sacral vertebral, just level with the 1st posterior sacral foramen.

Pangguangshu (BL28): 1.5 *cun* beside the spinous process of sacral vertebra, just level with the 2nd posterior sacral foramen.

Shangliao (BL31): On the 1st posterior sacral foramen and midway between the lower part of the posterior superior iliac spine and the median line.

Zhongliao (BL33): On the 3rd posterior sacral foramen.

Xialiao (BL34): On the 4th posterior sacral foramen.

Yinmen (BL37): 6 *cun* below BL36, and in the line of BL36 to BL40.

Weiyang (BL39): On the lateral side of the popliteal fossa, along the inner margin of the biceps femoris muscle.

Gaohuang (BL43): 3 *cun* beside the lower end of the spinous process of the 4th thoracic vertebra.

Shentang (BL44): 3 *cun* beside the lower end of the spinous process of the 5th thoracic vertebra.

Geguan (BL46): 3 *cun* beside the lower end of the spinous process of the 7th thoracic vertebra.

Zhishi (BL52): 3 *cun* beside the lower end of the spinous process of the 2nd lumber vertebra.

Feiyang (BL58): 7 *cun* above BL60, 1 *cun* inferior lateral to BL57.

Fuyang (BL59): 3 *cun* above BL60.

Pucan (BL61): Directly below BL60, lateral to calcaneus, at the junction of the red and white skin.

Shenmai (BL62): In the depression below the lateral malleolus.

Jinmen (BL63): Anterior and inferior to the lateral malleolus, in the depression on the lower border of the cuboid bone.

Jinggu (BL64): On the inferior part of the tuberosity of the 5th metatarsal bone, at the junction of the red and white skin.

Shugu (BL65): Posterior lateral to the head of the 5th metatarsal bone, at the junction of the red and white skin.

Zutonggu (BL66): In the depression on the anterior lateral part of the 5th metatarsal bone, at the junction of the red and white skin.

4. 3. 13 Ren Meridian (RN)

4. 3. 13. 1 General information

This meridian has 24 acupoints. The first acupoint is Huiyin (RN1) and the last acupoint is Chengjiang (RN24). The main indications include diseases of their relevant organs and tissues in abdomino-thoracic region respectively.

4. 3. 13. 2 The main course of the meridian

This meridian starts from the inside of the lower abdomen and emerges from the perineum. It goes anteriorly to the pubic region and ascends along the anterior midline to the throat. Ascending further, it passes through the neck, face and enters the orbital region (Fig. 4 -44).

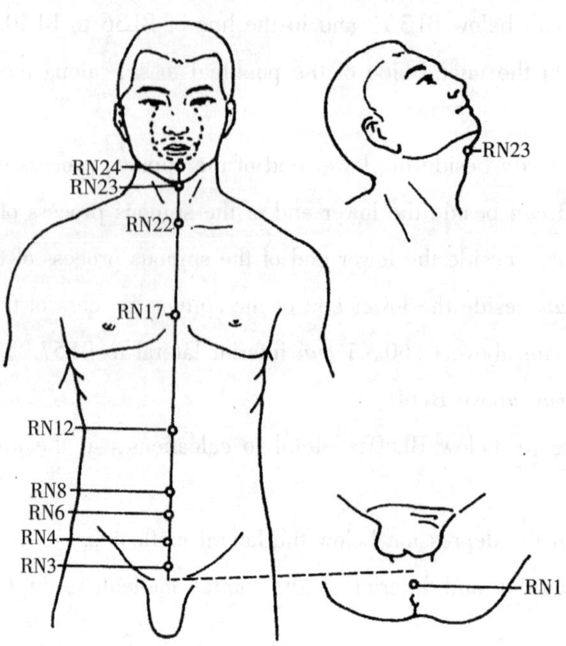

Fig. 4 – 44

4. 3. 13. 3　Commonly used acupoints

1. Guanyuan (RN4).

Location: 3 *cun* below the umbilicus, on the anterior midline (Fig. 4 – 44).

Layers of dissection: Skin→Subcutaneous tissue→Linea alba of abdomen→Transverse fascia→Extraperitoneal adiposity→Parietal peritoneum. There are anterior cutaneous branch of anterior branch of thoracic nerve Ⅻ and branches of superficial epigastric artery/vein in the superficial layer. In the deep layer are branches of anterior branch of thoracic nerve Ⅻ.

Indications: Nocturnal emission, impotence, irregular menstruation, pelvic inflammation, prolapse of uterus, retention of urine, enuresis, and weakness syndrome.

Manipulation: Perpendicular puncture for 0. 5 ~ 1. 2 *cun*. After the patient passing his water.

Reference: *Bian Que Heart Book*: This acupoint is chosen for moxibustion during the season changing between summer and fall to help people get used to the cold and hot weather. *Holy Peaceful Benevolent Prescriptions*: it is forbidden to puncture this acupoint in pregnant women. Modern studies in urine retention patients who received the acupuncture on RN4 Zhongji and Qugu show that in the patients whose vesical nerve was intact, when we twirled the needle, the vesical sphincter would contract, and the pressure in the bladder would increase; when we stopped twirling the needle, the sphincter would relax and the pressure would decrease. But in the patients who were in spinal shock stage and whose sacral nerves were injured, acupuncture on this acupoint had no effect. Qihai (RN6) and this acupoint have tonifying effects and can be used as health care acupoints.

2. Qihai (RN6).

Location: 1. 5 *cun* below the umbilicus, on the anterior midline (Fig. 4 – 44).

Layers of dissection: Skin→Subcutaneous tissue→Linea alba of abdomen→Transverse fascia→Extraperitoneal adiposity→Parietal peritoneum. There are anterior cutaneous branch of anterior branch of thoracic nerve Ⅺ and rete of umbilical part in the superficial layer. In the deep layer are branches of anterior branch of thoracic nerve Ⅺ.

Indications: Acute or chronic enteritis, dysentery, acute enteroparalysis, urethra infection, retention of urine, enuresis, impotence, prospermia, irregular menstruation, prolapse of the uterus, gastroptosis, prolapse of the rectum, weakness syndrome.

Manipulation: Perpendicular puncture for 0.5 ~ 1.2 *cun*. It is *forbidden* to use this acupoint in pregnant women.

3. Shenque (RN8).

Location: The center of the umbilicus (Fig. 4 –44).

Layers of dissection: Skin→Subcutaneous tissue→Parietal peritoneum. There are anterior cutaneous branch of anterior branch of thoracic nerve Ⅹ and rete of umbilical part in the superficial layer. In the deep layer are branches of anterior branch of thoracic nerve Ⅹ.

Indications: Gastroenteritis, collapse syndrome.

Manipulation: In ancient time, it was difficult to perform disinfection on the acupoint. Therefore, salt-partition moxibustion was commonly used on this acupoint.

4. Zhongwan (RN12).

Location: 4 *cun* above the umbilicus, on the anterior midline (Fig. 4 –44).

Layers of dissection: Skin→Subcutaneous tissue→Linea alba of abdomen→Transverse fascia→Extraperitoneal adiposity→Parietal peritoneum. There are anterior cutaneous branch of anterior branch of thoracic nerve Ⅷ and branches of superficial epigastric vein in the superficial layer. In the deep layer are branches of anterior branch of thoracic nerve Ⅷ.

Indications: Ulcers, gastrospasm, gastroptosis, gastritis, phrenospasm, anorexia, enteritis.

Manipulation: Perpendicular puncture for 0.5 ~1.2 *cun*.

5. Danzhong (RN17).

Location: Midway between the nipples, and in a level of the 4th intercostals space, on the anterior midline of the sternum (Fig. 4 –44).

Layers of dissection: Skin→Subcutaneous tissue→Body of sternum. There are anterior cutaneous branch of intercostals nerve IV and perforating branches of internal thoracic artery/veins in this area.

Indications: Asthma, phrenospasm, coronary heart disease, insufficient lactation, etc.

Manipulation: Perpendicular puncture for 0.3 ~0.5 *cun* or horizontal puncture.

6. Tiantu (RN22).

Location: In the center of the suprasternal fossa (Fig. 4 –44).

Layers of dissection: Skin → Subcutaneous tissue → between the left and right tendon of sternocleidomastoid muscle→up the jugular notch of manubrium sterni→left/right sternothyriod muscle→Pretracheal space. There are medial supraclavicular nerves, platysma and jugular venous arch in the superficial layer. In the deep layer is branchiocephalic trunk, left common carotid artery, arch of aorta and brachiocephalic vein.

Indications: Cough, asthma, faucitis, phrenospasm, and goiter.

Manipulation: First puncture perpendicular for 0.2 ~ 0.3 *cun*, and then insert the needle tip downward along the posterior aspect of the sternum 0.5 ~ 1 *cun*.

7. Lianquan (RN23).

Location: Depression of the upper border of the hyoid bone above the laryngeal prominence (Fig. 4 -44).

Layers of dissection: Skin → Subcutaneous tissue → between right and left digastrics muscle → Mylohyoid muscle → Geniohyoid muscle → Genioglossus. There are branches of cervical branch of facial nerve and superior branches of transverse nerve of neck. In the deep layer are branches of lingual artery/vein, branches of hypoglossal nerve and mylohyoid nerve.

Indications: Hoarseness of voice, motorial aphasia, chronic faucitis, difficulty in swallowing, etc.

Manipulation: Perpendicular puncture for 0.5 ~ 1 *cun*.

8. Chengjiang (RN24).

Location: In the center of the mentolabial groove (Fig. 4 -44).

Layers of dissection: Skin→Subcutaneous tissue→Orbicular muscle of mouth→Depressor muscle of lower lip→Mental muscle. There are mental nerve (the last branch of inferior alveolar nerve) and mental artery/vein in this area.

Indications: Facial paralysis, aphtha, toothache, hysterical aphasia, diabetes, etc.

Manipulation: Oblique puncture for 0.3 ~ 0.5 *cun*.

4.3.13.4 Less commonly used acupoints

Zhongji (RN3): 4 *cun* below the umbilicus, on the anterior midline.

Shimen (RN5): 2 *cun* below the umbilicus, on the anterior midline.

Yinjiao (RN7): 1 *cun* below the umbilicus, on the anterior midline.

Shuifen (RN9): 1 *cun* above the umbilicus, on the anterior midline.

Xiawan (RN10): 2 *cun* above the umbilicus, on the anterior midline.

Jianli (RN11): 3 *cun* above the umbilicus, on the anterior midline.

Shangwan (RN13): 5 *cun* above the umbilicus, on the anterior midline.

Juque (RN14): 6 *cun* above the umbilicus, on the anterior midline.

Jiuwei (RN15): Along the median line, 1 *cun* below the xiphoid process.

Xuanji (RN21): Along the median line, 1 *cun* below RN22.

4.3.14 Du Meridian (DU)

4.3.14.1 General information

The first acupoint is Changqiang, and the last acupoint Yinjiao. There are 28 acupoints. The main indications include febrile diseases, coma, mental disorder and corresponding splanchnopathies.

4.3.14.2 The main course of the meridian

The Du Meridian arises from the lower abdomen and emerges from the perineum. Then it runs posteriorly along the interior of the spinal column to Fengfu (Du16) at the nape, where it enters the brain. It further ascends to the vertex and winds along the forehead to the nasal column. It finally ends at the frenulum (Fig. 4 -45).

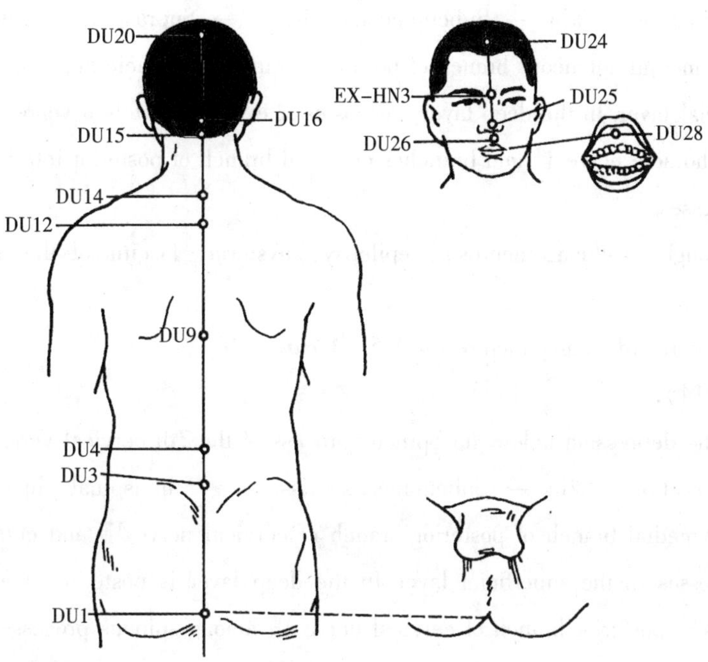

Fig. 4 – 45

4. 3. 14. 3 Commonly used acupoints

1. Yaoyangguan (DU3).

Location: Depression below the spinous process of the 4th lumbar vertebra (Fig. 4 – 45).

Layers of dissection: Skin→Subcutaneous tissue→Supraspinal ligaments→Interspinal ligament→Ligament flava. There are medial branch of posterior branch of lumbar nerve Ⅳ and following artery/veins in the superficial layer. In the deep layer are posterior external vertebral venous plexue, branches of posterior branch of lumbar nerve Ⅳ and branches of dorsal branch of lumbar artery/veins Ⅳ among spinous processes.

Indications: Nocturnal emission, impotence, irregular menstruation, pelvic inflammation, chronic lumbar pain, ankylosing spondylitis, rheumatoid diseases, polio, and paraplegia.

Manipulation: Perpendicular puncture for 0. 5 ~ 1 *cun*.

2. Mingmen (DU4).

Location: Depression below the spinous of the 2nd lumbar vertebra (Fig. 4 – 45).

Layers of dissection: Skin→Subcutaneous tissue→Supraspinal ligaments→Interspinal ligament→Ligament flava. There are medial branch of posterior branch of lumbar Ⅱ and following artery/veins in the superficial layer. In the deep layer are posterior external vertebral venous plexue, branches of posterior branch of lumbar nerve I and branches of dorsal branch of lumbar artery/veins I among spinous processes.

Indications: Nocturnal emission, impotence, prostatitis, irregular menstruation, pelvic inflammation, chronic diarrhea, chronic backache, chronic consumptive diseases.

Manipulation: Perpendicular puncture for 0. 5 ~ 1 *cun*.

3. Shenzhu (DU12).

Location: Depression below the spinous process of the 3rd thoracic vertebra (Fig. 4 – 45).

Layers of dissection: Skin → Subcutaneous tissue → Supraspinal ligaments → Interspinal ligaments. There are medial cutaneous branch of posterior branch of thoracic nerve Ⅲ and following artery/veins in the superficial layer. In the deep layer are posterior external vertebral venous plexus, branches of posterior branch of thoracic nerve Ⅲ and branches of dorsal branch of posterior intercostals artery/veins Ⅲ among spinous processes.

Indications: Cough, asthma, neurosis, epilepsy, hysteria, fascitis of the muscles in neck and back areas.

Manipulation: Perpendicular puncture for 0.5 ~ 1 *cun*.

4. Dazhui (DU14).

Location: At the depression below the Spinous process of the 7th cervical vertebra (Fig. 4 –45).

Layers of dissection: Skin → Subcutaneous tissue → Supraspinal ligaments → Interspinal ligaments. There are medial branch of posterior branch of cervical nerve Ⅷ and cutaneous venous plexus among spinous processes in the superficial layer. In the deep layer is posterior external vertebral venous plexus and branches of posterior branch of cervical nerve Ⅷ among spinous processes.

Indications: Fever, cough, asthma, Sunstroke, mental diseases, cervical spondylopathy, fascitis of the muscles in neck and back areas, etc.

Manipulation: Upward oblique puncture for 0.5 ~ 1 *cun*.

Reference: Study of inflammatory animal model have shown the acupuncture on DU14 could prevent the inflammation when it was not formed; quicken the disappearance of the inflammation when it occurred. When the inflammation was forming, acupuncture on DU14 could delay and relief the development of the inflammation. It is effective for acupuncture on DU14 with Hegu (LI4) and Zusanli (ST36) to treat leukopenia caused by radiotherapy or chemotherapy. Also these 3 acupoints can treat tropical acidophil leukocyte hyperplasia.

5. Yamen (DU15).

Location: Above 0.5 *cun* of middle of the natural line of the hair at the back of the head (Fig. 4 –45).

Layers of dissection: Skin→Subcutaneous tissue→between left and right trapezius muscle→Nuchal ligament (between left and right splenius muscle of head→between left and right semispinal muscle of head). There are occipital nerve Ⅷ and cutaneous veins in the superficial layer. In the deep layer are branches of posterior branch of cervical nerve Ⅱ, Ⅲ, posterior external vertebral venous plexue and branches of occipital artery/veins.

Indications: Post-apoplectic aphasia, hyoid muscle paralysis, deaf and dumbness, mental diseases, epilepsy.

Manipulation: Puncture toward the mandible for 0.5 ~ 1 *cun*.

This acupoint being near the medulla oblongata, don' t puncture too deep or lift or thrust the needle in big amplitude. Moxibustion is forbidden in this acupoint (Fig. 4 –46).

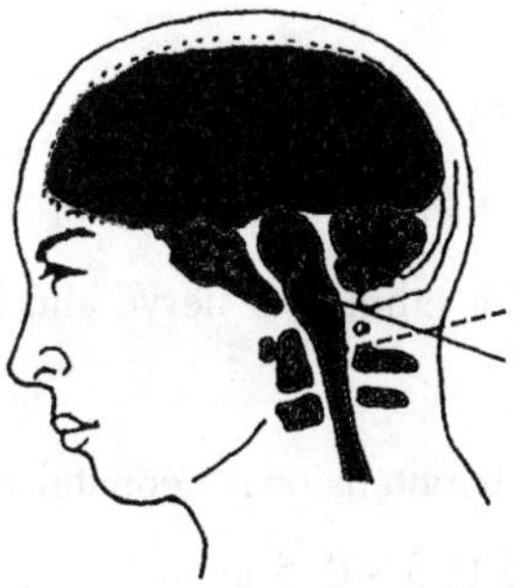

Fig. 4 – 46

6. Fengfu (DU16).

Location: In the depression above 1 *cun* of the midpoint of the posterior hairline (Fig. 4 – 45).

Layers of dissection: Skin→Subcutaneous tissue→between the left and right tendon of trapezius muscle→Nuchal ligament (between left and right semispinal muscle of head) →between left and right greater/lesser posterior straight muscle of head. There are branches of greater occipital nerve, occipital nerve Ⅲ and branches of occipital artery/veins in the superficial layer. In the deep layer are branches of suboccipital nerve.

Indications: Common cold, headache, vertigo, motor aphasia, hyoid muscle paralysis, cervical spondylopathy, mental disorder, epilepsy.

Manipulation: Puncture toward the mandible for 0.5 ~ 1 *cun*. Don' t puncture upwards, which can hurt medulla oblongata through the foramen magnum. Moxibustion is forbidden in this acupoint.

7. Baihui (DU20).

Location: 7*cun* directly above the midpoint of the posterior hairline, or directly above the apex auriculae, on the midline of the head (Fig. 4 – 45).

Layers of dissection: Skin → Subcutaneous tissue → Galea aponeurotica → porous tissue under aponeurosis. There are branches of greater occiptal nerve, frontal nerve and rete composed of left/right superficial temporal artery/veins in the area.

Indications: Headache, dizziness, hypertension, sequela of stroke, insomnia, neurosis, senile dementia, mental diseases, hysteria, visceroptosis (moxibustion), low immune function (moxibustion), shock.

Manipulation: Puncture horizontally for 0.5 ~ 1 *cun*, forwards or backwards.

8. Shenting (DU24).

Location: 0.5 *cun* behind the midpoint of the anterior hairline (Fig. 4 – 45).

Layers of dissection: Skin→Subcutaneous tissue→between right and left front belly of occipitofrontal muscle→loose connective tissue under aponeurosis. There are branches of supratrochlear nerve of frontal nerve and branches of frontal artery/veins in the area.

Indications: Headache, dizziness, insomnia, neurosis, mental diseases, epilepsy, rhinitis, conjunctivitis.

Manipulation: Horizontally puncture for 0.5 ~ 1 *cun*.

9. Suliao (DU25).

Location: On the tip of the nose (Fig. 4 – 45).

Layers of dissection: Skin → Subcutaneous tissue → cartilage of nasal septum and lateral nasal cartilage. There are lateral nasal branches of anterior ethmoidal nerve and lateral (dorsal) branch of nose of facial artery/vein in this area.

Indications: Rhinitis, nasal polyp, shock, hypotension, neonatal asphyxia, etc.

Manipulation: Oblique punctures upwards for 0. 3 ~ 0. 5 *cun*.

10. Shuigou (DU26).

Location: At the lower border of the upper 1/3 of the philtrum (Fig. 4 – 45).

Layers of dissection: Skin→Subcutaneous tissue→Orbicular muscle of mouth. There are branches of infraorbital nerve and superior labial artery/vein in this area.

Indications: Coma, respiratory failure, facial paralysis, mental diseases, hysteria, acute lumbar muscle sprain.

Manipulation: Oblique puncture upwards for 0. 3 ~ 0. 5 *cun*, or press the acupoint with a fingernail.

4. 3. 14. 4 Less commonly used acupoints

Changqiang (DU1): Below the tip of the coccyx, at the midway from the tip of the coccyx to the anal.

Yaoshu (DU2): On the posterior midline, in the middle process of the sacral hiatus.

Xuanshu (DU5): On the posterior midline, below the spinous process of the 1st lumber vertebra.

Jizhong (DU6): On the posterior midline, below the spinous process of the 11th thoracic vertebra.

Zhongshu (DU7): On the posterior midline, below the spinous process of the 10th thoracic vertebra.

Jinsuo (DU8): On the posterior midline, below the spinous process of the 9th thoracic vertebra.

Zhiyang (DU9): On the posterior midline, below the spinous process of the 7th thoracic vertebra.

Lingtai (DU10): On the posterior midline, below the spinous process of the 6th thoracic vertebra.

Shendao (DU11): On the posterior midline, below the spinous process of the 5th thoracic vertebra.

Taodao (DU13): On the posterior midline, below the spinous process of the 1st thoracic vertebra.

Naohu (DU17): 2. 5 *cun* above the middle of the posterior natural line of the hair (1. 5 *cun* above DU16).

Qiangjian (DU18): 4 *cun* above the middle of the posterior natural line of the hair (1. 5 *cun* above DU17).

Qianding (DU21): 3. 5 *cun* above the middle of the natural line of the hair on the forehead (1. 5 *cun* before DU20).

Shangxing (DU23): 1 *cun* above the middle of the natural line of the hair on the forehead.

Yinjiao (DU28): In the inner surface of the upper lip, on the conjunction of the lip chalaza and upper gums.

4.4 The Extraordinary Acupoints

Extraordinary acupoints refer to the effective acupoints found in practice and they are not included in the Fourteen Meridians. Many extraordinary acupoints were recorded in past dynasties. As many as 187 extraordinary acupoints were recorded in *Valuable Prescriptions for Emergency* of Tang Dynasty and only 19 of them will be introduced in this book. Among the acupoints, some of them lie outside the Fourteen Meridians; some of them have very special locations; sometimes several acupoints have the same name, which leads to the difficulty of assigning them to a specific meridian. And some of them lie in the courses of the Fourteen Meridians and it's difficult to distinguish them from the acupoints belonging to the Fourteen Meridians. The features of extraordinary acupoints imply that the existing meridian theories might be revised and supplemented, which may be insightful for innovation of modern meridian theory.

4.4.1 Acupoints of the Head and Neck (EX-HN)

4.4.1.1 Sishencong (EX-HN1)

Location: 1 *cun* in front of, behind, left and right to Baihui (DU20). There are 4 points in total (Fig. 4-47).

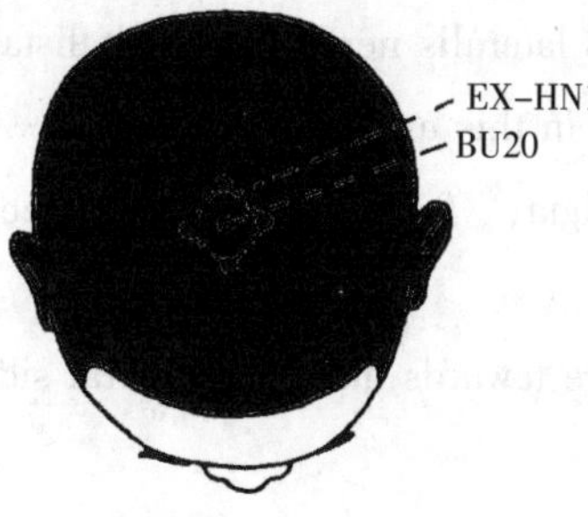

Fig. 4-47

Layers of dissection: Skin→Subcutaneous tissue→galea aponeurotica→loose connective tissue under aponeurotica. There are meshes of occipital artery/veins, parietal branch of superficial temporal artery/vein and supra-orbital artery/vein. There are also greater occipital nerve, temporal nerve and frontal branch of supra-orbital nerve.

Indications: Neurosis, headache, dizziness, insomnia, cerebral paralysis, cerebral dysgenesis, hemiplegia, epilepsy.

Manipulation: Horizontal puncture for 0.5 ~ 1 *cun*.

4.4.1.2 Yintang (EX-HN3)

Location: At the midway of the medial ends of the eyebrows (Fig. 4-48).

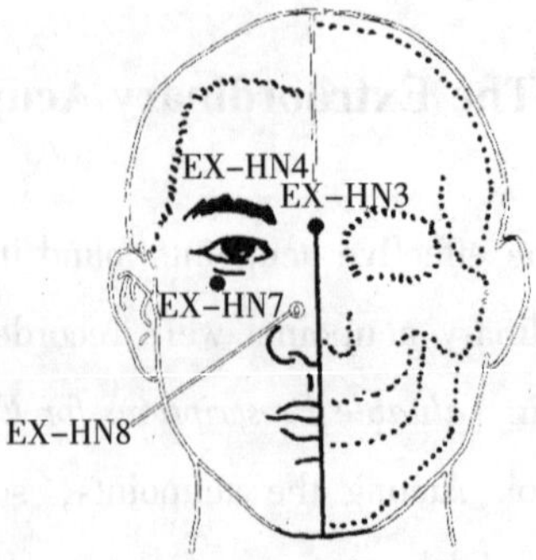

Fig. 4 – 48

Layers of dissection: Skin→Subcutaneous tissue→procerus muscle. There are nervus supratrochlearis, branches of ophthalmic arteries, and arteria. Arteria frontalis and its following veins in this area.

Indications: Headache, neurosis, dizziness, acute conjunctivitis, rhinitis, facial paralysis, hypertension, acne.

Manipulation: Horizontal puncture for 0.3 ~ 0.5 *cun*, downwards.

4.4.1.3 Yuyao (EX – HN4)

Location: At the midpoint of the eyebrow (Fig. 4 – 48).

Layers of dissection: Skin → Subcutaneous tissue → orbicularis oculi muscle → frontal belly of occipitofrontal muscle. There are ramus lateralis nervi supraorbitalista, branches of facial nerve and lateral branches of supra – orbital artery/vein in this area.

Indications: Trigeminal neuralgia, facial paralysis, facial spasm, eyelid drop, acute conjunctivitis, retinal hemorrhage.

Manipulation: Horizontal puncture towards medial or lateral side for 0.4 ~ 0.6 *cun*.

4.4.1.4 Taiyang (EX – HN5)

Location: In the depression about 1 *cun* behind the midpoint between the lateral end of the eyebrow and the outer canthus (Fig. 4 – 49).

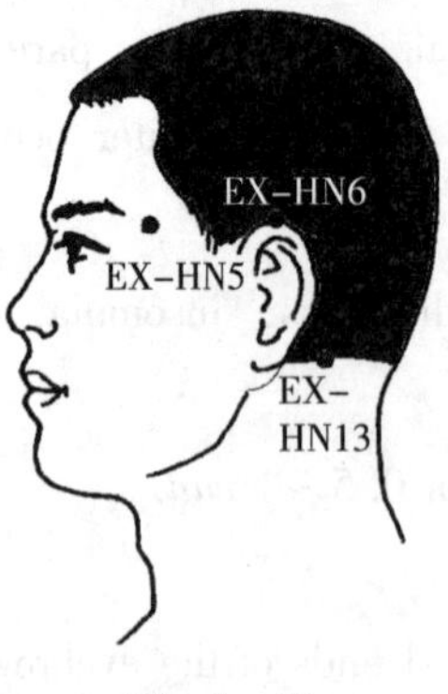

Fig. 4 – 49

Layers of dissection: Skin → Subcutaneous tissue → orbicularis oculi muscle → temporal fascia → temporal muscle. There are branches of zygomaticofacial nerve, temporal branches and zygomatic branch of facial nerve, zygomatic branch of mandibular nerve, and branches of superficial temporal arteries/veins in this area.

Indications: Headache, facial paralysis, trigeminal nuralgia, hypertension, vertigo, acute conjunctivitis, eyelid infection, optic atrophy, retinal hemorrhage, chalazion, toothache, etc.

Manipulation: Oblique puncture for 0.5 ~ 0.8 *cun*, downwards.

4.4.1.5 Erjian (EX - HN6)

Location: When you fold the auriculae forward, it locates on the apex auriculae (Fig. 4 - 49).

Layers of dissection: Skin→Subcutaneous tissue→auricular cartilage. There are anterior auricular branches of superficial temporal arteries/veins, posterior auricular branches of posterior auricular arteries/veins, anterior auricular branches of auriculotemporal nerve, posterior branches of lesser occipital nerve and auricular branches of facial nerve in this area.

Indication: Trachoma, acute conjunctivitis, keratitis, chalazion, migraine, acne, etc.

Manipulation: Perpendicalar puncture for 0.1 ~ 0.2 *cun*, or induce bleeding by Three-edged needle.

4.4.1.6 Qiuhou (EX - HN7)

Location: At the junction of lateral 1/4 and medial 3/4 of the inferior border of orbit (Fig. 4 - 48).

Layers of dissection: Skin→Subcutaneous tissue→orbicular oculi muscle→adipose body of orbit→between inferior oblique muscle and inferior wall of orbit. There are infraorbital nerve, branches of facial nerve, branches and tributaries of infraorbital artery/veins in the superficial layer. In the deep layer are inferior division of oculomotor nerve, branches and tributaries of Ophthalmic arteries/veins, branches and tributaries of infraorbital arteries/veins.

Indications: Acute conjunctivitis, myopia, glaucoma, retinitis, optic atrophy, optic neuritis, retinal pigmentolysis, cataract in early stage.

Manipulation: Push and fix the eyeball to the medial side of the orbit with your left thumb, slowly puncture for 0.5 ~ 1.5 *cun* through the inferior side of the orbit. Press the acupoint for 1 ~ 3 minutes to avoid bleeding after removal of the needle.

4.4.1.7 Shangyingxiang (Bitong) (EX - HN8)

Location: In the depression of the upper end of the nasolabial groove, at the juncture of nasal alar cartilage and turbinate (Fig. 4 - 48).

Layers of dissection: Skin→Subcutaneous tissue→Levator labii superioris alaerque nasi. There are nervus supraorbitalis, branches of nervus infratrochlearis, buccal branch of facial nerve, arteries and veins of inner canthus.

Indications: Acute or chronic rhinitis, sinusitis, nasal polyp, conjunctivitis, dacryocystitis, acne.

Manipulation: Oblique puncture toward upper and medial side for 0.3 ~ 0.5 *cun*.

4.4.1.8 Jingbailao (EX - HN15)

Location: 2 *cun* directly above Dazhui (DU14), 1 *cun* lateral to the posterior median line (Fig. 4 - 50).

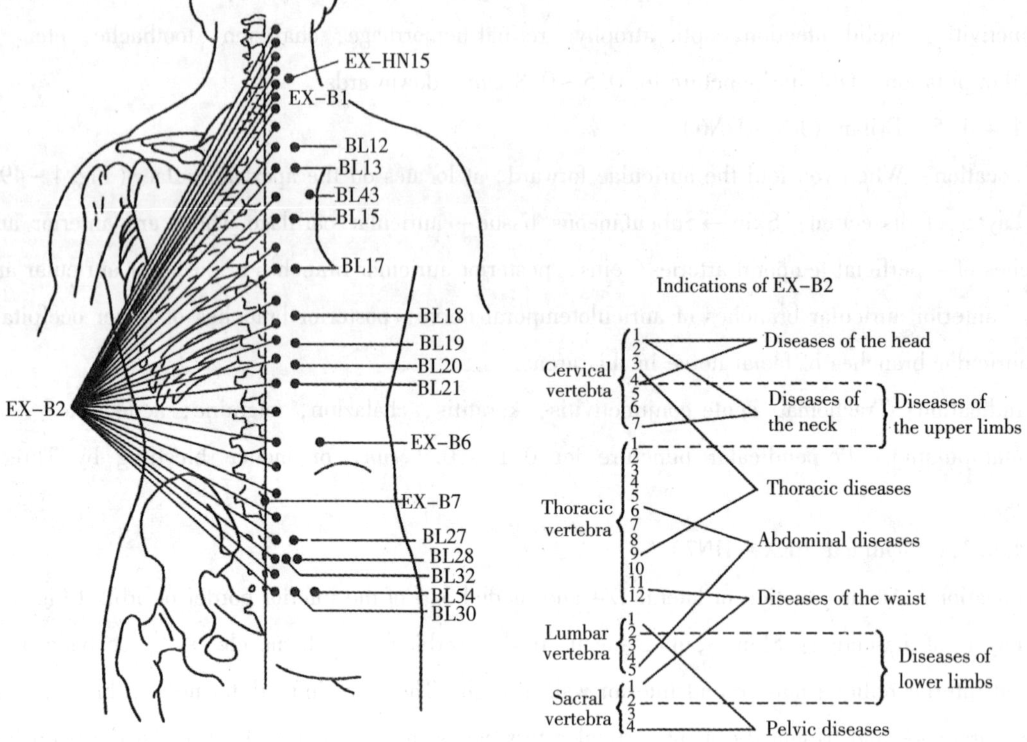

Fig. 4 – 50

Layers of dissection: Skin→Subcutaneous tissue→Trapezius muscle→Serratus posterior superior→Head and neck splenius→Semispinalis capitis muscle→Multifidus muscle. There are cutaneous branches of the 4th and 5th cervical dorsal rami nerve in the superficial layer. In the deep layer there are the branches of the 4th and 5th cervical dorsal rami nerve.

Indications: Asthma, whooping cough, stiff neck, fascitis of the muscles in the neck and back areas, cervical spondylopathy, cervical lymphadenovarix, neurosis.

Manipulation: Perpendicular puncture for 0. 5 ~ 1 *cun*.

4. 4. 2 Acupoints of the Back (EX –B)

4. 4. 2. 1 Dingchuan (EX – B1)

Location: 0. 5 *cun* lateral to Dazhui (DU14) (Fig. 4 – 50).

Layers of dissection: Skin→Subcutaneous tissue→Trapezius muscle→Rhomboid muscle→Serratus posterior superior→Neck splenius→Erector spinae. There are medial cutaneous branches of the 8th cervical dorsal rami nerve in the superficial layer. In the deep layer there are the branches and tributaries of transverse cervical arteries/veins, the 8th cervical dorsal rami nerve, the first rami posteriores nervorum thoracicorumta.

Indications: Chronic bronchitis, asthma, stiffneck, fasciitis of the muscles in the neck and back areas, cervical spondylopathy, nettle rash.

Manipulation: Perpendicular puncture for 0. 6 ~ 1. 2 *cun*.

4.4.2.2 Jiaji (Huatuo jiaji) (EX-B2)

Location: 0.5 *cun* beside the lower border of each spinous process from the 1st thoracic vertebra to the 5th lumbar vertebra (Fig. 4-50).

Layers of dissection: Because of different locations, different acupoints are related to slightly different muscles, blood vessels and nerves. The general layers of dissection are: Skin→Subcutaneous tissue→superficial muscles (Trapezius muscle, latissimus dorsi, Rhomboid muscle, Serratus posterior superior, Serratus posterior inferior) →deep muscles (Erector spinae, transversospinales). There are medial cutaneous branches and following arteries/veins of the first thoracic nerve to the fifth lumbar nerve. In the deep layer there are muscular branches of the first thoracic nerve to the fifth lumbar nerve, posterior intercostal arteries/veins, dorsal branches or tributaries of lumbar arteries/veins.

Indications: These points on the upper portion of the chest can be used to treat diseases of the heart and lung and diseases in upper limbs; the points on the lower portion of the chest, gastrointestinal diseases; the points in the lumbar region, diseases in the lumbar and abdominal regions and diseases in the lower limbs. All these points can treat diseases in the relevant spinal column respectively.

4.4.2.3 Yaoyan (EX-B6)

Location: In the depression 3 ~ 4 *cun* lateral to the lower border of the spinous process of the 4th lumbar vertebra (Fig. 4-50).

Layers of dissection: Skin→Subcutaneous tissue→Superficial layers of thoracolumbar fascia and aponeurosis of latissimus dorsi→musculus iliocostalis→deep layers of thoracolumbar fascia→quadratus lumborum. There are superior clunial nerves, posterior branch of the 4th lumbar nerve in the superficial layer. In the deep layer there are muscular branches of the 4th lumbar nerve, branches and tributaries of the 4th lumbar arteries/veins.

Indication: Acute or chronic lumbar sprain, iliolumbar ligament injury, irregular menstruation, prostatitis, nephritis, diabetes.

Manipulation: Perpendicular puncture for 0.5 ~ 1 *cun*.

4.4.2.4 Shiqizhui (EX-B7)

Location: Depression below the spinous process of the 5th lumbar vertebra (Fig. 4-50).

Layers of dissection: Skin → Subcutaneous tissue → Supraspinal ligament → Interspinous ligaments. There are posterior cutaneous branch of the 5th lumbar nerve and following arteries/veins in the superficial layer. In the deep layer there are posterior branches of the 5th lumbar nerve, and interspinal external vertebral veins.

Indications: Lower back pain, dysmenorrhea, prostatitis and enuresis.

Manipulation: Perpendicular puncture for 0.5 ~ 0.8 *cun*.

4.4.3 Acupoints of the Upper Extremities (EX-UE)

4.4.3.1 Wailaogong (EX-UE8)

Location: At the dorsum of the hand, between the second and third metacarpo-phalangeal joint, 0.5 *cun* behind the joint, also called stiff neck point (Fig. 4-51).

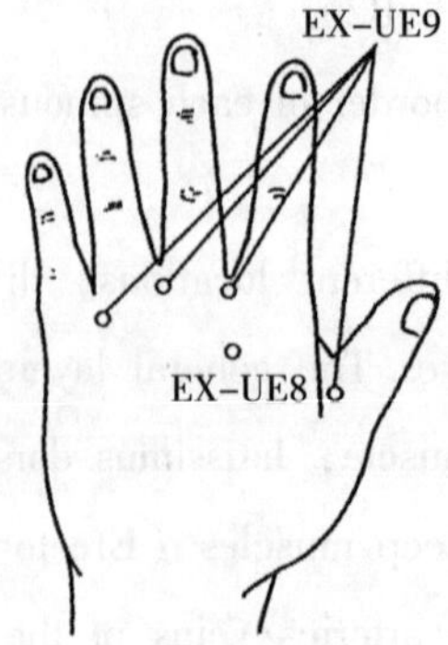

Fig. 4 – 51

Layers of dissection: Skin → Subcutaneous tissue → second dorsal interosseous → second dorsal interosseous. There are superficial branches of radial nerve (dorsal digital nerve), dorsal venous rete of hand and dorsal metacarpal artery in this area.

Indications: Stiff neck, numbness of fingers, stiff fingers.

Manipulation: Perpendicular puncture for 0. 5 ~ 0. 8 *cun*.

4. 4. 3. 2 Baxie (EX – UE9)

Location: At the junction of the red and white skin of the hand webs. There are 8 points at both hands, also called stiff neck point (Fig. 4 – 51).

Layers of dissection: Skin→Subcutaneous tissue→musculi interossei palmares→Lumbricales. In the superficial layer, there are dorsal metacarpal arteries/veins, dorsal digital arteries/veins and dorsal digital nerves. In deep layer, there are common palmer digital arteries/veins, proper palmar digital arteries/veins and proper palmar digital nerves.

Indications: Diseases of finger joint, swelling and numbness of the dorsum of the hand, snakebite, cervical spondylopathy, fasciitis of the muscles in the neck and back areas, pharyngitis, toothache.

Manipulation: Oblique punctures toward the area between the metacarpals for 0. 3 ~ 0. 5 *cun*, or induce bleeding.

4. 4. 3. 3 Sifeng (EX – UE10)

Location: At the palmar surface, on the midpoint of the transverse creases of the proximal interphalangeal joint of the index, middle, ring and small fingers. Each hand has 4 points (Fig. 4 – 52).

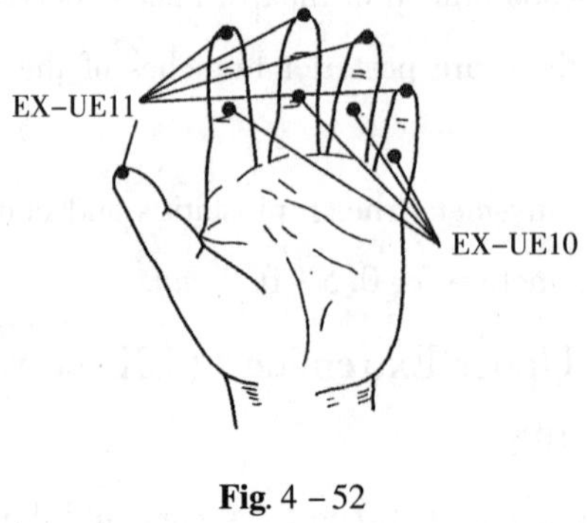

Fig. 4 – 52

Layers of dissection: Skin → Subcutaneous tissue → Finger sinew. Blood vessels of the acupoints:

branches and tributaries of proper palmar digital arteries/vines, subcutaneous veins of fingers. Nerves of the acupoints: there are proper palmar digital nerves in the Sifeng acupoints of the index finger and middle finger. For the ring finger Sifeng acupoint, at the radial side, there are proper palmar digital nerves from the median nerve and there are proper palmar digital nerves from ulnar nerve. In the Sifeng acupoint on the small finger, there are proper palmar digital nerves from ulnar nerve.

Indications: Malnutrition and indigestion syndrome in children, whooping cough.

Manipulation: Puncture superficially, squeeze out some yellowish viscous fluid.

4.4.3.4 Shixuan (EX-UE11)

Location: At the tip of each finger, about 0.1 *cun* behind the nail. There are ten points at both hands (Fig. 4-52).

Layers of dissection: Skin→Subcutaneous tissue. In the Shixuan acupoints on the thumbs, index fingers and middle fingers, there are median nerves. In the Shixuan acupoint on the ring finger, there are median nerves at the radial side and ulnar nerve at the ulnar side. There are ulnar nerves on the small finger.

Indications: Coma, fever, sunstroke, acute faucitis, numbness of fingers.

Manipulation: Induce bleeding by three-edged needle.

4.4.4 Acupoints of the Lower Extremities (EX-LE)

4.4.4.1 Xiyan (EX-LE5)

Location: In the depressions bilateral to the patella ligament, when knee is bent. Each knee has 2 points, lateral one is called Waixiyan and medial one is called Neixiyan (Fig. 4-53).

Layers of dissection: Skin→Subcutaneous tissue→between patellar ligament and medial patellar retinaculum→knee joint and alar fold. In the superficial layer there are the infrapatellar branch of the saphenous nerve and anterior cutaneous branches of the femoral nerve. In the deep layer there are arterial rete and rete venosum.

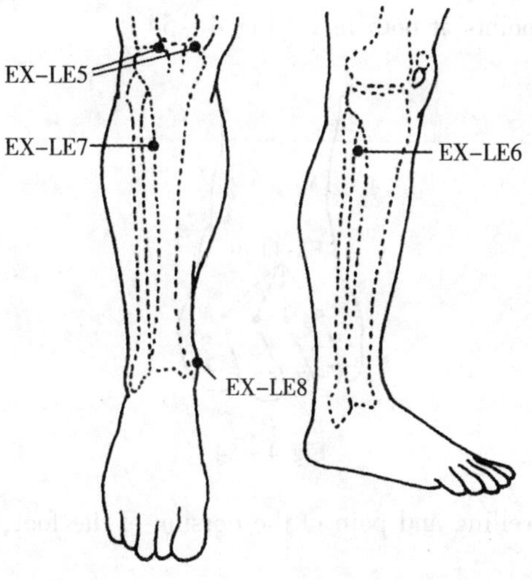

Fig. 4-53

Indications: Arthritis of knee.

Manipulation: Oblique puncture for 0.5~1 *cun* toward the center of the knee or toward opposite Xiyan.

4.4.4.2 Dannang (EX－LE6)

Location: 1～2 *cun* down to the point Yanglingquan (GB34) (Fig. 4－53).

Layers of dissection: Skin→Subcutaneous tissue→peroneus longus. In the superficial layer there are lateral sural cutaneous nerves. In the deep layer there are superficial peroneal nerve, deep peroneal nerve, anterior tibial arteries/veins.

Indications: Acute or chronic cholecystitis, cholelithiasis, biliary ascariasis, oppressed tibialis nerve syndrome.

Manipulation: Perpendicular puncture for 1～2 *cun*.

4.4.4.3 Lanwei (EX－LE7)

Location: About 2 *cun* down to the point Zusanli (ST36) (Fig. 4－53).

Layers of dissection: Skin→Subcutaneous tissue→Anterior tibial muscle→Interosseous membrane→Posterior tibial muscle. In the superficial layer there are lateral sural cutaneous nerves and superficial veins. In the deep layer there are deep peroneal nerve and anterior tibial arteries/veins.

Indications: Simple appendicitis, stomachache.

Manipulation: Perpendicular puncture for 1～1.5 *cun*.

4.4.4.4 Neihuaijian (EX－LE8)

Location: On the tip of the medial malleolus (Fig. 4－53).

Layers of dissection: Skin → Subcutaneous tissue → malleolus medialis. There are medial crural cutaneous branches of the saphenous nerve, malleolus medialis rete of anterior tibial artery, branches of medial anterior malleolus artery and medial malleolus branches of posterior tibial arteries.

Indications: Toothache.

Manipulation: Moxibustion. Acupuncture is forbidden.

4.4.4.5 Bafeng (EX－LE10)

Location: At the junction of the red and white skin of the web margin between the five toes on the dorsum of the foot. There are 8 points at both feet (Fig. 4－54).

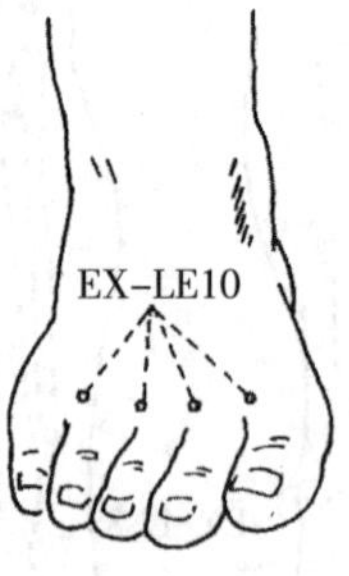

Fig. 4－54

Indications: Headache, swelling and pain of the dorsum of the foot, numbness of toes, snakebite, toothache.

Manipulation: Oblique puncture for 0.5～1 *cun*, upwards.

4.4.4.6 Duyin (EX－LE11)

Location: In the center of the distant phalangophalangeal joint of the second toe, on the sole side

(Fig. 4 – 55).

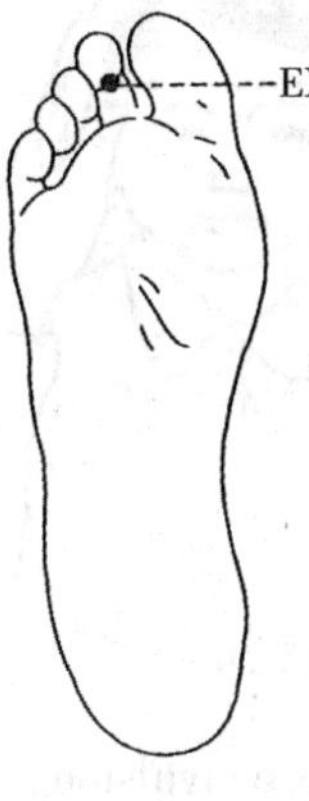

Fig. 4 – 55

Layers of dissection: Skin → Subcutaneous tissue → Long curved tendon and short curved tendon. There are proper planter digital nerves and toe inherent arteries/veins in this area.

Indications: Pain in the chest and hypochondriac region, vomiting, irregular menstruation, orchitis, angina pectoris, coma.

Manipulation: Perpendicular puncture for 0.1 ~ 0.2 *cun*.

4.5 Special Acupoints for Child Massage

Apart from the acupoints, there are some special acupoints used for children. These acupoints are not only in point form, but also in linear form and regional form. These acupoints belong to a group of Extraordinary Acupoints that have a distinctive effect on children. They are specially used for child massage.

4.5.1 Head and Face

4.5.1.1 Tianmen (MA – HF1)

Location: The part above the line between the eyebrows and up to the anterior hair line (Fig. 4 – 56).

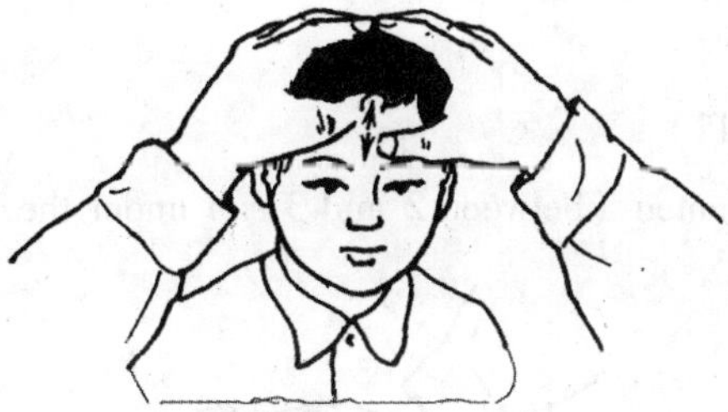

Fig. 4 – 56

Indications: Fever, common cold, headache, listlessness, vigilance and restlessness, etc.

Manipulation: Alternating pushing straight from below to above. The duration is usually 30 ~ 50 repetitions. Bottom-up pushing of the acupoint is also called "pushing Tianmen" or "pushing Zanzhu".

4.5.1.2 Kangong (MA – HF2)

Location: Along the entire length of the eyebrow (Fig. 4 – 57).

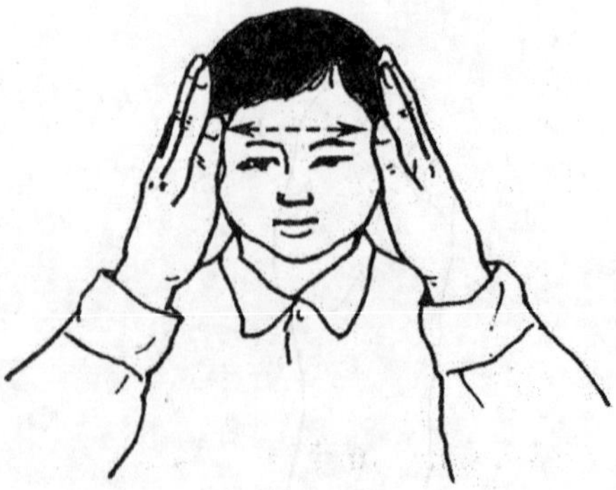

Fig. 4 – 57

Indications: Common cold, fever, infantile convulsion, and headache, etc.

Manipulation: Parting-pushing from the beginning to the end of the eyebrow with the thumbs. The duration is usually 30 ~ 50 times.

4. 5. 1. 3 Tianzhugu (MA – HF3)

Location: The straight line from the middle of the hairline to Dazhui (DU14) (Fig. 4 – 58).

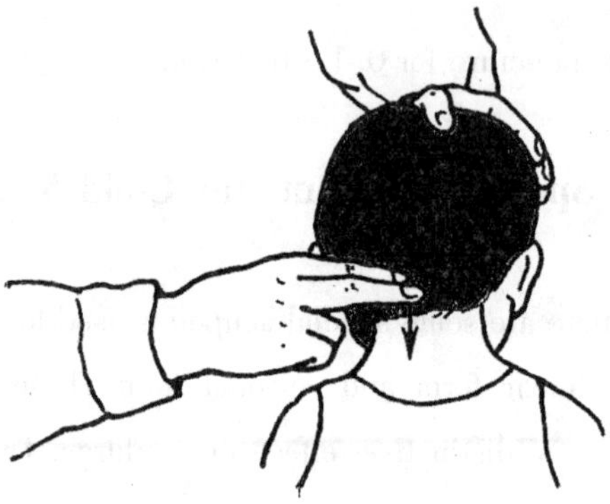

Fig. 4 – 58

Indications: Vomiting, nausea, fever, pharyngitis, infantile convulsion, stiff neck, etc.

Manipulation: Pushing Tianzhugu with the thumb or the index and middle fingers straight downward. The duration is usually 50 ~ 100 times.

4. 5. 2 Trunk

4. 5. 2. 1 Dantian (MA – T1)

Location: On the lower abdomen (between 2 and 3 *cun* under the umbilicus) (Fig. 4 – 59).

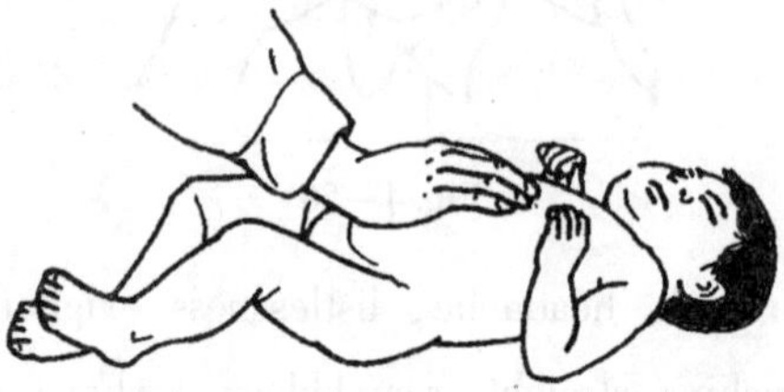

Fig. 4 – 59

Indications: Acute or chronic enteritis, enuresis, urine retention, hernia, and prolapse of the rectum, etc.

Manipulation: Kneading for 50 ~ 100 times, or robbing for 5 minutes.

4.5.2.2 Jizhu (MA – T2)

Location: The straight line from Dazhui (DU14) to Changqiang (DU1) (Fig. 4 – 60).

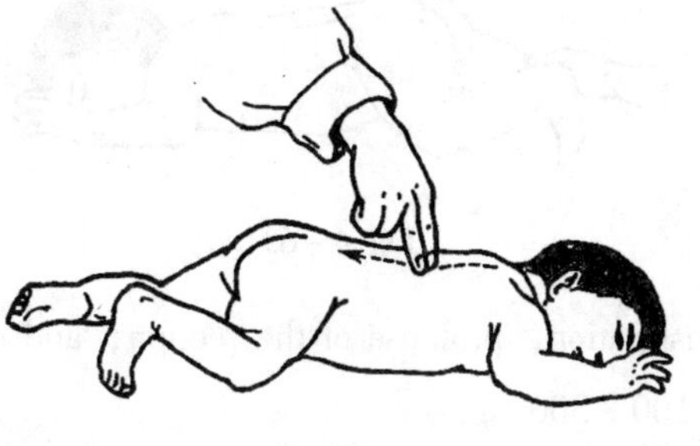

Fig. 4 – 60

Indications: Pushing Jizhu for fever and infantile convulsion. Pinching Jizhu for vomiting, enteritis, and constipation. Also used for children's health care.

Manipulation: Pushing with the palmar faces of the index and middle finger straight downward is called pushing Ji. The number of manipulations is usually 50 ~ 100 times. Pinching upward is called pinching ji, usually 3 ~ 5 times (Fig. 4 – 61).

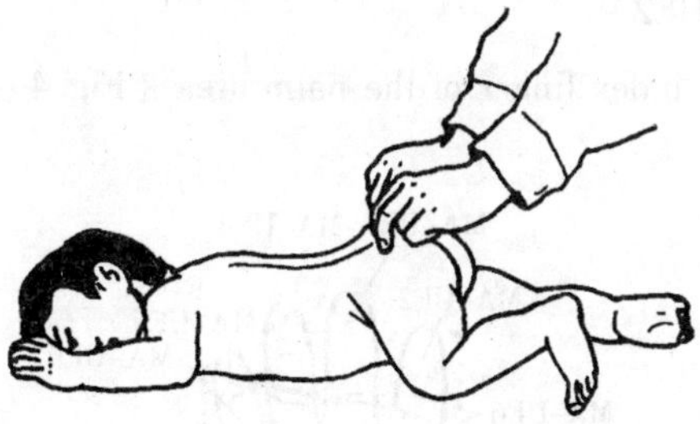

Fig. 4 – 61

4.5.2.3 Qijiegu (MA – T3)

Location: The line from the 4th lumbar vertebra to the caudal vertebra (Fig. 4 – 62).

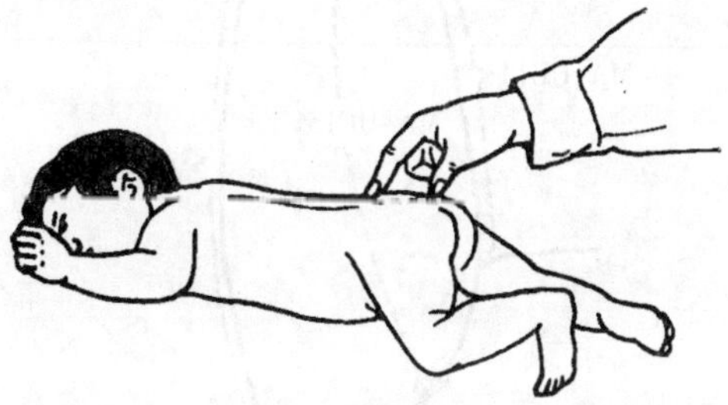

Fig. 4 – 62

Indications: Push-up Qijiegu for enteritis and prolapse of the rectum. Push-down Qijiegu for constipation.

Manipulation: Pushing straight upward with the palmar faces of index and middle fingers is called push-up Qijiegu. Pushing downward is called push-down Qijiegu. The quantity is usually 100 ~ 300 times.

4.5.2.4 Guiwei (MA – T4)

Location: At the end of the caudal vertebra (Fig. 4 – 63).

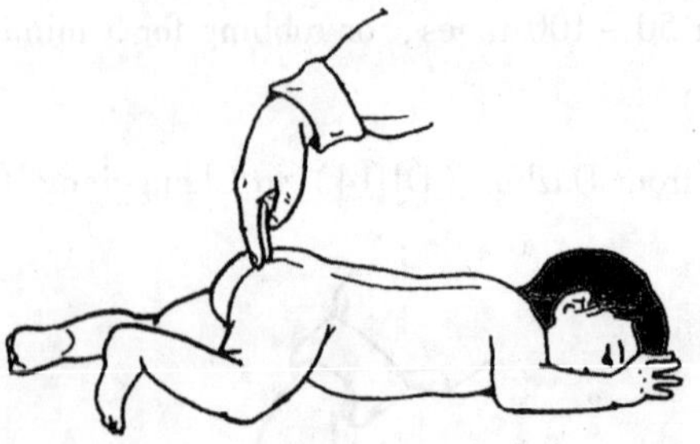

Fig. 4 – 63

Indications: Enteritis, constipation, prolapse of the rectum, and enuresis, etc.

Manipulation: Kneading, 100 ~ 300 times.

4.5.3 Upper Limbs

4.5.3.1 Pijing (MA – UE1)

Location: The palmar face of the thumb (Fig. 4 – 64).

Indications: Enteritis, constipation, and anorexia.

Manipulation: Pushing the thumb in a circular motion is called reinforcing Pijing, while pushing from the tip to the root of the thumb is called clearing Pijng. The frequency of both manipulations is 100 ~ 500 times.

4.5.3.2 Ganjing (MA – UE2)

Location: At the end of the index finger of the palm area (Fig. 4 – 64).

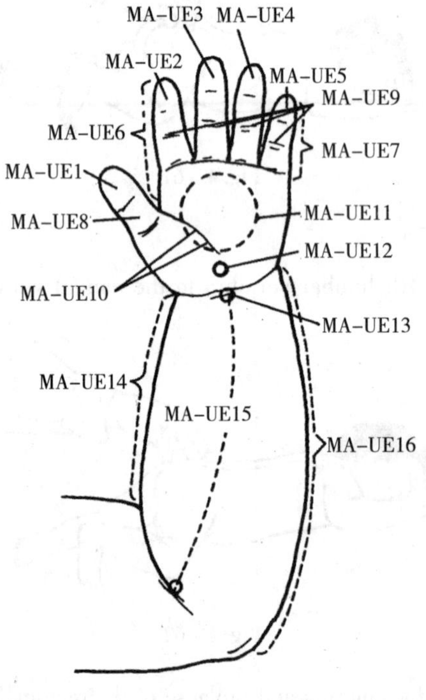

Fig. 4 – 64

Indications: Infantile convulsion, conjunctival congestion, bitter taste, and dry throat, etc.

Manipulation: Pushing the index finger in a circular motion is called "reinforcing Ganjing", while pushing from the tip to the root of the index finger is called "Clearing Ganjing". Always use clearing

Ganjing. Ganjing shouldn't be reinforced. The frequency is usually 100 ~ 500 times.

4.5.3.3 Xinjing (MA – UE3)

Location: At the end of the middle finger of the palm area (Fig. 4 – 64).

Indications: High fever with delirium and oral ulceration, etc.

Manipulation: Pushing the middle finger in a circular motion is called reinforcing, while pushing from the tip to the root of the middle finger is called clearing. The frequency is 100 ~ 500 times.

4.5.3.4 Feijing (MA – UE4)

Location: At the end part of the ring finger (Fig. 4 – 64).

Indications: Common cold, fever, cough, and asthma, etc.

Manipulation: The same as Xinjing.

4.5.3.5 Shenjing (MA – UE5)

Location: At the palmar surface of the end of the little finger (Fig. 4 – 64).

Indications: Reinforcing Shenjing can be used to treat congenital defect, weakness due to chronic disease, chronic diarrhea due to kidney deficiency, enuresis, and dyspnea, etc. Clearing Shenjing can be used to treat heat in the urinary bladder and dark urine, etc.

Manipulation: Pushing straight from the root to the tip of the little finger is reinforcing while pushing from the tip to the root is clearing.

4.5.3.6 Dachang (MA – UE6)

Location: The edge of the radial surface of the index finger (Fig. 4 – 64).

Indications: Enteritis, dysentery, and constipation, etc.

Manipulation: Pushing straight from the tip of the finger to the end is called reinforcing, pushing in the opposite direction is called clearing. Frequency is 100 ~ 300 times.

4.5.3.7 Xiaochang (MA – UE7)

Location: On the ulnar edge of the little finger, from the tip of the little finger to the end (Fig. 4 – 64).

Indications: Enteritis, enuresis.

Manipulation: Same as Dachang. Frequency is 100 ~ 300 times.

4.5.3.8 Weijing (MA – UE8)

Location: On the palmar surface of the first phalange of the thumb close to the palm. (Behind Pijing) (Fig. 4 – 64).

Indications: Vomiting, anorexia, etc.

Manipulation: Same as Xinjing. Frequency is 100 ~ 500 times.

4.5.3.9 Sihengwen (MA – UE9)

Location: On the cross-striation area of the first joint of the index, middle, ring and little fingers on the palmar side (Fig. 4 – 64).

Indications: Indigestion, acute or chronic enteritis.

Manipulation: Nipping with the nail of the thumb is called "nipping Sihengwen". Nipping 5 times for each finger.

Precaution: Sihengwen acupoints are partially overlapped with Sifeng (EX – UE10). Sifeng acupoints are located at the centers of cross-striation areas.

4.5.3.10 Banmen (MA – UE10)

Location: On the flat area of the major thenar eminence of the palm (Fig. 4 – 64).

Indications: Anorexia, indigestion and vomiting.

Manipulation: Kneading on this acupoint with finger tips is called kneading Banmen. Pushing from the end of the thumb to the cross striation of wrist is called pushing from Banmen to the cross striation. Otherwise, it is called pushing from the cross striation to Banmen. Frequency is 100 ~ 300 times.

4.5.3.11 Neibagua (MA – UE11)

Location: On the palm surface. Taking the center of the palm as the center of a circle and 2/3 from this center to the cross striation of the middle finger as the radius, draw a circle. This circle is Neibagua (Fig. 4 – 64).

Indications: Cough, asthma, anorexia, vomiting and abdominal distention, etc.

Manipulation: 100 ~ 300 times.

4.5.3.12 Xiaotianxin (MA – UE12)

Location: On the intersection point of the major thenar eminence and the minor thenar eminence (Fig. 4 – 64).

Indications: Infantile convulsion, night cry, and painful urination.

Manipulation: Kneading or nipping 100 ~ 300 times.

4.5.3.13 Zongjin (MA – UE13)

Location: On the middle of the transverse crease of the wrist, at the palm surface (Fig. 4 – 64).

Indications: Infantile convulsion, night cry, oral ulceration and toothache.

Manipulation: Kneading 100 ~ 300 times, pinching 3 ~ 5 times.

4.5.3.14 Sanguan (MA – UE14)

Location: The straight way from the transverse crease of the wrist to Quchi (LI11), on the radial aspect of the forearm (Fig. 4 – 64).

Indications: Weakness after chronic diseases, stomachache, common cold, etc.

Manipulation: Pushing from the transverse crease of the wrist to elbow is called pushing Sanguan. Frequency: 100 ~ 300 times.

4.5.3.15 Tianheshui (MA – UE15)

Location: The straight way form Zongjin to Quze (PC3), in the middle of the forearm (Fig. 4 – 64).

Indications: All kinds of heat syndromes such as fever due to cold.

Manipulation: Pushing from the wrist to the elbow is "clearing Tianheshui." Frequency is 100 ~ 300 times.

4.5.3.16 Liufu (MA – UE16)

Location: At the ulnar part of the forearm, the straight path from the Shenmen (HT7) to the elbow (Fig. 4 – 64).

Indications: All kinds of sthenic – heat syndromes such as high fever, infantile convulsion, acute tonsillitis, mumps, and constipation.

Manipulation: Pushing from the elbow to the wrist is called reducing Liufu. Frequency is 100 ~ 300 times.

4.6　Specific Acupoints

Specific acupoints refer to those of the Fourteen Meridians that have special therapeutic properties. They include Back – shu acupoints, Mu acupoints, Yuan acupoints, Luo acupoints, Xi acupoints, Lower-he acupoints, Eight Confluence acupoints, Eight Influential acupoints, etc.

4.6.1　Back Shu and Mu Acupoints

Back shu acupoints belong to the Bladder Meridian of the Foot – Taiyang, which is bilateral to the spinal column. These acupoints have a close relationship with the diseases of their associated organs. Mu acupoints are those on the chest and abdomen. They also have close relationship with the diseases of related organs. If the related organs are diseased, an abnormal reaction, such as tenderness, will often appear in the corresponding Shu or Mu acupoints. We choose these related Shu and Mu acupoints for acupuncture or moxibustion treatment. We call this Shu-Mu combination. The relationship between the acupoints and their related organs is shown in the following Table 4 – 3.

Table 4 – 3

Meridian Acupoint	Shu Acupoint	Mu Acupoint	Meridian Acupoint	Shu Acupoint	Mu Acupoint
LU	BL13	LU1	SP	BL20	LR13
PC	BL14	RN17	LR	BL18	LR14
HT	BL15	RN14	KI	BL23	GB25
LI	BL25	ST25	ST	BL21	RN12
SJ	BL22	RN5	GB	BL19	GB24
SI	BL27	RN4	BL	BL28	RN3

The neuroanatomy of the acupoints indicates that the neural segment distribution of the Back-Shu and Mu acupoints and their related organs are nearly the same. This is shown in the following Table 4 – 4.

Table 4 – 4

Organs and related neural segments		Shu Acupoint and neural segments		Mu Acupoint and neural segments	
Lung	C3 ~ T4	BL13	T1 ~ 3	LU1	T1
		BL14	T2 ~ 4	RN17	T4
Heart	T3 ~ 4	BL15	T3 ~ 5	RN14	
Liver	T7 ~ 10	BL18	T7 ~ 9	LR14	T8
Kidney	T12 ~ L1	BL23	T11 ~ L1	GB25	T11
		BL20	T9 ~ 11	LR13	T10
Stomach	T6 ~ 9	BL21	T10 ~ 12	RN12	T9
Large intestine	T11 ~ 12, L1 ~ 3	BL25	L3	ST25	T10
Gall bladder	T7 ~ 10	BL19	T8 ~ 10	GB24	T9
Bladder	T11 ~ L2	BL28	S 1 ~ 2	RN3	T12 ~ L1

4.6.2 Yuan and Luo Acupoints

Yuan and Luo acupoints are the main acupoints on the Twelve Meridians that are located distant to the elbow and knee. Yuan acupoints are located at the end of the limbs and have a close relationship with certain organs. Luo acupoints are the connecting points between the two exteriorly-interiorly related meridians. Yuan and Luo combination refers to the selection of Yuan acupoints on one meridian in combination with related Luo acupoints on the exteriorly-interiorly related meridians to reinforce the treatment effect for diseases on one meridian (Table 4 – 5).

Table 4 – 5

Meridian Acupoints	Yuan Acupoints	Luo Acupoints	Meridian Acupoints	Yuan Acupoints	Luo Acupoints
LU	LU9	LU7	SP	SP3	SP4
PC	PC7	PC6	LR	LR3	LR5
HT	HT7	HT5	KI	KI3	KI4
LI	LI4	LI6	ST	ST42	ST40
SJ	SJ4	SJ5	GB	GB40	GB37
SJ	SI4	SI7	BL	BL64	BL58

4.6.3 Xia-He Acupoints

Xia-He Acupoints are those acupoints located on the legs, which have close relationship with internal organs. For example, Shangjuxu (ST37) can treat diseases of the large intestine, and Yanglingquan (GB34), diseases of the gall bladder (Table 4 –6).

Table 4 –6

Meridian Acupoints	Xia-He Acupoints
Large Intestine Meridian of Hand-Yangming	ST37
Sanjiao Meridian of Hand-Shaoyang	BL39
Small Intestine Meridian of Hand-Taiyang	ST39
Stomach Meridian of Foot-Yangming	ST36
Gall bladder Meridian of Foot-Shaoyang	GB34
Bladder Meridian of Foot-Taiyang	BL40

4.6.4 Xi Acupoints

In ancient times, people thought that the Xi acupoints were the sites where the Qi and blood of the meridians converged. There are 16 Xi acupoints. Each of the Twelve Regular Meridians and the four extra meridians (Yinwei, Yangwei, Yinqiao and Yangqiao) has a Xi acupoint. In clinical practice, we use Xi acupoints to treat acute disorders and severe pain (Table 4 –7).

Table 4 – 7

Meridian	Xi Acupoints	Meridian	Xi Acupoints
LU	LU6	KI	K15
PC	PC4	ST	ST34
HT	HT6	GB	GB36
LI	LI7	BL	BL63
SJ	SJ7	Yinwei	KI9
SI	SI6	Yangwei	GB35
SP	SP8	Yinqiao	KI8
LR	LR6	Yangqiao	BL59

4.7 Ear Acupuncture Therapy

Ear acupuncture therapy treats and prevents diseases by stimulating certain points on the auricle with needles or other tools. This method is characterized by easy manipulation, wide indications, and good results.

4.7.1 Anatomy of the Auricle Surface

Fig. 4 – 65 shows the anatomy of the auricle surface.

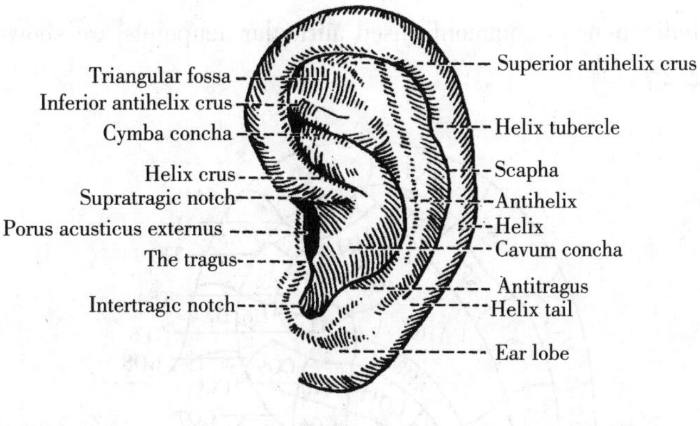

Fig. 4 – 65

4.7.1.1 Helix and Antihelix

Helix: Curling rim of the most lateral border of the auricle; Helix crus: Transverse ridge of the helix continuing backward into the ear cavity.

Antihelix: Medial aspect of the helix, an elevated ridge parallel to the helix. Its upper portion branches out into the superior antihelix crus and the inferior antihelix crus.

4.7.1.2 Ear lobe, Tragus, and Antitragus

Ear lobe: Lowest part of the auricle where there is no cartilage.

Tragus: Curved flap in front of the auricle.

Antitragus: Small tubercle opposite to the tragus and superior to the ear lobe.

4.7.1.3 Triangular fossa, Cymba concha, Cavum concha

Triangular fossa: Triangular depression between the two crura of the antihelix.

Cymba concha: Olive cavum between the helix crus and the inferior antihelix crus.

Cavum concha: Cavum inferior to the helix crus.

4.7.1.4 Scapha, Helix tubercle

Scapha: Narrow curved depression between the helix and the antihelix.

Helix tubercle: Small tubercle at the posterior – superior aspect of the helix.

4.7.1.5 Supratragic notch, Intertragic notch, Helix notch

Supratragic notch: Depression between the upper border of the tragus and the helix crus.

Intertragic notch: Depression between the tragus and antitragus.

Helix notch: Shallow depression between antitragus and antihelix.

4.7.2 Commonly Used Auricular Points

The auricle mirrors a fetus in the uterus with the head directed downwards and the buttocks upwards (Fig. 4 – 66). The distributions of the auricular points are as follows:

Acupoints located on the lobule are related to the head, those on the antitragus to the brain, those on the cavum concha to the chest, those on the helix crus to the diaphragm, those on the cymba concha to the belly, those on the triangular fassa to the pelvis, those on the antihelix to the trunk, neck, thorax waist, sacrum and coccygeal vertebra, those on the two crura of the antihelix to the lower limbs, those on the scapha to the upper limbs.

The locations and indications of commonly used auricular acupoints are shown in Fig. 4 – 66 and the following table (Table 4 – 7).

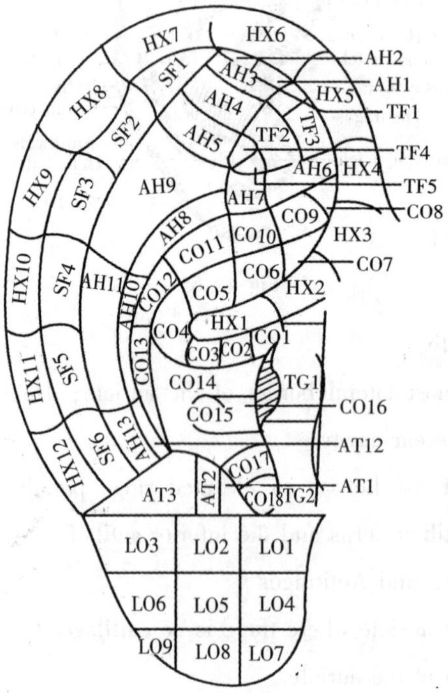

Fig. 4 – 66

Table 4 – 8 Location and Indications of commonly used auricular acupoints

Anatomy part	Acupoint	Location	Indications
Helix (11)	Ear Center (HX1)	Helix Crus	Hiccup, nettle rash, neurodermatitis, enuresis in children, hemoptysis
	Rectum (HX2)	Anterior and superior to Helix Crus	Constipation, diarrhea, rectum prolapse, hemorrhoid
	Urethra (HX3)	Superior to rectum	Urethrocystitis, urine retention
	External Genitalia (HX4)	Anterior to the inferior antihelix crus	Orchitis, epididymitis, external genitalia itching syndrome
	Anus (HX5)	Anterior o triangular fossa	Hemorrhoid, anal fissure
	Ear Apex (HX6)	At the tip of the helix	Fever, hypertension, acute conjunctivitis, chalazion
	Tubercle (HX7)	Helix tubercle	Dizziness, headache
	Helix 1~4 (HX9~12)	Under helix tubercle	upper respiratory tract infection
Scapha (6)	Finger (SF1)	At the top of scapha	Paronychia, finger pain and numbness
	Wrist (SF2)	Under SF1	wrist pain
	Fengxi (SF1, 2i)	Anterior to Helix tubercle, between SF1 and SF2	Nettle rash, neurodermatitis, allergic rhinitis
	Elbow (SF3)	Under SF2	Elbow pain
	Shoulder (SF4, 5)	Under SF3	Periarthritis of shoulder
	Clavicle (SF6)	Under SF4, 5	Periarthritis of shoulder
Antihelix (14)	Heel (AH1)	Anterior and superior part of the superior Antihelix Crus	Foot sprain, heel pain
	Toe (AH2)	Posterior and superior part of the superior Antihelix Crus	Paronychia, toe pain
	Ankle (AH3)	Under AH1 and AH2	Ankle sprain
	Knee (AH4)	Middle 1/3 of the superior antihelix Crus	Knee pain
	Coxa (AH5)	Inferior 1/3 of the superior antihelix crus	Hip pain, sciatica
	Sciatic Nerve (AH6)	Anterior 2/3 of the inferior antihelix crus	Sciatica
	Sympathetic Nerve (AH6a)	End of the inferior antihelix crus	Gastrointestinal colic, biliary colic, angina pectoris, urinary stone, vegetative nervous disorder

Continued

Anatomy part	Acupoint	Location	Indications
Antihelix (14)	Hip (AH7)	Posterior 1/3 of the inferior antihelix crus	Sciatica, hip fascitis
	Abdomen (AH8)	Superior 2/5 of the anterior part of the principal part of antihelix	Abdominal pain, acute waist sprain, dysmenorrheal, postpartum uterine pain
	Lumbosacral vertebrae (AH9)	Behind AH8	Pain at Lumbosacral area
	Chest (AH10)	Middle 2/5 of the Anterior part of the principal part of antihelix	Chest and hypochondria pain, chest tight, mastitis
	Thoracic Vertebrae (AH11)	Behind AH10	Chest and hypochondria pain, mastitis, premenstrual mammary distension and pain, insufficient lactation
	Neck (AH12)	Inferior 1/5 of the anterior part of the principal part of antihelix	Stiff neck, cervical spondylopathy
	Cervical vertebrae (AH13)	Behind AH12	Stiff neck, cervical spondylopathy
The triangular Fossa (5)	Superior triangular fossa (TF1)	Superior to the anterior 1/3 of triangular fossa	Hypertension
	Internal Genitalia (TF2)	Inferior to anterior 1/3 of triangular fossa	Dysmenorrhea, irregular menstruation, dysfunctional uterine bleeding, leukorrhagia, nocturnal emission, prospermia
	Middle triangular fossa (TF3)	Middle 1/3 of the triangular fossa	Asthma
	Shenmen (TF4)	Superior to the posterior 1/3 of triangular fossa	Insomnia, dream-disturbed sleep, dysmenorrhea, withdrawal syndrome
	Pelvic Cavity (TF5)	Inferior to the posterior 1/3 of triangular fossa	Pelvic inflammation
The tragus (9)	Supra tragus (TG1)	Upper 1/2 of the external aspect of the tragus	Pharyngitis, rhinitis
	Infra tragus (TG2)	Lower 1/2 of the external aspect of the tragus	Rhinitis
	External Ear (TG10)	Supra tragus notch close to the helix	Inflammation of the external auditory canal, otitis media, tinnitus
	Tragus Apex (TG1p)	Tip of the upper border of the tragus	Fever, toothache
	External Nose (TG1, 2i)	Middle of the external aspect of the tragus, between Supra tragus and Infra tragus	Rhinitis, sinusitis

Continued

Anatomy part	Acupoint	Location	Indications
The tragus (9)	Adrenal (TG2P)	Tip of the lower border of the tragus	Hypotension, rheumatic arthritis, mumps, streptomycin poisoning
	Pharynx-Larynx (TG3)	Upper half of the medial aspect of the tragus	Pharyngolaryngitis, tonsillitis, hoarseness
	Internal nose (TG4)	Lower half of the medial aspect of the tragus	Rhinitis, paranasal sinusitis
	Antero – intertragus (TG21)	Anterior to intertragus notch, the lowest point of the tragus	Stomatitis, pharyngitis
The antit-ragus (8)	Forehead (AT1)	Anterior part of the lateral aspect of the antitragus	Headache, dizziness, insomnia, dream – disturbed sleep
	Postero-intertragus (AT11)	Posterior to intertragus notch, anterior and inferior part of antitragus	Frontal sinusitis
	Temple (AT2)	Middle part of the lateral aspect of the antitragus	Migraine
	Occiput (AT3)	Posterior part of the lateral aspect of the antitragus	Headache, dizziness, asthma, epilepsy, neurosis
	Subcortex (AT4)	Medial aspect of antitragus	Painful disease, malaria, neurosis, pseudomyopia, insomnia
	Antitragus Apex (AT1, 2, 4i)	Tip of the antitragus	Asthma, mumps, neurodermatitis orchitis, epididymitis
	Middle border (AT2, 3, 4i)	Midpoint between the anti – tragic apex and helix – tragic notch	Enuresis, auditory vertigo
	Brain stem (AT3, 4i)	Helix – tragus notch	Occipital headache, dizziness, pseudomyopia
The concha (21)	Mouth (CO1)	Anterior 1/3 of inferior part of IIelix Crus	Facial paralysis, stomatitis, gallbladder stone, cholecystitis, withdrawal syndrome
	Esophagus (CO2)	Middle 1/3 of inferior part of Helix Crus	Esophagitis, esophagus spasm
	Cardiac Orifice (CO3)	Posterior 1/3 of inferior part of Helix Crus	Cardiospasm, nervous vomiting
	Stomach (CO4)	Area where the helix crus terminates	Gastrospasm, gastritis, gastric ulcer, indigestion, insomnia, toothache
	Duodenum (CO5)	Posterior to the superior aspect of the helix crus	Duodenal ulcer, gall-bladder stone, cholecystitis, pylorospasm

Continued

Anatomy part	Acupoint	Location	Indications
The concha (21)	Small Intestine (CO6)	Middle in the superior aspect of the helix crus	Indigestion, stomachache, tachycardia, arrhythmia
	Large intestine (CO7)	Anterior to the superior aspect of the helix crus	Diarrhea, constipation
	Appendix (CO6, 7i)	Between CO6 and CO7	Diarrhea, appendicitis
	Angle of Cymba Concha (CO8)	Anterior to the inferior part of inferiorantihelix crus	Prostatitis, urethritis
	Bladder (CO9)	Middle of the inferior part of inferior antihelix crus	Cystitis, enuresis, urine retention, occipital headache, backache, sciatica
	Kidney (CO10)	Posterior to the inferior part of inferior antihelix crus	Tinnitus, pyelonephritis enuresis, Noctural, emission, irregular menstruation, asthma
	Ureter (CO9, 10i)	Between CO9 and CO10	Ureter calculus
	Pancreas and Biliary Tract (CO11)	On the posterosuperior part of Cymba concha	Cholelithiasis, cholecystitis, biliary ascaris, migraine, pancreasitis, ear disease.
	Liver (CO12)	On the posteroinferior part of Cymba concha	Hypochondriac pain, hypertension, pseudomyopia, irregular menstruation, Climacteric syndrome
	Middle Cymba (CO6, 10i)	Between CO6 and CO10	Stomachache, abdominal distention, biliary ascaris
	Spleen (CO13)	Posterosuperior part of cavum concha	Abdominal distention, stomachache, constipation, anorexia, dysfunctional uterine bleeding, leukorrhagia, auditory vertigo
	Heart (CO15)	In the central depression of the cavum concha	Tachycardia, arrhythmia, angina pectoris, neurosis, stomatitis
	Trachea (CO16)	Between CO15 and the orifice of the external auditory meatus	Asthma, bronchitis
	Lung (CO14)	Around CO15 and CO16	Cough, hoarse voice, acne, constipation, nettle rash, withdrawal syndrome
	Sanjiao (CO17)	Posteroinferior part of the orifice of the external auditory meatus and CO18	Constipation, abdominal distention, stomachache
	Endocrine (CO18)	Anteroinferior part of cavum concha in the intertragus notch	Dysmenorrhea, irregular menstruation, climacteric syndrome, acne, malaria

Continued

Anatomy part	Acupoint	Location	Indications
The Ear Lobule (8)	Tooth (LO1)	Anterosuperior part of the ear lobule	Toothache, periodontitis, hypotension
	Tongue (LO2)	Superomedian part	Glossitis, stomatitis
	Jaw (LO3)	Posterosuperior part	Toothache, temporomandibular joint disorder
	Anterior of ear Lobe (LO4)	Anteromedian part	Neurosis, toothache
	Eye (LO5)	Center part	Acute conjunctivitis, chalazion, Pseudo myopia, electric ophthalmia
	Internal Ear (LO6)	Posteromedian part	Auditory vertigo, tinnitus, loss of hearing
	Cheek (LO5, 6i)	Between LO5 and LO6	Facial spasm, trigeminal neuralgia, Plane warts, acne
	Tonsil (LO7, 8, 9)	Inferior part	Tonsillitis, pharyngitis
The Back Auricle (6)	Back Heart (P1)	Superior part of the back auricle	Coronary heart disease, insomnia, dreaminess
	Back Lung (P2)	Medial to the central part	Asthma, neurodermatitis
	Back Spleen (P3)	Central part	stomachache, indigestion, anorexia
	Back Liver (P4)	Lateral to the central part	Cholelithiasis, cholecystitis, hypochondriac pain
	Back Kidney (P5)	Inferior part	Headache, dizziness, neurosis
	Back Groove (PS)	Backside of antihelix crus, superior, and inferior antihelix crus	Hypertension, neurodermatitis
Ear Root (3)	Superior Ear Root (R1)	Top of Ear Root	Epistaxis
	Mi Ear Root (R2)	Posterior groove of Helix crus	Cholelithiasis, cholecystitis, stuffy nose, tachycardia, diarrhea, stomachache
	Inferior Ear, Root (R3)	Bottom of Ear Root	Hypotension

4.7.3 Application of Auricular Points

4.7.3.1 Disciplines of acupoint prescription

1. Main acupoints are those on the ear areas that are related to the afflicted parts of the human body.

2. Assistant acupoints are those on the other areas of the ear that have abnormal reactions or have a relationship with the disease.

4.7.3.2 Manipulation

1. Finding the reactive acupoint: Make an acupoint prescription according to the disease and then locate the reactive acupoints in the chosen area of the ear; such as a tender point, or a point with low electrical resistance.

2. Treatment: After regular sterilization stimulate the acupoint with a 0.5 *cun* filiform acupuncture needle; or by applying pressure with magnetic balls or the seed of Vaccaria segetalis; or by imbedding a subcutaneous needle; or by acupoint injection. Penetrate the cartilage with the needle but avoid penetrating through the ear. The stimulation should always be within a patient's pain threshold. The needle can remain for 30 minutes or can be connected to electricity. Keep the seed or subcutaneous needle on one ear. Rotate to the other ear in 3 days. During the period of time, press it 2 ~ 4 times a day, 1 ~ 2 minutes each acupoint. During the summer the retention time can be shortened.

4.7.3.3 Precautions

1. Strict antisepsis and infection prevention is required. Avoid acupuncture or seed pressing on broken skin.

2. Acupuncture on the ear is forbidden in pregnant women who have a history of habitual miscarriage. Old people, who have hypertension or arteriosclerosis, need some rest before and after acupuncture.

3. Fainting may take place. Use preventative methods similar to those of filiform needle.

第五章　常见病治疗学

5.1　内科病症

5.1.1　头　痛

5.1.1.1　概况

现代医学的偏头痛、紧张性头痛、神经功能性头痛，以及高血压病、脑动脉硬化和眼、耳、鼻等所致的头痛均可参此治疗。但应注意与颅脑实质性病变鉴别，以便及时治疗原发病。中医学按疼痛部位分为阳明头痛（前额及眉棱骨痛）、少阳头痛（两侧颞部为主，可累及耳部）、太阳头痛（后枕部）、厥阴头痛（头顶及目）。

5.1.1.2　针灸治疗

主穴：风池、合谷。

配穴：前额头痛，印堂、头维、内庭；偏头痛，太阳、率谷、外关；头顶痛，百会、四神聪、通天、太冲；后头痛，天柱、风府、后溪。

随症配穴：伴发热，大椎、曲池；胸闷恶心，内关、中脘；眩晕，三阴交、行间或太溪。

操作：先针近部穴位，后针远道穴位，得气后留针 20～30 分钟，疼痛剧烈者可酌情延长至 1～2小时。可接脉冲电针治疗仪，用断续波中等刺激。

皮肤针：重点叩刺头痛的局部、后项部，体壮者叩刺可适当重些，以后项部皮肤微微渗血为度；妇女或体虚者叩刺宜轻，一般以皮肤出现红润、充血为度。

耳针：取枕、额、皮质下、神门、交感等穴，留针 20～30 分钟或用磁珠等贴压。

5.1.1.3　推拿治疗

1. 干浴头面：两掌轻摩面部，再翻转至后方下推颈枕部，约 5 分钟。十指微张，用指面从耳颞部开始由前向后做梳头动作。动作要轻柔，速度宜慢。

2. 用点、按揉法在穴位推拿，取穴同上，手法由轻到重，再由重逐渐到轻。以头顶痛为主者，重点按百会、四神聪；以偏头痛为主者，重点按揉太阳、率谷、角孙；以枕部后头痛为主者，重点按揉风池、天柱。共 5～10 分钟。

3. 结束治疗：轻叩头部结束。

5.1.2　失　眠

5.1.2.1　概况

失眠既是一个症状，又是一个病名。现代医学的神经衰弱症、贫血、绝经前后综合征等可参此治疗。中医学通常称为“不寐”“不得眠”“不得卧”“目不寐”。

5.1.2.2 针灸治疗

主穴：近取百会、风池；远取三阴交、神门。

随症配穴：多梦，心俞；腰酸耳鸣，肾俞、太溪；脘腹胀满，足三里、胃俞；急躁易怒，太冲。

操作：常规针刺，得气后留针20~30分钟，每日1次，10次为一疗程。针毕俯卧，在上背部脊柱两侧涂按摩乳，上下往返轻轻走罐，以皮肤略有潮红为度；或用皮肤针在脊柱两侧进行叩刺，尤其以心俞、肝俞附近为重点，以皮肤出现红润、充血为度。

耳针：取神门、心、脾、肾、额、枕、皮质下等穴埋贴，睡前按压5分钟左右。

5.1.2.3 推拿治疗

1. 患者仰卧，前额分推：先由中间向两侧分推，分上、中、下三部分完成，约3分钟；直推：再从印堂经神庭直推至百会穴，1~2分钟。颞部和头顶部轻揉、擦，1~2分钟。以一手掌托住患者后枕部，另一手用三指拿揉颈项部，2~3分钟。

2. 点揉百会、神庭、太阳、风池等穴各1分钟。然后患者双眼微闭，依次按揉睛明、攒竹、鱼腰、丝竹空、瞳子等眼周5穴，每穴各半分钟，至局部发热为好。点按上肢部神门、内关穴1~2分钟。

3. 结束治疗：轻叩头部，拿两肩井穴数次。

5.1.3 面　瘫

5.1.3.1 概况

现代医学的周围性面神经炎可参此治疗，中枢性面瘫应明确病因，非占位性所致者可配合头针治疗。中医学称为“口眼㖞斜”。

5.1.3.2 针灸治疗

主穴：近取攒竹、阳白、翳风、四白、迎香、地仓、颊车、颧髎；远取合谷、内庭、太冲。

操作：面部穴位一般取患侧，远部常取双侧。面瘫发病1周内局部慎用针刺，宜局部多针浅刺或常规针刺远部穴位，或翳风穴艾条灸15~20分钟。1周后病情稳定时，可用平刺透穴法。各穴得气后，配用脉冲电针仪断续波刺激20~30分钟，刺激量从小到大，以患者感觉舒适为度；超过1月未愈者，电针刺激量宜加大，以患者能耐受为度，并在患部配用艾条灸。

5.1.3.3 推拿治疗

1. 患者仰卧，以手掌或指腹轻轻揉抹整个患侧面部，以局部产生温热感为度，5~10分钟。

2. 用拇指按揉印堂穴，并沿眉弓推向患侧太阳穴；自印堂推至百会穴、神庭；眉毛中点推向阳白穴；睛明穴沿鼻旁推揉至迎香；迎香穴沿四白、颧髎、下关一线推揉；地仓向颊车一线推揉；人中向迎香一线推揉。以上每一步骤各需1~2分钟。按揉风池、曲池、合谷等穴各1分钟。

3. 轻弹患侧面部结束。

5.1.4 三叉神经痛

5.1.4.1 概况

本病相当于中医学的“面痛”“头风”。

5.1.4.2　针灸治疗

随症近取：额痛取攒竹、阳白；上颌痛取四白、颧髎、迎香；下颌痛取下关、颊车、大迎。远取：风池、合谷、外关、内庭、三阴交。

操作：下关针尖斜向对侧内眼角方向刺入2寸左右，患者同侧面、鼻、眼周、口唇等处出现电样感为佳；攒竹沿眶上切迹向上方刺入0.5～1寸，有触电样针感传到前额为佳；大迎向前下方刺入。其他穴位常规刺法，针感以重刺激为佳。

5.1.5　脑血管疾病后遗症

5.1.5.1　概况

脑血管疾病后遗症是指脑血管疾病急性期过后遗留的半身不遂、语言不利、口角㖞斜等症，现代医学的脑溢血、脑血栓、脑栓塞等后遗症属此范畴，其他脑部疾患手术的后遗症等也可参此治疗，小儿脑瘫可参此加减。中医学称为“偏瘫”“偏枯”等。

5.1.5.2　针灸治疗

上肢取穴：肩髃、曲池、手三里、外关、合谷；下肢取穴：环跳、风市、梁丘、阳陵泉、足三里、昆仑、解溪、太冲。

随症配穴：口角㖞斜，颊车、地仓、迎香；尿失禁，百会、曲骨、中极；吞咽困难，风府、哑门、风池、翳风；失语，廉泉、通里；肩关节运动障碍，肩髃透极泉、肩贞、肩井、天宗；膝关节屈曲困难，委中、委阳、膝阳关、殷门、承山；足内翻，悬钟、申脉、金门丘墟透照海；肌张力增高以肢体阴经穴位为主，如极泉、内关、孔最、曲泽、血海、曲泉、阴陵泉、三阴交等。另，小儿脑瘫智力低下，配百会、四神聪。

头针：顶颞前斜线、顶中线；感觉障碍加顶颞后斜线；失语者加颞前线；平衡障碍者加枕下旁线。

操作：体针常规操作，针刺得气后留针20～30分钟，可接脉冲电流。每日1次，10次1个疗程。头针多与皮肤成30°角斜刺，行抽气针法或捻转针法。顶颞前斜线、顶颞后斜线针刺时可采取由上而下的三针接力刺。

5.1.5.3　推拿治疗

1. 俯卧位，术者立于患侧，用揉法于患背、腰部或脊柱两侧自上而下反复3～5分钟；再点按肺俞、肝俞、脾俞、肾俞等穴。在患侧臀部至小腿后侧㨰、揉约5分钟，并点按环跳、委中、承山等穴。可配合腰后伸、髋过伸、膝屈伸、踝关节跖屈背伸。

2. 仰卧位，术者立于患侧，用揉法、㨰法于患侧上肢内侧、肩、肘、腕关节，下肢自髂前上棘沿大腿前面小腿外侧至踝部及足背，反复操作5～10分钟。点按患侧肩髃、曲池、尺泽、手三里、合谷、环跳、伏兔、梁丘、足三里、丰隆、解溪、悬钟穴，各约1分钟。配合做腕关节屈伸旋转、肘关节屈伸、肩关节屈伸内收外展旋转等被动运动，反复数次。

3. 拍打患肢结束。

5.1.6　多发性神经炎

5.1.6.1　概况

现代医学的多发性周围神经炎、格林·巴利综合征、周期性瘫痪、癔症性瘫痪、小儿麻痹后遗症、外伤性截瘫、急性脊髓炎、进行性肌萎缩、重症肌无力、进行性肌营养不良，均可参此治疗。中医学称为“痿证”。

5.1.6.2　针灸治疗

主穴：上肢取肩髃、肩髎、曲池、手三里、合谷；下肢取环跳、阳陵泉、悬钟、髀关、伏兔、足三里、解溪。

随症配穴：大便失禁，天枢、上巨虚；小便失禁或尿潴留，次髎、中极、三阴交、阴陵泉；截瘫，患部上下各取夹脊穴。

操作：每次选用4～8穴，交替轮换，一般针刺患侧，效差者可先针刺健侧。得气后中等刺激，留针20～30分钟，每日或隔日1次，10次为1疗程。休息3～5天后开始第2疗程。大小便失禁或尿潴留，可分别在天枢、中极行艾条灸，每日1次，20分钟左右。

穴位注射：双侧手三里、足三里，每穴注射弥可保注射液0.5mL，隔日1次，10天为1个疗程。

5.1.6.3　推拿治疗

1. 俯卧位：术者以㨰法、揉法于背部、腰部、脊柱两侧，自上而下反复7～12遍，左右交替进行，点按肺俞、肝俞、脾俞、胃俞、肾俞；然后用㨰法、揉法于患侧臀部至小腿后侧，点按环跳、委中、承山等穴，推拿时力量要均匀而有节律。

2. 仰卧位：术者位于一侧，用揉法、㨰法于上肢内侧、肩、肘、腕关节；下肢自髂前上棘沿大、小腿前外侧至足背反复7～12遍，左右交替进行，点按肩髃、曲池、尺泽、手三里、合谷、环跳、伏兔、梁丘、足三里、丰隆、解溪、悬钟穴，各约1分钟。继之做腕关节屈伸旋转、肘关节屈伸、肩关节屈伸内收外展旋转等被动运动，反复做7～12遍。

3. 拍打患肢结束。

5.1.7　咳嗽、哮喘

5.1.7.1　概况

现代医学的慢性气管炎、支气管扩张、哮喘等可参此治疗。中医学上它们属肺系疾病，临床表现虽异，但其病因为外感风、寒、湿、热、燥等邪气，内伤痰湿、肺脾肾脏虚弱，则多一致，治疗也多一致。

5.1.7.2　针灸治疗

主穴：肺俞、膻中、列缺、尺泽。

随症配穴：发热恶寒，大椎、曲池、合谷；鼻塞，印堂、迎香、合谷；痰多，内关、丰隆；哮喘，定喘、身柱、心俞等。

操作：肺俞，针尖向脊柱方向斜刺，膻中向下平刺，得气后留针20～30分钟，急性期每日1～2次，症状缓解后隔日1次，直至症状消失。慢性者10次为1疗程，疗程结束后休息3～5天，再开始下一疗程。也可接脉冲电针治疗仪，用断续波中等刺激。哮喘多采用天灸法，有显著疗法。还可配合在定喘穴、肺俞穴、膻中穴拔罐，每次10分钟。

耳针：在支气管、肺、平喘、肾上腺、皮质下、内分泌、肾等穴处找敏感点，选用2～3穴，留针20～30分钟或用磁珠等埋贴。

5.1.7.3 推拿治疗

1. 患者仰卧位，术者以一指推或揉法从天突穴缓慢推向膻中穴，往返推动2~3分钟；再做肋间梳理法，以两拇指从膻中穴向两旁分推2~3分钟。

2. 坐或俯卧位，术者拿揉颈项部3~5分钟，提拿肩井5~7下，然后平推肩背，斜推两胁，均以透热为度。点按风池、风府、肩井、肺俞、定喘、膈俞，以酸胀为度。按揉尺泽、合谷、丰隆、足三里，各约1分钟。

5.1.8 冠心病

5.1.8.1 概况

冠心病的早期不一定有明显症状，称为“隐性冠心病”。随着病情的发展，就会出现一系列临床症状，如胸闷、心悸、心绞痛等。中医学相当于“胸痹”。

5.1.8.2 针灸治疗

主穴：心俞、厥阴俞、通里、内关、膻中、巨阙。

随症加减：心血瘀阻加膈俞、阴郄；口唇发绀取少商、中冲、少冲点刺出血；肢冷加灸气海、关元；舌苔厚浊者加中脘、足三里、丰隆。

操作：内关、通里直刺0.5~1寸，捻转运针，使针感向远端放散；膻中向上平刺；巨阙直刺0.5~1寸，捻转运针；心俞、厥阴俞向脊柱方向斜刺，针感向深层放散。遇寒发作者，予加灸各穴。

耳针：心、小肠、交感、皮质下、神门、胸、降压沟，每次选用2~3穴，留针20~30分钟或用磁珠等埋贴。

5.1.8.3 推拿治疗

1. 仰卧位：分推胸胁部、摩胸，3~5分钟。点揉膻中、巨阙、内关、足三里穴，各1分钟。

2. 俯卧位：分推上背部、按压脊柱约5分钟。按揉或一指禅推心俞、厥阴俞、背部阿是穴，3~5分钟。

3. 轻拍胸部膻中区域结束。

5.1.9 急慢性胃炎

5.1.9.1 概况

现代医学的胃和十二指肠炎症、溃疡、胃肠神经官能症、胃下垂等疾病可参此治疗。中医学属“胃脘痛”“呕吐”“心腹痛”“痞证”“发痧”等范畴。

5.1.9.2 针灸治疗

主穴：中脘、内关、足三里。

随症配穴：肝气犯胃，太冲；气滞血瘀，公孙、膈俞；消化不良，梁门；便溏，脾俞、胃俞；脘冷喜暖，灸脾俞、胃俞；腹泻，天枢、上巨虚；便秘，天枢、支沟；腹胀，内庭。

操作：先取内关、足三里及随症配穴，得气后留针20~30分钟，可接电针疏密波中等刺激15分钟。疗效欠佳者再加中脘，温针灸2~3分钟，或艾条灸15~20分钟，温度以病人感觉舒适为宜。其他穴位采用常规刺法。每日或隔日1次，10次为1疗程。针毕可酌情配合中脘穴坐罐、背部走罐或皮肤针叩刺以增强疗效。

耳针：在胃、肝、膈、脾、十二指肠、神门等穴寻找敏感点，用磁珠等埋贴。

5.1.9.3　推拿治疗

1. 患者仰卧，微屈髋膝，医者在上腹部稍偏左处做掌摩法3～5分钟；从剑突向肚脐单方向推摩15～20次。中指振颤法振中脘穴1～2分钟，也可根据压痛点的情况酌选上脘或下脘与之交替进行。按揉内关、合谷穴，各做1分钟，按揉足三里穴2～3分钟。

2. 患者俯卧位，医者掌擦背部脊柱两侧，以肝俞至胃俞段为重点，发热为度。点按灵台、至阳、天宗、脾俞、胃俞等穴。

3. 空拳轻叩背部5～10下结束。

5.1.10　胆道疾患

5.1.10.1　概况

现代医学的胆道疾患包括急慢性胆囊炎、胆管炎、胆石症与胆道蛔虫病等，均参此治疗。中医学病名有黄疸、胁痛等，多为肝胆湿热或肝胆气郁所致。

5.1.10.2　针灸治疗

主穴：胆俞、肝俞、胆囊穴、阳陵泉、太冲。

随症配穴：发热，大椎、曲池、合谷；胆道蛔虫症，迎香透四白；黄疸，至阳、三阴交；恶心呕吐，内关、足三里。

操作：先取阳陵泉、胆囊穴、太冲，得气后接脉冲电强刺激，然后针刺其他穴位。胆俞、肝俞宜向脊柱方向斜刺，针感向深层放散。一般留针30分钟，每日1次，痛剧者可每日2次，必要时适当延长留针时间至1～2小时。

耳针：肝、胆、胃、交感、神门、内分泌等，磁珠贴压。胆囊泥沙样结石可在单侧耳穴埋针施治，三四天后交换，1个月为1疗程。治疗期间不必禁忌油腻，以利排石；疼痛发作时按压穴位4～5分钟，有良好的镇痛作用。

5.1.10.3　推拿治疗

1. 患者仰卧，医者做摩上腹2～5分钟，重点在右上腹及上腹中部。摩动宜轻，但局部要有轻微的温热感为好。按揉胆囊、足三里两穴，以酸胀感向下放射为好，各约1分钟。

2. 俯卧位，按揉肝俞、胆俞两穴，5～10分钟，穴位局部要有酸胀感。

5.1.11　急慢性肠炎

5.1.11.1　概况

现代医学的急慢性肠炎或肠功能紊乱、过敏性肠炎、溃疡性结肠炎、肠结核及细菌性痢疾或肠阿米巴病，均可参此治疗。中医学属“泻泄”“腹痛”范畴。

5.1.11.2　针灸治疗

主穴：近取天枢、关元、大肠俞、小肠俞；远取上巨虚、足三里。

随症配穴：发热，大椎、曲池、合谷；恶心呕吐，内关；里急后重，曲池、内庭；畏寒肢冷，百会、神阙；反复不愈、时作时止，脾俞、肾俞。

操作：先针上巨虚、足三里，针感向下肢放射；天枢、关元，针感向小腹部放射。然后随症配穴，诸穴得气后留针20～30分钟。腹泻经久不愈者，可在腹部进行排罐法拔罐。体虚久泻者，可在气海穴艾条灸10～20分钟。

5.1.11.3 推拿治疗

1. 患者仰卧，医者掌摩脐周2～5分钟。轻揉中脘、天枢、气海穴各1分钟，动作应轻柔缓和，不紧不慢，力达深部。按揉阴陵泉、足三里穴各2分钟，用力稍重，以有酸麻胀重感为好。

2. 患者俯卧位，医者双手用力搓擦腰骶部。

3. 双手叠掌轻轻振按脐周，一按一放，重复10次，每次之间停顿约10秒，此为振腹止泻法。

5.1.12 内脏下垂

5.1.12.1 概况

常见有胃下垂、子宫脱垂和脱肛。中医学中，子宫脱垂被称为“阴挺”；各内脏下垂均属阳气亏虚而不能升举的一类疾病，治疗以升阳举陷为总则。

5.1.12.2 针灸治疗

主穴：百会、关元。

配穴：胃下垂配中脘、提胃（中脘旁开4寸）、足三里；子宫脱垂配提托（关元穴旁开4寸）、三阴交；脱肛配长强（属督脉，位于尾骨尖处）、承山。

操作：百会、关元进针后，紧按慢提数次，留针20分钟，然后用艾条温和灸每穴10分钟。可两穴同时进行。

5.1.12.3 推拿治疗

1. 仰卧位，揉按百会穴5分钟。胃下垂者再以掌摩法自下腹向上腹部逆时针环形摩腹3～5分钟（当向上摩动时，应轻用力向上兜托），摩动的范围逐渐增大；然后以掌根自关元穴向中脘穴推摩3～5分钟，移动应缓慢。点按中脘、天枢、气海、关元穴，各1分钟。

2. 俯卧位，胃下垂者揉按脾俞、胃俞、肾俞各1分钟；然后擦背腰部，以热量深透为度。脱肛及子宫脱垂患者，先用温热水洗干净脱垂的子宫或直肠，医者戴一次性手套，用拇指指腹轻轻摩揉3～5分钟，再缓慢轻轻托入（患者也可自行操作）。

5.1.13 前列腺炎、尿潴留

5.1.13.1 概况

现代医学的尿潴留、遗尿、尿失禁、前列腺炎、前列腺肥大等病症，均可参此治疗。中医学将本病称为“癃闭”，认为与肾、膀胱功能失调有关。

5.1.13.2 针灸治疗

主穴：近取次髎、中极、关元；远取三阴交、阴陵泉。

随症配穴：腰膝疲软，肾俞、太溪。

操作：先针三阴交、阴陵泉，针感向足底放射；气海、关元与中极任取两穴，以针感向尿道口放射为佳。两组穴均在得气后接脉冲电针治疗仪，用断续波中等刺激20～30分钟。次髎穴不留针，针感向前阴放散为佳，行针2～3分钟。腹部和腰骶部的穴位可同时配用艾条灸。

耳针：膀胱、尿道、肾、外生殖器、交感等，每次选用3～4穴，留针或磁珠等埋贴。

5.1.13.3 推拿治疗

1. 医者以掌摩法摩下腹部，逆时针、顺时针各1~2分钟，以局部有微热感为度，并在气海、关元穴处重点按摩。

2. 点按气海、中极、关元、足三里、阴陵泉、三阴交等穴各1~2分钟。

5.1.14 遗精、阳痿

5.1.14.1 概况

遗精、阳痿均属男性性功能障碍的疾病，早泄、不射精、精血也可参此治疗。中医学认为，本病多责之于肾。

5.1.14.2 针灸治疗

主穴：近取中极、关元、次髎、秩边；远取三阴交、足三里。

随症配穴：失眠或有梦而遗，神门、心俞；滑精阳痿，肾俞、太溪；头晕目眩，风池。

操作：中极、关元选一，针感向尿道放射为佳；足三里、三阴交每次必取，针感向下放射为佳。得气后留针20~30分钟，腹部穴位可配合温针灸；次髎、秩边的针感应向前阴或会阴区放散为佳。

穴位注射：维生素B_1，注射液50mg分别注入中极、关元二穴，隔日1次，10次为1疗程。阳痿患者亦可用丙酸睾酮5mg，轮流注射关元或中极穴，隔2日1次，4次为1疗程。

耳针：外生殖器、皮质下、神门、内分泌，留针30分钟或磁珠贴压。

5.1.14.3 推拿治疗

1. 患者仰卧，微屈髋膝，医者掌摩下腹部3~5分钟。再从肚脐向耻骨联合处单方向推摩，以热深透为度。中指振颤法振神阙、气海、中极、关元、曲骨等穴各1~2分钟。点按足三里、三阴交、太溪、涌泉等穴各1~2分钟。

2. 患者俯卧，按揉肾俞、志室、腰眼各1~2分钟。掌根擦腰骶部，以热深透为度。点按肾俞、志室、大肠俞、秩边、次髎各1~2分钟。

5.1.15 中　暑

5.1.15.1 概况

中暑是由于高温环境而发生的一组急性疾病。中医学称痧症，俗称“发痧”。

5.1.15.2 针灸治疗

轻症：大椎、曲池、合谷、内庭；重症（晕厥）：水沟、十宣、曲泽、委中。

随症配穴：发热，十宣、大椎、合谷；恶心胸闷，内关；汗出肢冷、虚脱，灸关元、气海、神阙。

操作：中暑患者除虚脱者需用灸法外，其余均可用点刺出血，或用毫针中强刺激。

5.1.15.3 推拿治疗

1. 头、背部刮痧。刮头顶的百会穴，刮1~2分钟；刮背部的大椎、胸夹脊穴，皮下出现微紫红或紫黑色痧点、斑块即可。

2. 四肢刮痧。刮上肢的曲泽、内关穴以及下肢的委中穴，要求同上。

5.1.16 休 克

5.1.16.1 概况

休克是临床各科严重疾病中常见的并发症。中医学属“厥证”“脱证”“亡阴”“亡阳”等范畴。

5.1.16.2 针灸治疗

主穴：素髎、水沟、内关、关元、涌泉、足三里。

随症配穴：心源性休克，三阴交、合谷；感染性休克，十宣、尺泽、委中放血；出血性休克，灸百会、气海、人迎；过敏性休克，曲池、承浆；创伤性休克，耳神门、交感；神经性休克，合谷、太冲。

操作：素髎从鼻尖端斜向上方刺入 0.5 寸，持续运针；水沟向上以 45°角度斜刺，用中等刺激，严重者用强刺激，施以提插捻转手法。内关、涌泉直刺 0.5～1 寸，捻转持续运针。关元采用灸法；足三里中等刺激后加电针 30 分钟。

5.1.16.3 推拿治疗

以指尖掐按水沟、内关、涌泉等穴约 5～10 分钟，拇指指腹按揉合谷、足三里、太冲等穴 5～10分钟。

5.2 骨伤科病症

5.2.1 颈椎病（落枕）

5.2.1.1 概况

颈椎病临床一般分为 5 种类型，常见的有：

1. 颈型：颈椎关节囊松弛、韧带钙化、椎间盘退变、骨棘形成等，引起颈背部疼痛反复发作。

2. 神经根型：以颈神经根受累为主要临床表现。

3. 椎动脉型：颈椎的不稳定、椎间盘侧方的突出以及钩突关节的增生，均可直接刺激椎动脉使之痉挛，或压迫使之扭曲、狭窄、闭塞等，从而产生椎基底动脉供血不足而导致一系列临床表现。

4. 混合型：有两型以上症状者称为混合型，临床较常见。

中医学属“项筋急”“项肩痛”“眩晕”等范畴。

5.2.1.2 针灸治疗

主穴：近取风池、大椎、夹脊（与病变椎体相应）、阿是穴；远取悬钟、落枕穴、后溪。

随症配穴：肩部、上臂疼痛，肩髃、肩髎、条口；上肢麻木，曲池、手三里、外关；头痛眩晕，风池、印堂；视物模糊，睛明、风池；呕吐，内关、足三里。

操作：可先针悬钟或落枕穴，得气后，活动颈部，然后针刺近取穴位及阿是穴，时间 20～30 分钟，10 次 1 疗程。阿是穴可配用艾条灸 15～20 分钟，每日 1～2 次，疗效较佳。颈椎病患者如兼症多，每次一症取 1～2 穴。

5.2.1.3　推拿治疗

1. 病人坐位，用㨰、按、拿、一指禅推等手法在颈椎两侧及肩部治疗约10分钟。

2. 按揉各反应点，分颈部、肩部、肩胛内缘三部分进行。以拇指自枕下开始由上而下，两侧反复交替进行；时间为5～10分钟，以局部肌肉发胀或发热为好。远道取穴，按揉双侧手三里、悬钟各1～3分钟，以穴位局部有酸胀感或向下放射为好。

3. 病人仰卧，肩后用枕垫高，医生立于床头，右手紧托病人枕部，左手托住颏部，将病人头部自枕上拉起，使颈与水平面呈45°角，牵引持续1～2分钟。然后轻轻将头向左右旋转和前后摆动。此时往往可听到整复时的弹响声。

4. 结束治疗：用直擦法治疗颈椎两侧，以透热为度。可配合颈部热敷。

5.2.2　颞颌关节功能紊乱症

5.2.2.1　概况

颞颌关节功能紊乱症是由于颞下颌关节功能失调引起的关节疼痛、张口障碍、关节区弹响等综合征群。中医学属“痹症”范畴。

5.2.2.2　针灸治疗

主穴：近取下关、耳门或听宫、阿是穴；远取中渚、外关。

操作：可先针中渚或外关穴，得气后，轻轻张口以活动颞颌关节，症状减轻后再针刺近取穴位及阿是穴，时间约为20分钟，10次为1疗程。阿是穴可配用间接灸3～5壮，每日1次，疗效较佳。

5.2.2.3　推拿治疗

1. 病人坐位，用拇指按揉、一指禅推等手法在颞颌关节周围治疗约10分钟。

2. 按揉耳门或听宫，时间约为5～10分钟，以局部有轻微疼痛感为好。远道取穴，按揉对侧中渚、外关各1～3分钟，以穴位局部有酸胀感为佳。

3. 令患者做张、闭口运动，医生一手按揉患侧颞颌关节处，另一手托下颌帮助患者运动，反复5～10次。如有半脱位，则需更为复杂的手法操作。

4. 擦颞颌关节周围，以透热为度。可配合局部热敷。

5.2.3　肩关节周围病症

5.2.3.1　概况

现代医学的肱二头肌长头腱鞘炎、肱二头肌短头肌腱损伤、肩峰下滑囊炎、肩关节周围炎、冈上肌腱炎等参此治疗。中医学分属“伤筋”“痹症”“漏肩风”等范畴。

5.2.3.2　针灸治疗

主穴：根据病变的部位选取肩髃、肩髎、臑俞、天宗、阿是穴及抬肩穴；远取条口或阑尾穴。（抬肩穴为肩部病症经验穴，属经外奇穴，位于肩部锁骨连接的下方凹陷处。）

随症配穴：压痛点在肩部外侧者，外关；在肩前者，合谷。

操作：可先取条口或阑尾穴强刺激，并嘱病人同时活动患侧肩部，5～10分钟。再于肩关节周围部位电针，或温针灸。针刺留针一般20～30分钟，中强刺激。每日或隔日1次，10次为1疗程。可配合局部拔罐10～15分钟。

耳针：肩、锁骨、颈、枕等穴磁珠埋贴。

5.2.3.3 推拿治疗

1. 病人坐位，用㨰、揉、拿、一指禅推等手法在患部治疗，急性期宜手法轻柔，慢性期稍重，约10分钟。

2. 运用按揉、一指禅推及弹拨等手法进行穴位推拿（选穴同上），5~10分钟。

3. 上述推拿的同时，可配合肩外展活动。但急性期应禁用或慎用。

4. 摇、搓、抖患肩及上肢1~2分钟。

5.2.4 肘部疼痛

5.2.4.1 概况

现代医学的肱骨外上髁炎、肱骨内上髁炎、尺骨鹰嘴滑囊炎、旋后肌综合征、桡侧伸腕肌腱周围炎等参此治疗。中医学属“伤筋”“痹症”范畴。

5.2.4.2 针灸治疗

主穴：根据病变的部位选取阿是穴及曲池、手三里、小海、天井、外关。

操作：以阿是穴为主，可多向透刺其他穴位。得气后留针20~30分钟。亦可以阿是穴为中心，用皮肤针叩刺皮肤潮红后，隔姜艾炷灸10壮。每日或隔日1次，10次为1疗程。

耳针：肘、枕等穴磁珠埋贴。

5.2.4.3 推拿治疗

1. 病人坐位，用㨰、揉、一指禅推等手法在肘部患处治疗，急性期宜手法轻柔，慢性期稍重，约10分钟。

2. 运用按揉、一指禅推及弹拨等手法进行穴位推拿（选穴同上），5~10分钟。

3. 上述推拿的同时，可配合肘部拔伸、屈伸运动。

4. 搓、擦患肘关节1~2分钟。

5.2.5 腕部疼痛

5.2.5.1 概况

现代医学的腕关节损伤、腕管综合征、桡骨茎突部狭窄性腱鞘炎等参此治疗。中医学属“伤筋”“痹症”范畴。

5.2.5.2 针灸治疗

取穴：根据病变的部位选取阿是穴、阳溪、大陵、列缺、阳池等穴。

操作：阿是穴行针得气后，根据所在部位取其前后左右的穴位为配穴，静留针30分钟，或温针灸，每日1次。本部病症采用隔药饼灸较为有效。

5.2.5.3 推拿治疗

1. 用㨰、揉、一指禅推等手法在腕部患处治疗，可适当扩大范围至前臂下段，手法由轻到重，约10分钟。

2. 运用按揉、弹拨等手法穴位推拿（选穴同上），以局部酸胀感为佳，5~10分钟。

3. 牵拉拔伸、缓慢摇腕部关节。

4. 小鱼际擦患处1~2分钟。

5.2.6 腰腿痛

5.2.6.1 概况

现代医学的腰部软组织损伤、肌肉风湿病及腰椎退行性病变所致的腰痛及梨状肌综合征等所致的臀腿痛均可参此治疗；腰椎间盘突出症、椎管狭窄症可配合牵引治疗。

5.2.6.2 针灸治疗

主穴：根据不同的症状体征选取腰夹脊穴、肾俞、大肠俞、腰眼、次髎、秩边、环跳、委中、悬钟、阿是穴。急性腰扭伤远取人中、后溪。

操作：急性腰扭伤疼痛剧烈者，先针人中或后溪，得气后嘱患者活动腰部，常有立竿见影之效；疼痛缓解后针刺其他穴位，中强刺激，留针20~30分钟。风湿病者，可温针灸或电针配合艾条灸20分钟左右；梨状肌综合征臀部穴位针刺手法不宜过强过猛，以免损伤坐骨神经；腰椎间盘突出症、椎管狭窄症者，以相应节段的腰夹脊穴为主穴，配合牵引治疗。以上各病症均可局部拔罐10~15分钟，腰肌劳损者以走罐法为佳。

5.2.6.3 推拿治疗

1. 病人俯卧位，用㨰、按、揉法在腰骶臀腿患部治疗，用力要稍重，以力量渗透到深层为好，约10分钟。

2. 腰骶臀腿部阿是穴按揉2分钟；若痛点较多，先治最痛点，缓解后再治次痛点。宜先用轻手法，痛点减轻后逐渐加重手法。腰痛的远部穴位常取委中、昆仑和太溪等穴，各按揉1~2分钟，以酸胀麻木感为好。

3. 助手扶住患者腋部，医生握双踝部向下匀速牵拉数次；侧扳法：患者侧卧位，医生一手扶住患者肩部，另一手扶髋部，双手同时向相反方向用力扳动，常有清脆的关节活动声；屈晃法：患者仰卧位，屈髋屈膝，医生扶住其膝部，缓缓晃动腰椎关节数次。侧扳法和屈晃法对腰椎后关节滑膜嵌顿常较为有效，但棘上、间韧带损伤者禁用。

4. 拍、叩或擦腰骶患部。

5.2.7 髋部疼痛

5.2.7.1 概况

现代医学的髋关节扭伤、髋关节滑囊炎、退行性髋关节炎、弹响髋及髂胫束劳损、股外侧皮神经炎等参此治疗。中医学属“伤筋”“痹症”范畴。

5.2.7.2 针灸治疗

主穴：近取居髎、秩边、承扶、风市、阿是穴；远取悬钟。

操作：根据不同的病症选取3~5个穴位，各穴得气后中强刺激，留针20~30分钟。环跳宜侧卧屈膝取穴，针感传向足底。每日1次，10次为1疗程。髋关节扭伤或滑囊炎，可在局部刺络拔罐，每次15~20分钟。遇寒加重者可配合艾条灸15~20分钟。股外侧皮神经炎，在大腿外侧患部用皮肤针叩刺，再行走罐法。

5.2.7.3 推拿治疗

1. 用㨰、揉、一指禅推等手法在髋关节周围治疗，急性期宜手法轻柔，慢性期宜力量深沉有力，约10分钟。

2. 运用按揉、一指禅推及双拇指叠拨等手法进行穴位推拿（选穴同上），5～10分钟。

3. 上述推拿的同时，可配合髋关节轻柔的摇法，幅度由小到大。

4. 摇、抖患髋，并掌擦患部，以透热为度。

5.2.8 膝部疼痛

5.2.8.1 概况

现代医学的膝内外侧副韧带、十字韧带、半月板等损伤及髌下脂肪垫损伤、膝关节创伤性滑膜炎、膝关节骨性关节炎等参此治疗。中医学属“伤筋”“痹症”范畴。

5.2.8.2 针灸治疗

主穴：近取内膝眼、外膝眼、足三里、委中、阿是穴；远取三阴交、悬钟。

操作：内膝眼、外膝眼、阿是穴是针治膝关节疾病的常用穴，其他可酌情选取。各穴得气后留针20～30分钟。除创伤性滑膜炎积液严重者应穿刺抽液外，其余诸病均可在近取穴上配用温针灸，每日1次，10次为1疗程。

5.2.8.3 推拿治疗

1. 病人卧位，用摩法在髌周治疗，并可两手环抱膝部来回擦动，约10分钟。

2. 采用按揉、一指禅推及屈指点等手法进行穴位推拿（选穴同上），5～10分钟。

3. 上述推拿的同时，可配合膝关节屈伸、拔伸活动。

4. 掌擦膝部结束。

5.2.9 踝部疼痛

5.2.9.1 概况

现代医学的踝关节扭伤、踝管综合征、跟腱周围炎等参此治疗。中医学属“伤筋”“痹症”范畴。

5.2.9.2 针灸治疗

主穴：近取解溪、丘墟、商丘、昆仑、太溪、申脉、照海、阿是穴；远取阳池、阳溪等。

操作：以阿是穴为主，根据不同的病症每次选用2～3穴，得气后留针20～30分钟，或配用艾条灸20～30分钟。急性踝关节扭伤常取远道穴，并配合患踝即时轻微活动。

5.2.9.3 推拿治疗

1. 用㨰、揉、一指禅推等手法在踝关节周围治疗，急性期宜手法轻柔，慢性期宜力量深沉有力，约10分钟。

2. 采用按揉、一指禅推等手法进行穴位推拿（选穴同上），5～10分钟。

3. 上述推拿的同时，可配合髋关节轻柔的牵拉，幅度由小到大，以不引起局部疼痛为度。

4. 掌擦患部，以透热为度。

5.2.10 足跟痛

5.2.10.1 概况

本病病因有跟腱止点滑囊炎、跟骨下脂肪垫炎、跟骨骨骺炎、跖筋膜炎、跟骨骨刺等。

5.2.10.2 针灸治疗

主穴：近取仆参、昆仑、太溪、三阴交、阿是穴；远取大陵。

操作：以阿是穴为主，每次选用2~3穴，得气后留针20~30分钟，或配用艾条灸20~30分钟。

5.2.10.3 推拿治疗

1. 用掌根揉、一指禅推等手法在足跟部治疗，急性滑囊炎宜手法轻柔，慢性期宜力量深沉有力，约10分钟。

2. 采用按揉、一指禅推等手法进行穴位推拿（选穴同上），5~10分钟。

3. 掌擦患部使之透热。

5.3 妇科病症

5.3.1 痛　经

5.3.1.1 概况

痛经是指妇女经期或行经前后，出现少腹疼痛（有时可影响到腰骶部）的症状。现代医学将痛经分为原发性和继发性。前者见于生殖器官无明显异常者；后者见于子宫过度前倾或后倾、子宫内膜增厚、慢性盆腔炎、子宫内膜异位症，也见于卵巢囊肿等压迫生殖器官的病变中。两类痛经均可参此辨证治疗。

5.3.1.2 针灸治疗

主穴：近取气海、关元、十七椎；远取合谷、三阴交。

随症配穴：腹痛剧烈，次髎；呕吐，内关、足三里。

操作：先针合谷、三阴交，得气后行针5~6分钟，中等刺激；疼痛未见明显减轻者，针十七椎、关元或气海，针感向会阴部放射为佳，并配用艾条灸15~20分钟。腹痛仍不减者，加刺次髎。还可配合关元穴坐罐10~15分钟，或皮肤针叩刺腰骶部脊柱两侧，以皮肤出现红润、充血为度。子宫内膜异位症辨气虚血瘀或寒凝血瘀者，宜加灸。

耳穴：子宫、内分泌、神门、交感。用0.5寸毫针直刺，捻转泻法，或用磁珠贴压。

5.3.1.3 推拿治疗

1. 患者仰卧，下肢微屈膝髋，医者做摩腹2~3分钟。一指禅推法推气海、关元穴3~5分钟。按揉合谷、血海、三阴交穴各1~2分钟。

2. 患者俯卧，腰骶部涂以按摩乳，以手掌小鱼际擦腰骶部。

5.3.2 急性乳腺炎（缺乳）

5.3.2.1 概况

急性乳腺炎多见于哺乳期，可有发热、乳房红肿疼痛、硬结肿块和触痛等症状。本病相当于中医学的乳痈，由肝气郁结、热毒壅盛、乳汁排泌不畅而成。乳少即产后乳汁分泌量少，不能满足婴儿所需，中医认为多因肝气郁结或气血不足所致。

5.3.2.2 针灸治疗

主穴：膻中、期门、少泽、内关。

随症配穴：发热，大椎、曲池、合谷；食欲不佳，中脘、足三里。经验穴：肩井。

操作：膻中、期门针尖均向乳头方向平刺，针感向乳房扩散；少泽点刺出血；肩井稍向后斜刺1寸，只捻转不提插。膻中可加艾条灸，乳腺炎并可用艾条灸乳房肿块10～20分钟，每日2次。乳腺炎早期选大椎、第四胸椎夹脊、乳根（患侧）等穴拔罐，溃脓期局部用三棱针在所选的穴位处点刺出血后拔罐，每日或隔日1次。

5.3.2.3 推拿治疗

1. 乳腺炎患者仰卧，先在患侧乳房涂上少许按摩乳，医者可一手托住乳房，另一手以四指并拢由乳房四周轻轻向乳头方向推动，可沿着乳腺管的方向施以正压，把淤滞的乳汁逐步推出。在按摩的同时可用手轻轻揪乳头数次，以扩张乳头部的输乳管。每次操作10～15分钟。缺乳产妇操作同上，但手法更轻。

2. 医者以手掌顺时针方向摩腹5分钟，然后以拇指自中脘穴推至天枢穴，反复3～5分钟。

5.4 五官病症

5.4.1 目 疾

5.4.1.1 概况

现代医学的近视、斜视、视神经炎、视神经萎缩，可按以下针刺治疗；结膜炎、睑腺炎可按以下刺络放血法治疗。中医学中，目疾指以目赤肿痛或视物模糊为主证的眼科疾病。

5.4.1.2 针灸治疗

主穴：近取睛明、承泣、风池；远取合谷、养老。

操作：睛明与承泣交替应用，针刺时固定眼球，以细针沿眼眶内壁缓缓刺入，如针下有阻力或痛感，将针退出少许，稍微改变方向后再刺，不宜大幅提插、捻转；其他穴位可较强刺激，风池穴最好针感向眼区放散。各穴留针20～30分钟。结膜炎、睑腺炎刺络放血：耳尖、耳垂、太阳、中冲，每次选1～2穴放血，3次为1疗程。

耳针：近视或眼底病，可取眼、肝、肾、枕等区找敏感点用磁珠等埋贴。

5.4.1.3 推拿治疗

1. 患者仰卧位，医者以两拇指沿眼眶四周揉按5分钟，分推眉弓12～24次，点按睛明、太阳、鱼腰、攒竹、承泣等穴各1分钟。

2. 体位同上，医者一手托患者后枕部，另一手提拿颈项部5～7分钟，然后以拇指按揉风池穴、翳明穴各1～3分钟。

3. 体位同上，按合谷、阳陵泉、光明、太溪等穴各1分钟。

5.4.2 耳聋耳鸣

5.4.2.1 概况

耳聋耳鸣均为听觉异常的症状。中医学认为多由肝胆火热上逆或肝肾阴虚所致，后者常伴头痛眩晕、腰膝酸软等。

5.4.2.2　针灸治疗

主穴：翳风、听宫、听会、中渚、侠溪。

随症配穴：头痛眩晕，风池、印堂、百会、太冲、合谷；腰膝酸软，太溪、肾俞。

操作：听宫、听会在患侧任取一穴，远取穴位可取双侧，每次 1 ~ 2 穴，10 次为一疗程。

耳针：取心、内耳、肝、肾、皮质下，针刺或磁珠贴压，两耳交替使用。

穴位注射：取听宫、翳风、完骨、肾俞，用 654 – 2 注射液或维生素 B_{12}、维生素 B_1 注射液，每穴注射 0.2 ~ 0.5mL，隔日 1 次。

5.4.2.3　推拿治疗

1. 两掌心对患者两耳，一按一放，5 ~ 7 次。

2. 五指端自患侧率谷向后扫散（类似直推法，但速度较快）颞部 20 ~ 30 次，以拇指或中指自率谷向颊车揉按 20 ~ 30 次，然后搓揉耳尖、耳轮、耳垂，以患耳发热为度。点按合谷、中渚、足三里、光明、太溪等穴各 1 ~ 2 分钟。

5.4.3　鼻　炎

5.4.3.1　概况

现代医学的急慢性鼻炎、急慢性鼻窦炎、单纯性鼻炎、肥厚性鼻炎、过敏性鼻炎、萎缩性鼻炎可参此治疗。相当于中医学的“鼻渊”。

5.4.3.2　针灸治疗

主穴：印堂、迎香、通天、合谷。

随症配穴：发热，大椎、曲池；头胀痛，阳白、内庭。

操作：印堂宜向下平刺，使针感扩散至鼻部，迎香透鼻通，合谷强刺激。每日 1 次，留针 20 ~ 30分钟。

耳穴：内鼻、肺、额、肾上腺，多用磁珠贴压。

穴位注射：取印堂、迎香、合谷，用复合维生素 B 或川芎嗪注射液，每穴注射 0.3 ~ 0.5mL，隔日 1 次，10 次为 1 疗程。

5.4.3.3　推拿治疗

1. 干浴头面：两掌轻摩面部，再翻转至后方推摩颈枕部，约 5 分钟。十指微张，用指面从耳颞部开始由前向后做梳头动作。擦鼻梁：两手大鱼际沿鼻梁两侧上下往返用力擦动，向上至鼻根，下至双迎香穴，重复 30 ~ 50 次。

2. 按揉迎香、鼻通穴 2 ~ 5 分钟；两穴可交替使用。按揉合谷 1 ~ 2 分钟。按揉风池 1 ~ 2 分钟，以有酸胀感伴窜及脸部为佳。

3. 捏鼻法结束：拇食指相对捏住鼻翼，一捏一松，约 1 分钟，力量轻重应以无疼痛感为度。

5.4.4　牙　痛

5.4.4.1　概况

牙痛是口腔疾患中最常见的症状，现代医学的冠周炎、牙周炎、根尖周围炎、牙本质过敏等均可参此治疗。中医学将牙病分为虫病和火病，火病又有实火和虚火之别，实火多由胃火风热所致，虚火多由肾虚火旺引起。

5.4.4.2 针灸治疗

主穴：下关、颊车、合谷。配穴：太阳、颧髎。

操作：下关进针 1 寸；同侧下关、颊车可常规电针，用疏波刺激。颊车穴可加拔罐，留罐时间不超过 5 分钟。

耳针：三焦、神门、牙。

5.4.4.3 推拿治疗

1. 按揉患侧（或双侧）颊车穴 1～5 分钟，手法由轻逐渐加重，至疼痛缓解为止。若未见效，再以拇指较重地按揉下关穴 1～5 分钟。

2. 按揉合谷穴 1～2 分钟，先做患侧，若疼痛不能缓解加按对侧合谷穴。

3. 特殊疗法：将手洗干净，剪去指甲，以手指按摩牙龈，尤其在患牙处，重点按揉。手法可稍重一些，做 1～2 分钟。揉完后用淡盐水漱口。本法对于冠周炎及牙周炎有效。

5.5 单纯性肥胖 戒烟

5.5.1 单纯性肥胖

5.5.1.1 概况

单纯性肥胖症是指人体吸收的能量超过消耗量，使脂肪长时间的过剩，导致体重超过标准体重 20% 以上。中医学认为是脏腑功能失调所致。

5.5.1.2 针灸治疗

主穴：曲池、天枢、阴陵泉、丰隆、太冲。配穴：肥胖区域的穴位。

操作：针刺得气后接电针，可选择疏密波，留针 30 分钟。隔日或每日 1 次，10 次为 1 个疗程。

耳针：胃、内分泌、脾、三焦、缘中，可用毫针针刺或磁珠贴压，每天按压 7～10 次，有灼热感为宜，3～5 天换 1 次，10 次为 1 个疗程。

5.5.1.3 推拿治疗

1. 局部推拿。医者在需要减肥的部位做抹法或揉法 3～5 分钟，然后以掌摩法在腹部顺时针方向摩腹 3～5 分钟（可配用按摩乳）。再从剑突向关元单方向推摩 15～20 次。

2. 穴位推拿。医者用拇指点揉曲池、合谷、中脘、天枢、脾俞、胃俞、足三里、上巨虚、丰隆等穴各 1～2 分钟。

5.5.2 戒 烟

5.5.2.1 概况

吸烟危害人体健康，烟中有害物质，如尼古丁、烟焦油等多种化合物，与人类高血压、冠心病、慢性支气管炎、多种癌症以及胎儿畸形等多种疾病有关，对肺脏的损害更为突出。

5.5.2.2 针灸治疗

主穴：“甜蜜”穴（肺经列缺穴与大肠经阳溪穴之间的敏感点）、百会、神门。

随症配穴：烦躁不安，涌泉；欲眠，劳宫。

操作："甜蜜"穴向上斜刺1寸，产生酸、麻、胀感后接电针仪，用疏密波，强度以患者能忍受为度，留针30分钟。百会、神门常规针刺。每日或隔日1次，3次为1个疗程。

耳针：神门、肺、胃、口、交感。用针刺或磁珠贴压，两耳交替，3天换1次。平时还可在有吸烟欲望时便按压耳穴。

5.5.2.3　推拿治疗

医者以拇指按揉合谷、列缺、曲池、中脘、天枢、足三里、照海等穴各1～3分钟，局部产生酸胀重感。

Chapter 5 Common Disease Treatment

5.1 Internal Medicine Diseases

5.1.1 Headache

5.1.1.1 General information

Headache here means many different diseases in western medicine, such as migraine, tension headache etc, and headache caused by hypertension, arteriosclerosis of brain, diseases of the eye, ear and nose. But it should be differentiated from some sinister brain diseases such as space-occupying lesions, etc. These original diseases should be treated properly. Headaches are divided into different types according to the areas where they appear in Traditional Chinese Medicine. They are Yangming headache (frontal and eyebrow headache), Shaoyang headache (temporal headache, ears can be affected), Taiyang headache (occipital headache), Jueyin headache (parietal headache, eyes can be affected).

5.1.1.2 Acupuncture treatment

Main acupoints: Fengchi (GB20), Hegu (LI4).

Assistant acupoints: Frontal headache, Yintang (EX-HN3), Touwei (ST8), Neiting (ST44); migraine, Taiyang (EX-HN5), Shuaigu (GB8), Waiguan (SJ5); parietal headache, Baihui (DU20), Sishencong (EX-HN1), Tongtian (BL7), Taichong (LR3); occipital headache, Tianzhu (BL10), Fengfu (DU16), Houxi (SI3).

Acupoints chosen according to different symptoms: Fever, Dazhui (DU14), Quchi (LI11); Dyspnoea and nausea, Neiguan (PC6), Zhongwan (RN12); Dizziness, Sanyinjiao (SP6), Xingjian (LR2) or Taixi (KI3).

Manipulation: Puncture the local acupoints first, then the distant acupoints. Retain the needles for 20 ~ 30 minutes after arriving of Qi. Retain the needles for 1 ~ 2 hours for severe headache patients. Electrical impulse with moderate stimulation acupuncture can be used.

Skin Acupuncture: tap and puncture mainly the area where headache appears and in the nape. The stimulation can be strong in strong patients but should be stopped when nape skin mildly oozes blood. In women and weak patients, stimulation should be mild and only cause local flush.

Ear Acupuncture: Choose Occiput (AT3), Forehead (AT1), Subcortex (AT4), Shenmen (TF4), and Sympathetic Nerve (AH6a). Retain the needle for 20 ~ 30 minutes or press and paste the acupoints with magnetic pearls.

5. 1. 1. 3 Chinese massage treatment

1. Dry bath of the face and head: Mildly rub the face with two palms. Then rub neck and nape areas for about 5 minutes. Spread the ten fingers mildly and comb backward mildly and slowly, starting from the temporal areas.

2. Point-pressing, pressing and kneading acupoints from mild to strong then back to mild stimulation again. For parietal headache, mainly press Baihui (DU20), Sishencong (EX – HN1); For migraine, mainly press and knead Taiyang (EX – HN5), Shuaigu (GB8), Jiaosun (SJ20); For occipital headache, mainly press and knead Fengchi (GB20), Tianzhu (BL10). The treatment lasts for 5 ~ 10 minutes.

3. End of the treatment: Tap the head mildly to end the treatment.

5. 1. 2 Insomnia

5. 1. 2. 1 General information

Insomnia is both a symptom and a disease. Treatment for insomnia can also be used in treating neurosis, anemia, and menopause syndrome. In traditional Chinese Medicine, it is often referred to as "sleeplessness" and "being unable to sleep" etc.

5. 1. 2. 2 Acupuncture treatment

Local acupoints, Baihui (DU20), Fengchi (GB20); Distant acupoints, Sanyinjiao (SP6), Shenmen (HT7).

Acupoints chosen according to different symptoms: Dreaminess, Xinshu (BL15); waist soreness and tinnitus, Shenshu (BL23), Taixi (KI3); abdominal distention, Zusanli (ST36), Weishu (BL21); irritability, Taichong (LR3).

Manipulation: Puncture normally and retain the needle for 20 ~ 30 minutes after arrival of Qi once a day. One course consists of 10 treatments. After acupuncture, keep the patient in a prone position. Smear some massage lotion on both sides of the spine in the back. Then mildly cup up and down until a mild flush appears on the skin. Or tap and puncture both sides of the spine with a skin needle, especially areas near Xinshu and Ganshu until a mild flush appears on the skin.

Ear Acupuncture: Acupoints: Shenmen (TF4), Heart (CO15), Spleen (CO13), Kidney (CO10), Forehead (AT1), Occiput (AT3), Subcortex (AT4). Paste these acupoints and press them for about 5 minutes before sleeping.

5. 1. 2. 3 Chinese massage treatment

1. Keep a supine position. Press forehead from the middle to the lateral sides for about 3 minutes. This requires three – part manipulation: upper, middle and lower. Then push from Yingtang (EX – HN3) through Shenting (DU24) to Baihui (DU20) for 1 ~ 2 minutes. Mildly knead and rub temporal and parietal parts for 1 ~ 2 minutes. Hold a patients' occipital area with one palm, knead and grasp his nape with three fingers of the other palm for 2 ~ 3 minutes.

2. Digital – pressing and kneading at Baihui (DU20), Shenting (DU24), Taiyang (EX – HN5) and Fengchi (GB20) for 1 minute for each acupoint. Then ask the patient to close his or her eyes normally, and the doctor presses and kneads Jingming (BL1), Zanzhu (BL2), Yuyao (EX – HN4), Sizhukong

(SJ23), and Tongziliao (GB1) in turn for half minutes at each acupoint. Point – press and press acupoints Shenmen (HT7) and Neiguan (PC6) by hand for 1 ~ 2 minutes.

3. End of treatmeat: Mildly tap head and grasp Jianjing (GB21) acupoints on both shoulders several times.

5. 1. 3 Facial paralysis

5. 1. 3. 1 General information

Peripheral facial neuritis in western medicine can follow the treatment discussed here. In central facial paralysis patients, causes should be confirmed. Scalp acupuncture can be used to treat non-space-occupying lesions. The literal meaning of facial paralysis in TMC is "facial distortion".

5. 1. 3. 2 Acupuncture treatment

Local acupoints, Zanzhu (BL2), Yangbai (GB14), Yifeng (SJ17), Sibai (ST2), Yingxiang (LI20), Dicang (ST4), Jiache (ST6), Quanliao (SI18); distant acupoints, Hegu (LI4), Neiting (ST44), Taichong (LR3).

Manipulation: Usually, local acupoints on the paralyzed side and distant acupoints in bilateral sides are chosen for treatment. In the first week after onset of facial paralysis, avoid acupuncture on local acupoints. Undertaking moxibustion on Yifeng (SJ17) for 15 ~ 20 minutes is acceptable. One week after the onset, the condition will become stable. Horizontal acupuncture, which connects two acupoints at the same time, can be applied. After the arriving of Qi at each acupoint, stimulate the acupoints for 20 ~ 30 minutes with an electrical impulse stimulater. The stimulation should be mild to strong to make the patient comfortable. For patients who have not recovered after more than a month, the stimulation should be strong but not beyond the patient's endurance. Moxibustion is suggested to be used in these situations.

5. 1. 3. 3 Chinese massage treatment

1. Ask the patient to lie down horizontally, rub the paralyzed face mildly using the doctor's palm or fingers to cause local warmth for about 5 ~ 10 minutes.

2. Press and knead the Yintang (EX – HN3) acupoint using the doctor's thumb, and then advance to the Taiyang (EX – HN5) acupoint passing over the eyebrow. After that, proceed to Baihui (DU20) acupoint and Shenting (DU24) acupoint. At the same time, push from the middle-point of the two eyebrows to Yangbai (GB14). Then push downward and knead from the Jingming (BL1) to Yingxiang (LI20). Push and knead from the Yingxiang (LI20) acupoint to Xiaguan (ST7) pausing at Sibai (ST2) and then at Quanliao (SI18), from Dicang (ST4) to Xiache (ST6), from Renzhong (DU26) to Yingxiang (LI20). Each treatment requires about 1 ~ 2 minutes. Finally, press and knead Fengchi (GB20), Quchi (LI11), and Hegu (LI4) for 1 minute each.

3. Mildly tap the face to finish all the treatment.

5. 1. 4 Trigeminal neuralgia

5. 1. 4. 1 General information

In Traditional Chinese Medicine, trigeminal neuralgia is called "face pain" or "face wind".

5. 1. 4. 2 Acupuncture treatment

Acupoints chosen according to different symptoms: Frontal headache, Zanzhu (BL2), Yangbai

(GB14); maxillary Pain, Sibai (ST2), Quanliao (SI18), Yingxiang (LI20); mandibular Pain, Xiaguan (ST7), Jiache (ST6), Daying (ST5). Distant acupoints: Fengchi (GB20), Hegu (LI4), Waiguan (SJ5), Neiting (ST44), Sanyinjiao (SP6).

Manipulation: Puncture Xiaguan (ST7) towards inner canthus of the other part of the face for 2 *cun* to cause electrified feeling around nose, eye, lip area of the same side of the face. Puncture Zanzhu (BL2) upward along the supraorbital bridge for 0.5 ~ 1.0 *cun* to cause electrified feeling and cause the feeling to pass to the frontal area. Puncture Daying (ST5) downward. Use regular acupuncture on the other acupoints. It is preferable to make a strong needle sensation.

5.1.5 Cerebrovascular accidental sequela

5.1.5.1 General information

Cerebrovascular accidental sequela means hemiplegia, dysphasia, and deviation of the mouth after acute cerebrovascular diseases. Sequelae such as cerebral haemorrhaging or embolism, are all included in this topic. Other sequelae after cerebral operations and cerebral palsy in children can have similar treatment. In TCM, these sequelae are called "hemiplegia".

5.1.5.2 Acupuncture treatment

Acupoints on hands: Jianyu (LI15), Quchi (LI11), Shousanli (LI10), Waiguan (SJ5), Hegu (LI4); Acupoints on legs: Huantiao (GB30), Fengshi (GB20), Liangqiu (ST34), Yanglingquan (GB34), Zusanli (ST36), Kunlun (BL60), Jiexi (ST41), Taichong (LR3).

Acupoints chosen according to different symptoms: Deviation of mouth, Jiache (ST6), Dicang (ST4), Yingxiang (LI20); urine incontinence, Baihui (DU20), Qugu (RN2), Zhongji (RN3); dysphagia, Fengfu (DU16), Yamen (DU15), Fengchi (GB20), Yifeng (SJ17), aphasia, Lianquan (RN23), Tongli (HT5); movement Disturbance of shoulders, Puncture Jianyu (LI15) toward Jiquan (HT1), Jianzhen (SI9), Jianjing (GB21), and Tianzong (SI11); movement Disturbance of knees, Weizhong (BL40), Weiyang (BL39), Xiyangguan (GB33), Yinmen (BL37), and Chengshan (BL57); inward turning of ankles, Xuanzhong (GB39), Shenmai (BL62), Jinmen (BL63), and Puncture Qiuxu (GB40) toward Zhaohai (KI6); muscle Hypertonia, mainly the acupoints on Yin Meridians such as: Jiquan (HT1), Neiguan (PC6), Kongzui (LU1), Quze (PC3), Xuehai (SP10), Ququan (LR8), Yinlingquan (SP9), and Sanyinjiao (SP6), etc. Cerebral palsy in children, Baihui (DU20), Sishencong (EX-HN1).

Scalp Acupuncture: Mainly use the anterior oblique line of parietotemporal area and the mid-parietal line in scalp. For patients of sensory disturbance, superior posterior temporal oblique line should be added; for aphasiac, anterior temporal line is adopted; for equilibrium disorder patients, lower-lateral line of occiput is adopted.

Manipulation: Regular body acupuncture is adopted. The needle can remain in the body for 20 ~ 30 minutes and an electrical stimulator can be used. One time of treatment a day and 10 times of treatment form a course. The scalp needle forms an angle of 30° with the scalp, by using abstraction acupuncture or twirling acupuncture. When superior temporal oblique line and superior posterior oblique line are adopted in acupuncture, successive 3 acupuncture can be adopted from the top to the lower part of scalp.

5. 1. 5. 3 Chinese massage treatment

1. Keep the patient in a prone position. The doctor stands beside the paralysed side and kneads the patient's back and waist of bilateral sides along the spine for 3 ~5 minutes. Then apply digital-pressing on acupoints such as Feishu (BL13), Ganshu (BL18), Pishu (BL20), and Shenshu (BL23). The doctor should roll and knead from the hip to the back of the calf for about 5 minutes on the paralysed side and apply digital-pressing on acupoints such as Huantiao (GB30), Weizhong (BL40), and Chengshan (BL57), etc. The patient is encouraged to extend his waist, hips, knee and ankle at the same time.

2. Keep a patient in the supine position. The doctor stands beside the paralysed side and kneads, rolls for about 5 ~ 10 minutes on the medial side of the hand, shoulder, elbow, wrist and from the anterosuperior spine of iliac to the instep along the anterolateral side of the leg. Then apply digital-pressing on acupoints such as Jianyu (LI15), Quchi (LI11), Chize (LU5), Shousanli (LI10), Hegu (LI4), Huantiao (GB30), Futu (ST32), Liangqiu (ST34), Zusanli (ST36), Fenglong (ST40), Jiexi (ST41), and Xuanzhong (GB39) for 1 minute each. The patient is encouraged to do some passive movements several times on his wrist, elbow, and shoulder at the same time.

3. Tap the paralysed limbs to finish the whole manipulation.

5. 1. 6 Polyneuropathies

5. 1. 6. 1 General information

Treatment here can be used for many diseases in western medicine such as polyneuropathies, Gnillain-Barre syndrome, periodic paralysis, hysterical paralysis, sequela of poliomyelitis, trauma paraplegia, acute spinal cord inflammation, progressive muscular atrophy, myasthenia gravis, muscular dystrophies, etc. They are included in the flaccidity syndrome in Traditional Chinese Medicine.

5. 1. 6. 2 Acupuncture treatment

Main acupoints on the Hands: Jianyu (LI15), Jianliao (SJ14), Quchi (LI11), Shousanli (LI10), Hegu (LI4). Main acupoints Legs: Huantiao (GB30), Yanglingquan (GB34), Xuanzhong (GB39), Biguan (ST31), Futu (ST32), Zusanli (ST36), Jiexi (ST41).

Acupoints chosen according to symptoms: In continence of feces: Tianshu (ST25), Shangjuxu (ST37). In continence of urine or retention of urine: Ciliao (BL32), Zhongji (RN3), Sanyinjiao (SP6), and Yinlingquan (SP9). Paraplegia: Jiaji (EX – B2) acupoints, which are close to the affected area.

Manipulation: Choose 4 ~ 8 acupoints each time in turn. Usually the sick side is treated. If treatment is not effective, the healthy side can be recommended. After the arrival of Qi, retain the needle for 20 ~ 30 minutes with medium stimulation once a day or every other day. A full treatment includes 10 sessions. The second course can be started after a 3 ~ 5 day rest. Moxibustion on Tianshu (ST25) and Zhongji (RN3) for 20 minutes once a day is recommended in patients with urine incontinence or retention.

Acupoint Injection: Inject 0. 5mL of vitaminB_{12} in acupoints, such as Shousanli (LI10), Zusanli (ST36) once every other day. A full treatment is 10 days.

5.1.6.3 Chinese massage treatment

1. In prone position: Using rolling method and kneading from top to bottom on bilateral sides of the back, waist and spine for 7 ~ 12 times on right and left sides alternately. Then digital-pressing of Feishu (BL13), Ganshu (BL19), Pishu (BL20), Weishu (BL21), and Shenshu (BL23) is performed. After that, use the rolling method and kneading from hip to calf on the back of the sick side. Digital-pressing of Huantiao (GB30), Weizhong (BL40) and Chengshan (BL57). Massage with even force and rhythm.

2. In supine position: Doctor stands on the sick side of a patient and uses rolling method on the medial side of the hand, shoulder, elbow and wrist, also on the anterolateral side of the leg, from anterosuperior spine of iliac to the instep for 7 ~ 12 times, right and left sides alternately. Then digital - pressing Jianyu (LI15), Quchi (LI11), Chize (LU15), Shousanli (LI10), Hegu (LI4), Huantiao (GB30), Futu (ST32), Liangqiu (ST34), Zusanli (ST36), Fenglong (ST40), Jiexi (ST41), and Xuanzhong (GB39) for 1 minute each. After that, passively move wrist, elbow and shoulder 7 ~ 12 times.

3. Pat the sick limbs to finish the massage.

5.1.7 Cough and asthma

5.1.7.1 General information

Treatment here can be used for chronic bronchitis, bronchiectasis and asthma. They are all lung diseases in the Traditional Chinese Medicine and have many different clinical manifestness. However, they have similar causes such as exogenous wind-evil, cold-evil, wet-evil, hot-evil and dry-evil as well as endogenous wet-evil, and weak functioning of the lung, spleen and kidney. They also have similar treatments.

5.1.7.2 Acupuncture treatment

Main acupoints: Feishu (BL13), Danzhong (RN17), Lieque (LU7), Chize (LU5).

Acupoints chosen by symptoms: Fever: Dazhui (DU14), Quchi (LI11), Hegu (LI4); nasal Obstruction: Yingtang (EX - HN3), Yingxiang (LI20), Hegu (LI4); excessive saliva: Neiguan (PC6), Fenglong (ST40); asthma: Dingchuan (EX - B1), Shenzhu (DU12), Xinshu (BL15).

Manipulation: Puncture Feishu (BL13) obliquely toward spine and puncture Danzhong (RN17) subcutaneously in a downward manner. Retain the needle for 20 ~ 30 minutes after arriving of Qi. Acupuncture once or twice a day in the acute period. Then reduce it to once every two days after relief of the symptoms until the symptoms disappear. For chronic patient, 10 treatments are one series and the next series are started after 3 ~ 5 days' rest. Medium stimulation from the electrical impulse stimulater can be used in this treatment. Acupoint - plastering has an obvious effect in asthma treatment. Also cupping on Dingchuan (EX - B1), Feishu (BL13), Danzhong (RN17) can be applied at the same time. Each cupping needs to last for 10 minutes.

Ear acupuncture: Choose 2 ~ 3 sensitive acupoints among Trachea (CO16), Lung (CO14), Antitragus Apex (AT1, 2, 4i), Adrenal (TG2P), Subcortex (AT4), Endocrine (CO18), and Kidney (CO10). Retain needles for 20 ~ 30 minutes, or stick magnetic pearls on these acupoints.

5. 1. 7. 3 Chinese massage treatment

1. Keep a patient in a prone position. Pushing fingers or kneading from Tiantu (RN22) to Danzhong (RN17) slowly, to and fro for 2 ~ 3 minutes. Then do intercostal combing which means dividing and pushing from Danzhong (RN17) with both thumbs for 2 ~ 3 minutes.

2. Keep seated or supine position. Grasp and knead the neck for 3 ~ 5 minutes, and the shoulder for 5 ~ 7 times. Then flat-push the shoulder and back, obliquely push the hypochondrium until the diathermic purpose is reached. Digital-pressing Fengchi (GB20), Fengfu (DU16), Jianjing (GB21), Feishu (BL13), Dingchuan (EX - B1) and Geshu (BL17) until soreness and swelling are affected. Press and knead Chize (LU5), Hegu (LI4), Fenglong (ST40) and Zusanli (ST36) for 1 minute each.

5. 1. 8 Coronary atherosclerotic cardiopathy

5. 1. 8. 1 General information

At the early stages of this disease, there is no obvious symptom. So it is called latent coronary heart disease. With the development of the disease, many symptoms will appear such as chest tightness, palpitation, chest pain etc. In TCM, it is equal to "thoracic obstruction".

5. 1. 8. 2 Acupuncture treatment

Main Acupoints: Xinshu (BL15), Jueyinshu (BL14), Tongli (HT5), Neiguan (PC6), Danzhong (RN17), Juque (RN14).

Acupoints chosen by symptoms: Blood stasis in heart: Geshu (BL17), Yinxi (LI20); cyanosis: Shaoshang (LU1), Zhongchong (PC9), Shaochong (HT9); they can be punctured to bleed; cold limbs: Moxibustion on Qihai (RN6), Guanyuan (RN4); thick coating on tongue: Zhongwan (RN12), Zusanli (ST36) and Fenglong (ST40).

Manipulation: Perpendicular puncture Neiguan (PC6) and Tongli (HT5) for 0. 5 ~ 1. 0 *cun*, and twirl and rotate the needle to pass needle sensation. Subcutaneous puncture Danzhong (RN17) upward. Perpendicular puncture Juque (RN14) for 0. 5 ~ 1. 0 *cun*. Oblique puncture Xinshu (BL15) and Jueyinshu (BL14) toward spine and pass the needle sensation deeply inward. If the symptoms occur when it becomes cold, do moxibustion at each acupoint.

Ear acupuncture: Choose 2 ~ 3 acupoints each time from Heart (CO15), Small Intestine (CO6), Sympathetic Nerve (AH6a), Subcortex (AT4), Shenmen (TF4), Chest (AH10), Back Groove (PS). Retain the Paste magnetic pearls or needles for 20 ~ 30 minutes.

5. 1. 8. 3 Chinese massage treatment

1. Keep a patient in supine position. Then on each side (dividing) push and rub on chest and rib areas for 3 ~ 5 minutes. After that digital-knead Danzhong (RN17), Juque (RN14), Neiguan (PC6) and Zusanli (ST36) for 1 minute each.

2. Keep the patient in a prone position. Then on each side (dividing) push upper back area and press spine for 5 minutes. After that, press and knead or one-finger Zen push Xinshu (BL15), Jueyinshu (BL14), and Ashi acupoints on the back for 3 ~ 5 minutes each.

3. Mildly tap the Danzhong (RN17) area of the chest to end massage treatment.

5. 1. 9 Acute and chronic gastritis

5. 1. 9. 1 General information

Treatment here can be used for many diseases in western medicine such as gastritis, duodenitis, peptic ulcer, gastrospasm, gastrointestinal neurosis and gastroptosis. In Traditional Chinese Medicine, these diseases belong to the categories of epigastric pain, vomiting, pain in the chest, distention in the upper abdomen, heatstroke.

5. 1. 9. 2 Acupuncture treatment

Main Acupoints: Zhongwan (RN12), Neiguan (PC6) and Zusanli (ST36).

Acupoints chosen by symptoms: Attack on the stomach by the liver-Qi: Taichong (LR3); stagnancy of Qi and blood stasis: Gongsun (SP4), Geshu (BL17); dyspepsia: Liangmen (ST21); Thinstools: Pishu (BL20), Weishu (BL21); cold stomach, which can be relieved by warming, make moxibustion on Pishu (BL20), Weishu (BL21); diarrhea: Tianshu (ST25), Shangjuxu (ST37); constipation: Tianshu (ST25), Zhigou (SJ6); abdominal distention: Neiting (ST44).

Manipulation: First choose Neiguan (PC6), Zusanli (ST36) and other acupoints according to the different symptoms. Retain the needle for 20 ~ 30 minutes after arriving of Qi and medium stimulation from eletro-acupuncture for 15 minutes is encouraged here. If the effect is not satisfying, do extra moxibustion on Zhongwan (RN12) for 15 ~ 20 minutes. The temperature produced by the moxibustion should make the patient feel comfortable. Regular acupuncture can be performed in other acupoints, once everyday or every other day, 10 times of treatment for a course. Other acupuncture treatments, cupping on Zhongwan (RN12), move-cupping on the back and tapping by skin-needle can be chosen to enhance the treatment effect according to different situations.

Ear Acupuncture: Find sensitive acupoints from Stomach (CO4), Liver (CO12), Spleen (CO13), Ear Center (HX1), Duodenum (CO5), and Shenmen (TF4); paste magnetic pearls on these acupoints.

5. 1. 9. 3 Chinese massage treatment

1. Keep the patient in a supine position and mildly bend his knees and hips. The doctor rubs with palms on the upper abdomen (a little bit to the left) for 3 ~ 5 minutes. Then push-rub from xiphoid process to navel for 15 ~ 20 times. With the middle finger, the doctor vibrates Zhongwan (RN12) for 1 ~ 2 minutes. Shangwan (GB3) or Xiawan (RN10) can also be chosen for vibration in turn according to different stomachache situations. Press-knead Neiguan (PC6), Hegu (LI4) for 1 minute each, then Zusanli (ST36) for 2 ~ 3 minutes.

2. Keep the patient in a prone position. The doctor rubs with palms on the bilateral areas along spine. Especially rub the area from Ganshu (BL18) to Weishu (BL21) until it becomes warm. Point-press Lingtai (DU10), Zhiyang (DU9), Tianzong (SI11), Pishu (BL20), and Weishu (BL21).

3. Mildly tap the back 5 ~ 10 times with empty fists.

5. 1. 10 Biliary tract diseases

5. 1. 10. 1 General information

Treatment here can be used for many diseases in western medicine such as acute and chronic cholecystitis, cholangeitis, cholelithiasis, and biliary ascariasis. Jaundice, hypochondriac pain and so on are mostly caused by dampness-heat of liver and gallbladder and liver Qi depression.

5.1.10.2 Acupuncture treatment

Main Acupoints: Danshu (BL19), Ganshu (BL18), Dannangxue (EX - LE6), Yanglingquan (GB34), Taichong (LR3).

Acupoints chosen by symptoms: Fever: Dazhui (DU14), Quchi (LI11) and Hegu (LI4); biliary ascariasis: Puncture Yingxiang (LI20) toward Sibai (ST2); jaundice: Zhiyang (DU9), Sanyinjiao (SP6); nausea and vomiting: Neiguan (PC6), Zusanli (ST36).

Manipulation: First, puncture Yanglingquan (GB34), Dannangxue (EX - LE6) and Taichong (LR3). After arriving of Qi, give them strong electric impulse stimulation. Then puncture other acupoints. Obliquely puncture Danshu (BL19), Ganshu (BL18) toward spine to pass the needle sensation deep. Usually retain the needle for 30 minutes and give the treatment once a day. If the patient suffers severe pain, twice daily is allowed. Needle retaining time can be prolonged to 1 ~ 2 hours if necessary.

Ear Acupuncture: Prescription: Liver (CO12), Pancreas and Biliary Tract (CO11), Stomach (CO4), Sympathetic Nerve (AH6a), Shenmen (TF4), and Endocrine (CO18). Magnetic pearls can be pasted and pressed on these acupoints. For a gall-bladder sand stone patient, needles imbeded in a one-lateral ear can be used as treatment. Remove the needles to the other ear 3 ~ 4 days later. The total treatment takes one month. During treatment, greasy food is not forbidden since it can help discharge the stones. At the onset of severe stomachache, pressing these acupoints for 4 ~ 5 minutes can effectively relieve the pain.

5.1.10.3 Chinese massage treatment

1. Keep a patient in a supine position. Rub upper abdomen especially the right side and middle areas for 2 ~ 5 minutes. Rubbing should be mild but must make the local areas warm. Press and knead 1 minute on both Dannang (EX - LE6) and Zusanli (ST36) to pass the sour and swelling feeling downward.

2. Keep a patient in a prone position. Press and knead Ganshu (BL18) and Danshu (BL19) for 5 ~ 10 minutes each to make the local areas overcome the sourness and swelling.

5.1.11 Acute and chronic enteritis

5.1.11.1 General information

Treatment here can be used to treat many diseases in western medicine such as acute and chronic enteritis, intestinal function disorders, allergic enteritis, ulcerative colitis, intestinal tuberculosis, bacillary dysentery, and intestinal amebiasis. In traditional Chinese medicine, they belong to the categories of diarrhoea and stomachache.

5.1.11.2 Acupuncture treatment

Main Acupoints: Local acupoints: Tianshu (ST25), Guanyuan (RN4), Dachangshu (BL25) and Xiaochangshu (BL27); distant acupoints: Shangjuxu (ST37), Zusanli (ST36).

Acupoints chosen by symptoms: Fever: Dazhui (DU14), Quchi (LIll), Hegu (LI4). Nausea and vomitting: Neiguan (PC6); tenesmus: Quchi (LI11), Neiting (ST44); aversion to cold with cold limbs: Baihui (DU20), Shenque (RN8); chronic cases: Pishu (BL20), Shenshu (BL23).

Manipulation: First, puncture Shangjuxu (ST37) and Zusanli (ST36) to pass the needle sensation to the legs, puncture Tianshu (ST25) and Guanyuan (RN25) to pass the needle sensation to the lower abdomen. Then chose acupoints by symptoms and retain the needles in these acupoints for 20 ~ 30 minutes. Lined cupping can be used for chronic diarrhea patients. Do moxibustion 10 ~ 20 minutes on Qihai (RN6) for weak chronic diarrhea patients.

5.1.11.3 Chinese massage treatment

1. Keep a patient in a supine position. Palm-rub periumbilical area for 2 ~ 5 minutes. Mildly knead Zhongwan (RN12), Tianshu (ST25) and Qihai (RN6) for 1 minute each to pass the energy deep into the body. Press and knead Yinlingquan (SP9), Zusanli (ST36) for 2 minutes each with stronger stimulation to cause local soreness, numbness, swelling and heaviness.

2. Keep a patient in a prone position, strongly scrub lumbosacral area.

3. Put one palm on the other one and vibrate and press periumbilial area mildly for 10 times. There are 10 seconds breaks during each treatment.

5.1.12 Visceroptosis

5.1.12.1 General information

This includes some common diseases such as gastroptosis, uterine prolapse and rectum prolapse. In Traditional Chinese Medicine, visceroptosis is due to deficient Yang – Qi and organs cannot be raised in normal anatomical positions. The general guideline for treatment is to support Yang – Qi.

5.1.12.2 Acupuncture treatment

Main Acupoints: Baihui (DU20), Guanyuan (RN4).

Acupoints chosen by symptoms: Gastroptosis: Zhongwan (RN12), Tiwei which is 4 *cun* bilateral to Zhongwan (RN12), and Zusanli (ST36); uterine prolapse: Tituo which is 4 *cun* bilateral to Guanyuan (RN4), and Sanyinjiao (SP6); rectum prolapse: Changqiang (DU1), which is at the end of coccyx and belongs to the Du Meridian, and Chengshan (BL57).

Manipulation: Puncture Baihui (DU20) and Guanyuan (RN4), then thrust the needle strongly and lift it slowly several times. After that, retain the needle for 20 minutes. Finally, make moxibustion on each acupoint for 10 minutes. The treatment on both acupoints can be started at the same time.

5.1.12.3 Chinese massage treatment

1. Keep the patient in a supine position. Then knead and press Baihui (DU20) for 5 minutes. For gastroptosis patients palm-rub the belly counter-clockwise for 3 ~ 5 minutes beginning from the lower belly to the higher belly. Expand the rubbing area gradually. Then, palm-root push from Guanyuan (RN4) to Zhongwan (RN12) for 3 ~ 5 minutes slowly. Finally, Point – press Zhongwan (RN12), Tianshu (ST25), Qihai (RN6) and Guanyuan (RN4) for 1 minute each.

2. Keep a patient in a prone position. For gastroptosis patient, knead and press Pishu (SL20), Weishu (BL21) and Shenshu (BL23) for 1 minute each. Then scrub the back and loins to pass the energy deep into the body. For patients who suffer from prolapse of the uterine or rectum, first clean the prolapsed uterine or rectum area with warm water. Then rub and knead them mildly for 3 ~ 5 minutes with

the underside of the doctors' thumb covered by a clean glove. Finally, softly push the organs back into the body and this can be done by the patients themselves.

5.1.13 Prostatitis, uroschesis and urinary incontinence

5.1.13.1 General information

Treatment here can be used for many diseases in western medicine such as: uroschesis, enuresis, urinary incontinence, prostatitis and prostatauxe. In Traditional Chinese Medicine, the diseases belong to "retention of urine", caused by disorder of kidneys and bladder.

5.1.13.2 Acupuncture treatment

Main Acupoints: Local acupoints: Ciliao (BL32), Zhongji (RN3), and Guanyuan (RN4); distant acupoints: Sanyinjiao (SP6), Yinlingquan (SP9).

Acupoints chosen by symptoms: When the patient has soreness and weakness of the loins and knees, choose Shenshu (BL23) and Taixi (KI3).

Manipulation: First, puncture Sanyinjiao (SP6) and Yinlingquan (SP9) to pass the needle sensation to the bottoms of the feet. Then chose two acupoints from Qihai (RN9), Guanyuan (RN4), and Zhongji (RN3), and pass the needle sensation to the urethral orifice. After arriving of Qi, give medium electric impulse stimulation for 20 ~ 30 minutes. Do not retain needle on Ciliao (BL32) and manipulate this acupoint for 2 ~ 3 minutes to pass the needle sensation to the anterior orifice. Moxibustion can be used on the acupoints located on the belly and lumbosacral areas.

Ear Acupuncture: Choose 3 ~ 4 acupoints from Bladder (CO9), Urethra (HX3), Kidney (CO10), External Genitalia (HX4), and Sympathetic Nerve (AH6a). Retain needles or paste magnetic pearls for treatment.

5.1.13.3 Chinese massage treatment

1. Palm rub the lower belly anticlockwise and clockwise for 1 ~ 2 minutes each to keep the local area warm. Then strongly press and rub on Qihai (RN6) and Guanyuan (RN4).

2. Digit press Qihai (RN6), Zhongji (RN3), Guanyuan (RN4), Zusanli (ST36), Yinlingquan (SP9) and Sanyinjiao (SP6) for 1 ~ 2 minutes each.

5.1.14 Seminal emission and impotence

5.1.14.1 General information

Nocturnal emission and impotence belong to sexual disorder of males. Treatment here can also be used to treat diseases such as premature ejaculation, ejaculation obstruction, and bloody ejaculation. In Traditional Chinese Medicine, these diseases are mostly caused by kidney problems.

5.1.14.2 Acupuncture treatment

Main Acupoints: Local acupoints: Zhongji (RN3), Guanyuan (RN4), Ciliao (BL32), Zhibian (BL54); distant acupoints: Sanyinjiao (SP6), Zusanli (ST36).

Acupoints chosen by symptoms: Insomnia or wet dreams: Shenmen (HT7), Xinshu (BL15); spermatorrhea or impotence: Shenshu (BL23), Taixi (KI3); vertigo: Fengchi (GB20).

Manipulation: Choose one acupoint between Zhongji (RN3) and Guanyuan (RN4) and pass the needle sensation toward urethral meatus. Zusanli (ST36) and Sanyinjiao (SP6) must be chosen and the needle sensation should be passed downward. Retain the needles for 20 ~ 30 minutes after arriving of Qi. Moxibustion can be used for the acupoints, which are located on the belly. The needle sensation from Ciliao (BL32) and Zhibian (BL54) should be passed toward anterior orifice of the perineum.

Acupoint Injection Treatment: Inject 50mg of vitaminB_1 into Guanyuan (RN4) and Zhongji (RN3) once every other day. One course consists of ten treatment repetitions. Inject 5mg of testosterone propionate into Guanyuan (RN4) or Zhongji (RN3) alternating once every other day for impotent patients. One course consists of four treatments.

Ear Acupuncture: Retain needles for 30 minutes or paste magnetic pearls on acupoints such as External Genitalia (HX4), Subcortex (AT4), Shenmen (TF4), and Endocrine (CO18).

5.1.14.3 Chinese massage treatment

1. Keep a patient in a supine position and mildly bend his hips and knees. Palm rub the lower abdomen area for 3 ~ 5 minutes. Then rub from navel to pubic symphysis in one direction to pass the warmth deep into the body. Middle finger vibration on Shenque (RN8), Qihai (RN6), Zhongji (RN3), Guanyuan (RN4) and Qugu (RN2) for 1 ~ 2 minutes each. Digit press Zusanli (ST36), Sanyinjiao (SP6), Taixi (KI3) and Yongquan (KI1) for 1 ~ 2 minutes each.

2. Keep a patient in a prone position and press and knead Shenshu (BL23), Zhishi (BL52) and Yaoyan (EX – B6) for 1 ~ 2 minutes each. Palm root scrub lumbosacral area to pass the warmth deep into the body. Digitaly-press Shenshu (BL23), Zhishi (BL52), Dachangshu (BL25), Zhibian (BL54) and Ciliao (BL32) for 1 ~ 2 minutes each.

5.1.15 Sunstroke

5.1.15.1 General information

Sunstroke is a group of acute diseases caused by heat dissipation difficulty in a hot environment. It is called "Fasha" (heatstroke) in Traditional Chinese Medicine.

5.1.15.2 Acupuncture treatment

Main Acupoint: Dazhui (DU14), Quchi (LI11), Hegu (LI4), Neiting (ST44) for mild cases; Shuigou (DU26), Shixuan (EX – UE10), Quze (PC3), Weizhong (BL40) for severe cases.

Acupoints chosen by symptoms: Fever: Shixuan (EX – UE10), Dazhui (DU14), Hegu (LI4); nausea and chest oppression: Neiguan (PC6); sweating with cold limbs and physical collapse: Moxibustion on Guanyuan (RN4), Qihai (RN6) and Shenque (RN8).

Manipulation: Prompt prick to cause bleeding or medium to strong acupuncture are usually used in sunstroke patients. Only patients with total collapse need moxibustion.

5.1.15.3 Scraping treatment

1. Scraping on head and back: Scrape Baihui (DU20) on the top of the head for 1 ~ 2 minutes. Then scrape Dazhui (DU14) and Xiong jiaji (EX – B2) acupoints on the back until pink or black skin eruptions or bruises appear.

2. Scraping of limbs: Scraping Quze (PC3) and Neiguan (PC6) on the hand, Weizhong (BL40) on the leg until a similar situation appears.

5.1.16 Shock

5.1.16.1 General information

Shock is an acute situation caused by severe neurogenic, metabolic, endocrine and circulation failures after a strong attack of pathogenic factors.

5.1.16.2 Acupuncture treatment

Main Acupoints: Suliao (DU25), Shuigou (DU26), Neiguan (PC6), Guanyuan (RN4), Yongquan (KI1), Zusanli (ST 36).

Acupoints chosen according to symptoms:

Cardiogenic: Sanyinjiao (SP6), Hegu (LI4); septic: Shixuan (EX – UE10), Chize (LU5), Weizhong (BL40); bleeding can be caused in this treatment; Haemorrhagic: Moxibustion on Baihui (DU20), Qihai (RN6), Renying (ST9); anaphylactic: Quchi (LI11), Chengjiang (RN24); traumatic: Shenmen (TF4), Sympathetic Nerve (AH6a); neurogenic: Hegu (LI4), Taichong (LR3).

Manipulation: Obliquely puncture the tip of the nose upward to Suliao (DU25) for 0.5 *cun*. Then continuously manipulate the needle. Obliquely puncture Shuigou (DU26) upward in 45°angle. Then give medium stimulation. In severe cases strong stimulation can be used combined with lifting, thrusting, twirling and rotating. Perpendicular puncture Neiguan (PC6) and Yongquan (KI1) for 0.5 ~ 1.0 *cun*. Then continuously twirl the needle. Take moxibustion in Guanyuan (RN4). Puncture Zusanli (ST36) with medium stimulation, plus pulse electrotherapy for 30 minutes.

5.1.16.3 Chinese massage treatment

Nip and press Shuigou (DU26), Neiguan (PC6), and Yongquan (KI1) for 5 ~ 10 minutes using fingertips. Then press and knead Hegu (LI4), Zusanli (ST36), Taichong (LR3) for 5 ~ 10 minutes with the underside of the thumb.

5.2 Orthopedic Diseases

5.2.1 Cervical spondylopathy (stiff neck)

5.2.1.1 General information

Cervical spondylopathy includes 5 different categories. The most common ones are:

1. Cervical category: repetitive occurring of neck and back pain caused by flaccidity of vertebral joint capsule, calcification of ligament, regression of intervertebral disc and formation of bone etc.

2. Nerve root category: the main clinical manifestations is cervical spondylopathy of nerve root.

3. Vertebral artery: unstable cervical vertebra, protrusion of intervertebral disc and hyperplasia of the hook joint can directly stimulate vertebral artery and lead to its spasm, distortion, narrowing and blocking, which in turn may lead to a series of symptoms caused by the shortage of blood supply in intervertebral basilar artery.

5.2.1.2 Acupuncture treatment

Main Acupoints: Local acupoints include Fengchi (GB20), Dazhui (DU14), Ashi acupoint, and

Jiaji (EX – B2), which are directly related to the affected vertebra, while distant acupoints include Xuanzhong (GB39), Luozhen (EX – UE8), and Houxi (SI3).

Acupoints are chosen according to the symptoms: Shoulder or the upper arm pain: Jianyu (LI15), Jianliao (SJ14) and Tiaokou (ST38); Upper arm numbness: Quchi (LI11), Shousanli (LI10) and Waiguan (SJ5); headache and dizziness: Fengchi (GB20), Yintang (EX – HN3); blurry Vision: Jingming (BL1), Fengchi (GB20); vomiting: Neiguan (PC6), Zusanli (ST36).

Manipulation: First puncture Xuanzhong (GB39) or Luozhen (EX – UE8) acupoint until the arrival of Qi occurs. Then ask the patient to move his neck by himself. Finally puncture the local acupoint and Ashi acupoint for 20 ~ 30 minutes; one (series) course consists of 10 treatments. Moxibustion can be used on the Ashi acupoint for 15 ~ 20 minutes, once a day or on alternate days. If one patient has several symptoms at the same time, 1 ~ 2 acupoints can be chosen for each symptom.

5.2.1.3 Chinese massage treatment

1. Keep the patient seated. Treat the bilateral sides of the cervical vertebra and shoulders for 10 minutes by Rolling, pressing, grasping and one-finger Zen.

2. Press and knead the sensitive points along the neck, shoulder and medial sides of scapulas using the thumb. Starting from the occipital area, treat the bilateral sides in turns, up and down until local swelling and warmth are felt. The treatment lasts for 5 ~ 10 minutes. For distant acupoints, press and knead Shousanli (LI10), Xuanzhong (GB39) on bilateral sides for 1 ~ 3 minutes until local soreness and swelling are felt. It is preferable if the sensation is directed downwards.

3. Keep a patient in a supine position and put big pillows behind his or her shoulders. Hold and support the occipital area with the doctor's right hand and support the chin with the left hand. Pull the head upward to make a 45°angle between the neck and the bed. The traction time lasts for 1 ~ 2 minutes. Then rotate the head from left to right, forward and backward mildly. Usually a click can be heard at this moment.

4. End of treatment: Straight scrubbing of the bilateral sides of the cervical vertebra until local warmth is felt. Hot compresses at the neck can be matched up.

5.2.2 Function disorder of temporomandibular joint

5.2.2.1 General information

This disorder is manifested by joint pain, difficulty in opening the mouth, clicking around the joints. It belongs to arthralgia syndrom in Traditional Chinese Medicine.

5.2.2.2 Acupuncture treatment

Main Acupoints: Local acupoints include Xiaguan (ST7), Ermen (SJ21), Tinggong (SI19) and Ashi, while distant acupoints include Zhongzhu (SJ3), Waiguan (SJ6).

Manipulation: First puncture Zhongzhu (SJ3) or Waiguan (SJ6) until the arrival of Qi. Then ask the patient to open his or her mouth to move his temporomandibular joint mildly. After the relief of symptoms, puncture local acupoints and Ashi acupoints. The treatment lasts for 20 minutes. One series consists of 10 treatments. Moxibustion can be used on Ashi acupoints once a day with 3 ~ 5 indirect moxibustion applied.

5. 2. 2. 3 Chinese massage treatment

1. Keep a patient seated. Treat the joint area by thumb pressure, kneading, and one-finger Zen for 10 minutes.

2. Press and knead acupoints Ermen (SJ21) or Tinggong (SI19) for 5 ~ 10 minutes until mild pain is felt locally. For distant acupoint, press and knead Zhongzhu (SJ3), Waiguan (SJ6) on the opposite side for 1 ~ 3 minutes each, until local soreness and swelling are felt.

3. Ask the patient to open and close his or her mouth. Press and knead the sick joint area with one hand, hold and support his jaw with the other hand to help keep his mouth moving for 5 ~ 10 times. For subluxation cases, more complicated manipulations are needed.

4. Scrub the joint area until local warmth appears. Hot compress may be used to match up with the treatment.

5. 2. 3 Periarthritis of shoulder

5. 2. 3. 1 General information

Treatment here can be used to cure diseases such as brachial biceps tenosynovitis, brachial biceps breviflexor tendon injury, sub-acromial bursitis, and tendonitis of the suprascapular muscle. They belong to tendon injury, arthralgia syndrom and leakage of shoulder wind in Traditional Chinese Medicine.

5. 2. 3. 2 Acupuncture treatment

Main Acupoints: Local acupoints include Jianyu (LI15), Jianliao (SJ14), Naoshu (SI10), Tianzong (SI11), Ashi, and Taijian acupoint, while distant acupoints include Tiaokou (ST38) and EX - LE7. (The Taijian acupoint is an experience acupoint, which belongs to the extraordinary acupoints. It is located in the indentation under the union of clavicles.)

Acupoints chosen according to symptoms: When Ashi acupoints are located on the lateral side of the shoulder, Waiguan (SJ5). When Ashi acupoints are located on the anterior part of the shoulder, Hegu (LI4).

Manipulation: First, strongly stimulate Tiaokou (ST38) or EX - LE7 acupoint for 5 ~ 10 minutes and at the same time, ask the patient to move his affected shoulder. Then give electric or warm needling stimulation. The needle is retained for 20 ~ 30 minutes. The treatment can be once a day or on alternate days. One course consists of ten treatments. Local cupping for 10 ~ 15 minutes can also be used.

Ear Acupuncture: Paste magnetic pearls on acupoint such as Shoulder (SF4, 5), Clavicle (SF6), Neck (AH12), Occiput (AT3).

5. 2. 3. 3 Chinese massage treatment

1. Keep a patient seated. Treat the sick area with rolling, kneading, grasping, and one-finger Zen. Give mild stimulation during acute stage and give stronger stimulation during the chronic stage for abnut 10 minutes.

2. Treat acupoints with pressing-kneading, one-finger Zen and plucking for 5 ~ 10 minutes.

3. Ask the patient to do some abductive movements during Chinese massage treatment. This movement is forbidden during acute stages.

4. Rotate and shake the sick shoulder and limb for 1 ~ 2 minutes.

5. 2. 4 Elbow pain

5. 2. 4. 1 General information

The treatment here can be used for diseases such as external or internal humeral epicondylitis, olecranon process bursitis, supinator syndrome, and extensive carpal radial muscle tenontitis, etc. They belong to tendon injury and arthralgia syndrom category.

5. 2. 4. 2 Acupuncture treatment

Main Acupoints: Ashi, Quchi (LI11), Shousanli (LI10), Xiaohai (SI8), Tianjing, Waiguan (SJ5).

Manipulation: Mainly Ashi acupoints are treated. Puncture them in relation to other acupoints. After the arrival of Qi, retain the needle for 20 ~ 30 minutes. Or tap the sick area with skin needle until local skin flushes. Then give moxibustion with ginger once a day or every other day. One course consists of ten treatments.

5. 2. 4. 3 Chinese massage treatment

1. Keep a patient seated. Treat the sick with rolling, kneading and one-finger Zen for 10 minutes. The manipulation should be mild during the acute stage; while during the chronic stage, it can be stronger.

2. Treat the acupoints for 5 ~ 10 minutes with pressing, kneading, one-finger Zen pushing and plucking.

3. Ask the patient to make some extension and flexion movements during Chinese massage treatment.

4. Scrub the sick elbow for 1 ~ 2 minutes.

5. 2. 5 Wrist pain

5. 2. 5. 1 General information

Treatment here can be used for diseases such as wrist injury, carpal tunnel syndrome, and tenosynovitis stenosis. They belong to tendon injury and arthralgia syndrom category in Traditional Chinese Medicine.

5. 2. 5. 2 Acupuncture treatment

Main Acupoints: Ashi, Yangxi (LI5), Daling (PC7), Lieque (LU7), and Yangchi (SJ4).

Manipulation: After the arrival of Qi on the Ashi acupoint, choose some related acupoints for further acupuncture. Retain needles for 30 minutes once a day. Moxibustion with herbal medicine is quite effective here.

5. 2. 5. 3 Chinese massage treatment

1. Treat the sick area with rolling, kneading, and one-finger Zen pushing for 10 minutes. The treated area can be extended to the lower part of the upper arm. The massage can be done from mild to strong.

2. Treat the acupoints with pressing, kneading and plucking for 5 ~ 10 minutes until local soreness and swelling are felt.

3. Tract, stretch and rotate the wrist slowly.

4. Scrub the sick area for 1 ~ 2 minutes with the minor thenar.

5.2.6 Waist and leg pain

5.2.6.1 General information

The treatment here can be used for diseases such as lumbago caused by waist soft tissue injury, rheumatic diseases or lumbar vertebra degeneration, and piriform muscle syndrome. Traction treatment can be used to treat lumbar intervertebral disc prolapse.

5.2.6.2 Acupuncture treatment

Main Acupoints: Lumbar Jiaji (EX – B2), Shenshu (BL23), Dachangshu (BL25), Yaoyan (EX – B6), Ciliao (BL32), Zhibian (BL54), Huantiao (GB30), Weizhong (BL40), Xuanzhong (GB39) and Ashi. For acute waist strain cases, the distant acupoints can be Renzhong (DU26), Houxi (SI3).

Manipulation: For an acute waist strain case with severe backache, first puncture Renzhong (DU26) or Houxi (SI3). After the arrival of Qi, asking the patient to move his waist can be very effective. After the relief of pain, give medium stimulation to the other acupoints. Retain the needle for 20 ~ 30 minutes. For rheumatic cases, give warm needle moxibustion or electric acupuncture combined with moxibustion for 20 minutes. For piriform muscle syndrome cases, don't give strong stimulation on acupoints which are located around the hip area to avoid sciatic nerve injury. For lumbar intervertebral disc prolapse cases, choose lumbar jiaji (EX – B2) related to the sick area as the main acupoints for treatment. Traction can be combined for treatment. All the diseases mentioned here especially chronic lumbar muscle strain can receive 10 ~ 15 minutes' cupping treatment.

5.2.6.3 Chinese massage treatment

1. Keep the patient in a prone position. Treat the sick area with rolling, pressing and kneading for 10 minutes. The force should be strong enough to pass deep into the body.

2. Press and knead Ashi acupoints for 2 minutes. If there are many Ashi acupoints, treat the most painful ones first. The force should be from mild to strong. Distant acupoints such as Weizhong (BL40), Kunlun (BL60) and Taixi (KI3) can be pressed and kneaded for 1 ~ 2 minutes until local soreness and numbness are felt.

3. Traction treatment: The assistant should hold and support the axillary area, while the doctor presses the ankles and tract downward several times at an even speed. Lateral Turning Treatment: Keep the patient lying in a lateral position. Hold the patient's shoulder with one hand, turn his hip with the other hand in the opposite direction. Clicks can often be heard at this moment. Bending and Shaking Treatment: Keep the patient in a supine position with bent hips and knees. Hold his knees and slowly shake the lumbar vertebra joints several times. Lateral turning, bending and shaking treatment are effective for cases with incarceration of the synovium at the lumbar vertebrae's posterior articulation. They should not be used to treat cases with supraspinal or interspinal ligament injury.

4. Pat, tap or scrub the lumbosacral area.

5.2.7 Hip pain

5.2.7.1 General information

The treatment here can be used for diseases such as hip strain, hip bursitis, retrograde arthritis of the hip, clicking hip, strain of tractus iliotibialis, and neuritis of the nervus cutaneus femoris lateralis, which belong to the category of tendon injury and arthralgia syndrom in Traditional Chinese Medicine.

5.2.7.2 Acupuncture treatment

Main Acupoints: Local acupoints include Juliao (GB29), Zhibian (BL54), Chengfu (BL32), Fengshi (GB31) and Ashi, while distant acupoints include Xuanzhong (GB39).

Manipulation: Choose 3 ~ 5 acupoints according to different symptoms. After arrival of Qi, give medium to strong stimulation. Then retain the needle for 20 ~ 30 minutes. Keep the patient in a recumbent position with a bent knee in order to locate acupoint Huantiao (GB30). Pass the needle sensation to the bottom of the foot. The treatment should be once a day and one course consists of 10 treatments. Cupping for 15 ~ 20 minutes each time can be used to treat hip strain and hip bursitis. Moxibustion for 15 ~ 20 minutes can be used to treat patients whose symptoms aggravate when it becomes cold. Tapping with skin needle followed by cupping can be used to treat patients with neuritis of the nervus cutaneus femoris lateralis.

5.2.7.3 Chinese massage treatment

1. Treat the hip area with rolling, kneading, and one-finger Zen pushing for 10 minutes. Treatment should be milder at the acute stage.

2. Treating acupoints for 5 ~ 10 minutes with pressing, kneading, one finger Zen pushing and two-thumb – overlapping plucking, etc.

3. Rotate the hip mildly at the same time. The movement should be limited at first.

4. Rotate and shake the hip. Then scrub the sick area until it turns warm.

5.2.8 Knee pain

5.2.8.1 General information

The treatment here can be used for diseases such as injury of the lateral collateral ligament of the knee, cross ligamenta, or meniscus; injury of infrapatellar fat pad, traumatic bursitis of the knee, and knee osteoarthritis. These problems belong to the categories of tendon injury and arthralgia syndrom in Traditional Chinese Medicine.

5.2.8.2 Acupuncture treatment

Main Acupoints: Neixiyan (EX – LE4), Waixiyan (EX – LE5) and Ashi acupoint are the most commonly used acupoints for knee disease treatment. Other acupoints are chosen according to the symptoms, such as Zusanli (ST36), Weizhong (BL40), Sanyinjiao (SP6), and Xuanzhong (GB39).

Manipulation: After arrival of Qi, retain the needles for 20 ~ 30 minutes. Except for traumatic bursitis of the knee with severe effusion, which needs drainage, all the other diseases of the knee can be treated by moxibustion with a warm needle once a day. One treatment consists of ten repetitions.

5.2.8.3 Chinese massage treatment

1. Keep a patient in a horizontal position. Rub the patella. Then hold the knee with two palms and scrub it back and forth, for 10 minutes.

2. Treat the acupoints by pressing, kneading, one-finger Zen pushing and Digital-pointing with a

bent finger for 5 ~ 10 minutes.

3. At the same time, exercise the knee.

4. Palm scrub the knee to finish the treatment.

5.2.9 Ankle pain

5.2.9.1 General infomation

The treatment here can be used for diseases such as ankle strain, ankle tunnel syndrome, and achillobursitis, etc. These problems belong to the categories of tendon injury and arthralgia syndrom in Traditional Chinese Medicine.

5.2.9.2 Acupuncture treatment

Main Acupoints: Local acupoints include Jiexi (ST41), Qiuxu (GB40), Shangqiu (SP5), Kunlun (BL60), Taixi (KI3), Shenmai (BL62), Zhaohai (KI6), Ashi acupoint, while distant acupoints include Yangchi (SJ4), Yangxi (LI5).

Manipulation: Mainly treat Ashi acupoints. Choose 2 ~ 3 acupoints according to the diverse symptoms. After arrival of Qi, Retain the needle for 20 ~ 30 minutes. Moxibustion for 20 ~ 30 minutes can also be used at the same time. For acute ankle strain cases, distant acupoints are more commonly used for treatment. Mild simulaneous exercise of the sick ankle is part of the treatment.

5.2.9.3 Chinese massage treatment

1. Treat the ankle area with rolling, kneading and one-finger Zen pushing. During the acute stage, the manipulation should be mild. While at the chronic stage, strong stimulation is encouraged. The treatment lasts for 10 minutes each time.

2. Acupoint massage with pressing, kneading and one finger Zen pushing for 5 ~ 10 minutes each time.

3. At the same time, mildly tract the ankle starting with small amplitudes. This is not supposed to cause local pain.

4. Palm scrub the sick area until it is warm.

5.2.10 Heel pain

5.2.10.1 General information

The treatment here can be used for diseases such as achillobursitis, fat inflammation under calcaneus tendon, calcaneus epiphysitis, metatarsal aponeurositis and calcaneal spur etc.

5.2.10.2 Acupuncture treatment

Main Acupoints: Local acupoints include Pushen (BL61), Kunlun (BL60), Taixi (KI3), Sanyinjiao (SP6), and Ashi acupoint while distant acupoints include Daling (PC7).

Manipulation: Mainly treat Ashi acupoints and choose 2 ~ 3 other acupoints according to the symptoms each time. After arrival of Qi, retain the needle for 20 ~ 30 minutes. Moxibustion for 20 ~ 30 minutes can also be used at the same time.

5.2.10.3 Chinese massage treatment

1. Palm kneading, one-finger Zen pushing is used in heel disease treatment. Acute bursitis needs mild manipulation, while during chronic stages, strong stimulation is encouraged. The treatment lasts for

10 minutes each time.

2. Treat the acupoints with pressing, kneading and one-finger Zen pushing, etc. The treatment lasts for 5 ~ 10 minutes each time.

3. Palm scrub the sick area until it turns warm.

5.3 Gynecological Diseases

5.3.1 Dysmenorrhea

5.3.1.1 General information

Dysmenorrhea refers to the severe pain appearing in the lower abdomen or sometimes lumbosacral region during, before or after menstruation. In western medicine, it is divided into two categories, primary and secondary dysmenorrhea. The former category indicates that there is no obvious abnormality in genital organs while the latter one implies genital organ abnormity such as over bending of uterus, chronic pelvic inflammatory disease, hyperplasia, endometriosis and ovarian cyst. Treatment here can by used in both categories.

5.3.1.2 Acupuncture treatment

Main point: Local acupoints include Qihai (RN6), Guanyuan (RN4), Shiqizhui (EX - B7), while distant acupoints include Hegu (LI4), Sanyinjiao (SP6).

Acupoints chosen according to symptom: Severe stomachache: Ciliao (BL32); vomiting: Neiguan (PC6), Zusanli (ST36).

Manipulation: First, puncture Hegu (LI4), Sanyinjiao (SP6). Give medium stimulation for 5 ~ 6 minutes after arriving of Qi. If the pain is not obviously relieved, puncture Shiqizhui (EX - B7), Guanyuan (RN4) or Qihai (RN6). It is better to pass the needle sensation toward perineum. Moxibustion (RN4) for 15 ~ 20 minutes can be used at the same time. If the pain is still not relieved, puncture Ciliao (BL32) and cup Guanyuan for 10 ~ 15 minutes. The lumbrosacral area can be tapped by skin needle until it flushes. Moxibustion can be used in endometriosis patients who are diagnosed as Qi deficient or with Blood stagnation or stagnation of Blood caused by cold-evil.

Ear Acupuncture: Internal Genitalia (TF2), Endocrine (CO18), Shenmen (HT7) and Sympathetic Nerve (AH6a). Perpendicular puncture, then reduce by twirling and rotation. Or magnetic pearls can be pasted and pressed here.

5.3.1.3 Chinese massage treatment

1. Keep a patient in a supine position, and mildly bend her knees and hips. Rub the belly for 2 ~ 3 minutes. Then one-finger Zen push Qihai (RN6) and Guanyuan (RN4) for 3 ~ 5 minutes each. Press and knead Hegu (LI4), Xuehai (SP10) and Sanyinjiao (SP6) for 1 ~ 2 minutes each.

2. Keep a patient in a prone position. Smear lotion on his or her lumbrosacral. Then scrub it with the doctor's minor thenar.

5.3.2 Acute mastitis

5.3.2.1 General information

Acute mastitis is often found during lactation period. Fever, swelling and pain of breast, indurated lump and tenderness are the main symptoms. The disease is called "Ruyong" (acute mastitis) in traditional Chinese Medicine, caused by stagnation of liver Qi, excessive toxic heat and galactostasis. Shortage of milk refers to insufficiency of milk secretion after delivery and can not meet babies' demand for milk. According to Traditional Chinese Medicine, it is caused by stagnation of liver *qi* or shortage of Qi and blood.

5.3.2.2 Acupuncture treatment

Main Acupoints: Danzhong (RN17), Qimen (LR14), Shaoze (SI1), Neiguan (PC6).

Acupoints chosen according to symptoms: Fever: Dazhui (DU14), Quchi (LI11), Hegu (LI4); dyspepsia: Zhongwan (RN12), Zusanli (ST36); acupoints chosen from experience: Jianjing (GB21).

Manipulation: Horizontally puncture Danzhong (RN17) and Qimen (LR14) toward the nipple and pass the needle sensation toward the breast. Promptly prick Shaoze (SI1) to cause bleeding. Obliquely puncture Jianjing (GB21) backward for 1 *cun*. Do not lift and thrust the needle but only twist and twirl the needle. Moxibustion can be used on Danzhong (RN17) or on the abscess for 10 ~ 20 minutes, twice a day for mastitis cases. During the early stage of mastitis, cupping can be used on Dazhui (DU14), Jiaji (EX - B2) of T4 and Rugen (ST18) etc. During the pus drain stage, three-edged needles can be used to cause bleeding on local acupoints. After that, cupping can be used. This treatment can be daily or every other day.

5.3.2.3 Chinese massage treatment

1. Keep a patient in a supine position. First, smear some massage lotion on the sick breast. Then hold the breast in one hand and push from peripheral area of the breast toward the nipple by four closed fingers of the other hand. Press following the direction of mammary ducts to squeeze the stagnant latex out gradually. Mildly pull the nipple several times during massage to dilate the mammary ducts in the nipple area. The treatment can last for 10 ~ 15 minutes each time. The manipulation should be milder when there is lack of lactation.

2. Rub the belly clockwise for 5 minutes using the doctor's palms. Then move from Zhongwan (RN12) to Tianshu (ST25) repeatedly for 3 ~ 5 minutes using the doctor's thumb.

5.4 Five Sense Organs Diseases

5.4.1 Eye diseases

5.4.1.1 General information

Treatment here can be used to treat diseases such as myopia, strabismus, optic neuritis or atrophy, etc. Bleeding treatment can be used in diseases such as conjunctivitis and chalazion. In Traditional Chinese Medicine, eye diseases refer to diseases which have main symptoms of swelling and pain of eye or blurring vision.

5.4.1.2 Acupuncture treatment

Main Acupoints: Local acupoints include Jingming (BL1), Chengqi (ST1), and Fengchi (GB20), while distant acupoints include Hegu (LI4), Yanglao (SI6).

Manipulation: Puncture Jingming (BL1) or Chengqi (ST1) alternately. First fix the eye-ball. Then slowly puncture with a slim needle following the intra side of the orbit. If resistance is felt through the needle or the patient feels painful, withdraw the needle a little bit, change its direction a little, then puncture it again. It is not advisable to twirl or lift and thrust the needle with amplitude. Strong stimulation can be used in other acupoints. It is preferable to pass the needle sensation to the eye area of Fengchi (GB20) acupoint. Retain the needle for 20 ~ 30 minutes at each acupoint. Bleeding treatment for conjunctivitis and hordeolum. Choose 1 ~ 2 acupoints from Ear Apex, Ear lobe, Taiyang (EX-HN5) and Zhongchong (PC9) to cause bleeding. One series consists of three treatments.

Ear Acupuncture: Myopia or fundus diseases: Paste magnetic pearls on sensitive points in areas such as Eye (LO5), Liver (CO12), Kidney (CO10) and Occiput (AT3).

5.4.1.3 Chinese massage treatment

1. Keep a patient in a prone position. Knead and press around the orbit for 5 minutes with the doctor's two thumbs. Divide-push the eyebrows 12 ~ 24 times. Digital press Jingming (BL1), Taiyang (EX-HN5), Yuyao (EX-HN4), Zanzhu (BL2) and Chengqi (ST1) for 1 minute each.

2. Keep the same position as above, hold the occipital part of the patient in one hand, grasp the nape of the patient in the other hand for 5 ~ 7 minutes. Then press and knead Fengchi (GB20) and Yiming (EX-HN14) for 1 ~ 3 minutes each using the doctor's thumb.

3. Keep the same position. Press Hegu (LI4), Yanglingquan (GB34), Guangming (GB37) and Taixi (KI3) for 1 minute each.

5.4.2 Deafness and tinnitus

5.4.2.1 General information

These are symptoms of abnormal hearing. In Traditional Chinese Medicine, these problems are thought to be caused by ascending of hepatobiliary heat or liver-kidney Yin deficiency, and the latter is often accompanied by headache, dizziness, soreness and weakness of waist and knees.

5.4.2.2 Acupuncture treatment

Main acupoints: Yifeng (SJ17), Tinggong (SI19), Tinghui (GB2), Zhongzhu (SJ3) and Xiaxi (GB43).

Acupoints chosen according to symptoms: Headache and dizziness: Fengchi (GB20), Yintang (EX-HN3), Baihui (DU20), Taichong (LR3) and Hegu (LI4); lassitude of the loins and knees: Taixi (KI3), Shenshu (BL23).

Manipulation: Choose one acupoint from Tinggong (SI19) and Tinghui (GB2) on the sick side. 1 ~ 2 distant acupoints can be chosen from both sides during each treatment. One series consists of 10 treatments.

Ear Acupuncture: Acupuncture or magnetic pearl pasting on acupoints such as Heart (CO15),

Internal Ear (LO6), Liver (CO12), Kidney (CO10), Subcortex (AT4). The two ears can be treated in turn.

Acupoint injection: Choose acupoints Tinggong (SI19), Yifeng (SJ17), Wangu (SI4) and Shenshu (BL23). Inject 0.2 ~ 0.5mL anisodamine, vitaminB_{12} or vitaminB_1 into each acupoint every other day.

5.4.2.3 Chinese massage treatment

1. Press the doctor's palm centers on the ears for 5 ~ 7 times.

2. Push from Shuaigu (GB8) backward to the temple on the sick side using the doctor's fingertips for 20 ~ 30 minutes. Then, knead and press from Shuaigu (GB8) toward Jiache (ST6) 20 ~ 30 times using the doctor's thumbs or middle fingers. After that, foulage and knead ear apex, helix and lobe until the ear becomes warm. Finally, digital-press Hegu (LI4), Zhongzhu (SJ3), Zusanli (ST36), Guangming (GB37) and Taixi (KI3) for 1 ~ 2 minutes each.

5.4.3 Rhinitis

5.4.3.1 General information

Treatment here can be used to treat diseases such as acute or chronic rhinitis, acute or chronic sinusitis. Simple rhinitis, hypertrophic rhinitis, allergic rhinitis and atrophic rhinitis. It equals to "nasosinusitis" in Traditional Chinese Medicine.

5.4.3.2 Acupuncture Treatment

Main Acupoints: Yintang (EX - HN3), Yingxiang (LI20), Tongtian (BL7), Hegu (LI4).

Acupoints chosen according to symptoms: Fever: Dazhui (DU14), Quchi (LI11); headache: Yangbai (GB14), Neiting (ST44).

Manipulation: Horizontally puncture Yintang (EX - HN3) downward to pass the needle sensation to the nose. Puncture Yingxiang (LI20) towards Bitong. Hegu (LI4) needs strong stimulation. The treatment should be once a day and the needle should be retained for 20 ~ 30 minutes.

Ear Acupuncture: Paste magnetic pearls on acupoints, such as internal nose (TG4), Lung (CO14), Forehead (AT1), and Adrenal (TG2P).

Acupoint Injection Treatment: Inject 0.3 ~ 0.5mL of vitaminB complex or Chuanxiongqin into acupoints such as Yintang (EX - HN3), Yingxiang (LI20) and Hegu (LI4) once every other day. One series consists of 10 treatments.

5.4.3.3 Chinese massage treatment

1. Mildly rub face with two palms. Then push and rub nape occipital area for 5 minutes. Finally mildly open the ten fingers to comb the head backward starting from the ear and temporal area. Scrub the bridge of the nose: The bilateral sides of the bridge of the nose should be strongly scrubed up and down by the two major thenars of the two palms. Begin at the root of the nose and end at the Yingxiang (LI20) Acupoint. The scrubing can be repeated as many as 30 ~ 50 times.

2. Knead and press Yingxiang (LI20) and Bitong for 2 ~ 5 minutes in turn. Knead and press Hegu (LI4) for 1 ~ 2 minutes. Knead and press Fengchi (GB20) for 1 ~ 2 minutes until local soreness and swelling are felt or are passed to the face.

3. Pinch and release the nostrils by using thumb and an index finger for about 1 minute, without feeling painful.

5.4.4 Toothache

5.4.4.1 General information

Toothache is the commonest in oral diseases. Treatment here can be used to treat diseases such as pericoronitis, periodontitis, periapical periodontitis and hypersensitive dentin etc. In Traditional Chinese Medicine, dental diseases can be classified into bacterial diseases and fire diseases. Fire diseases can be further classified into excess fire and deficiency fire. Excess fire is mostly caused by stomach fire and wind-heat. Deficiency fire is mostly caused by kidney deficiency and hyperfire.

5.4.4.2 Acupuncture treatment

Main Acupoints: Xiaguan (ST7), Jiache (ST6), Hegu (LI4). Assistant acupoints: Taiyang (EX-HN5), Quanliao (SI18).

Manipulation: Puncture Xiaguan (ST7) for 1 *cun*. Electric stimulation can be used on Xiaguan (ST7) and Jiache (ST6) on the same side. Cupping can be used on Jiache (ST6), but the treatment cannot last more than 5 minutes.

Ear Acupuncture: Sanjiao (CO17), Shenmen (TF4), Tooth (LO1).

5.4.4.3 Chinese massage treatment

1. Press and knead Jiache (ST6) for 1 ~ 5 minutes. The manipulation should be mild at first, then it could be stronger and stronger until the toothache is relieved. If it does not occur, work strongly with pressing and kneading Xiaguan (ST7) for 1 ~ 5 minutes with the thumb.

2. Press and knead Hegu (LI4) for 1 ~ 2 minutes beginning with the sick side. If the toothache cannot be relieved, press Hegu (LI4) on the other side.

3. Special Treatment: Wash the hand and clip the nails. Then press the gums with fingers and after that strongly press and knead the sick area for 1 ~ 2 minutes. Finally rinse the mouth with salt water. This treatment is effective for pericoronitis and periodontitis.

5.5 Simple Obesity and Abstention of Smoking

5.5.1 Simple Obesity

5.5.1.1 General information

Simple obesity means excessive adipose tissues caused by a caloric intake exceeding caloric consumption. Usually the body weight exceeds the standard body weight by 20%. In Traditional Chinese Medicine, simple obesity is thought to be caused by dysfunction of Zang organs and Fu organs.

5.5.1.2 Acupuncture Treatment

Main Acupuncture: Quchi (LI11), Tianshu (ST25), Yinlingquan (SP9), Fenglong (ST40), Taichong (LR3). Assistant Acupoints: Acupoints in the obese area.

Manipulation: Give electric stimulation after arriving of Qi. Retain the needle for 30 minutes. The treatment can be once a day or every other day. One series consists of 10 treatments.

Ear Acupuncture: Acupuncture or paste magnetic pearls on acupoints such as Stomach (CO4), Endocrine (CO18), Spleen (CO13), Sanjiao (CO17), and Middle Border (AT2, 3, 4i) 7 ~ 10 times a day. The pearls can be changed in 3 ~ 5 days. One series consists of 10 treatments.

5.5.1.3 Chinese massage treatment

1. Wipe or knead the obese area for 3 ~ 5 minutes. Then Palm-rub the belly clock wisely for 3 ~ 5 minutes. Finally, push-rub from xiphoid process to Guanyuan 15 ~ 20 times in one direction.

2. Thumb digital – press and knead acupoints such as Quchi (LI11), Hegu (LI4), Zhongwan (RN12), Tianshu (ST25), Pishu (BL20), Weishu (BL21), Zusanli (ST36), Shangjuxu (ST37) and Fenglong (ST40) each for 1 ~ 2 minutes.

5.5.2 Abstention of smoking

5.5.2.1 General information

Smoking is harmful to health. Chemicals in tobacco, such as nicotine and tar are related to many diseases such as hypertension, coronary heart disease, chronic bronchitis, cancer, and foetus abnormality. They are especially harmful to lungs.

5.5.2.2 Acupuncture treatment

Main Acupoints: Baihui (DU20), Shenmen (HT7), and Sweet acupoint, which is the sensitive point locating between Lieque (LU7) and Yangxi (LI5).

Acupoints chosen according to symptoms: restlessness: Yongquan (KI1); sleepiness: Laogong (PC8).

Manipulation: Obliquely puncture Sweet acupoint upward for 1 *cun* until soreness, swelling and numbness are felt. Then give electric stimulation for 30 minutes. Puncture Baihui (DU20), Shenmen (HT7) once a day or every other day for 30 minutes. One course consists of three treatments.

Ear Acupuncture: Puncture or paste magnetic pearls on acupoints on each ear such as Shenmen (HT7), Lung (CO14), Stomach (CO4), Mouth (CO1), Sympathetic Nerve (AH6a) in turn. One ear needs 3 days of treatment. The ear acupoints can be pressed whenever people want to smoke.

5.5.2.3 Massage treatment

Thumb press and knead Hegu (LI4), Lieque (LU7), Quchi (LI11), Zhongwan (RN12), Tianshu (ST25), Zusanli (ST36) and Zhaohai (KI6) for 1 ~ 3 minutes each until soreness, swelling and heaviness are felt.

第六章　灸推疗法应用

6.1　保健灸

艾灸保健法历史悠久，宋《扁鹊心书》记载："保命之法，灼艾第一，人至三十，可三年一灸，脐下三百壮；五十可二年一灸，脐下三百壮；六十可一年一灸，脐下三百壮，令人长生不老。""灼艾"即艾灸法，古多用艾炷灸，一炷称"一壮"，脐下指关元穴。现代实验显示，艾灸相应穴位能使白细胞增加，网状内皮系统活跃，吞噬功能增强，还可使肾上腺功能增强。以下介绍几种常用保健灸法。

6.1.1　慢性病体质灸法

取穴：气海、中脘、曲池、足三里，女性加三阴交穴。

方法：每穴艾条灸3~5分钟，或艾炷灸10壮，两天灸1次，10次为1疗程。疗程结束可休息3~5天。有不适反应者，可配合针刺调理。一般坚持几个疗程，可逐步改善慢性病体质，加速疾病的治愈。

6.1.2　预防感冒灸法

取穴：风门、肺俞、足三里。

方法：每穴艾条灸3~5分钟，每日1次，连灸7日。

6.1.3.　预防脑血管病灸法

取穴：足三里、悬钟。

方法：每穴艾炷灸100~300壮，每日1次，连灸10日为1疗程。一般灸1~3疗程。

6.2　保健推拿

6.2.1　头面保健推拿

受术者仰卧位，施术者坐于其头部前方，搓热两掌后开始推拿。要求用力宜缓慢、均匀而有力，推摩时以局部温热感为度；揉穴位时应有适度的酸胀感。

1. 敞开天门（加点百会）：两拇指交替，自印堂穴直推到神庭穴，反复操作10~30次；再点按印堂、神庭、百会穴各1~2分钟。

2. 分抹双柳（加揉太阳）：两拇指指端掐双侧攒竹穴约半分钟，再以指腹从攒竹沿眉弓自内向外推至太阳穴（不可逆行），10～30次；揉太阳穴1～2分钟。

3. 轻揉眼眶：两拇指指端掐双侧睛明穴约半分钟，再以指腹自睛明穴始，由内向外轻揉上、下眼眶，10～30次。

4. 轻揉耳郭：两拇指与食指揉捏双侧耳郭1～2分钟，再向下方拉耳垂数次。

5. 分推鼻颧（加揉双香）：两手拇指从迎香经巨髎推至颧髎穴，重复10～30次。按揉迎香、上迎香穴各1～2分钟。

6. 推揉颌颊：两手拇指从两耳前下方听会穴处沿下颌外缘，经颊车到大迎穴，反复推动10～30次。按揉双颊车穴1～2分钟。

7. 搓掌浴面：两手掌心相搓产生温热，随即掌摩面部10～30次。

8. 勾点风池：掌心朝上，双食指向上托住中指，中指指端勾点双风池穴，向上用力点揉1～2分钟。

9. 干洗头法：双手十指自然屈曲，以指端及指腹着力于头部，对称进行搓动，如洗头状，反复操作10～30次。

6.2.2　胸腹部保健推拿

受术者仰卧位，施术者站于其头部前方或身侧，要求术时腹部肌肉有牵拉微胀感，术后全腹轻松而有轻微的温热感。饭后半小时内不宜按摩上腹部；按摩下腹部前应排空小便。

1. 按压双肩：双掌同时压双肩5～15次，双侧用力均匀，由轻到重逐渐加力。

2. 分推胸胁：两手掌根分别放在胸骨两侧边缘，从第一肋开始由内向外分推至腋中线；逐渐下移分推至胸剑联合水平（女性乳上方止）。反复10～30次。

3. 腹部横抚：以一手掌心，放在受术者的上腹部左或右侧端，掌指均匀用力，反复横向抚摩上腹部10～30次；然后反复横向抚摩下腹部10～30次。抚法比摩法更轻；手法宜徐缓而轻柔。

4. 腹部旋摩：以一手掌心，放在左或右季肋下，从上向对侧内下方摩动，掌指均匀用力，双手交替抚摩各5～15次。

5. 狮子滚球：一手握空拳放在脐部，另一手以全手掌贴于拳上滚揉，形如狮子滚绣球状。先后进行顺、逆时针旋转滚揉，逐渐扩大范围，连续操作各5～15次。

6.2.3　颈部保健推拿

受术者俯卧位或坐位，施术者站于其头前或身侧。颈上段手法操作以指为主，颈背交界处以掌为主。

1. 横推颈肩：一手扶前额部，另一手以掌指紧贴颈枕部，来回用力推擦，并缓缓下移至大椎穴水平止。1～2分钟。

2. 按压颈肩：双手拇指指腹并置于受术者的颈1棘突上，自上而下沿督脉经按压3～5次，至胸2棘突止；再分别沿两侧夹脊穴、两侧横突，自上而下逐节按压3～5次，至胸2水平止。

3. 按揉颈肩：一手扶前额部，另一手拇指指腹置于受术者的颈1棘突上，其余四指自然扶放颈侧，拇指先后沿督脉经两侧夹脊穴、两侧横突自上而下按揉，至胸2水平止。要求揉动快、移动慢。3～5分钟。

4. 提拿颈肩：一手扶前额部，一手拇指与食、中指对合，提拿颈项部肌肉 5～10 次。再以双手拇指指腹放在受术者两肩（以肩井穴处为重点），其余四指放在锁骨上窝，双手同时着力提拿，反复提拿 5～10 次。

5. 颈肩滚透：沿颈下段与肩背交界处，由外向脊柱侧施滚法 3～5 分钟。要求沉肩垂肘，力量渗透至深层组织。

6. 穴位按揉：点按或按揉风府、风池、夹脊、肩井、天宗、阿是穴等穴各半分钟。

7. 掌叩颈肩：双手合掌，掌心相对，五指略分开，以掌指尺侧缘叩打颈肩部约半分钟。

6.2.4 背腰部保健推拿

受术者俯卧位，双手置于身体两侧，施术者站于其头前或身侧。背部用力稍轻，腰骶部宜稍重。体瘦者穴位可用按揉法，体胖者可用肘点法。

1. 平推背腰：以单掌或双掌，分别沿受术者背腰部督脉经、膀胱经从上到下平推，至骶骨裂孔水平止。各 10～30 次。

2. 分推背腰：两手掌并置于脊柱两旁与大椎穴平高处，由脊中线向两侧分推至腋中线。自上而下至腰阳关穴水平止。1～3 分钟。

3. 按压背腰：以拇指或肘尖置于脊柱两侧竖脊肌处，自上而下逐节均匀按压 5～10 次。

4. 掌揉背腰：以掌心或掌根，放在受术者背部大椎穴，自上向下按揉至命门穴止。再于脊柱两侧的竖脊肌，自上向下反复按揉 2～4 分钟。

5. 背腰滚透：第五掌指关节吸贴于选定部位，施滚法 3～5 分钟。根据受术者的当时情况选取施术部位，多选用肩胛内侧缘、腰三横突、腰骶关节、骶髂关节等易疲劳损伤处，注意手法的力量、角度和方向。

6. 穴位按揉：点按或按揉肾俞、志室、大肠俞、环跳、承山等穴各半分钟。

7. 叩击背腰：双手握空拳，腕关节一起一落带动双拳心或拳眼叩打背腰部，由上而下 3～5 次。

6.2.5 上肢部保健推拿

受术者仰卧或坐位，施术者站于其身侧。要求操作灵活而富有节奏。按揉穴位时有明显的酸胀感，点按穴位一点一松，持续时间不宜过长。

1. 双手揉球：双掌心对合放在肩关节，一前一后相对旋转揉动肩部，如球在手中揉动，连续操作 10～30 次。然后双掌心对合用力挤压肩关节，最后提拿三角肌结束。随后点按或按揉肩髃、肩髎等穴各半分钟。

2. 拿揉臂部：一手托住受术者腕部，另一手拇指和其余四指相对如钳状，从肩峰部沿上臂、前臂至腕部，自上而下拿揉 10～30 次。随后点按或按揉曲池、手三里、外关等穴各半分钟。

3. 揉腕推掌：一手握住受术者手指，另一手四指托住腕部，拇指轻揉腕关节 1～2 分钟。随后一手托起受术者手掌，另一手拇指沿受术者掌骨及骨间肌由下向上直推，每一部位各做 3～5 次。再点按或按揉合谷、内关等穴各半分钟。

4. 摇肩关节：一手扶住受术者肩关节上部，另一手托起肘部，缓缓环转摇动肩关节，顺、逆时针各 6～8 次。

5. 拔理指节：先用食指与拇指夹合，分别顺受术者手指的四面自上而下理捋；然后食指与中指夹合，稍用力捏住受术者的指骨关节，从上向下捋而滑动到指端，产生清脆的滑响声。十指依次一一操作，手法要灵活，不要干扯。

6. 双手搓（抖）臂

双手搓臂：术者先一脚踏于方凳上，膝半屈位，受术者一侧上肢置于术者大腿；然后两手相对分别放在臂内、外侧，一上一下同时着力，由肩至腕往返搓动，反复操作3~5次。

双手抖臂：双手分别握住受术者手掌，先上下，后左右，交替抖动双臂。

以上两法均为上肢按摩的结束手法，可根据具体情况任选其一。

6.2.6 下肢前保健推拿

受术者仰卧或坐位，施术者站于其身侧。要求受术者下肢肌肉放松，施术时有微热舒适感。穴位按摩要求同上肢部。

1. 掌推下肢：双手掌分别紧贴大腿内外侧，自上而下平推至足踝部，随后点按或按揉足三里、阴陵泉、三阴交等穴各半分钟。

2. 抱擦膝关：两手环抱左膝，用力来回擦动；然后换做右膝，各10~30次。两手心紧按膝盖，同时向外旋转摩动10~30次，然后向内旋转摩动10~30次。

3. 推搓足背：受术者微屈膝，足底紧贴床面，施术者一手扶住小腿下端，另一手由上向下快速推搓足背。随后捏揉昆仑、太溪各1~2分钟，点按或按揉太冲半分钟。

4. 摇踝关节：一手托住受术者足跟部，另一手握足趾部，缓缓环转摇动踝关节，顺、逆时针各6~8次。

5. 抖动（拍叩）双肢

抖动双肢：两手握受术者足趾部，同时用力向左右方向抖动3~5次。

拍叩双肢：两手以空掌有节奏地自上而下拍打下肢前、内、外侧或以两手握空拳叩击3~5次。

以上两法均为下肢按摩的结束手法，可根据具体情况任选其一。

6.2.7 下肢后保健推拿

受术者俯卧，施术者站于其身侧。要求同上。

1. 掌推臀腿：双手掌沿大腿后侧，自上而下平推至足踝部10~30次。随后点按或按揉承山委中、承筋等穴各半分钟。

2. 叩击足底：以空拳有节奏地叩击足底3~5次。

6.2.8 小儿保健推拿

小儿保健推拿具有健脾和胃、增进食欲、行气活血、强壮身体的作用，能有效促进小儿生长发育，提高小儿的身体素质。

6.2.8.1 操作方法

1. 腹部：先仰卧位，摩腹3分钟，摩中脘5分钟，揉丹田3分钟。

2. 四肢部：先补脾经，医者用拇指旋推小儿的拇指末节螺纹面2~5分钟；再推三关，用中指从腕背横纹正中央，推向肘部的曲池穴，做3分钟；再退六腑，用中指推前臂尺侧，从神门穴至肘部，做3分钟；最后按揉足三里约半分钟。

3. 背脊部：俯卧位，按揉脾俞、胃俞各约半分钟；捏脊5～7次。

以上操作每天1次或早晚各1次（间隔6小时以上）。每周为1疗程，休息3～5天后，可继续进行第2疗程。

6.2.8.2　注意事项

1. 应在小儿空腹时操作，如饭后做，必须间隔1小时后。

2. 急性传染病或其他急性病，包括感冒发热可暂时停做，等痊愈后再做。单纯性消化不良、腹泻等则不必停做。

Chapter 6 Health-care Applications of Moxibustion and Massage

6.1 Health – care moxibustion

Moxibustion has been used in health care for a long time. In *Bian Que Heart Book* (a classic book of Traditional Chinese Medicine written in Song Dynasty), it says that "Moxibustion is the best for longevity. When people grow into their thirties, they can have one course of moxibustion every three years and each course includes 300 moxa cones moxibustion just below the umbilicus. When they grow into their fifties, they can have one course of moxibustion every two years and each course consists of 300 moxa cones moxibustion just below the umbilicus. In their sixties, they can have one course of moxibustion every year and each course consists of 300 moxa cones moxibustion just below the umbilicus. This kind of practice will make people live longer". "Moxibustion" here refers to the moxibustion with dried mugwort. In ancient time, people usually used moxa cones and one moxa cones is called "one cone". "Just below the umbilicus" refers to the acupoint of Guanyuan (RN4). Modern experiments have shown that moxibustion on corresponding acupoints can increase white blood cells, make reticuloendothelial system (RES) more active, improve phagocytic function and improve the functions of adrenal gland. Several commonly used health-care moxibustion treatments are introduced as follows.

6.1.1 Chronic disease

Acupoints: Qihai (RN6), Zhongwan (RN12), Quchi (LI11), and Zusanli (ST36). Add Sanyinjiao (SP6) in female patients.

Manipulations: Treatment for each acupoint is about 3 to 5 minutes. If moxa cone moxibustion is used, then 10 cones are used each time and the treatment can be once every 2 days. The whole course includes ten times treatment. 3 to 5 days' rest between two courses is encouraged. Acupuncture can be used at the same time when the patient has any discomfort from the Moxibustion treatment. Usually, the constitution improvement will be made in the chronic cases after several courses of treatment.

6.1.2 Cold prevention

Acupoints: Fengmen (BL12), Feishu (BL13), Zusanli (ST36).

Manipulations: 3 to 5 minutes treatment for each acupoint with moxa-roll. Once a day, 7 days for one course.

6.1.3 Stroke prevention

Acupoints: Zusanli (ST36), Xuanzhong (CB39).

Manipulations: 100 to 300 moxa cones are used for each acupoint. Once a day, 10 days for one course. Usually, 1 ~ 3 courses are needed for one case.

6.2 Health – care Massage

6.2.1 Massage on the face

Keep the patient in a supine position. The doctor sits in front of the patient's head, rubs his hands and begins to massage when the hands are warm. The force should be slow, even and forceful enough. The massage should not stop until the massaged area becomes warm. When acupoints are kneaded, the patients should have the sense of soreness and swelling.

1. Push the midline of the forehead (and press Baihui): Push from Yintang (EX – HN3) to Shenting (DU20) by both thumbs in turn, repeat 10 to 30 times, and then press Yintang (EX – HN3), Shenting (DU20) and Baihui (DU24), each point for 1 to 2 minutes.

2. Push two sides of the forehead (and knead Taiyang): Nail Zanzhu (BL2) for about half a minute, then push with each thumb-pulp from Zanzhu (BL2) to Taiyang (EX – HN5) along the brows for about 10 to 30 times, and knead Taiyang (EX – HN5) for 1 to 2 minutes.

3. Knead eye orbit: Nail both Jingming (BL1) by both tips of the thumbs for half minutes. Then starting from this acupoint, knead the upper and lower eye orbits from inner side to outer side by both thumb pulps for 10 to 30 times.

4. Pinch the ear: The thumbs and index fingers of both hands are used to pinch, knead, and pull the ears, for about 1 to 2 minutes.

5. Push nose and cheek: Push with two thumbs from Yingxiang (LI20), Juliao (GB29) to Quanliao (SI18) for 10 to 30 times, press Yingxiang (LI20), Shangyingxiang (EX – HN8) for 1 to 2 minutes.

6. Push and knead jaw and cheek: Push with two thumbs along outline of jaw from Tinghui (GB2), Jiache (ST6) to Daying (ST5) for 10 to 30 times; press and knead Jiache (ST6) for 1 to 2 minutes.

7. Palm-rubbing on face: Rub face with the two palms for 10 to 30 times, which has been scraped each other hot.

8. Digital-press Fengchi (GB20): With both hands upward, support the middle finger with index finger in each hand to digital press Fengchi (GB20) with the finger pulp and knead for 1 ~ 2 minutes.

9. Dry-clean hair: Flex the index fingers naturally, forcefully put finger tips and finger pulps on the scalp, rub the scalp symmetrically with the finger pulps (like washing the hair) for 10 ~ 30 minutes.

6.2.2 Massage on chest and abdomen

Keep the patient in a supine position. The doctor stands in front of the patient's head or beside the patient. When manipulation is done, muscles at the abdomen should feel slight pulling and swelling. After manipulation, the whole abdomen should feel relaxed and slightly warm. Massaging upper abdomen is not allowed until half an hour after having dinner. Urination is necessary before massaging lower abdomen.

1. Press the shoulders: Press the shoulders with the two palms for 5 to 15 times. The force should be

even and from mild to strong.

2. Pushing chest rib: Put two palm roots on the two sides of the sternum. Starting from the first rib, push from the sternum to midaxillary lines. Then repeat the manipulation from the second rib to xiphisternal joint (for females, stop just above the breast). Repeat the manipulation for 10 ~ 30 times.

3. Stroke the abdomen transversely: Put the palm center of one hand on one side of the upper abdomen, stroke the upper abdomen transversely for 10 ~ 30 times; then repeat the manipulation at the lower abdomen for 10 ~ 30 times. Stroking is gentler than rubbing. Therefore, the manipulation should be slow and gentle.

4. Rub the abdomen circlewise: Put the center of one palm on the left or right hypochondrium, then rub to the opposite hypochondrium. The palm and fingers should rub evenly and two hands should rub in turn.

5. Knead abdomen: One hand grasps like a ball, the other hand put on the ball and roll it for 5 to 15 times, clockwise and anticlockwise in turn while the treating area is enlarged on the abdomen at the same time.

6.2.3 Massage on the neck

Keep the patient in a supine position. The doctor stands in front of the patient's head or beside the patient. Manipulation on the upper neck is done mainly by using fingers and manipulation on the neck – back juncture is mainly performed by using palm.

1. Push the neck and back transversely: Support the forehead with one hand, put another hand closely on the neck, rub the neck heavily. Then gradually lower the rubbing area down to Dazhui (DU14). The manipulation lasts for 1 ~ 2 minutes.

2. Press the neck and back: Put the pulps of both thumbs on the first spinous process of neck, press the spinal processes following Du meridian until the second thoracic process for 3 ~ 5 times. Then press along Jiaji (EX – B2) and transverse process at both sides down to T2 for 3 ~ 5 times.

3. Press and knead the neck and shoulder: Support the forehead with one hand, put the thumb pulp of the other hand on the first spinous process while the other four fingers put on the side of the neck naturally. Then use the thumb to press and knead along Du meridian, two Jiaji (EX – B2) and transverse process at both sides down to T2 for 3 ~ 5 minutes. Pressing and kneading action should be quick while shifting movement should be slow.

4. Grasp neck and shoulder: Support the forehead with one hand, the thumb, index finger and middle finger of the other hand grasp the muscles at the neck and back for 5 ~ 10 times. Then put the thumbs on both shoulders [focusing on Jianjing (GB21)] and other fingers on supraclavicular fossa to grasp the muscles with force for 5 ~ 10 times.

5. Roll the neck and shoulder: In the area from the lower part of the neck to the conjuncture of the neck and back, roll from the lateral side to the spine for 3 ~ 5 minutes. The patient should relax his/her shoulders and elbows so that the force can penetrate into deep tissues.

6. Press and knead acupoints: Press and knead Fengfu (DU16), Fengchi (GB20), Jiaji (EX – B2), Jianjing (GB21), Tianzong (SI11), and Ashi acupoint, each point for half a minute.

7. Put both palms together and spread all fingers apart naturally, then pat the neck and shoulder with ulna sides of the closed two palms for half a minute.

6. 2. 4 Massage on the back and waist

Keep the patient in a supine position, with his hands at both sides of the body naturally. The doctor stands in front of the patient's head or beside the patient. When the manipulation is done, force at the back should be mild but force at the lumbosacral region can be stronger. Pressing and kneading can be adopted for thin patients and elbow point pressing can be adopted for obese patients.

1. Push the back and waist: Push the back and waist along DU and Bladder meridian in downward direction to sacral hiatus with one palm or both palms for 10 to 30 times.

2. Part-push the back and waist: Put the palms at Dazhui (DU14) and the spine, part－push from spine to midaxillary line at both lateral sides. Repeat the manipulation gradually from Dazhui down to Yaoyangguan (DU3) and the manipulation lasts for 1 ~ 3 minutes.

3. Press the muscles along the spine: Press muscles along the spine with the thumb or elbow tip in downward direction for 5 to 10 times.

4. Palm-knead muscles along the spine: Put the center or root of the palm on Dazhui (DU14), press and knead downward to Mingmen (DU4). Then press and knead the vertical spinalis at both sides of the spine top-down for 2 ~ 4 minutes.

5. Roll the back and waist: Cling the 5th metacarpophalangeal joint on the selected area and roll for 3 ~ 5 minutes. The area should be selected according to the condition of the patients. The fatigable and vulnerable areas, such as medial margin of shoulder blade, the third lumbar transverse process, lumbosacral joint and sacroiliac joint, are usually chosen. Attention should be paid to the force, angle and direction of manipulation.

6. Press and knead acupoints: Press and knead Shenshu (BL23), Zhishi (BL52), Dachangshu (BL25), Huantiao (GB30) and Chengshan (BL57), each point for half a minute.

7. Pat the back and waist: The hands are formed into empty fists that are used to pat the back and waist in downward direction for 3 to 5 times.

6. 2. 5 Massage on the upper limbs

Keep the patient in a supine position. The doctor stands beside the patient. The manipulation should be flexible and rhythmic and the patient will feel obvious soreness and swelling at the acupoints. Pressing and relaxing should be done alternatively and manipulation should not last too long.

1. Knead with two hands: One palm is put before the shoulder, and the other is put behind it to face the first palm. Then roll the two hands around the shoulder for 10 to 30 times. After that, press the shoulder with the two palms face to face, and grasp the deltoid muscle. Finally, press Jianyu (LI15) and Jianliao (SJ14), each for half a minute.

2. Grasp-knead upper limbs: Hold the wrist with one of the doctor's hand, grasp－knead the upper limb like a plier, from acromion, upper arm to wrist, for 10 to 30 times. Then press or knead Quchi (LI11), Shousanli (LI10), Waiguan (SJ5), and each point for half a minute.

3. Hold all the fingers of the patient with one hand and support the wrist with the other. Then mildly

knead the wrist with the thumb for 1 ~ 2 minutes. After that, support the patient's palm with one hand and push upwards along each metacarpal bone for 3 ~ 5 times. Finally, digital – press or press and knead Hegu (LI4), Neiguan (PC6), and each point for half a minute.

4. Rotate shoulder: Hold the shoulder with one hand, and support the elbow with the other. Then rotate the shoulder clockwise and anticlockwise, each way for 6 to 8 times.

5. Pinch phalangeal joints: First pinch the fingers of the patient with the manipulator's index finger and thumb and knead each finger top-down. Then clamp the patient's finger with flexed index finger and middle finger of the manipulator and slide from bottom to the tip of finger quickly. A clear light sound is heard every time. Manipulations should be done on all the ten fingers and they should be flexible.

6. Rub (and shake) the arms.

Rub the arm: The manipulator treads one foot on a stool and flexes his knee. The manipulated person puts one arm on the lap of the manipulator. Then the manipulator put his hands on lateral side and medial side of the arm to rub the arm from the shoulder to the wrist for 3 ~ 5 times.

Shake the arms: Hold the manipulated person's palms respectively with two hands and then shake them up – down first and then horizontally.

These two manipulations are the ending manipulations for massage on the upper limbs. One of them can be chosen according to proper situation.

6.2.6 Massage on the anterior part of the leg

Keep the manipulated person in a supine or sitting position and the manipulator stands beside him/her. The legs of the manipulated person should be relaxed and feel comfortably warm in manipulation. Pressing the acupoints on legs is similar to pressing the acupoints on upper limbs.

1. Push the leg: Push both medial and lateral sides of one leg with palms in downward direction, then digital-press or press and knead the acupoint Zusanli (ST36), Yinlingquan (SP9), and Sanyinjiao (SP6), each point for half a minute.

2. Embrace and rub the knee joint: The palms of both hands firmly embrace the knee joint and scrub each knee joint for 10 to 30 times, then rub on the knee clockwise by both palms for 10 to 30 times, and counter – clockwise for 10 to 30 times.

3. The manipulated person slightly flexes the knee so that the sole of the foot cling to bed surface closely. The manipulator holds the shank with one hand, and the other hand pushes and scrubs dorsum pedis top – down quickly. Then press Kunlun (BL60) and Taixi (KI3), each for 1 to 2 minutes. Then point – press or press and knead Taichong (LR3) for half a minute.

4. Rotate the ankle joint: The manipulator holds the manipulated person's foot heel with one hand, and the other hand holds the toes and rotates the ankle joint slowly, clockwise and counterclockwise for 6 ~ 8 times each.

5. Shake and tap the legs

Shake the legs: Grasp the toes of the feet with two hands to shake the legs in left – right and right – left direction for 3 ~ 5 times.

Pat and tap the legs: Close the hands to form empty fists to pat and tap the anterior, median and lateral parts of the legs; or use empty fists to pat and tap the legs for 3 ~ 5 times.

Both of the manipulations can be used as the ending manipulations for leg massage. The manipulator can choose one of them according to the situation.

6.2.7 Massage on the posterior part of the leg

Keep the manipulated person in supine position and the manipulator stands beside him/her. Other requirements are the same as above section.

1. Push buttocks and legs with palms: Push the posterior part of the leg in downward direction with two palms for 10 to 30 times, then point-press or press and knead Chengshan (BL57), Weizhong (BL40), Chengjin (BL56), each acupoint for half a minute.

2. Tap the sole: Tap the sole of the foot with empty fists for 3 to 5 times.

6.2.8 Health-Care Massage for children

Health-care massage for children has the functions of strengthening the spleen and stomach, improving appetite, promoting Qi to activate blood, strengthening the body, promoting growth and improving physical quality of children.

6.2.8.1 Manipulation

1. Massage on the abdomen (supine position): Rub the abdomen for 3 minutes, rub Zhongwan (RN12) for 5 minutes, knead Dantian (MA – T1) for 3 minutes.

2. Massage on the four limbs: Firstly, Reinforcing Pijing (MA – UE1) by circle-pushing with the pad of one thumb for 2 to 5 minutes, then push Sanguan (MA – UE14) by pushing to Quchi (LI11) with the middle finger for 3 minutes; after that Reduce Liufu (MA – UE16) by pushing from Shenmen (HT7) to elbow on the ulna side of the forearm for 3 minutes; finally press and knead Zusanli (ST36) for half a minute.

3. Massage on the back (prone position): Press and knead Pishu (BL20), Weishu (BL21), each for half a minute, then knead along spine for 5 to 7 times.

The above manipulations can be practiced once a day, or twice a day (once in the morning and once in the evening, at least 6 hours apart). One week's manipulation forms a course of treatment. After 3 ~ 5 days' rest, the second course of treatment can begin.

6.2.8.2 Notice

1. Massage should be applied at least 1 hour after meal or on an empty stomach.

2. When children catch acute infectious diseases or other acute diseases, including cold and fever, the manipulation should not resumed until recovery. If children suffer from simple indigestion and diarrhea, the manipulation does not need to be stopped.

附 录

砭石疗法

一、砭石的历史

砭石疗法即砭术是一种中国古针灸术，以中医经络穴位理论为宗旨，不口服、不刺破皮肤、不用介质，可直接在皮肤上操作，也可隔着棉织物操作，在无痛苦的前提下使用“刮、推、抹、摩、擦、缠、凉、划、拔、点、按、振、拿、拍、扣、剁、温、清、感、电热温烫”砭术法，充分发挥砭石的场效应和“无形针”的作用，内病外治，以疏通经络、调理气血为根本，排除经络中阻气血运行，尤其是皮肤深部经脉中的病理产物，标本兼治，在短时间内极大地缓解临床症状，达到痊愈的目的。对脑血管病，颈、肩、腰腿病及对广大的亚健康状态的人群都有治疗效果。

据《黄帝内经》，砭、针、灸、药是我国古代四种独立并存的医术，砭起源于新石器时代，东汉前逐渐消失，至今失传已两千年。砭是一种石制尖刀，它是针灸术器具针的前身，专门用来切开痈肿或穿刺脓包，排除毒血脓水。

出自《尚书》的泗滨浮石是制作磬与砭具的材料，这种石头在古籍中一直蒙着神秘的面纱。大禹帝时期，用泗滨浮石制作的磬是贡品，是神器（虎纹磬）。佛、道、儒出现后，磬是庙、观里的法器（古代的磬是石制），儒家养生、陶冶情操的乐器、礼器，孔子当年就以击磬作为养生的方法。《黄帝内经》中说“砭从东方来”，这里说的“东方”指的是山东；《路史》中说“伏羲尝草制砭，以治民疾”。伏羲是太昊部落的酋长，太昊是东夷的一支，东夷是古代山东沿海的民族，也就是说伏羲是山东人；在山东出土了大量的砭具，也可为证；而仿制作砭具的泗滨浮石也产自山东。20 世纪 80 年代，我们找到并采集完毕仅存的 200 余吨珍贵的泗滨浮石，还在中国科学院、核工业部、国家地震局、北京中医药基础医学院等权威实验室进行了严格的检测，结果如下：

1. 有一奇异的能量场，作用在人体可产生红外热像并循经而行。
2. 摩擦或敲击此石可发出极丰富的超声波脉冲。
3. 此石无放射性，对人体无害。
4. 含有三十几种微量元素，其中锶的含量甚高。
5. 接触人体表皮，在监视器中可清楚地看到小血管及毛细血管中被改善而加速的血液流动状态。
6. 饮用泗滨浮石浸泡的水可降低血中的甘油三酯、胆固醇，提高高密度脂蛋白，有明显的调节血脂作用。

7. 用砭石（砧或尺最明显）叩、拍人体有明显的针刺感（无形针）。应该说用泗滨浮石制作的砭具是正宗的砭石，我们所开发的砭术是古籍中所述的真正的砭。

二、常用砭石疗法十六法

砭石疗法十六法包括感、压、滚、擦、刺、划、叩、刮、拍、揉、振、拔、温、凉、闻、扭。现分别叙述如下：

（一）感法

感法即感应法，是指接近和接触泗滨砭石，达到保健和调治的目的。其中它又分直接接触和间接接触两种方式。直接接触指用泗滨砭石直接触及人体。间接接触指泗滨砭石与人体之间有一定距离或隔着专门敷设的棉布类织物。因为泗滨砭石有一奇异的能量场，接触人体可使人体产生红外热像，可显著加快人体微循环血流速度，所以泗滨砭石无论直接还是间接接触人体，均可以对人体健康起到很好的调节作用。一般来说，质量大的砭具，如泗滨浮磬、砭球、砭棒、砭砧、砭尺等，实施感法效果较好。

砭术感法广泛应用于砭术各种调治方法之中，是砭术十六法之母。从某种意义上来说，由于砭术感法存在良好的调治效果，才有了砭术特殊存在的价值。

（二）压法

压法的施行是将砭具与人体接触后，再加以一定的压力，使砭具压迫人体，以达到更强的效果。实施压法，可以使泗滨砭石的场能和砭术师的作用力更好地作用于经络。在砭术的实施过程中都必须用压法。

在砭术调治的过程中，压法贯穿于各种手法之中。在砭术治疗中实施压法，是砭术的特点，也是取得较好疗效的关键。

（三）滚法

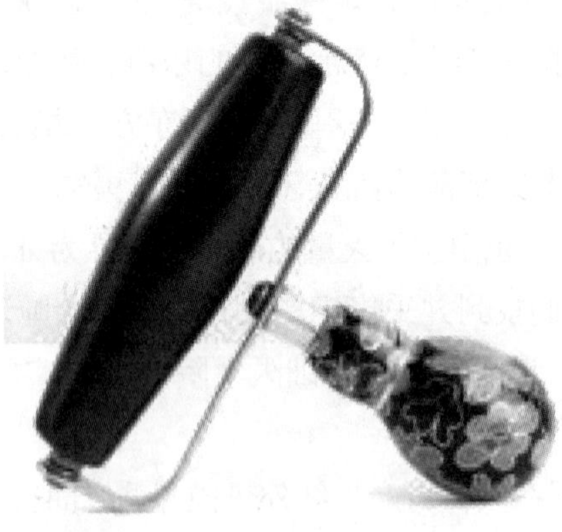

砭石磙

滚法是用砭具直接作用于人体体表部位，施加一定的压力，并沿着经络方向进行滚动的一种方法。滚法作用强度比较缓和，面积比较大，有利于调和经络之气。滚法可广泛应用于全身，所用的砭具有砭棒、砭磙、砭球等。

（四）擦法

擦法是指用泗滨砭石在体表进行摩擦的一种方法。直接作用于人体皮肤的擦法，一般作用强度较轻，有利于调和经络气血。用于砭术调治时，一般都施加一定的压力，隔一层棉织物作用于机体上，这样更有利于放松机体，疏通经络，调畅气血，活血化瘀，达到更好的调治目的。擦法使用的砭具有砭砧、砭棒和多功能砭板。

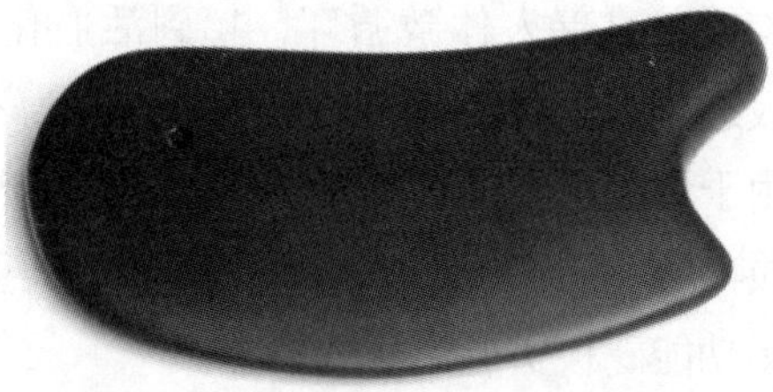

砭石刮痧板

擦法的应用比较广，经常结合揉法一起应用，常贯穿于整个砭术调治过程中。擦法对人体的刺激比滚法强，但仍属于弱刺激，常用于人体比较薄弱的部位。

（五）刺法

刺法是指用砭具点穴的方法。实施砭术刺法所使用的工具有砭锥、多功能砭板、砭砧、砭棒和砭球。其方法是利用砭具的尖部刺激人体的相关穴位以达到调治疾病的目的。砭术中的刺法不是机械刺激，而是利用泗滨砭石本身所固有的场能，达到调治目的，故不可盲目追求刺激强度。

（六）划法

划法是指用砭具沿着体表经络方向划动的一种方法。施行砭术划法的工具是砭锥和带有锥状尖端的多功能砭板。划法实施方法与擦法不同的是使用了尖锐的砭锥，触及皮肉的面积小、压力大、刺激强，因而在调畅经络、排泄热毒等方面较之擦法有较好的效果。

（七）叩法

利用砭具连续地叩击人体的砭术方法称作叩法。

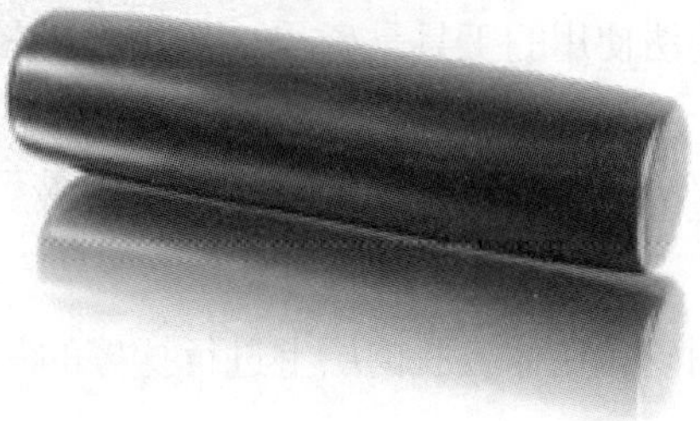

砭石按摩棒

几乎所有的砭具都可以用来实施叩法，最常用的有砭砧、砭棒、砭锥、多功能砭板等。叩击的力量不宜过大，叩击的频率最好与患者的脉搏相同。这样，实施叩法能有助于人体内的气血流动，帮助人消除疲劳、消除体内的热毒。扣法最常用的工具是砭砧，叩击在人体上有明显的针刺感，能作用于经络穴位上，激发循经感传，促进经络脏腑气血流动，活血化瘀，达到较好的调治效果。

实施叩法时，肩背部和四肢部肌肉丰厚的部位力度可大一些，在躯体上要轻，头部做叩法时要极轻。

（八）刮法

利用砭具刮拭人体的砭术手法叫作刮法。实施刮法的砭具很多，如砭砧、砭棒等，最适用的是多功能砭板。砭术中的刮法是砭术十六法中应用最广的方法，在民间已经发展成独立的一种医疗保健方法，俗称刮痧疗法。因此，各种用于刮法的多功能砭板常被称作刮痧板。

需要注意的是砭板和刮痧板的概念不完全相同。首先，砭板是用泗滨浮石制作，具有特殊的能量场，直接或间接接触人体均可以改善人体微循环，起到活血化瘀、治疗疾病的作用；再者，由于泗滨浮石的特性，使用砭板进行治疗时，并不要求出痧，因为不出痧就能达到较好的疏通经络、排出热毒的作用。另外，由于泗滨浮石具有微晶结构，质地光滑细腻，作用于人体有非常舒服的感觉，不需要润滑油等介质再隔一层棉织物作用于人体。因而受术者在接受治疗以后，皮肤不会有不适反应。这就是使用多功能砭板实施刮法的特点。

日本最新研究发现，人体后背有大团免疫细胞，平时处于休眠状态，经常刮拭后背，可以激活这些免疫细胞，提高人体免疫力。砭术治疗以刮拭后背、调畅五脏六腑之经气为基础，疏通心肾经络为轴心，达到保健、提高免疫力、治疗疾病的作用，是一种值得推广应用的全民健康保健医疗方法。

（九）拍法

拍法是指砭术师手持砭尺拍击人体体表经络穴位的一种治疗方法。

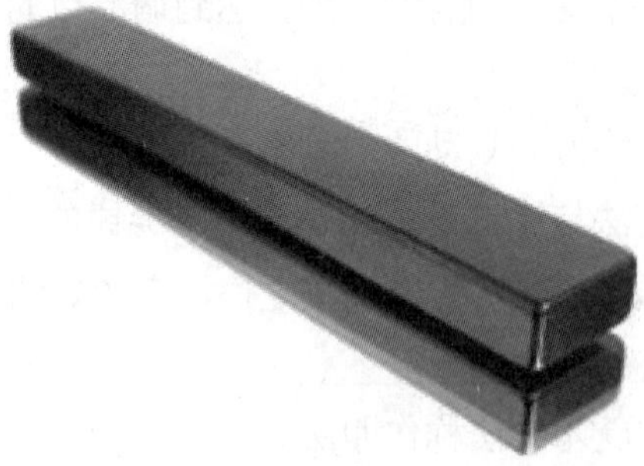

砭尺

拍法与叩法的不同在于：拍法使用的工具是砭尺，作用力比较集中，针刺感更明显，渗透层次更深，能更有效地疏通经络、活化气血循环。故砭尺是最常用的治疗方法之一，广泛用于疏通四肢各大经络、拔毒祛瘀、软坚散结，治疗各种顽固性疾病。

（十）揉法

揉法是指在一定压力下使用砭具在体表肌肉层上进行揉擦的一种方法。

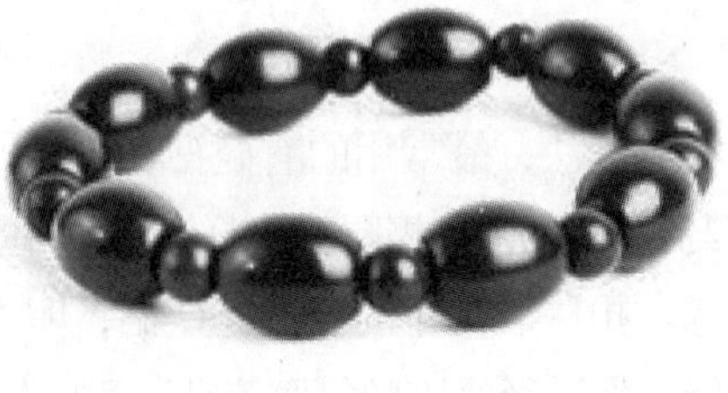

砭石手链

应区别于擦法：揉法使用一定的压力，作用于肌肉层，比擦法层次较深，作用强度较大，渗透层次更深，能更有效地激励气血、活化气血循环、放松肌肉，更有利于实施进一步的治疗。

使用揉法的作用要点是：使用一定压力，达到所需层次，在同一层次上按逆时针方向均匀、柔和、渗透地实施揉法，由点到面、由轻到重，持续地作用于机体上。

（十一）振法

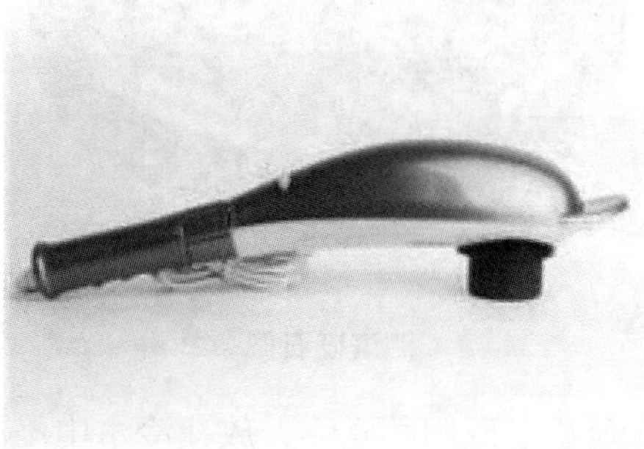

捶式砭震（按摩仪）

在压法和刺法的基础上，砭术师手持砭具，有节奏地上下振动，这种做法称为振法。在压法和刺法中加以振法，可以将压法和刺法对人体的作用传向人体的内部深处，有助于对人体内部脏腑的调理。

（十二）拔法

在压法和刺法中，当压力与刺力达到最大时，砭术师迅速沿相反方向将砭具撤离人体，这种做法称拔法。拔法的要领在于缓压速拔或缓刺速拔。这种做法的机理是当砭砧缓压入体或砭锥缓刺入体时，人体局部压力增高，气血向受压区深部或四周流动。拔法的施行，使人体局部压力增高的区域压力骤减，受压区深部和四周的气血快速向原受压区回流，使原受压区以及周围区域内人体的气血一时处在极度活跃的状态，有利于疏通气血的通道，并能排除人体内的热毒邪气。负压拔罐也属此法。

（十三）温法

将砭具加热以后置于人体体表部位，用温热治疗疾病的方法称作温法。温法最常使用的砭具是砭砧，有时也可用砭板。使用砭具做温法时，可以在热水中加热或晴天在日照下加热后，再把它置于施治部位。

温法在治疗中是最重要的治疗方法之一，这是由泗滨砭石的特性所决定的。将泗滨砭石接近人体以后，人体微循环会明显改善，能起到很好的调节气血的作用，而将泗滨砭石加热以后，这种补气活血、疏通经络、扶正祛邪、温阳祛寒的作用就更为明显了。将加热的砭具置于人体身上，患者可以明显感觉热气往身上走，并渗透到脏腑深处，有非常舒服的感觉。

（十四）凉法

凉法的做法与温法相反。将砭具放在冷水中浸泡良久，然后取出擦干，再把它置于人体患部，这种做法称为凉法。凉法的作用在于消减人体内的热毒。应用凉法要注意掌握分寸，不能过度，过度则会使患者受寒。特别是对年老体弱者。

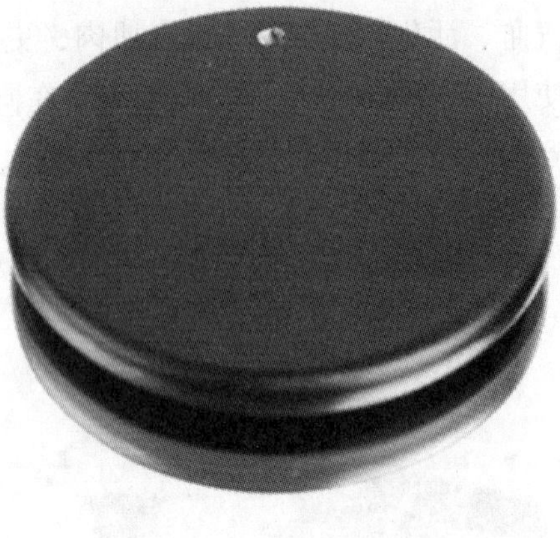

泗滨砭石佩

近来，有人将小型砭具，如砭板、砭佩和砭棒，放在冷水中浸凉，应用凉法做美容砭术。这样有助于消除面部皱纹及皮下多余脂肪。

（十五）闻法

闻是听的意思。闻法就是听磬。

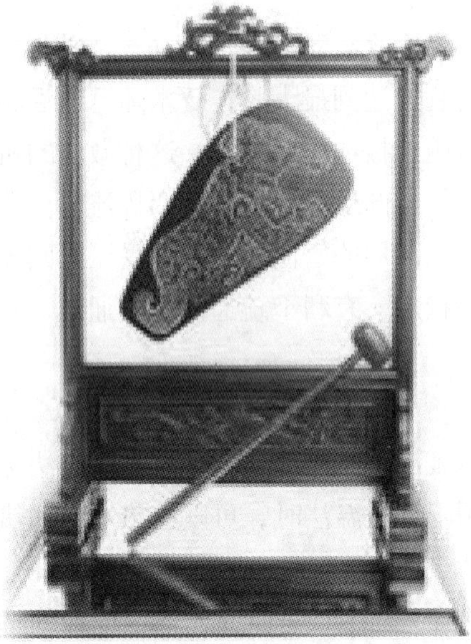

泗滨砭石磬

听泗滨浮磬声有益于人的健康。过去有人听到古砭术十六法中有闻法，认为是诊断的方法。这显然是受了中医四诊——望、闻、问、切的影响。中医中的闻，是四诊之一，是诊断方法。砭术中的闻，是十六法中的乐音疗法。泗滨浮磬的出土，泗滨砭石的发现，泗滨浮磬的重新开发，泗滨砭石和浮磬的声学、超声学性质的科学检测，泗滨浮石和浮磬具有医疗保健作用这一系列事物被揭示、被认识，使人们终于解开了砭术闻法的谜团。闻法就是听泗滨浮磬，现在已成为砭术研究者的共识。

现代科技检测揭示出砭术优良的超声性能，产生一种新砭术方法，即乐音超声砭术。

（十六）拊法

拊法即自己亲自击磬的砭术方法，并列于砭术的十六法中。孔夫子就曾以击磬来修养身心。《论语·宪问》记载：“子击磬于卫。有荷蒉而过孔氏之门者。曰：‘有心哉，击磬乎。’”泗滨浮磬，其乐音（包括超声波）有极强的穿透性，能穿透人体。所以无论是闻磬还是亲手击磬都有益于人的健康。闻磬时，磬发出的声波通过空气介质传到人体。击磬时，由于磬与人直接接触，或通过固体磬锤与人体相通，磬发出的声波传到人体时带来的声能大于闻磬的场合。正因为如此，闻法与拊法是与泗滨浮磬相关，但又有所区别的两种砭术方法。

三、砭石保健法

砭术作为一种医疗方法，对它的评价不仅要看它的医疗效果，也要看它的保健效果。保健对防病有重要的意义。古人强调治“未病”，今人主张防患于未然，都是希望在疾病未发生时注意保健，使疾病不发生。砭石疗法在保健方面有很好的效果。现列举部分如下：

（一）头部砭石保健法

1. 前额感应：

【方法】将砭板的板面贴在前额上做感法。在感应过程中还可以用手按砭板，使砭板压紧前额，感法和压法并施。

【功效】促进头部气血流畅。预防和治疗头痛、目眩、记忆力减退、阿尔茨海默病、感冒、高血压等症，减缓额部皱纹发展。

2. 刮印堂：

【方法】用砭板的外弧形板刃，以印堂为起点交替向左、右两方刮拭。

【功效】预防和治疗头晕、头疼、眼病、鼻病、感冒、高血压等症。

3. 理眉：

【方法】用砭板的外弧形板刃由两眉之间起，分别向左、右两方梳理眉毛。

【功效】预防和治疗头痛、眼病、耳病、鼻病和面部神经麻痹等症。

4. 拭目：

【方法】闭目，用砭板的外弧形板刃轻轻地刮拭眼部，刮拭的方向由内向外。

【功效】预防和治疗偏头痛、眼病和面部神经麻痹等症。减缓额部皱纹发展。

5. 梳头：

【方法】将砭石的外弧形板刃当作梳子，像梳头一样梳理头上长头发的部位。

【功效】促进头部气血流畅。预防和治疗感冒、头晕、头痛、高血压、脑血管疾病、记忆力减退、阿尔茨海默病。延缓白发、脱发等症的出现。

（二）颈部和肩部砭石保健法

1. 刮颈部后方：

【作法】用砭板的外弧形板刃自上而下刮颈部后方。

【功效】预防和治疗感冒、发热、支气管炎、哮喘、项强和颈椎病等。

2. 刮颈部两侧：

【作法】用砭板的板背自上而下刮颈部两侧。

【功效】预防和治疗耳鸣、咽喉肿痛、扁桃体炎、项强等。

3. 刮颈部前方：

【作法】用砭板的板面自上而下刮颈部前方。

【功效】预防和治疗高血压、咽喉肿痛、哮喘、支气管炎、甲状腺肿大等症。

4. 拍打肩部：

【作法】手持砭板的板尾，用砭板前部的板面，自内向外拍打左、右两肩的上部。

（三）四肢砭石保健法

1. 刮上肢内侧：

【方法】用砭石的砭背自上而下刮上肢内侧。

【功效】促进手三阴经（手太阴肺经、手厥阴心包经和手少阴心经）的通畅。预防和治疗心、肺疾病，手臂疼痛、麻木。

2. 刮上肢外侧：

【方法】用砭石的外弧形板刃自上而下刮上肢外侧。

【功效】促进手三阳经（手阳明大肠经、手少阳三焦经和手太阳小肠经）的通畅。预防和治疗便秘、泄泻、手臂不能举、疼痛。

3. 刮下肢内侧：

【方法】用砭石的板背自上而下刮下肢内侧。

【功效】促进足三阴经（足太阴脾经、足厥阴肝经和足少阴肾经）、阴跷经脉、阴维脉的通畅。预防和治疗肝、肾疾病，腿痛麻木、行动不便。

4. 拍打四肢：

【方法】四肢放松，用砭板的板面拍打四肢肌肉部分。

【功效】消除疲劳、清热解毒。

芳香疗法

一、芳香疗法的简介

芳香疗法系指使用植物芳香精油来舒缓压力与增进身体健康的一种自然疗法，其以芳香精油为物质基础，以芳香疗法学为理论指导，依不同的方法如香熏、按摩、吸入、沐浴、热敷等，让精油作用于人体上，而通过调节人体的各大系统，激发人类机体自身的治愈平衡及再生功能，达到强身健体、改善精神状态的目的。

数千年前，人们引用天然植物达到保健、治病、增进性趣的功效，历经时代的淬锑改良，演变成今天的芳香疗法。其中最主要的成分即是自花朵、树叶、果实、枝干等部分萃取而来，因具有镇静、杀菌、收敛的特性，长久以来被广泛运用在沐浴、护肤、按摩当中，甚至到今日，现代人承受种种来自环境、情绪、身体、精神的压力，导致“文明病”的产生。专家研究发现，采用植物源作为日常保健，可有效且无副作用地改善人们的压力及促进健康。芳香疗法，就是利用芳香植物的纯净精油来辅助医疗工作的另类疗法，就是人们从大自然中的各种芳香植物的不同部位中提炼出有不同气味和颜色的精油，如桉树的叶、玫瑰的花、佛手柑的果皮等。精油又萃取于多种具有“草药”性能的植物，具有杀菌、消炎、调节内分泌、改善机体代谢水平与免疫能力等作用，同时还有局部理疗、治疗的作用。利用纯天然植物精制油的芳香之气和治愈能力，以特殊的按摩手法，经由嗅觉器官和皮肤的吸收管道，到达神经系统，促进血液循环，以帮助人身心获得舒解，并达到皮肤保养、改善身体健康的功效。

中国是世界上最早使用芳香植物的国家之一，并在数千年前就有详细的研究。在距今 3000 多年前的黄帝、神农时代，人们采集树皮草根来驱疫辟秽，这是利用植物的香气来杀虫治病。那时人们对天然花卉的香气就有好感，用来敬神拜佛，清净身心，还用于祭祀、敬天、丧葬等。中医自古就有“芳香开窍”的理论，并在临床上被普遍运用。有资料表明，名医扁鹊、华佗等都有用芳香物质寮香让病人“起死回生”的本领。而中国第一本专述各种药草的目录书籍，相传是由距今 2800 年前的神农氏所著的《本草》。著名的《本草纲目》则是李时珍于 1578 年写成，书中记载了两千多种药用植物，其中包含大量的芳香植物的药效。

二、芳香疗法的特殊按摩手法

芳香疗法的特殊按摩手法包含了淋巴引流、神经肌肉按摩法，以及穴道指压三种手法，是结合了“精、气、神”三者合一的健康平衡之道，其效用有三：

精——激发人体潜在的生命活力（平衡疗法）

气——运用嗅觉使心灵舒畅（气息疗法）

神——解脱负担后的心旷神怡（意识疗法）

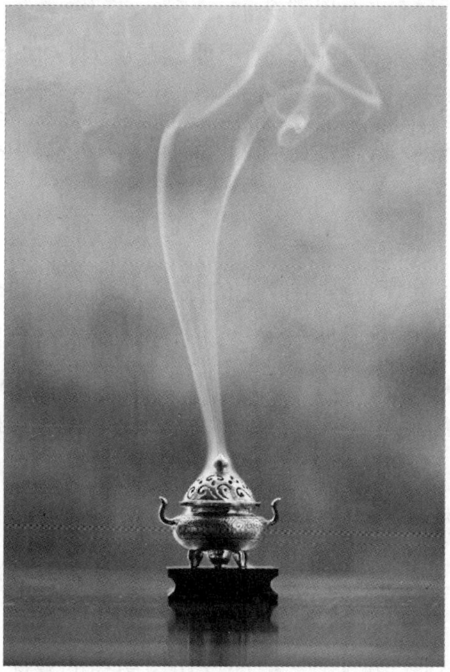

芳香疗法

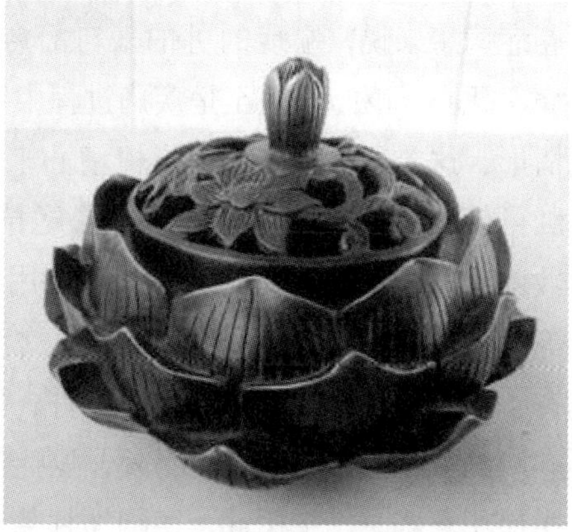

古人常用的香炉

三、芳香疗法的疗效

芳香疗法是运用芳香植物蒸馏萃取出的精油，以获得身、心、灵之整合性疗效，是一种辅助疗法。精油含酮、酯等 100 多种化学成分，这些成分决定它的治疗特性，可直接通过吸入、沐浴、按摩等方式来使用，改善焦虑、疼痛、疲倦及促进伤口愈合等。萃取出的精油，以获得身、心、灵之整合性疗效。由于芳香分子非常细微，很容易自皮肤渗透入血液、组织及分泌系统，所以迅速就有疗效，更因为若干精油的微粒分子作用类似荷尔蒙，与人体自身的荷尔蒙交相作用后，直接影响调理身心的反应，运用天然植物精华，透过皮肤、经络到神经系统、荷尔蒙系统、血液系统、免疫系统，帮助人体纾解身心、调理新陈代谢，达到促进身体健康和心理愉悦的功效。

四、芳香疗法的应用

（一）芳香疗法在保健美容方面的应用

芳香疗法有益于护肤，护肤效果明显的精油有花梨木、薰衣草、苦橙柑、甘菊、胡萝卜籽、鼠尾草、天竺葵、百里香、柠檬、橙花、玫瑰等。

精油有三个特性：第一，杀菌。精油不但对细菌有效，对一般之病毒及微生物亦有良好的杀灭抗力，如将精油加热，使精油分子挥发进入空气中，可达到杀菌和除臭的双重功效。第二，促进细胞再生。精油不但可以促进细胞再生能力，帮助伤口愈合，且具有延长细胞生命和使细胞延迟老化的能力。第三，解毒。一旦精油进入人体细胞，可以帮助细胞新陈代谢，促进有效呼吸作用之进行，排除细胞代谢后之废物及毒素，使细胞保持健康状态。

所以，芳香疗法有其强大的护肤功效：（1）促进皮肤的血液循环；（2）加强淋巴系统的排毒功能；（3）增强免疫力；（4）激活细胞再生能力；（5）调理细胞的呼吸代谢正常；（6）防止及治疗微生物的感染；（7）舒解身心，稳定情绪；（8）加速表皮的代谢，清洁皮肤；（9）增进皮肤吸收养分。比如：玫瑰，气味甜而沉的纤细花香，其精油不仅对头痛、失眠、神经紧张有其精神心理的效用，还可清血、利肝、利脾、健胃等，对身体有效用，更重要的是，对皮肤有消炎、抗菌、收敛的功效。玫瑰香清油，适用于所有的皮肤，特别有益于成熟、干燥、硬化或敏感的皮肤，其紧实、舒缓的特性，对发炎很有帮助。由于它能收缩微细血管，所以是治疗皮肤中微细血管扩张、破裂的神奇之宝。

（二）芳香按摩疗法用于减轻癌症患者的症状

对癌症病患来说，癌症的可怕来自治愈的难度及治疗过程中产生的诸多不适，例如全身无力、疼痛、恶心、呕吐，甚至是疾病过程中所带来的焦虑及情绪低落。许多癌症病患常会出现食欲降低情形，这个问题可以使用甜橙精油来改善。口腔及伤口的异味能用茶树纯露或薄荷纯露。身体水肿可使用葡萄柚、柠檬、快乐鼠尾草、杜松等精油，再配合淋巴结按摩，会有不错的功效。多数癌症患者不能忍受的疼痛，则可用快乐鼠尾草、甜马郁兰、罗马洋甘菊、德国洋甘菊、薰衣草等精油。让癌症病患煎熬的焦虑、忧郁等情绪低落问题，可用橙花、快乐鼠尾草、佛手柑、乳香、檀香、葡萄柚、甜橙、迷迭香、甜马郁兰等精油，改善心灵及心情的疲惫，让癌症病患敞开心胸，放松紧张的情绪。另外，癌症病患因免疫力下降，常会导致伤口的不易恢复，此时可以考虑使用薰衣草、茶树油、德国洋甘菊等精油涂抹于伤口上，会促进伤口组织的复原。而如果因为化疗而造成恶心呕吐，则可使用柠檬、甜橙、薄荷、姜等精油，用薰香的方式让病患吸入，可以改善病患的恶心呕吐情形。因疾病或药物造成的肠胃便秘或腹胀，可用橙花、甜橙、乳香、葡萄柚、佛手柑、柠檬等精油按摩腹部。

芳香疗法是温和的辅助疗法，无法用来消灭癌细胞，但看似简单的精油若能适当地使用于癌症病患身上，也能在一定程度上减缓病患身体不适及促进心灵缓和，促使疾病治疗过程的顺利，提高病患生活品质，进而能积极面对癌症治疗，对癌症病患来说，是一举数得的好帮手。

近年来，大多数人处于繁忙、紧张的生活状态中。生活节奏加快，人的身心压力也加大，便希望有一些能放松肌肉、消除疲劳、有助于身心健康的天然产品，使疾病得到治疗或减轻。芳香疗法正好能满足人们的这种需要。芳香疗法不仅能护肤、护发和去除表皮上的一些瑕疵，而且能让人在舒适、芳香的环境里使身心松弛下来，得到休息，激发人体免疫力，使人体身心的一些不适或病痛得到治疗或减轻。因此，芳香疗法受到了人们的喜爱，并逐渐在世界各地流传开来。

Appendices

Bian Stone Therapy

Ⅰ. The history of Bian stone

Bian stone therapy is one kind of ancient Chinese acupuncture. It is guided by the theories of meridians and acupoints of Traditional Chinese Medicine. When the therapy is performed, no oral taking, no piercing of the skin and no medium is needed. The Bian stone can be used directly on skin, or used with the separation of cotton fabrics. Without bringing any suffering, its manipulations include "scraping, pushing, wiping, rubbing, scratching, tangling, cooling, paddling, pulling, point-pressing, pressing, shaking, stroking, patting, knocking, cutting, warming, cleaning, induction, electric heating and warming", which can give full play to its field effect and "invisible needle" functions. It can help to treat internal diseases with external treatment, by dredging the meridians, regulating Qi and blood, eliminating pathological substances that hinder flow of Qi and blood (especially the pathological substances deep in the meridians under skin). Therefore, it can help people to treat both symptoms and root causes of diseases, greatly relieve clinical symptoms in a short period of time and meet the purpose of healing. It has good treatment effect for cerebrovascular diseases, neck, shoulder, waist and leg diseases and sub-health status of the masses.

According to the records of *Huang Di's Canon of Internal Medicine*, Bian stone therapy, acupuncture, moxibustion and medicine are four competing treatment branches in ancient China. Bian stone therapy originated in the Neolithic Age and got lost before East Han Dynasty. It had been lost for over two thousand years when it was rediscovered again. Bian is one kind of stone knife and predecessor of Bian needle, which can be used to cut carbuncle and pierce pustule to discharge blood and pus.

Sibin pumice, mentioned in *Shang Shu* (an ancient Chinese book), is the material for making Bian chimes and Bian tools. This kind of stone was covered with a mysterious veil in ancient documents. In the period of Yu the Great, chimes made from Sibin Bian stone were tributes and holy artifacts (chimes with tiger stripes). After the appearance of Buddhism, Taoism and Confucianism in China, chimes made from Sibin Bian stone were musical instruments in temples (ancient chimes were made from stones). They were also Confucianists' musical instruments for life cultivation and taste cultivation. Confucius used chime beating as one of his means of life cultivation. It is said in *Huangdi Neijing* (*The Inner Canon of Huangdi*) that "Bian stones come from the east". "The east" here refers to Shandong. It is said in *The History of the Road* that "Fu Hsi tasted herbs and made Bian stone devices to treat the people's illness". Fu Hsi was the chief of Tai Hao tribe, one branch of Dongyi (Eastern Barbarian) who lived in the coastal area of Shandong in ancient time. That is, Fu Hsi was born in Shandong. A lot of chimes have been excavated in Shandong, which can be regarded as references too. Sibin pumice, which is used to make Bian stone devices, is also from Shandong. In 1980s, all the existing precious Sibin pumice was found and collected. Sibin pumice was meticulously examined in labs of some authoritative agencies, such as Science Academy of China, Ministry of Nuclear Industry, State Seismological Bureau of China, and School of Basic Medicine of Beijing University of Chinese Medicine and the results of the examinations are as follows:

1. Bian stones have an odd energy field which can produce infrared image in human body and flow along meridians.

2. When rubbed or knocked on, Bian stones can produce rich ultrasonic pulses.

3. Bian stones do not have any radiation and they are not harmful to health.

4. They contain over thirty kinds of trace elements, and their content of strontium is quite high.

5. When they touch human skin, it can be clearly found from monitors that blood flow in small blood vessels and blood capillaries are improved and accelerated.

6. After drinking water soaked with Sibin pumice, people's triglyceride and cholesterol are reduced and high-density lipoprotein is improved, which means that Sibin pumice can obviously regulate blood fat.

7. When people use Bian stones (especially Bian stone anvil and ruler) to knock human body, people will feel obvious needling sensation (hence called invisible needle). Therefore, Bian devices made from Sibin Bian stones are the original Bian tools. The Bian stones we are talking about are the true Bian stones recorded in ancient documents.

Ⅱ. Sixteen manipulations of Bian stone therapy

Bian stone therapy has 16 kinds of manipulations which include induction, pressing, rolling, scratching, piercing, paddling, knocking, rubbing, patting, kneading, shaking, pulling, warming, cooling, hearing and seizing and they will be narrated as follows:

1. Induction manipulation.

Induction refers to touching or being close to Sibin Bian stones to realize the purpose of health care and regulation. Contact can be divided into direct contact and indirect contact. Direct contact means that Sibin Bian stones are used to touch human bodies directly. Indirect contact means that there are some distances or cotton fabrics between Sibin Bian stones and bodies. Sibin Bian stones have one kind of special energy field. When they touch or are close to human bodies, human bodies can produce infrared images and micro blood circulation is improve. Therefore, they have very good regulating functions to health whether they have direct or indirect contact with human bodies. Generally speaking, big Bian stone tools, such as Sibin Bian chimes, Sibin Bian balls, Sibin Bian anvils and Sibin Bian rulers, etc. have better effects for induction treatment.

Induction treatment is widely used in all kinds of manipulations and it is the origin of the remaining 15 manipulations. To some extents, it is because of very good regulating and treatment effect of induction that Bian stone therapy has its special value.

2. Pressing.

The manipulation of pressing is performed when it has direct contact with human body and the therapist exerts some pressure on human body so as to achieve better effect. When people perform pressing, the field energy of Bian stones and the therapist's pressing force are combined to work on meridians. In the process of pressing manipulation, pressure will last from beginning to the end of manipulation.

In all kinds of Bian stone manipulations, pressing exists in all of them. Therefore, pressing manipulation is one of the characteristics of Bian stone therapy and it is also a key to achieve good treatment effects.

3. Rolling.

Rolling is using Bian stone devices to press on human surface and roll along meridians. The intensity of rolling manipulation is mild but its coverage is wide, which is helpful for regulating meridians. Rolling manipulation can be extensively used on the whole body. Suitable Bian stone devices for rolling include Bian stone sticks, Bian stone rollers and Bian stone balls etc.

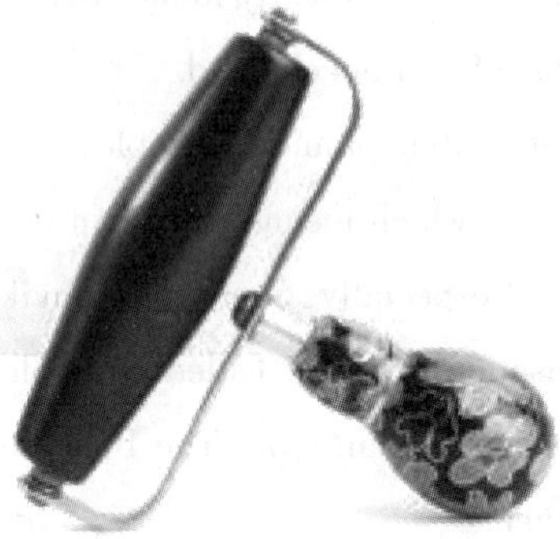

Bian Stone Roller

4. Scratching.

In scratching manipulation, the therapist uses a Sibin Bian stone to scratch and rub the surface of human body. When scratching is used, its intensity should be small, which will be helpful for reconciling meridians, Qi and blood. In the process of Bian stone therapy, a certain degree of pressure on human body, sometimes with the separation of cotton fabrics, can help to relax the body, dredge meridians, reconcile Qi and blood to realize the purpose of better treatment and reconciliation. The devices used for scratching include Bian anvil, Bian stick and multifunctional Bian plate.

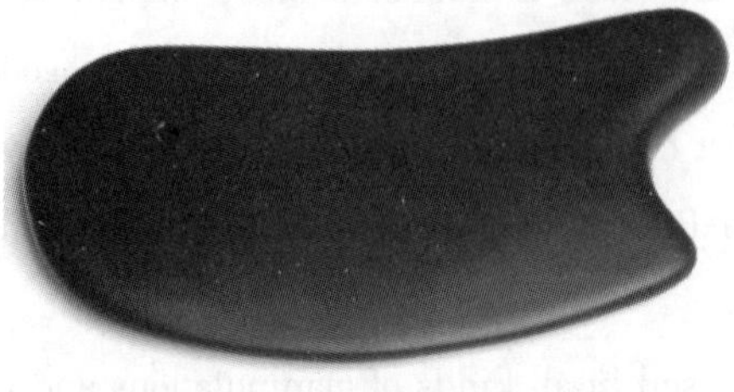

Guasha Plate

5. Piercing.

Piercing manipulation refers to pointing acupoints with Bian stone tools, which include Bian stone awls, multifunctional Bian stone plates, Bian anvils, Bian sticks and Bian balls. The therapist uses the pointed end of Bian stone devices to stimulate corresponding acupoints to treat diseases and tone the body. Piercing of Bian therapy is using the inherent field energy of Bian stones to treat diseases and tone the body, rather than mechanical stimulation. Therefore, the therapist should not pursue stimulating intensity blindly.

6. Paddling.

Paddling refers to the manipulation of using Bian devices to paddle along meridians. The devices for paddling manipulation are Bian awls and pointed multifunctional Bian plates. Unlike scratching manipulation, paddling manipulation adopts pointed Bian awls, whose contact area with skin is small but its pressure and stimulation at the skin is big. Therefore, it has very good effects for dredging meridians and heat toxin.

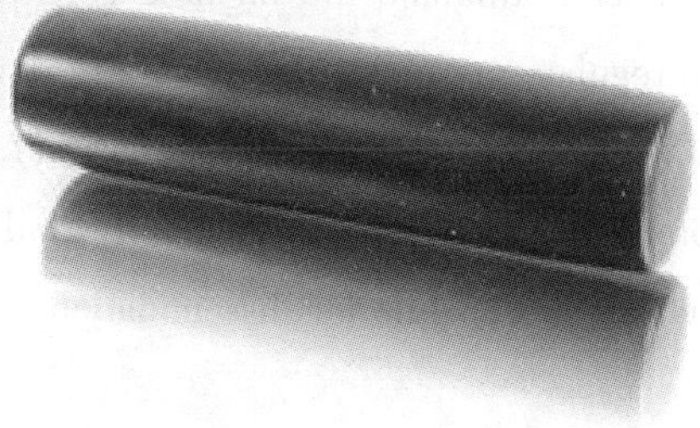

Bian Stone Massage Stick

7. Knocking.

Nearly all Bian stone devices, including Bian stone anvils, Bian stone sticks, Bian stone awls and multifunctional Bian plates etc. , can be used for knocking manipulation. Knocking force should not be too strong, and it would be better if the frequency of knocking is the same as the frequency of pulse. Knocking manipulation can help to promote flow of Qi and blood, get rid of fatigue and heat toxin in the body. The best device for knocking manipulation is Bian stone anvil. When Bian stone anvil is knocking on the body, the manipulated person has a clear sense of needling. Knocking can impact meridians, promote the spread of needling sensation, promote the flow of Qi and blood in meridians, Zang organs and Fu organs, activate blood circulation to dissipate stasis and realize the purpose of treatment and reconciliation.

When the therapist knocks on the back and the areas of limbs with thick muscles, knocking force can be strong. While knocking on the trunks, the knocking force should be mild. When knocking on the head, the knocking force should be extremely mild.

8. Scraping.

In scraping manipulations, Bian stone devices are used to scrap human bodies. Many Bian stone tools, such as Bian stone anvils, Bian stone sticks etc. can be used for scraping manipulation. However, the best device for scraping is multifunctional Bian anvil. Scraping is probably the most widely used manipulation among 16 manipulations of Bian therapy. In the folk, scraping has developed into an independent health care branch, which is called Guasha in Chinese. Therefore, the multifunctional Bian plate is often called Guasha plate.

It should be noticed that Bian plate and Guasha plate are two definitions that are not completely the same. First of all, a Bian plate is made from Sibin pumice, which has special energy field and its direct or indirect contact with the skin can improve micro circulation of the body and has the functions of activating blood circulation to dissipate stasis and treat diseases. Second, because of the special properties of Sibin pumice, when a Bian plate is used for treatment, very good effect of activating dredging meridians and dissipating heat toxins without actual diseases. Furthermore, Sibin pumice has a microcrystalline structure and very fine and smooth texture. When it is used to have contact with human body, people feel very comfortable. Medium or lubricant is not necessary. A piece of cotton fabric is usually used if people insist. After treatment, there is no uncomfortable reaction in the skin. These are some characteristics of using multifunctional Bian plate for Guasha.

Some latest researches in Japan show that there are a lot of dormant immune cells at the backs of people. Regular scraping at the back can stimulate the immune cells and improve people's immunity. In Bian therapy, scraping the back to regulate meridians and blood of the five Zang organs and six Fu organs serves as the basic. Dredging the channels of heart meridian and kidney meridian serves as the focus. Scraping the back can improve health, improve immunity and treat diseases. It is one kind of nationwide fitness manipulations that are worthwhile for dissemination.

9. Patting.

Patting is one kind of treatment that the therapist uses a Bian ruler to pat on meridians and acupoints.

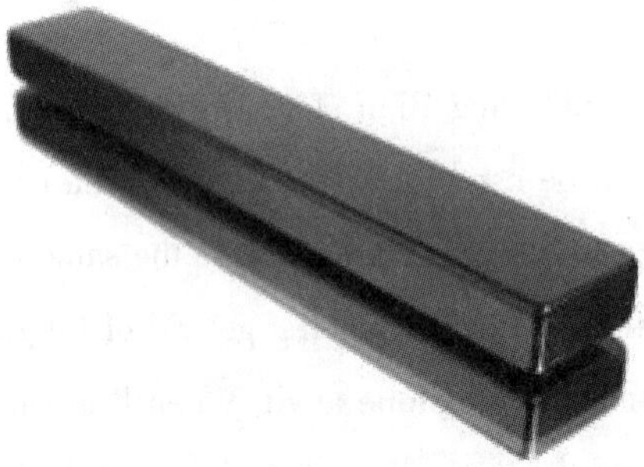

A Bian Stone Ruler

The differences between patting manipulation and knocking manipulation: the device used in patting is a Bian ruler. Its impact is comparatively concentrated. Its needling sensation is stronger and can penetrate deeper. It can dredge meridians, activate blood and qi circulation more effectively. Therefore, patting with a Bian ruler is one of the most commonly used manipulations. It is widely used for dredging meridians along four limbs, drawing out pus, removing stasis, removing hard lumps and treating all kinds of intractable diseases.

10. Kneading.

Kneading refers to the manipulation that Bian devices are used to knead the surface muscles.

Kneading should be differentiated from scratching: kneading needs a certain degree of pressure to impact on muscles. It has impact on deeper layers, bigger strength and depth of penetration than scratching. Therefore, it stimulates Qi and blood better, promotes Qi and blood circulation better and relaxes muscles better and it is more beneficial for further treatment.

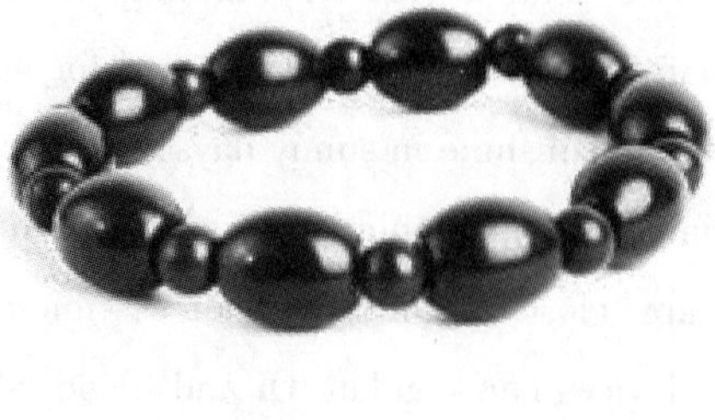

A Bian Stone Bracelet

The key point of kneading manipulation is: Exert corresponding force to reach needed layers of muscles. At the same level, adopt clockwise and anticlockwise even mild and penetrating kneading manipulation. The kneading manipulation should be done continuously from a point to an area, from mild force to strong force.

11. Shaking.

On the basis of pressing and piercing manipulation, the therapist can adopts shaking manipulation by holding a Bian device to shake up and down on human body. Add shaking manipulation to pressing and piercing manipulation can help to transmit the functions of pressing and piercing manipulation into deeper parts of human body, which is helpful for regulating internal human Zang organs and Fu organs.

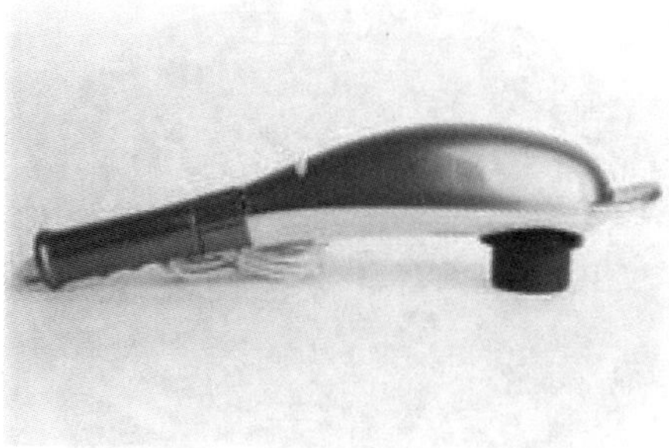

A Bian Stone Massage Device

12. Pulling.

In the process of pressing and piercing manipulation, when the pressing force and piercing force reach their maximum, the therapist removes Bian device quickly in the opposite direction, such manipulation is called pulling manipulation. The key point of pulling manipulation lies in slow pressing and fast pulling, and slow piercing and fast pulling. The mechanism of the manipulation is: When a Bian anvil presses on human body, or when a Bian awl pierces human body, pressure at the impacted area increases and Qi and blood flow to deeper area or surrounding areas. When pulling manipulation is performed, pressure at the impacted area drops immediately. Blood and qi in deeper area and surrounding areas flow to the impacted area quickly. This manipulation makes blood and Qi at the impacted and surrounding areas become extremely active very quickly, which is helpful for dredging Qi and blood channels, and getting rid of heat toxin and pathogenic factors. Negative pressure cupping also adopts the same mechanism.

13. Warming.

Warming a Bian device and putting it on human body to treat diseases is called warming manipulation. The most commonly used Bian device for warming manipulation is Bian anvil. Sometimes Bian plates are also used. When Bian devices needs to be warmed for manipulation, they can be warmed by soaking in warm water, or leaving in sunshine in sunny days, before putting them on the treated areas.

Warming is one of the most important manipulations, which is due to the properties of Sibin Bian stones. When Sibin Bian stones are close to human bodies, micro blood circulation is obviously improved. It means that Sibin Bian devices can regulate Qi and blood very well. When Sibin Bian devices are warmed, their functions of enriching qi, activating blood, dredging meridians, strengthening body resistance, eliminating evil, warming yang and dispelling cold are more obvious. When warmed Bian devices are placed on human bodies, the patients can feel that warmth is flowing in their bodies and penetrates into their Zang organs and Fu organs. It's very comfortable to receive such treatment.

14. Cooling.

Cooling manipulation is just the opposite of warming manipulation. Put a Bian device in cold water for some time. Take it out, wipe it dry and place it on the treated area. This kind of manipulation is called cooling. The function of cooling is to dispel heat toxins in the body. While adopting cooling manipulation, the therapist should pay attention to proper degree of cooling. Over cooling is forbidden because it may lead to patient's catching cold, especially the old and the weak.

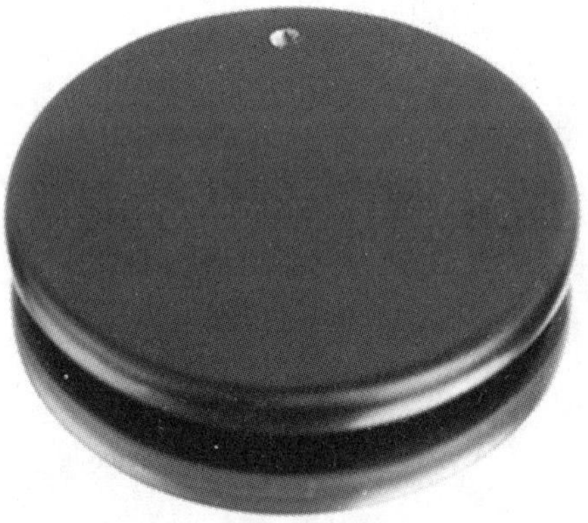

A Bian Pendant

In recent years, some people soak small Bian devices, such as Bian plates, Bian pendants and Bian sticks etc. in cold water for beauty therapy. Such manipulation can help to remove wrinkles and redundant subcutaneous fat.

15. Listening.

Listening manipulation here refers to listening to Bian chimes.

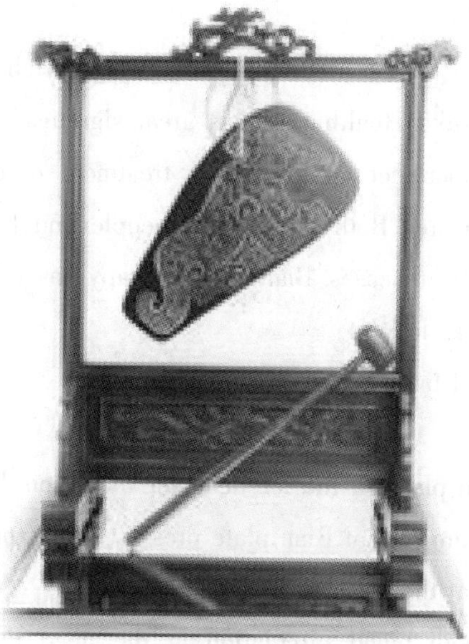

A Sibin Bian Stone Chime

Listening to the sound of Bian stone chimes is beneficial to our health. In the past when people read of 16 manipulations of ancient Bian therapy, they supposed that it was one kind of diagnosis, which is obviously influenced by the Four Diagnostic Methods of Traditional Chinese Medicine (observation, listening, interrogation and pulse-taking). "Listening" in Traditional Chinese Medicine is one kind of diagnostic methods while "listening" in the 16 manipulations of Bian therapy belongs to music therapy. The excavation of Sibin pumice chimes, rediscovery of Sibin Bian stones, redevelopment of Sibin pumice chimes, acoustic and ultrasonic examinations of Bian pumice chimes and the discovery of medical and health-care functions of Sibin pumice and Bian pumice chimes finally solve the mystery of listening manipulation. Listening manipulation is just listening to Sibin pumice chimes and this is the consensus of Bian therapy researchers.

Scientific examinations of Sibin pumice and disclosure of its excellent ultrasonic properties lead to the birth of one kind of new Bian therapy method, that is, ultrasonic Bian music therapy.

16. Beating.

Beating refers to beating Bian chimes, which is listed as one of the sixteen Bian therapy manipulations. Confucius once beat Bian chimes for self-cultivation. It is recorded in Questions Raised by Yuan Xuan in *The Analects of Confucius that* "Confucius beat chimes in Wei Kingdom. One person carrying a grass basket passed by Confucius' gate and said: 'He has something on his mind, so he beats the chime to release his pent-up feelings'". Sibin pumice chimes and their sound (and their ultrasonic waves) have very strong penetrating power and they can penetrate human bodies. Therefore, both listening to Bian chimes and beating Bian chimes are beneficial to health. When listening to Bian chimes, acoustic waves of chimes reach people via the medium of air. When people beat Bian chimes, chimes have direct contact with people, or indirect contact with people via hammers. Their acoustic energy is bigger than that of listening to Bian chimes. Though both listening manipulation and beating manipulation are related to Bian chimes, they are two different Bian therapy manipulations.

Ⅲ. Bian stone health care

As one branch of Traditional Chinese Medicine, its evaluation should include not only its medical results but also its health care results. Health care has great significance for disease prevention. Ancient Chinese people attached great importance to preventive treatment of diseases. Present people also pay attention to taking preventive measures. Both the ancient people and present people hope that they can make preventive measures to prevent diseases. Bian stone therapy has very good effect for health care and some manipulations are described as follows:

(Ⅰ) Health care of the head by using Bian stones

1. Induction at the forehead:

【Manipulation】Place a Bian plate on the forehead for induction. In the process of induction, some pressure may be exerted on the plate so that Bian plate presses closely on the forehead. That is, induction and pressing can be manipulated at the same time.

【Functions】Promoting smooth blood circulation at the head. Preventing and treating headache, dizziness, hypomnesis, Alzheimer disease, cold, hypertension and mitigating wrinkles at forehead.

2. Scraping ophryon:

【Manipulation】Using the external arc of a Bian plate to scrape from the ophryon to right side and left side of the forehead alternatively.

【Functions】Preventing and treating dizziness, headache, eye diseases, nasal diseases, cold and hypertension etc.

3. Combing eyebrows:

【Manipulation】Using the external arc of a Bian plate to scrape the right and left eyebrows alternatively.

【Functions】Preventing and treating headache, eye diseases, ear diseases, nasal diseases and facial nerve numbness, etc.

4. Wiping eyes:

【Manipulation】After closing the eyes, using the external arc of a Bian plate to wipe the eyes from internal side to external side.

【Functions】Preventing and treating migraine, eye diseases and facial nerve numbness; mitigating wrinkles at forehead.

5. Combing hair:

【Manipulation】Using the external arc of a Bian device to comb the hair, as if using a comb to comb the hair.

【Functions】Promoting the flow of qi and blood at the head; preventing and treating cold, dizziness, headache, hypertension, cerebrovascular diseases, lapse of memory, and Alzheimer; delaying appearance of white hair and losing of hair;

(Ⅱ) Health care for the neck and shoulder by using Bian devices

1. Scraping the posterior neck:

【Manipulation】Using the external arc of a Bian plate to scrape posterior neck in top-down direction.

【Functions】 Preventing and treating cold, fever, bronchitis, asthma, stiff neck and cervical spondylosis.

2. Scraping both sides of the neck:

【Manipulation】 Using the back side of a Bian plate to scrape both sides of the neck.

【Functions】 Preventing and treating rhinitis, swollen and sore throat and amygdalitis and stiff neck etc.

3. Scraping anterior neck:

【Manipulation】 Using the surface of a Bian plate to scrape the anterior neck.

【Functions】 Preventing and treating hypertension, swollen and sore throat, asthma, bronchitis and thyroid enlargement etc.

4. Patting on the shoulder:

【Manipulation】 Holding the tail of a Bian plate to pat on the right and left shoulder from inner side to outer side with the other end of the Bian plate.

(Ⅲ) Health care for the limbs by using Bian devices

1. Scraping medial upper limbs:

【Manipulation】 Using the back of a Bian stone to scrape the medial side of upper limbs in top-down direction.

【Functions】 Promoting the smoothness of 3 Yin meridians of hand (Lung Meridian of Hand-Taiyin, Pericardium Meridian of Hand-Jueyin and Heart Meridian of Hand-Shaoyin); preventing and treating heart diseases, lung diseases, numbness and pain of arms.

2. Scraping lateral upper limbs:

【Manipulation】 Using the external arc blade of a Bian stone to scrape the lateral side of upper limbs in top-down direction.

【Functions】 Promoting the smoothness of 3 Yang meridians of hand (Large Intestine Meridian of Hand-Yangming, Sanjiao Meridian of Hand-Shaoyang and Small Intestine Meridian of Hand-Taiyang); preventing and treating constipation, diarrhea, incapability to raise arms and pain of arms.

3. Scraping medial lower limbs:

【Manipulation】 Using the back of a Bian stone to scrape the medial limbs in top-down direction.

【Functions】 Promoting the smooth flow of 3 yin meridians (Spleen Meridian of Foot-Taiyin, Liver Meridian of Foot-Jueyin and Kidney Meridian of Foot-Shaoyin), Yinqiao Meridian and Yinwei Meridian; preventing and treating liver diseases, kidney diseases, pain and numbness of legs and mobility difficulty.

4. Patting on limbs:

【Manipulation】 Relaxing the limbs and then using the surface of a Bian plate to pat on muscles of four limbs.

【Functions】 Dispelling fatigue and clearing away heat and toxic materials.

Aromatherapy

Ⅰ. A brief introduction to aromatherapy

Aromatherapy refers to one kind of natural therapy that uses essential oils to relax pressure and enhance health. Fragrant essential oils are the material foundation of aromatherapy and it is guided by aromatherapy theory. Different methods such as fragrance activity, massage, bathing and hot compress help essential oils to function on human body to regulate different systems of human body, activate immune function and regenerating function of human body, so as to realize the purpose of building body and improving mental status.

Thousands of years ago, people began to use natural plants for health care, treatment of diseases and improve sexual interest. After refinement and improvement of ages, they have evolved into present aromatherapy. The main ingredients of essential oil come from extraction of flowers, leaves, fruits and branches of trees etc. Because of their calming, disinfecting and convergent properties, they have long been used in bathing, skin products and massage products. Nowadays, people suffer from various kinds of environmental, emotional, physical and mental stress, which lead to the occurrence of "modern diseases". Experts' studies show that using botanic materials for daily health care activities can effectively solve people's stress problems and promote health without side effect. Aromatherapy is one kind of therapy that adopts essential oils extracted from fragrant plants to aid medical treatment. People extract essential oils with different flavors and colors from different parts of plants from the world, such as eucalyptus leaves, rose flowers and peels of bergamot etc. Some essential oils are extracted from medical herbs. When such essential oils function on human bodies, they have the functions of disinfection, anti-inflammation, regulating endocrine, enhancing metabolism and immunity, local physiotherapy and treatment. The fragrance and healing properties of natural essential oils, through special massage manipulations and absorption via olfactory organ and skins, can reach nervous system and blood circulation system of human body. This will help people to gain physical and mental relaxation, care for skin and enhancement of health.

China is one of the earliest countries to use fragrant plants, which were studied carefully thousands of years ago. 3000 years ago in Yellow Emperor and Shennong Era, people collected barks and grass roots to dispel epidemic and evil because fragrance from plants can kill insects and bacteria. At that time, people were fond of fragrance of natural flowers. They used flowers and their fragrance for worshiping gods and Buddha, purifying their body and mind, sacrifice, worshiping heaven and funeral ceremonies. Since long time ago, Traditional Chinese Medicine has been holding the idea that "fragrance can enlighten people", which is also widely used in clinical practice. Documents indicate that ancient famous doctors such as Bian Que and Hua Tuo, had the ability to bring the dying back to life by using Lao Xiang (one kind of fragrant material). *Chinese materia medica*, the first Chinese book that recorded nearly all kinds of medical herbs, was said to have been written by Shennong 2800 years ago. *Compendium of Materia Medica*, a famous book, was written by Li Shizhen in 1578. More than 2000 kinds of medical herbs, including many fragrant herbs and their efficacy, were recorded in the book.

Ⅱ. Special massage manipulations of aromatherapy

Manipulations of aromatherapy include lymphatic drainage, massage of nerves and muscles and finger massage. Because of their healthy and balanced integration of "vitality, smell and mind", their functions include the following three kinds:

Vitality—stimulating the potential vitality in human body (balance therapy)

Smell—olfactory organs are adopted to make people happy both physically and mentally (smell therapy)

Mind—exhilaration after liberation from all worry

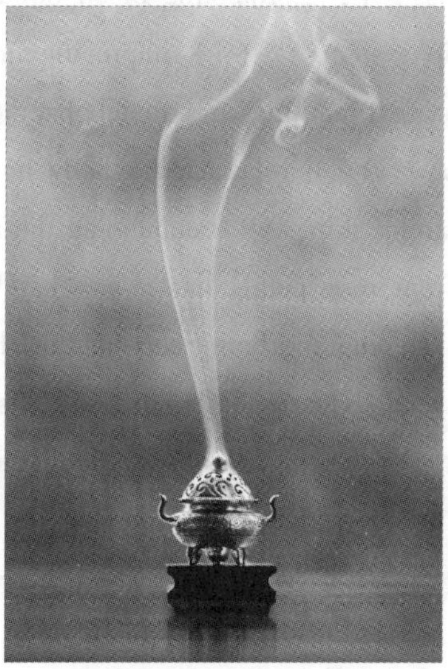

Aromatherapy Activity

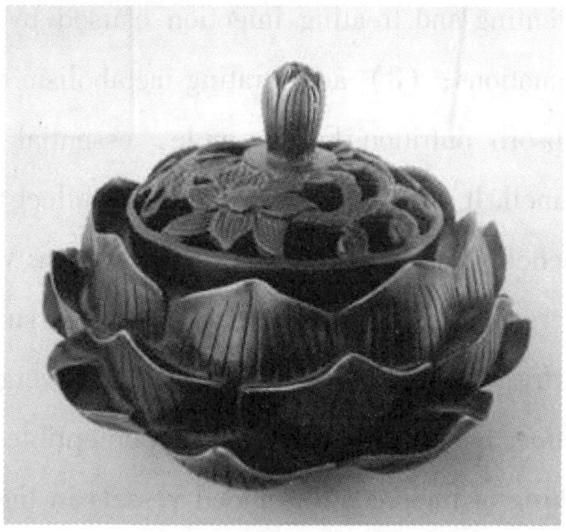

One Incense Burner of Ancient People

Ⅲ. Efficacy of aromatherapy

Aromatherapy, one kind of complementary therapy, is the use of essential oils extracted from aromatic plants to obtain integrated effects of body, mind and spirit. Essential oils contain more than 100 kinds of chemical components such as ketones and esters. These ingredients determine the therapeutic properties and essential oils can be used by direct inhalation, bathing, massage, etc. to improve anxiety, pain, fatigue and wound healing. Extracted essential oils can achieve an integrated effect of body, mind and spirit. Because the aromatic molecules are very fine, they are easy to penetrate into the blood, tissue and secretion system from the skin, so they have rapid curative effect. Moreover, because the micro-particles of several essential oils act like hormones, they directly affect the conditioning of body and mind after interacting with the body's own hormones. The use of natural plant extracts, through skin and meridians into nervous system, hormonal systen, blood system and immune system, helps the body to ease the body and mind and adjust metabolism, to achieve the function of promoting physical health and psychological pleasure.

Ⅳ. Application of aromatherapy

(Ⅰ) Application of aromatherapy in health care and cosmetics

Aromatherapy is beneficial to skin. The essential oils that are beneficial to skin are extracted from rosewood, lavender, bitter orange, citrus, carrot seeds, sage, thyme, lemon and rose etc.

Essential oils have three properties: First, killing bacteria. Essential oils are not only effective to bacteria but also effective to ordinary virus and microorganism. For example, when essential oils are heated, molecules of essential oils are vaporized into air, which has dual functions of disinfection and deodorization. Second, promote regeneration of cells. Essential oils can not only promote regeneration capacity and healing of wounds but also extend cell life and delay cell aging. Third, detoxification. When essential oils penetrate into human cells, they can enhance metabolism of cells, promote effective breathing, eliminate wastes and toxins left by cell metabolism to maintain health of cells.

Therefore, aromatherapy has very strong skin care functions: (1) promoting blood circulation of skin; (2) enhancing the detoxification function of lymphatic system; (3) improving immunity; (4) stimulating regenerating capacity of cells; (5) regulating breathing and metabolism of cells; (6) preventing and treating infection caused by microorganism; (7) relaxing the body and mind, calming emotions; (8) accelerating metabolism of skin and cleaning skin; (9) enhancing the ability of skin to absorb nutrition. For example, essential oil extracted from rose petals has a sweet, deep and delicate smell. It not only has psychological effect to headache, insomnia and being nervous but also clears blood, benefits the liver and tonify the spleen. More importantly, it has anti-inflammation, disinfection and convergent functions. Rose essential oil is suitable for all kinds of skin. It is especially beneficial to mature, dry, hard or sensitive skin. Its convergent and calming properties is also beneficial for anti-inflammation. Because it can shrink imperceptible blood vessels, it is a treasure for treating the expansion and breaking of imperceptible blood vessels in the skin.

(Ⅱ) Application of aromatherapy massage to alleviate syndromes of cancer patients

For cancer patients, the terror of cancer lies in difficulty to cure and much discomfort caused in the process of treatment, such as general weakness, pain, sickness, vomiting and even anxiety and depression occurring in the process of treatment. Many cancer patients have the problem of low appetite, which can be solved by using sweet orange essential oil. Smell of the mouth and odor of wounds can be overcome by using tea tree hydrolate or peppermint hydrolate. Edema patients can use grapefruit, lemon, Clary Sage and Juniper essential oils. With the support of lymphatic massage, they have very good effect. When cancer patients have to endure great pain, they can use Clary Sage oil, sweet Marjoram oil, Roman chamomile oil, German chamomile oil and lavender oil etc. When cancer patients suffer from anxiety and depression, they can use orange flower oil, Clary Sage oil, bergamot oil, frankincense oil, sandalwood, grapefruit oil, sweet orange oil, rosemary and sweet Marjoram to improve their mental and emotional tiredness and help them open their mind and be relaxed. In addition, due to the drop of immunity, cancer patients' wounds can not recover easily. Lavender oil, tea tree oil and German chamomile oil can be used to smear on wounds, which will promote the healing of wound tissues. If chemotherapy leads to sickness and vomiting, vaporization of lemon essential oil, sweet orange essential oil, peppermint essential oil and ginger essential oil can be adopted to improve the condition of sickness and vomiting. Orange flower essential oil, sweet orange essential oil, frankincense essential oil, grapefruit essential oil, bergamot essential oil and lemon essential oil can be adopted for constipation or abdominal distention caused by diseases or drugs.

Aromatherapy is one kind of complementary therapy. Though they can not be used to kill cancer cells, if essential oils are properly used, they can definitely relieve patients' physical discomfort and increase mental ease. This will promote smooth treatment of diseases, improve patients' life quality and help patients to face cancer treatment actively. For cancer patients, essential oils can serve multiple purposes.

Nowadays, most people are living busy and nervous lives. They have fast pace of life and increasing physical and mental stress. Many people hope that they have some natural products that can help them to relax muscles, remove fatigue, treat or alleviate diseases. Aromatherapy can just meet such demands. Aromatherapy can not only provide skin care, hair care and eliminate some flaws on the skin, but also help people to calm down physically and mentally in comfortable and fragrant environment, to have rest and stimulate their immune system, so that people's physical and mental discomfort and diseases are treated or alleviated. Therefore, more and more people are fond of aromatherapy and it has gradually spread in the world.

参考文献

［1］沈国权、严隽陶：《推拿手法图解》，上海科学技术出版社 2004 年版。

［2］蒋松鹤、楼新法：《汉英对照针推精要》，人民卫生出版社 2004 年版。

［3］王旭东：《中医养生康复学》，上海中医药大学出版社 2003 年版。

［4］王玉川：《中医养生学》，上海科学技术出版社 1999 年版。

［5］丁悦森、毛湄、潘慧敏、施安丽：《施氏砭术综合疗法治疗颈源性眩晕 40 例》，载《中医外治杂志》2012 年第 5 期。

［6］《古代芳香疗法》，载《身心灵在线》，网址：http：//www. sxl – online. com/a_ zrly/fxlf/2011/0719/5400. html。

［7］石小峰：《芳香植物学》，载《芳香疗法的起源与发展》，网址：http：//wenku. baidu. com/view/96ff688cec3a87c24028c4fe. html。

References

[1] Shen Guoquan & Yan Juntao. *Illustrations of Tuina*. Shanghai Scientific and Technical Publisher, 2004.

[2] Jiang Songhe & Lou Xinfa. *Chinese Acupuncture and Massage: A Concise Annotation*. People's Medical Publishing House, 2004.

[3] Wang Xudong. *Life Cultivation and Rehabilitation of Traditional Chinese Medicine*. Publishing House of Shanghai University of Traditional Chinese Medicine, 2003.

[4] Wang Yuchuan. Life Cultivation of Traditional Chinese Medicine. Shanghai Scientific and Technical Publisher, 1999.

[5] Ding Yue, Mao Mei, Pan Huimin & Shi Anli. 40 *Cases of Using Shi's Comprehensive Bian Stone Therapy to Treat Cervicogenic Vertigo*. Journal of External Treatment of Traditional Chinese Medicine: 1999 (10).

[6] "Ancient Fragrance Treatment" in *Online Body, Heart and Soul* (Website: http://www.sxl-online.com/a_zrly/fxlf/2011/0719/5400.html).

[7] Shi Xiaofeng. *The Origin and Development of Fragrance Therapy* (https://wenku.baidu.com/view/96ff688cec3a87c24028c4fe.html).

References